Spas of England

AND
PRINCIPAL SEA-BATHING PLACES

BY A. B. GRANVILLE, MD, FRS
WITH A NEW INTRODUCTION BY GEOFFREY MARTIN

1: *the North*

ADAMS & DART

First published in 1841
This edition published in 1971 by Adams & Dart
40 Gay Street, Bath, Somerset
SBN 239 00085 4
Printed in Great Britain by Redwood Press, Trowbridge

Introduction

THE rise of the English spas and their intensive development
in the eighteenth and early nineteenth centuries is a substantial but comparatively neglected part of modern social
history. The history even of individual resorts has been
unevenly investigated, and their collective contribution to
our national patterns of behaviour has never been thoroughly
assessed. The spas are ancient and hard-wearing institutions.
From being places of pilgrimage and health resorts they
became places of amusement, centres of social education,
and then the models for resorts of a new kind, the sea-side
watering places. The early sea-side resorts were at first crude
and derivative, but they were adaptable, and were able to
meet the demands which the new industrial society made for
formal amusement and recreation. The older spas may seem
anachronisms in the Victorian and twentieth-century world,
but they did it a great service in their time. The interest of
Granville's *Spas of England* derives as much from the date of
its appearance as from its content: it is a landmark in the
development of that vital and deeply interesting institution,
the holiday.

The Spas of England is a survey of English resorts compiled in the early years of Victoria's reign, the work of a
fashionable and widely-experienced London doctor. It was
published in three parts in 1841, as a sequel to its author's
influential book *The Spas of Germany* (1837), and it is a
substantial and measured contribution to the topographical,
medical, and social literature of its age. It did not, however,
run to a second edition, and has remained ever since the only
work of its kind. Granville believed firmly in the efficacy
of natural mineral waters, and he found the spas in
what seemed to be an assured state of prosperity. His

commentaries upon them are often critical, for he was a
shrewd observer, but he wrote always with a conviction that
their fortunes and their general usefulness could be greatly
increased. In fact it was the sea-side resorts that prospered
and multiplied during the rest of the century, while the
inland watering-places were able at best only to hold their
ground. Granville's survey therefore showed them still in
their prime, but on the eve of a slow and relative, but
unmistakable decline. In consequence, despite its authorita-
tive tone and evident good sense, his work took on an
old-fashioned air, like its subject, as the century advanced.
Even so, the book would have an historical interest, but its
value is greatly increased by the far-sighted view that its
author took of the sea-side resorts, which he also visited and
carefully assessed. The relationship of the inland and the
coastal resorts just at that time, and Granville's own
personal history and interests, gave a distinctive quality to
his observations. A proper appreciation of his work depends
upon our knowledge both of the previous history of the spas
and of Dr Granville.

The origins of the spas are lost in time. The springs at
Bath and Buxton were used by the Romans, who may have
found healing cults already established at both places.
The high temperature of the waters at Bath, 120° Fahrenheit
at the surface, must certainly have attracted attention at the
earliest period of human settlement. Although resorts at
thermal and saline springs took their generic name from
Spa in Belgium in the sixteenth century, wells and rising
streams have their own fascination, and religious and magical
cults attach to them everywhere. In the Middle Ages it is not
possible to distinguish medical centres from pilgrims'
shrines; the springs at Bath were managed by the abbey,
where medical skills were cultivated, but Buxton's reputation was maintained by the simple invocation of St Anne's
well. There were shrines famous for healing, like those
of St Thomas at Canterbury or St Alban's, where the presence of the saint's body or other relics was sufficient, but at

Walsingham, where pilgrims sought the Virgin Mary's house, two holy wells were associated with her cult. All these, and many other celebrated and obscure shrines in England and abroad, were places of resort, to which pilgrims travelled and where they sought accommodation. They were also, we may note, centres of a rudimentary trade in souvenirs, cap-badges and similar mementos, and occasionally the subject of literature which sought or served to publicise them. To the ordinary purposes of pilgrimage, religious devotion, and a divine aid to health, there was added at least on occasion a quest for diversion and for such gratification as travel affords.

At the Reformation the cult of the saints was proscribed and their shrines demolished. The monasteries were dissolved between 1536 and 1540, and images removed from all churches and chapels under an act of 1550. Pilgrimage was no longer a respectable and legitimate activity; those wells which survived as objects of devotion, and they were many, did so on the strength of local superstition. It was at this point, however, that science intervened to justify instinct. Physicians perceived that not all waters were alike, and began to ascribe curative powers to chemical solutions rather than to faith. It was a verdict from which present medical science would have to dissent, but it served. The first work in English on medical bathing, *A booke of the natures and properties of the bathes in England . . . Germany, and Italy* by Dr William Turner, was published in 1562. It praised Bath, but deplored its neglect by English physicians and their patients, saying that mineral springs on the Continent were better appointed and patronised. Granville in his day said much the same thing. Ten years later Bath and Buxton were both mentioned in the Poor Law Act of 1572 as places to which the sick resorted; the corporation of Bath had secured possession of the baths after the dissolution of the abbey, and at Buxton, where the wells had been closed by Thomas Cromwell's agent, the Earl of Shrewsbury had begun to build a bath-house and other amenities for visitors. In

1613 Anne of Denmark, James II's queen, visited Bath, and the citizens spent £1,000 on her entertainment; the town was already well established as a health resort, but there was no patronage like royal patronage.

Buxton was overshadowed by Bath in the early seventeenth century and developed more slowly, but the best indication of their joint success lay in the search for and discovery of mineral springs in other places. Of subsequently famous resorts, Harrogate was publicised in the late sixteenth century, the springs at Tunbridge Wells discovered in 1606, and the well under the cliff at Scarborough identified about 1625. Tunbridge Wells, which grew up at the junction of three ancient parishes and had no settled name until after the Civil War, was patronised in 1629 and 1630 by Charles I's queen, Henrietta Maria, but she also led her ladies to Wellingborough in Northamptonshire, which is not now celebrated for its waters. The most important of the new discoveries was that at Scarborough, where the accident of the spring flowing out of the cliff made an amenity of the beach and foreshore long before sea-bathing was in fashion. The promenade was not to everyone's taste: Celia Fiennes observed tartly in 1697 'all the diversion is ye walking on this sand twice a day at ye ebb of the tide and till its high tide and then they drink', but the habit survived. There were also horse races on the sands.

The rise of the spas testifies both to a demand for medical services and to a social need that they satisfied. Except in so far as the warm springs of Bath soothed the skin and relieved the pain of rheumatism, or other mineral waters served as aperients, the malady for which the spas catered best was hypochondria. Faith might work wonders at any resort, but the simple amenities which were offered to the convalescent and the ambulant patient were accepted gratefully by those whose real search was not so much for health as for diversion. The evolution of pleasure resorts was a long process, and one never fully accomplished at the spas themselves, but a substantial start was made in the seventeenth century. The reputation that several springs, and especially Bath's, enjoyed for curing sterility in women probably referred to the same facts. Cynics had their own explanation, but relaxation, a sense of well-being, and the stimulus of new scenes and company might well have benefited more marriages than they harmed.

That the spas survived the Civil War and the Interregnum shows clearly that their informal attractions still took a second place to their medical régimes. The republican governments regarded them morosely as centres of Royalist intrigue, which they were, but like gambling, idle conversation, and adultery, that could be considered a by-product, not the central purpose of their existence. The rule of the Saints and of Cromwell's major-generals would certainly have borne harder upon the watering-places if they could have been shown to be mere pleasure resorts. Even in the more self-indulgent society after the Restoration, when the country began to taste the benefits of colonial trade and there were dividends to be spent on pleasure, the spas were by no means transformed. Bath was visited by companies of actors from London, as it had been before the war, but it had no permanent theatre. The whole equipment of Epsom spa was a pair of small wooden huts. The chief diversion at Tunbridge Wells was to walk along the promenade from the springs that later became the Pantiles, but was only a path in the fields until 1676. There was a good deal of building and re-building in England in the later seventeenth century. Brick, stone and tiles replaced timber and thatch, and the elements of the agreeably self-assured style that we call Georgian were imposed upon a variety of local practices, but the spas were still modest places, the majority of them rustic rather than urban, and they did not attract more of that activity than was their due.

At the same time, some hundreds of new mineral springs were discovered and promoted in various parts of the country, some of them old holy wells refurbished, and others the reward of diligent tasting. They were particularly and

naturally abundant round London, where places like
Islington, within walking distance of the city, or Richmond
or Epsom, a comfortable drive away, had a ready clientèle.
Mr Sadler's wells at Islington survived as a resort in an age
with other tastes; the springs at Streatham enjoyed a longer
popularity for their own sake, but less enduring fame. What
was plain in the late seventeenth century was that taking
the waters, or affecting to do so, was as much a fashionable
amusement as a medical fad, and that it could be gratified
upon a very small outlay of capital was part of its general
attractiveness.

A crucial change took place at Bath in the opening years
of the eighteenth century. Mary of Modena, James II's
queen, took the waters there in 1687, and then there were no
royal visits until 1702, when Queen Anne came. The corporation appointed a master of ceremonies to supervise the
arrangements made to entertain her, and no doubt feeling
that the experiment had justified itself when she returned
the following year, kept him as a permanent official. The
post had an evident affinity with that of a twentieth-
century festival manager, and some also with that of a
nineteenth-century American sheriff. The first incumbent
survived only until 1705, when he was killed in a duel.
He was succeeded by Richard Nash, a professional gambler
who had some experience of staging formal entertainments,
and who now revealed an extraordinary talent for social
organisation. Nash had some able associates, but his
legendary fame does no more than justice to his career.
He disciplined the visitors into a community, instilling an
elementary but effective code of good behaviour, and
inducting newcomers with irresistible ceremony. His
autocratic rule served both to soften the manners of those
who were sure of themselves, and to instruct those who were
uncertain and who had come, whether they knew it or
not, to learn. The lesson was of great general significance,
one which worked with other accidents of English history
to make a ruling class which was not as exclusively recruited

as most of its contemporaries, and was less brutal in tone, more sensibly intelligent, than its predecessors. Nash was only one of its instructors, but a powerful one. His academy was the Assembly Rooms, which he helped to establish, and in which his gratified pupils first displayed what they had gathered of urbanity before they took it home with them.

It was now no longer enough for a successful spa to have a well, or even a pump-room, and a promenade: formal manners deserved a formal setting. While Nash refined Bath's society, the city's appearance was remodelled by a combination of two gifted architects and a far-sighted business-man. The elder and the younger John Wood, encouraged and supported by Ralph Allen, devised a brilliant series of architectural spectacles, through the Parades and Queen Square to the Circus and the Royal Crescent, that enlarged and transfigured the old walled town. The strong but disciplined originality of their work was a perfect setting for the transformed society of the spa, matching it with an unsurpassed display of architectural elegance. The whole device was the urban equivalent of the great country house and its park, laid out to flatter transient but demanding residents. It had little enough to do with medical draughts and therapeutic bathing, but much to do with assimilating wealth and other disruptive forces in society, and with establishing canons of taste.

The new Bath offered a pattern that other spas copied and developed according to their means and opportunity. Public buildings of more or less elaboration, a hall for assemblies as well as a pump-room, better accommodation than rustic cottages afforded, a circulating library, all became necessities, and their appearance a mark of success. A new resort could presume upon a little patience from its visitors, but not for long. The cult of the picturesque was only nascent, and still an intellectual rather than a practical taste: urban sophistication was not yet well enough established for many people to seek systematic relief from it. Tunbridge Wells, which had begun to take shape as a town at the end of the seventeenth century, borrowed Nash in the summer, between Bath's spring and autumn seasons, from 1735 onward. At Buxton the Duke of Devonshire commissioned John Carr to build the Crescent in 1781, providing an assembly room, a news-room, and hotel accommodation as well as better-appointed baths. John Carr's was the first crescent outside Bath, and the precursor of many less ingenious adaptations of the device. It gave Buxton the new lease of life that its patron hoped for, closing the gap that had opened between it and its upstart rivals. By that time, however, there was more than the challenge of other inland spas for a resort to meet.

As Bath and Buxton have thermal springs, they began as bathing establishments, with the internal use of the waters as a secondary, though subsequently important practice. Elsewhere it was usual to drink the chalybeate waters, but cold baths were offered in spartan tribute to the older resorts. It had occurred to some physicians by the early years of the eighteenth century that the sea was a natural saline bath of unlimited potentiality, but we have no record of its regular use for several decades longer. The earliest instances come appropriately enough from Scarborough, where the first marine promenade was a natural adjunct to the spa, and where there was regular provision for sea-bathing by 1735. At the same time, however, other hardy souls were visiting Brighton, then a small fishing port, and with the encouragement of physicians who recommended bathing and the drinking of sea-water as a supplement or alternative to treatment at the spas, a score of similar places were patronised in the early years of George III's reign. By the end of the century, the Prince Regent's liking for Brighton had made it a resort as celebrated and as expensive as, though still less well-appointed than Bath, and the king himself had raised hopes of similar fame and riches in Weymouth by his visits there. Together with Scarborough, the sea-bathing resorts were in the same position as the inland spas a century earlier, and that after only a few decades' growth.

There was one important difference, however, between the two groups at this stage of their development. The seventeenth-century spas in their own time had no rivals: the sea-side resorts, if they aspired to fashionable patronage, had to meet a formidable challenge. The contest looked an unequal one for some time; Brighton flourished during the French wars, but its rise was matched by that of Cheltenham, and the Regent's patronage, even after his accession as king, was not a universal commendation. The wars benefited all British resorts by inhibiting travel abroad, but even in the 1830s the advantages still seemed to lie with the spas. It is true that a wider taste for the picturesque and the cult of Romanticism lent a dramatic quality to the sea—it is interesting to compare Charlotte Brontë's reactions to Scarborough with Celia Fiennes's dry assessment—but in general the sea-side was a place for simple pleasures, including those of savouring makeshift accommodation. Brighton's amusements were raffish, and its lodgings extremely expensive; sober, even self-indulgent visitors were as likely to seek Bath or Cheltenham as Brighton or Sidmouth, and northern manufacturers, like the neighbouring gentry, looked to Scarborough before Blackpool. That was still the position when Dr Granville began to commend hydropathic cures to his patients.

Augustus Bozzi Granville was born in Milan in 1783, the third son of Carlo Bozzi, post-master general of the Austrian province of Lombardy. He was educated at the Collegio de Merati and at the University of Pavia, where he read medicine and received his doctoral diploma in 1802. His student days therefore coincided with Napoleon's invasion of Italy and the establishment of the republican régime, events which excited patriotic and radical sympathies in him, and led eventually to his renunciation of the Roman Catholic faith. Those sympathies, however, did not incline him to accept military service as a conscript in the French armies, and after some adventures reminiscent of those of Fabrice in *La Chartreuse de Parme* not long afterwards, he escaped by way of Genoa and Piacenza to Venice, where his brother, an Austrian civil official, helped him to take ship for Corfu. There he fell in with William Richard Hamilton, secretary to Lord Elgin, and later British minister at Naples. Hamilton offered the young man a post as physician to the British Embassy in Constantinople, and they travelled together through Albania and Greece.

Granville's subsequent career sustained the promise of these exciting but restless beginnings. Hamilton was recalled to England when they reached Athens, and although Granville took up his appointment in Constantinople, where he caught bubonic plague, he was induced by the accidents of friendship to apply for a commission as second surgeon to the Turkish fleet. After a brief tour of service in the eastern Mediterranean, he resigned and made his way to Spain. There he lived for three years, adding Spanish to his languages and learning to play the guitar, an accomplishment which, as he confesses, later proved a hindrance rather than an aid to his professional advancement in England. Having assumed the name of Granville upon his mother's death, at her wish, to commemorate his Cornish great-grandfather, he removed to Lisbon in 1806, and the next year was commissioned as an assistant surgeon on a British sloop in the Tagus. That his ship immediately took a prize in its way to Portsmouth, and that before settling in England in 1812 he should have been shipwrecked off Oporto and served in the West Indies, returning with Simon Bolivar's dispatches to the British government, was in no way out of character. He eventually retired from the Navy on half-pay in 1812, having married an English wife in 1809, and after a short stay in Manchester, where he was received into the Literary and Philosophical Society by John Dalton, he moved to London to establish himself in medical practice. In the process he lectured in chemistry at the Westminster Medical School, studied and practised for a year at *La Maternité* in Paris, and was eventually elected physician-accoucheur at the Westminster Dispensary. In the meantime he had acted as an interpreter at the Foreign Office, carried British dispatches to Italy in 1814, and fallen under the justifiable suspicion of the Austrian authorities during his travels in Lombardy, where he was arrested and detained as a spy. It was his belief, and that of some of his fellow physicians, that he might have saved the life of the Princess Charlotte in 1817, if he had returned sooner from his residence in Paris. It is a matter of which he wrote with some diffidence later, in Queen Victoria's reign, but one which he felt bound to mention.

For the rest of his long life Granville lived and practised in London, though he travelled extensively abroad, and paid a professional visit to the spa at Kissingen every year from 1840 to 1863. He retired after his last visit there, and began to write his autobiography, which was edited and published by his daughter in 1874. He died at Dover in March 1872. His self-confidence and vigorous spirit had roused some jealousies and made him enemies, but they were outweighed by the friends who admired his warm enthusiasms. He enjoyed a large practice, which he maintained with skill and vigour. In his early years in England he was befriended and encouraged by Sir Humphry Davy and Sir Joseph Banks, and his obliged patients included Palmerston, a man not readily blinded with science. Granville was elected Fellow of the Royal Society in 1817, and was among the first members chosen for the Athenaeum. His published works, which between 1812 and 1865 ranged over medicine, chemistry, public health, literature, travel, and politics, fill two-and-a-half columns of the British Museum catalogue; *The Spas of England*, therefore, falls near the middle of his professional and literary career.

Granville's particular interest in spas dated from the 1830s, although his taste for chemical analysis and what would now be called biochemistry went back to his student days. He was moved in 1836, following the success of a popular essay on the principal German spas by Sir Francis Head (*Bubbles from the Brunnens of Nassau*, 1835), to plan a comprehensive work on the German watering-places. *The Spas of Germany* appeared in 1837; its author showed himself much impressed with the professional competence of the German régimes, and the great popularity of the spas, and although he had some rivals to contend with, he impressed his readers. John Murray's first *Handbook for travellers on the Continent* (1839) cites Granville on diet as a matter of course, assuming that tourists who wish to take the waters will recognise the English authority upon them. There may therefore have been others than the handsome manageress of the Grand Hotel at Buxton who reproached him for his neglect of the English spas (*Midlands, p. 25*) and it was natural that he should turn his attention next to them. He travelled extensively in England in the summer and autumn of 1839, and again in the autumn of 1840. He seems to have made these tours much as he describes them in his book, traversing northern England from Liverpool to the Tyne, returning by Shap to the Fylde coast and the Mersey, and then having worked from Buxton to Lincolnshire, passing into the south-west via Cheltenham and Bath, to cover the south coast from Torquay to Brighton. The resorts of the Thames estuary, including the newly-discovered and short-lived mineral spring at Hockley, are then treated before Tunbridge Wells, but these were all places within easy reach of London. Granville's work on the book was interrupted by his treatment of Joseph Bonaparte, formerly King of Naples and of Spain, and elder brother of Napoleon I, whom he had attended regularly in 1838 and whom he accompanied to Wildbad in the summer of 1840. That was the urgent professional business to which he referred in his preface, and which resulted in the sheets of the first volume, printed in 1839–40, being held over until 1841, when the whole work was issued.

The Spas of England is a single-minded but leisurely book, abounding in discursive detail. As Granville says in his preface, his object was to describe 'things as they are', and he quite rightly supposed that his own experiences in

compiling the work were as consequential as the things
that he discovered. The result is not just a medical treatise,
which would now have a very limited interest, but also a work
of travel, topography, and social comment. Granville was a
busy, inquisitive man, used to making his way in strange
company, and sustained by the kind of self-confidence that
contrives to engage other people's interest in his affairs. His
belief in the medicinal value of the spa waters was ill-
founded, so far as we can answer for it, but it gives the
book a unifying theme and helps to direct his other observations. The modern reader may chafe at the stately
introductory dialogue and at some of the asides, and will
find the longer reported conversations incredible. Granville
himself had occasional misgivings, and at Shotley Bridge,
for which he mistakenly foresaw a glorious future as a
resort, he closed his notebook, 'lest I should be betrayed
into greater prolixity' (*Northern, p. 304*), but even his
undisciplined flourishes have an appeal of their own. There
are also many pungent reflections to set against them:
on the shortcomings of English hotels, for example, inspired
by the coffee room at the New Inn, Derby, or the realisation
that the popularity of Teignmouth as a resort for invalids
'does not seem to have much enriched its inhabitants'
(*Southern, p. 469*). Common sense and a wide experience were
valuable qualities in a physician; there are occasions when
Granville is able to compress the whole pattern of his life
into a single sentence. One such opportunity occurred in
Dorset: 'for a mere blow of sea air, such as one may get on a
quarter-deck, I know of no better place for an idler in these
parts than Weymouth' (*Southern, pp. 508–9*).

The most striking of Granville's general reflections are
those upon the railways. His journeys are in any case a real
and vivid part of the book, and he seized upon travel by rail,
not just as a dramatic and exciting novelty, but as a matter
of great social significance. His comments upon the management of the railways, on the difference in tone between
different companies or between stations ('as compared' to

London, all the officers and servants at the Liverpool
terminus are perfection' [*Northern, p. 15*]) are as illuminating as his descriptions of the night train's departure, or the
bustle of the travelling post-office. His strictures upon the
early companies were all justifiable, although some improvements had been made by the time the book was published.
The legislative regulation of the railways, for which Granville called, proved to be a continuing and exacting charge
upon nineteenth-century government, and a unified control,
with all the advantages that a standardised policy promised,
has been achieved only in recent times. The general tenor of
Granville's discussion would be creditable if he had had a
much longer time to sample travel by rail and to consider its
significance: as a judgment upon the experiences of something less than a decade it was most shrewd and far-sighted.

The Spas of England is consistently and soundly informed
by its author's own experience. Granville was a natural
experimenter, always anxious to enlarge his knowledge, and
his solemn records of his pulse and physiological sensations
when he entered a bath were to him as much part of assessing
a spa as was analysing its waters. It followed that he should
also interest himself in the whole organisation of a resort,
and in everything that its visitors were likely to do. Much
of his detail is practical and eminently sensible: he comments
as a matter of course upon the nature and cost of accommodation, not forgetting the cost of wax candles where
charges were not inclusive (*Northern, p. 72*), and upon social
life and provision of amenities as well as upon the ordering
of baths and pump-rooms. He notices where people walk,
and when and how they eat. The effect of the Blackpool air
upon the appetite is well-observed, but Granville kept a
sharp eye upon public dining-rooms at all times, and his
strictures upon the ill manners displayed at the Half Moon
Inn at Exeter conjure up the scene very convincingly
(*Southern, pp. 458–9*).

Details of that kind are of more consequence now than
the constituents of spa water, or the ill-advised use of metal

pipes, but it is precisely the wide scope of Granville's interests that makes his observations valuable. One matter on which he would have been more precise if he had been able was the régime of the spas, but we can see from his testimony, as we might suspect on other grounds, that there was a laxness in the English that defied exact classification. German spas were undoubtedly better-ordered, but then their patrons were more amenable. Granville felt and said that the English started their day too late, and were apt to arrange it self-indulgently. He seems likely to have been right.

It is significant that Bath, which Granville praised highly and justly as a town, should have disappointed him in several details as a spa. There as elsewhere the patrons came too late to the pump-room, and they neither drank the waters nor used the baths as intensively as they might. The baths themselves were inferior to, at least in the sense that they were less ingeniously contrived than, those that a Continental resort of the same quality would have offered. The implication is that Bath, as agreeable and impressive by night, with 'the twinkling of all the gas-lights' (*Southern, p. 365*), as it was by day, was in the eyes of its visitors as much a place for idle diversion as it was a health resort.

Like the other inland spas, Bath was about to be sharply challenged by its upstart rivals on the coast. Granville himself could hardly be aware of the fact, but he sensed the potentiality of the sea-side resorts as he had already assessed that of the railways, and his comments upon them are particularly interesting. It was his impression that the English bathed less assiduously than other Europeans, yet the rise of the coastal resorts told its own story. The amenities that they offered were few and simple, and Granville was not deeply impressed by them as resorts for the sick and convalescent. His remarks upon the short-comings of Torquay, with its one level walk for invalids, varied according to the direction of the wind, and the hills that outfaced its 'asthmatic ... and pulmonic and ... phthisical' visitors (*Southern, p. 482*), are sharper in tone than most of his comments upon the inland spas. The contrast implied is a natural one, for if such places were judged as health resorts, then the superior amenities and experience of the older centres must have told in their favour. Only Bournemouth, in which Granville took a particular and markedly intelligent interest, really satisfied him in that respect. He deplored the thoughtless speculative building that he found elsewhere, and considered that if the new resort was properly planned it promised to be 'a perfect discovery', such a place as 'we vainly thought to have found elsewhere on the south coast of England' (*Southern, p. 512*). In the event, Bournemouth was developed much as Granville hoped, and the prescription proved a great success, but the real strength of the sea-side resorts lay in their freedom from the historic patterns of the spas. The only amenity that the new resorts needed to borrow from the old ones was the promenade, and even that was soon dominated by the beach. With the rapid extension of holiday-making through the middle classes and among the working classes in the nineteenth century, the most important qualities in a resort were accessibility and the capacity to grow: the railway provided the one, and the beach the other. Having no other models, the sea-side was likely to imitate the buildings and institutions of the spa, but its chief business was to range its visitors along the edge of the sea. By the end of the century the patrons had forgotten that it was a mineral water that they had come to seek, although the memory of ozone stayed long in their collective mind.

The chief interest of Granville's work therefore lies not in the matters that first engaged its author, such as the presence of iodine in the newly-discovered waters of Woodhall Spa, or the appointment of the baths at Buxton, but in its juxtaposition of two different styles of life. The tradition of the spas, for all their popularity, was aristocratic; the tradition of the sea-side, for all the distinction of its early patrons, was to be popular. The two institutions were closely connected, both before and after Granville's day, but their inter-dependence was particularly striking at that time, when travel overseas was once again drawing off aristocratic patronage from the English resorts, and when the great popular holiday trade, which depended upon the steamboat and the Thames wherries even before the railways were built, had begun to transform the resorts of the south-east.

Granville brought some notable qualifications to his work. His professional experience enabled him to speak authoritatively to his contemporaries on the central functions of the spas, and also to look at their clientèle with an informed eye. His upbringing and his cosmopolitanism saved him from parochial judgements, although his attachment to England was warm and complete. One personal preoccupation emerges in the long discussion on the Roman Catholic and Protestant churches that is attached to the passage on St Mary's College at Oscott, in the section on the Midland spas (*Midlands, pp. 192–217*). His Anglican faith was part of Granville's Englishness, and to his original readers his disconcertingly sudden excursion into Christian apologetics would have been remarkable only for its studied mildness. To Granville and his contemporaries it was an intelligent man's business to concern himself with what was significant in his world, a category of topics to which St Mary's College belonged as naturally as the harbour works at Hartlepool, the rocks on Brimham Moor, or the uses and shortcomings of gas-lighting. In that, as in all other respects, the work is a faithful portrait of its time, a reminder, like the history and personality of its author, of the richness and variety that characterised nineteenth-century England.

BIBLIOGRAPHY

A. B. Granville, *The spas of Germany*, London, 1837, 2 vols. (illus.).

Paulina B. Granville, *ed.*, *Autobiography of A. B. Granville*, London, 1874, 2 vols. (illus.).

R. C. Hope, *The legendary lore of the holy wells of England*, London, 1893. (illus.).

R. V. Lennard, *ed.*, *Englishmen at rest and play: some phases of English leisure, 1558-1714*, Oxford, 1931. (illus.).

G. H. Martin, *The town*, London, 1961, bibl. (illus.).

J. A. R. Pimlott, *The Englishman's holiday: a social history*, London, 1947, bibl. (illus.).

SCARBOROUGH NEW SPA.

THE

SPAS OF ENGLAND,

AND

PRINCIPAL SEA-BATHING PLACES.

BY

A. B. GRANVILLE, M.D., F.R.S.

AUTHOR OF "THE SPAS OF GERMANY," "ST. PETERSBURG," &c.

NORTHERN SPAS.

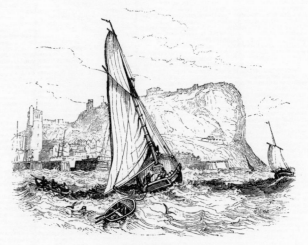

SCARBOROUGH.

LONDON:

HENRY COLBURN, PUBLISHER,

GREAT MARLBOROUGH STREET.

1841.

TO

HER MOST GRACIOUS MAJESTY,

QUEEN

VICTORIA,

WHO

HAS CONDESCENDED

TO

ACCEPT THEIR DEDICATION,

THESE VOLUMES

ARE,

WITH THE DEEPEST FEELINGS

OF

LOYALTY AND RESPECT,

INSCRIBED BY

THE AUTHOR.

PREFACE.

Siste Viator!—was the emphatic phrase of olden times, by which the attention of the casual passenger was suddenly arrested, when the writer of an epitaph desired to secure to himself a succession of readers, and engage their sympathy in behalf of the subject of his composition.

I wish I could use an equally successful mode of checking, in those who may be inclined to peruse my present volumes, the proneness so prevalent nowadays to pass by the preface and proceed at once to the subject-matter; for in no case has the author of a work of facts stood more in need than I do of being heard preliminarily, owing to circumstances which were not contemplated when the present book was first undertaken.

Therefore it is that I most respectfully request my readers not to refuse their attention, for a few moments, to the contents of this Preface; inasmuch as without the knowledge of them, some part of the narrative, and a few of the arguments and descriptions that follow, would seem incomprehensible and defective.

And first it is important that it should be stated that the TOUR of which my two volumes purport to give an account, was made principally during the summer and autumnal months of 1839, and not completed until the summer months of 1840.

Those readers who are aware of the heavy responsibilities and duties that attach to a London physician of twenty-three years' standing, as well as of the importance of the inquiry I had undertaken, will readily comprehend the motives for this division of labour, in the performance of one and the same task; they will recollect that such an author cannot command his own time for any extra-official occupation he may undertake, and has often to abide the will of others and of many.

In the second place I am bound in justice to myself to declare, that nearly the whole of the First Volume was written and *printed* soon after the completion of the first or principal part of the TOUR—that is, in the spring of 1840. As it was my intention to send it forth immediately, the sheets were printed as soon as written, and were ready before the concluding information I required for the second volume was personally collected.

At this conjuncture my personal attention to the continuation of the work was suddenly and most effectually prevented, by a professional engagement of such honour and importance, that it could not be refused without derogating from the character of an upright, consistent, and humane practitioner.

That engagement necessarily required my absence from England for several weeks in the early part of the summer of 1840; and on my return, the season for publication, according to the technical arrangements of the trade, was passed. I therefore profited by this species of recess, and devoted a few leisure days in the autumn to the completion of my materials for the second volume.

It is these explanations which I am naturally anxious the reader should peruse, ere he proceed to look into the work itself. They will enable him to understand that, in whatever part (if any) of the present volume I may seem to him to have been anticipated by other writers, the fact is not really so, since the contents of the following pages were not only written, but actually printed, more than a year ago ; and that wherever he may imagine that I have omitted facts or observations concerning some of the Spas, it is because those facts have only come into existence since these sheets were printed.

Without trespassing too long on the patience of my readers, I will, with their permission, illustrate each of my positions by a suitable reference.

The subject of railway-travelling had never, before the year 1839, that I know of, been treated *ex-professo*, in a medical point of view. Being about to describe a very extensive tour through nearly the whole of England, the principal object of which was the consideration of certain natural agents, capable of assisting in the recovery of health,—and railway-travelling having entered largely into that tour, and being likely to do so with many of the invalids whom the perusal of my work may induce to perform the whole or any part of the same tour,—I deemed the subject not only a legitimate but a most appropriate point of consideration ; for which reason I began my work with the introduction of two Chapters upon that mode of travelling.

Subsequent events have proved how accurately I had calculated on its importance; and writers of every class

and degree—particularly those in the public journals—
have been teeming with discussions on the same subject, drawn from them by the too-frequent occurrence of
those very multifarious dangers and accidents, which will be
found fully descanted upon, deprecated, and described, in
the present volume. Nay, the legislature itself has since
been roused (though but partially and imperfectly) to the
real state of the case, as between speculators and the public,
and something like the remedial measure which I have stoutly
demanded (and I may appear to have demanded *ex post facto*
in these sheets) has been adopted.

But neither in the arguments of the writers alluded to,
nor in my recommendation of a remedial measure,—still less
in my descriptions of the intolerant impertinence and shameful neglect prevalent on certain railroads, and of their rapacity also,—have I been anticipated by a single writer; for the
two Chapters I here offer to the public were written almost
immediately after my return from the Northern Spas of England, in July, August, and September, 1839, and sent to
press soon after,—as the gentlemen connected with my publisher's establishment can testify. At that time, neither
journalist, specific author, member of government, or member of parliament, had grappled with the subject; and it
was not until a twelvemonth afterwards, subsequent to a committee of inquiry upon it, that the legislative measure which
was proclaimed in these sheets a year before, to be both necessary and absolutely called for, as well as consistent with
the usual practice of the country in analogous institutions,
was partially adopted.

I do not dwell upon this explanation from a disposition to
attach any importance to such a claim of priority, since,

after all, the consideration of the subject is so natural, and so forced upon every one by what we see daily to occur before us, that there is hardly any merit in being one among the first to discuss it. But I bring the explanation forward, lest I should be accused by all those writers who, in reality, have come after me, of having taken up a portion of my volume with a repetition of what had already been stated and re-stated by them; and by my readers, of having ridiculously insisted upon the necessity of a controlling power over rail-ways, after such a controlling power had been established by parliament.

I only wish, in common with all my fellow-men, that such a controlling power had been more efficient, and just the thing that was wanted. And still more do I heartily wish that subse-quent events, and the further experience of myself and others, had enabled me to qualify the condemnation of the system pursued on certain railroads, but particularly on that which is more specifically alluded to in my first and second Chapter.

Unfortunately the reverse is the case; the more I have examined that establishment during the many occasions I have had since of travelling by it, to visit patients on different points of the railway—the more reasons have I seen for allow-ing my reflections upon it, written more than a twelvemonth ago, to remain unaltered. But what stronger argument can I add in confirmation of those reflections, than the able and timely remarks brought forward at the close of a late me-morable coroner's inquest by the foreman of the jury, in their presentment?

Thus much in illustration of my first position.

With regard to the second; namely, that if I should seem in the following pages to have omitted any facts connected with certain Spas herein described, it must be because the facts themselves did not exist when these pages were printed, but have come to light since;—I may illustrate it by what has occurred at Shotley Bridge, where a second and a very important mineral spring has been discovered since my visit to that Spa; or by what has been done at Scarborough, where the whole extent of the ground behind the Spa,—which in my description I lamented was not decked out with plantations and promenades,—has since been converted into a most charming garden and shrubbery; or lastly, by the many improvements that have taken place in one or two other Spas, which did not exist when my account was written. Had my volume appeared at the epoch for which it was intended and nearly ready, no such apparent omissions would have existed.

It is precisely because the delaying any longer the publication of the first part of my TOUR, referable to the NORTHERN SPAS, which forms as it were a work of itself,—with a view of affording me time to complete the second part, relating to the Spas of the Midland Counties, and of the South, including the most popular sea-bathing places, as well as those which in my professional opinion are the most desirable,—would inevitably produce further appearances of deficiencies on my part, and anticipations by others, that it has been determined to lay at once before the public the first volume, without waiting for the completion of the second; although it will follow in a very few weeks.

A few lines more and I conclude. To those who are acquainted with my previous work on the Spas of Germany, it is needless to observe that I have followed, as nearly as it was possible, the same arrangement of matter in the present publication which I adopted in the other; and that I have endeavoured to treat the subject likewise in that same general, miscellaneous, and popular manner, which public opinion has largely sanctioned by their countenance of the former production. In this manner I thought I could best evince my desire to be perfectly impartial in my account of the Spas of the two nations. My motto has been "Things as they are," without instituting invidious comparisons. By following this determination on many previous occasions, I have invariably reaped the reward which ought best to please an author—the satisfaction of those whose places I described, because I did so impartially; and the approbation of the visiters to the same places, because they had found the descriptions accurate, and had not been disappointed.

Lastly, I must add that I have taken every pains to supply each volume with a correct table of analyses of the several mineral waters, (as in the case of the Spas of Germany) which may be referred to with confidence in the respective authorities, without interrupting the perusal of the narrative, or the account of the several Spas: and I have in a similar manner introduced a general skeleton map of all the English Spas that have come within my own knowledge; as nothing of importance has been admitted into this work from mere hearsay, or at secondhand, or which is not the result of my own observations.

Although the form of the present is smaller than that of the previous volumes, it is not because less pains have been taken with the Spas of England than with those of the continent: the contrary, I trust, will be found to be the case; as a much greater *quantity* of matter has, by typographic contrivance, been compressed into the present form.

The Illustrations, of which there is a greater number in the

present than there was in my former work, are, with three
exceptions, executed in wood by Mr. Orrin Smith, who,
entering into the spirit of the author, and anxious that the
Spas of his own country should not lag behind those of
Germany, has omitted no exertion to render his share of these
volumes deserving of the patronage of the public.

109, Piccadilly.   **A. B. GRANVILLE, M.D.**
Dec. 1840.

POPULAR CONSIDERATIONS

ENGLISH MINERAL WATERS.

---

1. INTRODUCTORY REMARKS.

CONSIDERING the great indifference which prevails among the reading classes of society in this country for any description or systematic account of their own native land, its natural beauties, its many striking objects, and local advantages, and even some of the most interesting of its natural productions,—I am perhaps imprudent and ill-advised in attempting to draw attention to a work, such as I venture now to offer to the public.

Had it been written in a foreign language, or by a total stranger to England, on his return to the continent, after a brief and rapid run, *de longue en large*, through this country —as in the case of the illustrious Pückler Muskau, and Mine Herr Waagen—curiosity, perchance, or the expectation of having a hearty laugh at many anticipated blunders, would have induced people to look into the book, and place it for a season on the drawing-room table.

But neither the author nor the work in the present instance being in that predicament, my chance of being accepted with

indulgence as a new candidate in the field of graphic delineation of the fairest and largest portion of England, must depend on the importance of the principal object of my volumes,
and the strict accuracy of the descriptions they are to contain.

Novelty, as one of their elements of attraction, must at
once be admitted to be out of the question. Yet, as there is
a novelty of manner, as well as of matter,—and as, where the
latter is impossible, the former may reasonably be received
as a substitute,—I would fain hope, that in having treated an
old subject in the manner I have done—(a manner I am not
aware to have been adopted before on the like subject)—
I have taken the most proper course for securing the attention
of my readers.

That subject is the examination of the principal Spas, or
Mineral Waters of England. My former work on the mineral waters of Germany having been received with great kindness by the English public, I was almost bound in return
to make known as extensively those of this country.

The study of mineral waters, after having formed the
object of my leisure moments, has since engaged a large
portion of my professional time. From the extensive researches I have been able to make into their nature and
power, and the numerous occasions I have had of witnessing
their effect in a variety of diseases, I have been led, very naturally, to form enlarged views of the subject. These are
not only applicable to foreign waters, but to those of this
country as well; and although, as we shall have occasion to
see in the following pages, the latter are neither so various nor
so potent, yet their claim to the serious consideration of the
profession and the public are sufficiently strong to authorize
me to bring them forward in a parallel publication to " The
Spas of Germany."

That the latter has had the effect of sending thousands

abroad, many of whom would probably have remained at home, and drank at the fountains of health in England, had a work of a general and popular character upon them existed, like " The Spas of Germany," there is much reason to believe. But still more firmly do I believe that such a result will now proceed from a publication of that description, when so many thousands of English people, having returned from the foreign baths, will be able to compare with them those of their own country, provided they can find in a professed work on the subject, the same prominent features which first attracted their attention in " The Spas of Germany," and subsequently determined them to proceed thither.

This is what I have felt, and what I have endeavoured to accomplish. I undertook the task with no other view. I entered into it earnestly, and executed it consecutively, even at considerable personal inconvenience, and some detriment to my professional practice, owing to my absence from London during three or four months, though not all at one time. The means I adopted for securing success was to admit nothing in my notes, but what I had myself seen and could vouch for. In the few instances where that could not be so, from obvious or unavoidable reasons, I have quoted the authority, and leave to my informant the responsibility of having stated the truth.

What I have recommended, I recommended from a conscientious impression that the object deserved recommendation ; and where, on the contrary, the result of my own unbiassed observations has been to induce me to withhold praise, or to decline to join in the praises given by others, or I have been obliged to censure or criticise, I have done so from precisely similar conscientious motives.

In following my researches, and examining such a variety of establishments, I felt anxious to keep aloof from all possibility of a bias. I have therefore abstained almost always, from making myself or my errand known, when on the spot, to proprietors of mineral waters, Spas, hotels, and other establishments; and in a few cases even to some of the medical faculty resident at the Spa, when I knew that they were either obstinately against, or extravagantly in favour of, their own mineral spring—when, in fact, some made the using of mineral waters the butt of their discourse, and others the hobby of their professional life.

Yet I have been too happy in receiving at the hand of some, that degree of assistance which would facilitate the object of my researches; and to the few who have so aided me I gladly avail myself of the present opportunity of acknowledging generally their kindness.

That there were but few of my medical brethren who assisted me in the pursuit of my present inquiries, is neither to be attributed to any want of notice they might have had of my intention, nor to be explained by the little interest which the inquiry might be supposed to have excited.

With regard to the latter supposition, I know the contrary to have been the case; since in almost every leading provincial paper of the time, my visit to the several Spas of the country has been noticed with satisfaction: and as to the first of the two suppositions, I can declare that every legitimate means was adopted by myself, at no inconsiderable expense, of informing the profession in each separate county I intended to visit, of the object of my visit, by an advertisement in the principal county journals. In it I stated that I should receive with great thankfulness any information which medical men, or proprietors of, or other persons connected with, mineral watering-places, or insulated springs, would feel disposed to communicate to me, particularly with regard to those which were less known or of recent discovery, and all of which I offered to proceed to examine without any charge whatever.

For a month previous to my departure from London, and

during the whole course of my inquiry, not more than a dozen answers worthy of notice reached me; the rest of the correspondence, and it was voluminous enough, being manifestly dictated by selfish motives, and not from professional persons;—and out of that small number, five only were from medical persons honourably interested in the success of some mineral spring in their own immediate neighbourhood.

True, I did receive, after my return to London, when it would have been exceedingly inconvenient for me, as well as unjustly burdensome to my purse, again to quit my post in search of a mineral spring—and after the expiration of the period to which I had limited my readiness to undertake the inquiry at my own risk—several accounts of mineral waters I had not seen in my tour, or had only heard of accidentally; but those accounts were from self-interested persons, who called upon me to introduce the same into my volumes.

Such, however, was not the line of conduct I had chalked out to myself in my present inquiry, and the admitting any description of places or springs into my volumes, which I had not drawn up myself on the spot, was what I had determined not to do. The accounts, therefore, remained unnoticed; nor do I regret it, except in the case of two or three minor Spas which I have admitted and dotted in my map, but of which no description will be found in these volumes; because upon my offering to proceed to examine them, ere I could admit any account of them in my intended publication, provided my necessary expenses were defrayed, the offer was declined, and the mere copying of their own printed descriptions and commendations politely requested.

These explanations argue no doubt great apathy among the different classes of persons to whom I have alluded, respecting an inquiry to accomplish which I had myself undertaken an arduous and expensive task, and for the completion of which I used all means in my power; flinching from no difficulty, and disregarding personal fatigue and incon-

venience; travelling upwards of three thousand miles of
ground, and committing to paper, invariably on the spot,
every fact, statement, or description, which the contemplation of the various places or objects before me elicited and
rendered necessary. In executing this, I have sometimes
come in contact with lukewarm or hostile medical brethren
(otherwise amiable and respectable), on the subject of the
treatment of disease by mineral waters, whom I have had
the great satisfaction of rousing to a due sense of the importance of the question, and of converting to my views on
the subject. They are looking forward with anxiety for the
appearance of the present publication; and the consideration
of this one pleasing fact makes me forgetful of the little I
have encountered that was the reverse of agreeable.

Such is the origin, the motive, and the scope of "The
Spas of England," and such are the bases on which they have
been constructed. That I have adopted the popular style
rather than the professional in their composition—that I have
chosen the form of a continuous narrative or a tour, rather
than a stiff, systematic classification of English mineral
waters, learnedly discussed—that I have mingled the jocose
with the serious—the grave with the gay—that amidst descriptions of naturally medicated waters, I have inserted delinea-
tions of many other subjects—all this is not to be wondered
at, since to precisely such a course do I ascribe the good fortune of having been extensively read and extensively consulted on the subject of the German waters. That which
has succeeded once may succeed again; and, at all events,
English readers will not blame me for having assumed a
manner of treating matters so immediately interesting to
them, which they have already approved in regard to matters
to them only of indirect importance.

As I wrote "The Spas of Germany" for the information
of English readers (although translations into foreign languages have since been made of that work abroad), so I write

the present work on "The Spas of England," not without
some hopes and expectation that the information they contain may be of use to foreigners, who will probably evince
sufficient curiosity to know what there is of analogous between their own establishments of that sort and those
of this country. It is for this reason that I have deemed it
expedient to introduce many details, much collateral information, and several descriptions of localities and institutions,
with which the English reader is no doubt already familiar,
but the omission of which would have rendered my present
performance almost unintelligible to continental readers;
thereby defeating one of the objects I had in view in writing
it—that of exhibiting in their true light the English Spas
abroad, as I endeavoured to exhibit those of Germany at
home.

II.—Remarkable Change that has taken place in England, in regard to the Knowledge and Use of Mineral Waters, in the last Two Years.

In the second section of the "Popular Considerations on
the Use and Power of Mineral Waters," published in "the
Spas of Germany," I had occasion to descant on the indifference and want of knowledge that prevailed at the time
in this country in respect to that subject, and pointed out
how little medical men, in great practice in London, were
conversant with it:—nay, how hostile most of them appeared to be to the recommendation of foreign baths. I
proved the assertion by numerous facts and illustrations, and
its truth was never denied or called in question by that part
of the press which undertook to give an account of the
volumes containing the assertion.

During the London season which followed immediately
after the appearance of the first edition (1838); I could
already perceive a gradual change working in this respect,

first among the public—the middle as well as the upper classes—and next among some of the leading physicians and surgeons, whom I met in consultation, at the request of patients determined to give foreign mineral waters a trial in their own complaints, after having perused the work in question.

The season of 1839 was even more triumphant for the German waters, and the cause of mineral waters in general—including those imitated by Struve's process at Brighton, which I had been in the habit of recommending ever since their first introduction into this country in 1825, and respecting which I had published my opinion as far back as 1828. Not only the converts to the belief in the power of the German mineral waters, amongst the better classes of society, had prodigiously increased in that year, but the incredulous practitioner had ceased to be so—had become suddenly the advocate of the cause I had strenuously contended for—and, lastly, had taken the lead with his own patients, in recommending a journey to some German Spa, without the necessity of consultation, but with such knowledge of the subject as he himself had gathered from reading.

The year just about to close has supplied me with evidence of this almost sudden and favourable change in public opinion on the subject of mineral water, many degrees stronger than that of the two preceding seasons—and I may at present confidently assert, that the utility, safety, and importance of the treatment of chronic and painful diseases by foreign mineral waters,—to encourage which I had exerted my utmost zeal and humble abilities,—are very generally acknowledged and likely so to continue.

Nay, the tide would seem now to be about to turn the other way; and we are probably destined to see this particular point of medical practice ridden to death as a hobby, —if one is to believe in the variety of new spas which people are discovering in all directions,—and consider the number of publications that are promised on the same subject, both at home and abroad—as well as those that have appeared since " The Spas of Germany."

Thus, a gentleman, whose previous slender account of *all* the mineral waters of Europe I had occasion to notice, by pointing out some mistakes, and the many omissions found in his book—has reproduced part of that same book, for the purpose of repeating, on a somewhat larger basis, his previous account of a few of the Nassau Spas, so fully described in my own publication, and has entitled his *ri-faccimento*, " The Baths of Germany" !

In it the author has exhibited some little degree of ill-humour that is quite amusing, at my having praised Kissingen and Wildbad above some of the Nassau *baths*. But in return he has made the admission, and with a *naïveté* which enhances its merit, that when in his former little work he had himself written slightly of Wildbad, he had *not then seen that Spa*

I had suspected as much when I referred to that work in my own ; and, further, I had occasion to hint, that Wildbad was not the only place that author had described without having examined or seen it.

As the writer in question has thought it necessary, notwithstanding my extended account of Baden, Wisbaden, Ems, and Schwalbach, the four principal Nassau Spas, to publish separately a more enlarged description of those places, by himself, than he had previously written,—I concluded that he had something new to say respecting them, and gladly referred to the work, in hopes of finding therein fresh arguments in support of my favoured subject—the use of mineral water in disease ; or some novel description of the places which might have escaped my attention. If those readers who have done me the honour of perusing my account of the Nassau Spas, in " The Spas of Germany," will also refer to

" The Baths of Germany" for a description of the same places, they will see at once if there was any need for the latter performance, in which nothing appears more conspicuous than a desire to lower the principal medical man in one of the most popular of those Spas, by statements and insinuations beyond the limits of fair criticism.

The English work I have just referred to has been written abroad. At home we hear only of works to come, on the subject of foreign mineral waters. One, it is understood, is to be entitled, " The Pilgrim to the Spas of Germany," or some such title. If it proceed from the pen which has been hinted at to me, the public will have reason to be satisfied with the performance, and I shall have to rejoice in an able coadjutor in maintaining the cause of mineral hydro-medical practice ; a coadjutor, too, who is an old friend, and was once a brother officer in the naval service. If this author should, perchance, introduce into his intended work an account of Pyrmont, Aix-la-Chapelle, and Kreuzenach, three important Spas, with which I am personally as well acquainted as with the rest, (but my description of which was omitted, from a desire of my publisher to avoid the necessity of .a third volume to " The Spas of Germany,")—he will have assisted in completing the medical history of the Spas of that country, drawn up for the information of English readers.

A second work is also announced, from a gentleman at Brighton, whose name the medical profession has not had the pleasure, I believe, of hearing before ; but who, in a small pamphlet on the subject of the artificial mineral waters sold at " the German Spa" at that place, written in such a manner as if no one else had ever written upon them before *ad satietatem*, states, that " considering that there is not in the English language a standard work on the mineral waters of Germany" (!) he had been induced to prepare, and was preparing for the press, an extensive work on that subject; founded, of course, upon as enlarged an experience and personal knowledge of it, as he has had of the artificial waters at Brighton.

Besides these striking instances of the interest created in the medical world by the publication of " The Spas of Germany," both in England and on the Continent,—the re-publication of that work in France, in Belgium, and in two different cities of Germany,—its translations, and the many original works on mineral waters, in German, as well as French, which have appeared within the last three years, and are constantly issuing from the press,—together with the great attention which practitioners and the medical press in this country are beginning to pay to the subject—serve to prove to conviction the assertion with which I set out; namely, that a great change has taken place in, and a new and favourable turn been given to, the public opinion in England, respecting the efficacy of foreign mineral waters.

This is as it should be: and if such is the case, with regard to foreign mineral waters, shall it not be so also with respect to those of this country? I hope so, and believe so. In endeavouring, by the present work, to bring about the real-ization of such a happy result, I do not pretend to take the lead of my professional brethren. Many have distinguished themselves in the same good work already, by treating of some of the leading mineral springs; and many more are at work in their respective districts to promote the success of the mineral-water treatment in their own neighbourhood. With such coadjutors, and a publication like the present, embracing a much larger field of information on all the mineral springs of note, the use of mineral waters in the cure of diseases in Eng-land may be expected to become deservedly popular.

III. —Principal and striking Differences between the English and German Mineral Waters.

The mineral waters of Germany principally employed in the treatment of disease, and of which I have given a full description upon another occasion, differ, chemically, from those of England in a most remarkable manner. I am bound to state this at once, and without reservation, of all the principal mineral waters of the two countries.

In the first place, all the cold mineral waters of Germany abound in carbonic-acid gas. Of twenty-one such waters, given in my analytical table, not fewer than seventeen yield from *five-and-twenty* to *forty* cubic inches of carbonic-acid gas in a pint, and are consequently highly effervescent. The others have not less than an average quantity of fourteen cubic inches of the same gas in a pint; and even two of the thermal or hot springs, Ems and Carlsbad, boast, the one of seventeen, the other of eleven and one-half cubic inches of gas in the before-mentioned proportion of water.

Now, the reader who is familiar with the agreeable taste of Seltzer or of soda water; or who knows how much more pleasant it is to drink a fizzing solution of the so called Seidlitz powders, than a flat mixture of Epsom salts and water; or how much more agreeably one drinks off a dose of magnesia with lemon-juice and soda-water, instead of its simple suspension in ordinary water—such a reader, I say, must be aware that those pleasing effects are owing to the presence of a large quantity of carbonic-acid gas in the liquids he has taken. Just so it is with the German mineral waters of a low temperature, as contrasted with the English mineral waters of the same or analogous temperature usually drunk medicinally.

In looking at the analytical tables which accompany the present volumes, the reader will at once perceive, in the column headed " free carbonic gas in cubic inches," that the quantity of that gas in the eighth part of an imperial gallon (a little more than a pint), of twenty-three different waters of low temperatures, out of thirty-two English mineral springs, is under two cubic inches ; that in five only it a little exceeds two inches ; and in one other it is stated to be as much as eight cubic inches. As for the thermal or warm waters, they contain little or no gas of this kind.

This striking deficiency is of the utmost consequence to those patients who are ordered to drink day by day, and for some time, a succession of glasses of a mineral water generally endowed with a saltish, or bitter, or soapy, or astringent, or nauseous taste, whether they drink it with the agreeable sensation of a pleasantly sub-acid effervescence, or without it. In the former case not only is the natural unpleasant taste of the water masked at the time of drinking it, but the water also sits more lightly on the stomach, and is not likely to produce nausea.

But there is another and much more important reason for deprecating so great a difference between the cold mineral waters of the two countries, in respect to carbonic-acid gas, and its deficiency in those of England ; and that is, the much greater degree of solvent power which the said gas imparts to a mineral water containing it ; whereby not only a larger proportion of the active ingredients are constantly kept in solution in the water than would be the case without it, but the said proportion receives an additional as well as beneficial energy in its action on the system.

This, in the case of chalybeate or steel waters in particular, is of incalculable advantage—an advantage that may easily be noticed while drinking Tunbridge water at home, or the Bruckenauer water abroad, each of which contains nearly the same weight of steel, but differs in the quantity of carbonic gas as one to thirty-six and one-half.

The next most remarkable difference between the German

and English mineral waters—one indeed which the mere inspection of the respective chemical tables will at once point out—is that which exists in the total quantity of the saline ingredients in equal measures of the water. It will be seen at once that in this respect not only are the English mineral waters totally deficient in some of the salts to be found in those of Germany, which give to a mineral water virtues in the cure of certain disorders that one would seek in vain in waters not endowed with the same salts ; but that the total or absolute quantity of the saline ingredients altogether— particularly of those of a solvent or purgative character—is inferior in the mineral springs of this country.

Thus it will be observed, that whereas in the German table there are columns for phosphates and fluates of lime and of magnesia—of nitrate of magnesia—of muriate, sulphate, and carbonate of potash, and of oxide and carbonate of manganese ; no such columns are to be found in the English tables of analyses. And again it will be noticed, that most of the German waters hold in solution a much larger proportion, than do the English waters, of muriate and sulphate of soda, of sulphate and carbonate of magnesia, and of the salts of lime : and finally, that whereas a pint of most of the more active and esteemed German mineral waters contains never less than from 200 to 350 grains of active ingredients ; corresponding mineral springs in England do not hold more than half that quantity.

With all these admitted differences, however, there still remain a number of mineral waters in this country, presenting a happy combination of certain ingredients, which render them sufficiently active and efficacious in the cure of special disorders, and in respect to some of which they are even superior to the German springs I have described in my previous publication. Such is the case, for example, with regard to the large proportion of iodine found in the Woodhall and Tenbury waters. The Germans have also an iodine

Spa *par excellence*, Kreuzenach, a description of which I did not include in my former work, for reasons already alluded to in the preceding section, and the nature of whose water approaches somewhat to the Iodine Spas at home : so that in this respect the two countries may be said to be on an equality.

One only ingredient, and that of the gaseous kind, is found (as it seems) in almost every one of the English mineral waters I have inquired into, obtained authentic analyses of, and admitted in the tables of the present volumes, which has hardly ever been detected in the mineral waters of Germany. I allude to Azote, or that principle so abundantly entering into the composition of our atmosphere or common air, which will be observed to be present in twenty-nine out of thirty-six springs inserted in the English tables.

This remarkable discrepancy in the constitution of the mineral waters of the two countries,—this constant finding of azote in those of England and never in those of Germany, leads one to suspect that some false result is probably obtained during the analysis of the gaseous parts of a mineral water under examination, through the adoption of some peculiar mode of operating for the detection of gases. It is not impossible that common or atmospheric air, either intimately and naturally mixed with the mineral water under examination, or collected with the water about to be analyzed, may have, in the course of the several manipulations, lost its oxygen and left the *azote* behind, which has been falsely ascribed to the mineral water itself.

The almost invariable finding of that peculiar gaseous substance, by the English analysts of modern times, in the springs of this country, would seem to countenance such a surmise. At the same time I am not prepared to gainsay its existence as an insulated ingredient in those waters ; for it is just as possible that the German chemists themselves may have overlooked the azote in their own mineral springs, or may have set it down as common air accidentally mixed with

them. Yet considering the immense reputation of such men
as Berzelius, Sigwart, Kœlreuter, Gmelin, Federhaff,
Kastner, Vogel, Struve, Bischof, and others who have
analyzed those waters, such an oversight can scarcely be
credited.

Admitting, however, for the present, that azote, in proportions such as I have quoted in the analytical table at the
end of each volume,—proportions which are by no means de-
spicable, and which certainly do constitute a marked difference in the English waters,—actually exists; the question
would be—what influence, if any, the presence of such a
gaseous principle can have, in giving new properties to the
mineral waters ; in modifying those which they might otherwise possess through their other component parts; or, lastly,
in annihilating certain of those medical properties altogether ?

Of azote, as a medical agent, we know nothing, except
that it will not support life. We are, on the contrary, perfectly conversant with the physiological as well as medical
effects of carbonic-acid gas, and sulphuretted hydrogen gas,
so frequently found in mineral waters, both at home and
abroad. On this point, therefore, we have probably much,
or nothing at all, to learn ; for it may turn out that the presence of azote in water does materially affect it; or that, in
almost constantly proclaiming its presence, the analytical
chemists of this country have been led into error.

The question must rest there for the present, and with it
I terminate what I had to offer respecting the differences between the mineral waters of the two countries.

IV.—POSSIBILITY OF CURING ACUTE, AS WELL AS CHRONIC DISEASES, BY EITHER NATURAL, ARTIFICIAL, OR STRUVE-MINERAL WATERS.

HAD I not so recently addressed the public " on the mode in which mineral waters act, and how they ought to be employed," in one of the sections of my introduction to a former work, this would have been the place for bringing forward the notions which long experience has induced me to entertain on the subject. To do so, however, would be a mere repetition, and I pass, therefore, to the brief consideration of the important proposition placed at the head of this section.

It is assumed that a mineral water taken inwardly, acts on the system, through the stomach, in the first instance, by the agency of its own peculiar ingredients. A pill, or a draught, or any other form of internal medicine administered to a patient by his physician, in no wise differs from this supposed preliminary mode of action. By the stomach is meant, of course, the whole of the digestive tube; and by the *mode of action*, is understood, the first or *direct* effect produced. What the second, or indirect, or reflected effect, may consist in, and on what part of the organization the mineral waters produce that effect, is not so readily surmised; except from some consequences or other which may have been observed to follow frequently, if not invariably, the use of the same mineral waters in individuals affected by a similar disease. It is not otherwise with regard to all artificial medicines, whether simple or compounded, which are exhibited to cure that same disease. Mineral waters, therefore, are medicines, and they are medicines prepared in a laboratory, the constant accuracy of whose results is so certain, that we ourselves cannot be sure of success in any of our chemico-medical compositions, except in as far as we follow the laws which seem to regulate the laboratory in question, namely, that of nature.

These premises being granted, for they admit of no dispute, wherefore shall we not consider mineral waters as capable and sufficient to combat and remove diseases which other compound medicines, imperfectly put together as compared to fluids naturally medicated, are expected to combat successfully and remove?

We will suppose, for example, that a happy combination of sulphate of soda, or glauber salts, with some sulphate, carbonate, and subphosphate of lime, besides muriate, sulphate, carbonate, and nitrate of magnesia, sulphate of potash (the general reader will forgive me, I trust, this introduction of technical names, that are *untranslatable*), and minute proportions of alumine, silica, iron, and manganese, be required to remove a severe disease of the kidneys, and the consequent derangement of its peculiar secretion, accompanied by its inevitable concomitants—an impaired digestion, and weak stomach; it having been ascertained from long practice, and empiric observations of the effects of such chemical agents on that region, that the result, by employing them, would be the one desired; what better course could we adopt than to prescribe, either all conjointly, or separately, the said agents, in the most convenient and least disagreeable form? Now, *long practice*, as well as empiric observation, has shown that the Seidschütz water of Bohemia, containing all those very agents, has been pre-eminently useful in the removal of the diseases in question, and I can most conscientiously vouch for the fact. Are we not then authorized to take those chemical or medical agents where we find them already happily combined, rather than to attempt to combine them ourselves in the chemist's shop? when, the attempt being made, we shall discover that some of those agents or salts will not apparently dissolve and combine, and the mixture will continue thick or opake, as well as unpleasant to taste; whereas, in the Seidschütz we shall meet with nothing but a brilliantly clear and almost sparkling water, having a moderate degree of bitterness in the taste.

I could multiply cases and analogies to a considerable extent. In the treatment of fevers—particularly those of the bilious or inflammatory character—we often require saline combinations, first, to assist other and more potent as well as expeditious agents, such as mercury and bleeding; and, secondly, to dilute, promote perspiration, and other fluid secretions,—quench thirst, lower the pulse, and in fact abate irritation.

For the production of the last-mentioned effects, Riverius, an Italian physician, invented the never-to-be-forgotten " saline draught," either mute or effervescent, into which modern practitioners not unfrequently dissolve some aperient salts, whereby they have obtained very happy results.

But frequently such a draught is found insufficient—or after a few times it disagrees with the stomach, or becomes inert. Often other ingredients are rendered necessary in the draught, to make a more effectual " fever draught;" and yet, by the ordinary laws of human chemistry, such ingredients would be deemed *incompatible* with those already entering into the composition of the saline draught.

Well then, where man is at fault, nature triumphs; and if on such occasions, and in such conjunctures, small two-ounce draughts of one of the many saline mineral waters of this or any other country were used, containing the requisite ingredients which we ourselves know not how to combine,— we should obtain all the desired effect, and benefit largely our patient smarting under fever.

Led by considerations and persuasions of this kind, I have often prescribed in fevers some of the German or English saline waters, alternately with other necessary medicines and auxiliaries,—to the simplification of the treatment, the hastening of the recovery, and the satisfaction of the patient.

But the class of diseases not of the chronic sort, in which the appropriate and daily use of mineral waters has more eminently succeeded than any ordinary compound medicine in my experience, is that which embraces all the varieties of indigestion, and a disturbed state of the functions of the liver and intestines—under which a very large number of men in the prime of life in this vast metropolis labour.

Such disorders generally begin abruptly, and after a succession of years, during which, the individual having enjoyed the best of health, has indulged in all the pleasures of the world, thinking himself invulnerable, or has applied too earnestly and continuously to too fatiguing and exhausting occupations.

In the former class will be found your young noblemen, and eldest sons of people of wealth, leading an independent life—your club-men—your young unmarried bankers—your officers of the household troops—and, finally, the *viveurs*, as the French call those who look out for exquisite cookery and high living.

In the latter class, much more to be pitied and more numerous,—we reckon the professional people of sedentary life, such as lawyers—men of letters who are at their desk all day, eat a hearty dinner, and sit up again late at night at the desk once more—artists—merchants devoted to their counting-house—and above all, clergymen without number.

It is curious how few females suffer from the dyspeptic and biliary disorders under which all these people suffer. The latter are seldom attacked before thirty years of age. But it is between the ages of thirty-five and forty-two or forty-three, that the disturbance in the general health begins : and when it does so, it is generally accompanied by symptoms which seldom fail to alarm or disquiet the patient, who thinks himself lost. For he has frequent palpitations at the heart—or his pulse intermits—or he has a constant noise and swimming in the head—or a beating at the pit of the stomach—or a sudden shortness of breath—or a disposition to faint—and other symptoms too many to enumerate.

Hence despondency; hence a misanthropic or gloomy view of the world ; hence a change from an even and amiable, to an irritable and morose temper; hence a desire to seek relief in medicine, a flying from one medical man to another, without any firm reliance on any, or a fair trial given to their prescriptions ; and finally, perhaps, an entire surrender into the hands of a quack, who very speedily brings the disease to an unwished-for termination.

These cases are not, properly speaking, instances of chronic, but of acute or recent disease. They are often, very often cured by being sent to an appropriate Spa; and in that respect I have reason to be highly satisfied with the numerous examples of perfect recovery which followed the recommendation I have given to patients of that description, when consulted by them. But I contend that they may, are, and have been cured at home also, by combining with the appropriate treatment which most medical men know how to apply to them, the use of such mineral waters as are suitable to the case, instead of the *black* doses and *soi-disant* strengthening draughts that are made to follow.

Pullna water is one of those ; the Seidschütz another; the waters of Kissingen ; those of Marienbad ; the Woodhall Spa water; the real Cheltenham ; the Tenbury; the newly-discovered waters of Shotley Bridge ; all these mineral waters may be employed with success in the cases under consideration, provided a proper choice be made, and the necessary rules, imperative in the use of mineral waters, be observed.

That such mineral waters will expedite the cure they are intended to perform (far more than some of the means generally employed) in combination with mercury and other necessary medicines, I can with confidence promise.

It is almost incredible, for example, the number of persons, principally of the better and higher classes of society, who have been benefited by substituting Pullna water for every other sort of physic. M. Schweitzer, of the German Spa, at Brighton, has sent me word that this water, which after my recommendation of it in the first edition of the work on " The Spas of Germany," began to be drunk, and went on increasing in sale, so that on the appearance of the second edition in 1839, I had his authority for stating that it had then doubled; has, since that time, more than quadrupled in its circulation, which continues on the increase.

Many other practitioners in the metropolis now recommend it to their patients, in which they evince their good sense; while many more patients take it of their own accord, from what they have learned upon the testimony of others.

In fact, mineral waters, whether of home or foreign origins, including those so ably imitated by Struve's process, and by that only—properly selected, and accompanying alterative and prudent doses of some mercurial preparation, or other apt substitute, suitable to the individual constitution of the patient—also, regimen and above all a proper diet, which should invariably be well explained to, and insisted upon with, the patient; these will be found to cure recent diseases better than a farrago or a never-ending change of medicaments.

I have entered into this subject (which to most of my general readers will appear new), because I am not aware that any of my brethren have before publicly recommended the adoption of the plan explained in this section, and in order to do away with the common error of supposing that mineral waters are only effectual in the treatment of chronic diseases.

V.—Reasons of the recent Disfavour of English Mineral Waters, and of the Decline of most of the
once-fashionable Spas.

No one can deny, who is acquainted with the social and
medical history of this country, that mineral waters have, for
the last thirty years, been growing out of fashion ; that those,
even, which were most in repute have become nearly forgotten;
and that if one or two mineral watering-places of recent
formation have, during that period, started into existence,
their temporary elevation has been due to causes alien to the
intrinsic and legitimate object of mineral waters; while their
continuing or not in the enviable position they occupy is becoming every day more and more problematical.

Need I quote Bath and Tunbridge to illustrate the first,
and Cheltenham and Leamington to illustrate the second
part of my proposition ?

There is probably no modern literature in Europe that can
supply a larger collection of works, of different degrees of
merit, on the subject of mineral waters, than that of England.
Not only have general treatises on that subject been written at
various epochs, from the time of Dr. Short in 1734, to that of
Dr. Saunders at the beginning of the present century; but
many monographs and very curious accounts have been published from time to time, both before the first, and since the
second of those authors, on separate mineral springs or baths.

Most of their works would be of little use now ; for neither their chemistry, nor their principles of medical doctrine
and physiological inferences, are on a par with the advance-
ments that each of those branches of knowledge (so essentially necessary in the true estimation of mineral waters) has
made in our days. They, however, ended all, as might be

expected, in praising their favourite or respective *Spa*, or mineral spring.

In more recent times, publications on the subject under consideration have been of a different and more influential character ; and I need only mention the respected names of some of their authors, to medical as well as non-medical readers, to prove that the publications in question are entitled to confidence. Pearson, Babington, Falconer, Gibney, Murray, Hunter, Scudamore, and others whose names do not at this moment occur to my mind, are the writers on special mineral waters who in our days have most attracted the attention of patients. Their writings, like those of their predecessors, conclude by recommending the virtues and efficacy of their respective Spas.

As far, therefore, as writing and descanting on each and every particular mineral spring, and forcibly introducing them to the notice of the public, the Spas of England have not lacked advocates and supporters within the last quarter of a century, and ought not, therefore, to have fallen into an almost total disuse, as the greater number of them have done. Where, then, lies the cause ?

When a once highly-fashionable Spa fails in popularity, and gradually sinks into " a thing that has been," the causes of such a change may be traced either to the virtues of its spring having been originally exaggerated or altogether misrepresented ; or to the mismanagement of its water ; or, lastly, to the interference of some extraneous circumstances, inimical, if often repeated, to the quiet enjoyment of the benefit of mineral water.

Where neither misrepresentation nor exaggeration of the virtues of a mineral water has taken place, no such falling off in popularity has ever been observed. Look to Carlsbad and Aix-la-Chapelle abroad. Are they not now what they always have been—most valuable (as they have ever been represented), and therefore most frequented ? And look to the Hot

Wells at Bristol, and to Tunbridge Wells, at home—are they not now deemed much less valuable than they were formerly? (because they had originally been misrepresented), and are they not therefore much less attended?

When I visited both those Spas, in the autumn of 1839, and summer of 1840, I had full proofs of the facts of such an untoward change having taken place in both, from finding that not above a hundred people of any consequence had, during that season, drunk of the tepid stream at the former, and not more than double that number of the steel water at the latter; while, moreover, at the only bathing-establishment with mineral water in the latter place, one or two baths daily were administered, " and no more," as the omnibus legend has it.

The reason of these dismal truths is manifest. The effect derived from using those Spas had not answered the expectations raised among invalids, by those who, conscientiously or otherwise, had strongly recommended them to the public attention. Hence their decay.

And how is it with Bath in our days? Where is the splendid era of the " king of the feast;" of him whose portrait is even now suspended as a decoration in the Great Assembly Rooms cf that city—Beau Nash, the *arbiter elegantiarum*, whose history is the most eloquent eulogium of the palmy days of that Spa? Can we compare that with the present epoch, or even with the history of Bath as a watering-place during the last twenty-five years? Has not the falling off there been as great as it is indisputable?

And what has been the cause of such a disaster? First, mismanagement of the waters. What, for example, would my readers think of the propriety of sending Bath water to every part of the country, in bottles, at the recommendation of medical men, and of raising the expectation of cure by them with such invalids as were unable to attend the Spa from a distance? Could they bottle, along with the water, its *natural* heat, in which consists the most powerful of its virtues?

Oh! but the bottle was heated by being immersed into ordinary hot water previously to its being drunk. If such a process be sufficient to realize the true Bath water, then Carlsbad salts, which are the residue of Carlsbad water after evaporation, would be as efficacious as the far-famed Sprudel from which they are taken, when drank, dissolved in common hot water, at 162 degrees of Fahrenheit.

But who pretends to assert as much? Certainly not those best acquainted with the nature and intrinsic virtues of the waters in question.

Here, then, mismanagement had damaged the reputation of the Bath waters when drank.

Mismanagement of another sort, but still mismanagement, though dependent only on ignorance of chemistry, damaged, no doubt the fame of the water at Tunbridge. This water owes its virtues to the presence of iron. As there must have been thousands of people who could not leave home to travel thither, the water, with all its virtues—that is with the iron—was sent carefully bottled and corked; but when the water came to be drunk, it failed of its effect. How could it have been otherwise? Those medical readers who may happen to have perused the twenty-first volume of the Medical and Physical Journal, edited by myself some eighteen years ago, will have found in a note, that Wurza, an eminent continental chemist, on examining some bottles of chalybeate water, was surprised to find no sign of iron in them; and that, on seeking the cause of that circumstance, he discovered it in the astringent nature of the corks, which had combined with the metallic substance. And so it was with the Tunbridge water in bottles; the iron was gone, and with it its virtues, and therefore was Tunbridge Wells gradually damaged.

These are only the two instances of mismanagement which I can introduce in this place; more will be found under their proper head, in the second volume.   For the present they suffice to show the effect they had of completely annihilating the reputation of Bath and Tunbridge waters, when sent out in bottles to distant patients.

Secondly, the turmoils of electioneering for the choice of that most preposterous of all offices, a master of the ceremonies; which, in the case of Bath, as it is well known, was carried on with the same violence, acrimony, and disturbance of the city, that a disputed election of an M. P., by the Westminster Rump, used to give rise to in days not far remote from us; when brickbats and cabbage-stalks were as numerous as votes, and broken heads as plentiful as speeches; all for the sake of exhibiting the *freedom* of election, and the independence of the citizens of Westminster!

Another cause of the falling off of Bath has been its very unnatural growth and extension, as the result of its pristine splendour, thus converting a Spa with a town, into a town with a Spa—a state of things seldom favourable to the duration of the latter.

Lastly, much of the decline of that as well as of other English Spas, may be ascribed to the great proneness of successive medical men,—established, and invariably found to multiply in a city which possesses a mineral spring in great vogue,—to interfere with the natural action of its waters.   In such a case two inevitable effects are produced.   The patients become soon disgusted with, or are disappointed at, the mineral water; and the medical practitioner ultimately disregards the said waters altogether, and becomes incredulous of their power; a condition of things, in which, as was elsewhere observed, I found mineral-water practice in this country, when I published " The Spas of Germany."

When any or all of these deteriorating and destructive causes are in operation, the several appliances and establishments connected with the Spa become neglected, and cease to be worthy of the patronage of the public.   In some respects this has been the case at Clifton, Tunbridge, Gilsland, Bath, and many other Spas.

But a new era, I am happy to say, is dawning for the last-mentioned beautiful city, whose mineral water is, indeed, the spring *par excellence* of these islands, and whose bathing and drinking establishment ought to constitute it the Sovereign Spa of England. It will not be any lack of desire on my part, in doing justice to that most important source—or any shrinking from the exercise of my usual exertions in the cause of a genuine mineral water like that, as will be seen when I come to treat of Bath in the second volume,—if that Spa be not speedily restored to the highest rank it formerly occupied in this country.

The same resuscitating effect I hope to witness in the case of other Spas; while the examples quoted will be a warning in time to Cheltenham and Leamington, where all the said deteriorative and destructive causes have been silently operating for some years, in spite of the many efforts made by some spirited and well-intentioned inhabitants of the former, to retain a renown which is escaping from their hands.

To the newly-discovered Spas now forming, the lesson also will, I trust, not be thrown away. Matters, in respect to treating diseases, particularly with those wonderful gifts of Providence " Medicated Waters," must be managed differently nowadays. The public have their eyes open; the *prestige* of a mysterious art no longer binds them; and the intercourse between physician and patient, in order to be successful, must be marked by candour, explicitness, straightforwardness, and the absence of all intentional delusion.

As far as the humble efforts of the author of " The Spas of England," and " The Spas of Germany," could contribute to foster and maintain such an improved state of things in medical practice—at which all respectable physicians must equally rejoice—they have been placed at the service of the public, with a frankness that none will deny, and a total absence of technicalities and unintelligible jargon, which every one will perceive.

One concluding remark on a further cause of the progressive decay of some of the English Spas before I have done. It refers to the exorbitance of the charges, and consequently to the enormous expense which families of the middle classes have to encounter at these places of public resort, when they desire to live according to their station in society, at some of the principal hotels. I have alluded, in treating of Harrogate, to the weekly expense of a gentleman and his lady, with three daughters, and two men and a woman servant, who while living at one of the principal hotels at that Spa, and using the public rooms, was disbursing seldom less than twenty guineas a week ; and had he desired a private sitting-room, the charge would have been three guineas more.

Now mark the difference in this respect at the Spas in Germany. The same number of persons would have been magnificently lodged, and sumptuously fed, in the New Hotel at Wildbad, called the BELLEVUE (which has started into existence since my first commendation of that Spa, and is one of the most showy and comfortable establishments of that kind in Germany, and much to be recommended), for 189 florins a week, including every possible expense for master and servant, instead of 281, which are the representatives of twenty-three guineas. Again, a single gentleman, with a servant, who desires to pass his allotted time at the crack hotel of " The Dragon," at Harrogate, must consent to pay five guineas a week, using the *table d'hôte*, and the public sitting-room. But at the same Spa of Wildbad, in the comfortable hotel of Mine Herr Klumpp, I have known a dignitary of the church, during the last season, occupy an extremely neat room, with another for his valet, and to have two excellent repasts, besides breakfast and the board of his domestic, for forty-five florins, or one-third less than the charge at the English Spa.

VI.—Concluding Observations, touching the Auxiliaries of Mineral Waters—Rules of Diet—and
Sea-bathing.

Among these preliminary and popular considerations, I
must find a place for the consideration of the " auxiliaries
to the powers and virtues of mineral waters ;" of the " special
object in using mineral waters ;" and, lastly, of the " regimen
and diet proper during the use of mineral waters, with rules
for taking the same." But these are *general* considerations,
applicable, not to one, but to all Spas ; not to the Spas of a
particular nation only, but to those of any nation. They are,
in fact, generalities, and not specialities.

Now, as I have entered fully into them, under the very
heads quoted above, in the Introduction to my former work
on the German Spas, which is especially devoted to English
readers, and for their guidance, it is not necessary so soon
after their publication to reproduce in this place the observations they contain. To that work, therefore, must I
beg leave to refer my readers, for a more extended information on these essential points in the management of mineral
waters, whether considered as medical aids to cure, or merely
as preventives to impede the coming on of disease.

The auxiliaries alluded to are all those several circumstances which attend the use of mineral waters taken at their
source. One must travel thither. The air is naturally
changed in so doing. The mode of living is no longer the
same at a Spa as at home. There is, moreover, an end to
all ordinary or fatiguing or worrying occupations. Business
and anxiety are equally thrown on one side ; and the daily
rounds of amusements that people seek in general at a
Spa, and the gaiety for which some of them are remarkable,

are all circumstances which assist in hastening the recovery of
the patient, under treatment by mineral waters, and render
that treatment more pleasant.

That such adjuvants are essentially necessary, will be admitted by all; but none will contend, for a moment, that
they are absolutely required when a cure is to be performed
by means of mineral waters; since many such cures, and by
such means, are daily effected at home, in the very heart of
the metropolis, and under circumstances neither of gaiety nor
amusement, but rather the reverse, as I have stated in a previous section.

It is, however, always desirable, when the complaints are
of a protracted or chronic character, and likely to require the repetition of the mineral waters for two or
three successive seasons, (which is the case in many of the disorders of the articulations, in palsy, liver complaints, and in
nervous disorders) to send the patient in search of health to
the source itself, and thereby place him in a condition to
profit by the auxiliaries alluded to.

Of these several auxiliaries, travelling and change of air
are probably the most important; and these the English Spas
offer to a sufficient extent. There is hardly one of those
establishments that does not require the former, as they are
all more or less at a distance from the metropolis and principal towns; although the journey be not so long, nor so
interesting from local circumstances, as that undertaken
by an invalid who has to proceed to any, even the nearest,
of the German Spas. It is, however, possible, when a longer
period of travelling is necessary, to facilitate its accomplishment by judicious *détours*, which in England, perhaps, better
than on the continent, may be rendered easy to the patient as
well as useful, owing to the superior facilities and comforts
one meets in almost every part of the country, provided one
is prepared with a well-filled purse.

Under our present view of travelling, the railroad is out of the question, for the patient would be presently whisked from his home to his destination, ere he knows how that has been done; whereby the object of travelling, as an auxiliary to the mineral water, would be defeated. Posting, therefore, in his own easy carriage, open or otherwise according to the weather, is the mode which would best attain the object in view. But here, unlike the posting in Germany, this mode of travelling involves an expense which a very large number of invalids would rather not encounter, and which, with the much higher charges made for every thing at the Spas, raises the total amount of expenditure for the one single object of trying mineral waters as a means of cure, too high for, or beyond the reach of, the majority of persons requiring such a mode of treatment.

If, for instance, any one out of that number of patients, after having for some weeks sojourned in the character of a quiet bachelor at St. Leonard's for the sake of sea-bathing and excellent houseroom, desired to try the effect of the vaunted steel-water of Tunbridge, and proceeded thither in a posting carriage, he would find that a sum of money sufficient to have enabled him to continue where he was a fortnight longer, would pass from his pocket into those of three postmasters and postboys, and not fewer than *twelve* turnpikemen, upon his line of distance, nominally of thirty, but in reality only of twenty-seven and a half miles.

This is only one of the many examples of this class I could cite from experience. Now the same distance performed by similar means, whether in Nassau, Bavaria, Würtemberg, or Austria, would cost exactly one-third of that sum. Hence the adjuvant of travelling is more easily attained abroad than at home, both with regard to private as well as public means of conveyance.

Change of air, another of the adjuvants, this country offers abundant ways of obtaining, and of a very marked character also. The transition from the southern and sea-girt countries to the midland ones, or from these to the upland regions of Yorkshire and Northumberland; the passing from the bracing and dry north-west or north-east corners of England, to the south-west and south-angles—warmer, but moist and relaxing; together with many other changes that may be suggested to patients by a medical man conversant with the several topographies of the country, and above all with the general aspects of their towns and villages—these are the ways by which an invalid requiring mineral waters may obtain the adjuvant of a change of air.

I attach great importance, and have always paid great attention to the topographical climate of a Spa, or a sea-bathing place; and even to the particular exposition of the dwelling houses for invalids. The medical man who has neglected that study is incapable to advise a patient rightly.

As to the contemplation of a beautiful country, in many parts equal, and even superior, to what one beholds near some of the Spas abroad; or the view of interesting objects, particularly those of human industry and agriculture; or the display of country residences and superb domains; or the sight of neatness, comfort, and order, in general prevailing among the country villages and country towns;—in all these things, supposing them to act, as there is no doubt they do, influentially and beneficially on the invalid who journeys to his allotted Spa—England affords them all to a degree that leaves no room for envying those of continental nations.

It has been one of my particular objects throughout the following pages to put those things forward in the most prominent manner; and in so doing I hope I have done professional as well as general service to my readers,—all of whom cannot have been travellers, even in their own country; inasmuch as by following such a method I have exhibited to them many of the auxiliaries said to be necessary in the cure of diseases by mineral waters.

Those who, never having left their fireside, or not having

traversed the country in all directions as I have done, shall peruse the present volumes, will perceive and admit that none of the auxiliaries thus far discussed, are wanting in England, save and excepting that of a genial climate. But even in regard to the latter, as the season for travelling to and from the Spas is at the most favourable part of the year, the natural inferiority of the climate of this country at all times will not interfere much at that particular period of the year; especially if, in recommending a Spa to a patient, the medical adviser takes care to select it with such a climate, and such local advantages, as will suit the case and constitution of that patient.

Hence, and from all that has been stated on the subject, it will be seen that in order to prescribe successfully to an invalid a treatment by mineral waters, it is not sufficient that the medical attendant should be acquainted with the precise composition and declared virtues of those waters from reading—he ought also, if possible, to be personally conversant with every minute particular, and distinguishing characteristics of every sort, of the place to which he is about to send his patient.

The want of knowledge like this has led people into fatal errors, and sometimes into ludicrous mistakes. I remember a gentleman residing not many miles from Stanhope Gate, telling me one day last summer, that upon a friend of his, a baronet, asking a leading physician, who had been long in attendance upon his lady, whose health had been for some time in a very indifferent state, whether any of the German Spas would suit her case,—the reply had been that the patient might very likely be benefited by drinking the waters of Ems for ten days; then for as many days those of Wisbaden; and lastly those of Kissingen for the same length of time.

Now, setting aside the somewhat ludicrous character of such a recommendation, *per se*,—which would be somewhat as judicious as that of a physician in London who should send a fair lady for ten days to Bath, then for ten days to Buxton, and lastly for as many days to Cheltenham; and disregarding also the important chemical as well as medical facts, that no three mineral waters can differ more than the three before-mentioned German Spas do; there is the climate to be considered, which is again as diverse as the water is in each of those places, as well as its exposure or aspect, the nature of its soil, and the character of vegetation around it; all influential points in a question of adjuvants or auxiliaries.

That people in this country should have been unacquainted with the peculiar climate of Kissingen, the last of the three Spas recommended by the medical gentleman in question, is not surprising, seeing that even the name of that Spa, and much more its peculiar virtues, were unknown to the English until my description and recommendation of the place appeared in this country; since which time many hundred patients from hence have gone thither to try the effect of that water. Had the patient in the case of our anecdote asked her physician, who recommended the three places, whether he knew well how far the air, the climate, and the aspect of those places, together with any other peculiarities for which the place might be remarkable, were likely to suit her constitution, she would have soon seen, by the sort of answers he had given her, whether she could place any confidence in his recommendation.

Patients in their own interest would do well to put a question or two of that sort to their own medical advisers. One often hears that such a person has been ordered to Nice, and such another to Madeira, and so forth. It is no trifling matter for a patient smarting under disease to be torn from home, sent upon a difficult and expensive journey, and deprived at once of his daily and customary comforts—to meet perhaps with nothing but disappointment after all. In order to prevent this, the patient should endeavour to become thoroughly convinced, from the lips of the very man who suggests the expedient, that he is himself perfectly acquainted with the

many peculiarities (particularly of situation) of the two mentioned places,—of Nice, for example,—where many patients
would be seriously injured by a mistake in the choice of the particular region (of which there is more than one there) the most
suited to their case. When Dr. Pitcairne returned from Lisbon
with the tracheal disease to which he ultimately fell a victim,
he told Dr. Baillie, whom he had left in charge of his London
patients, that he had gone thither because he had been told
to do so, upon the general but loose impression then prevalent among the leading medical men of the town—who had,
however, no practical knowledge of the place. " But," added
the eminent and amiable physician, " now that I have been
there I will take care not to send a patient of my own with
the same complaint, if I am spared."

Another, and a very striking illustration of the truth and
accuracy of the principles laid down in the two preceding
paragraphs, occurred in my practice last summer, when in the
case of an illustrious foreign prince, the application of thermal
baths was deemed necessary, through the effect of which he
ultimately recovered from the distressing results of a most
sudden, and at one time very threatening attack of illness.
Various warm mineral baths had been named in consequence,
and ·recommended by friends, relatives, and even medical
persons; but the one which was finally selected, and
which produced the happy and wished for result of a complete restoration to health, was that recommended by myself,
in consultation with the two eminent and leading physicians
who had attended the case with me; simply because being
on the one hand well acquainted with the patient's constitution, and at the same time with the local peculiarities and
advantages of the Spa I recommended—peculiarities exactly
suitable to such a constitution—the medical attendants called
upon to decide adopted the course most likely to be successful, and eschewed the hazard of a mere experiment, as the
sequel has proved.

I will not trespass for the present on the time of my readers, with the consideration of the minor auxiliaries to be expected at the Spas for the quicker recovery of health, such as amusement and gaiety. Unfortunately these are but sparingly to be found at the Spas of this country, as will be seen in the perusal of the description I have given of each of them in the following volumes; and, unless invalids themselves, and their friends, who congregate together at those public resorts of health, exert themselves more than they have of late years done in such places, these are likely to continue, as I have found them almost every where, in regard to gaiety and amusement, " flat, and un-profitable." It is a pity it should be so, and still more a pity because true.

Of diet and regimen suitable to the employment of mineral waters in the treatment of disease, I have spoken at such great length in my Introduction to " The Spas of Germany," that I must simply refer those of my readers who are likely to avail themselves of any of the counsels contained in my present work, and desire to know how they are to live and what they should eat, to the pages of that Introduction : inasmuch as the rules of diet and regimen there fully laid down for such as are likely ro require the use of foreign mineral waters, will serve admirably, under similar circumstances, in using the mineral waters at home. In that respect, mineral and medical hydrology admits of but one system, the particu-lars of which have been embodied in the essay in question ; in the same manner that all the chemical analyses of the mineral waters described have been embodied in a general table ;—for the purpose of not interrupting the continuous thread of the narrative by stopping at each Spa to tell the invalid of what his breakfast and dinner should consist, or of what particular ingredients the mineral water he is to drink is composed, and in what proportions he should drink it.

If it should appear, after the perusal of these volumes,

that the English Spas, take them all in all, are not quite so excellent as those of Germany, the reading of my description of the principal sea-bathing places in this country will, on the other hand, show that England excels all other nations, in the possession of some of the very first-rate establishments of that sort. This I have taken care, in the following pages, to bring prominently forward; and as, in the consideration of the treatment of disease by the system which I advocate, the operation of cold and sea bathing of every form and degree is, to a great extent, naturally and essentially included, it is satisfactory to find that, in this one point, England out-rivals every other nation in the north and west of Europe.

CONTENTS.

CHAPTER IV.

ROAD TO HARROGATE.

CHAPTER V.

HARROGATE.

CHAPTER VI.

HARROGATE CONTINUED.

CHAPTER VII.

HARROGATE CONTINUED.

CHAPTER VIII.

HARROGATE CONCLUDED.

CHAPTER IX.

KNARESBOROUGH AND ALDFIELD.—ENVIRONS OF HARROGATE.

CHAPTER X.

ENVIRONS OF HARROGATE CONTINUED.

CHAPTER XI.

THORPE ARCH—NEW MALTON SPA—ROAD TO SCARBOROUGH.

CHAPTER XII.

SCARBOROUGH.

CHAPTER XIII.

SCARBOROUGH CONTINUED.

CHAPTER XIV.

SCARBOROUGH CONCLUDED.

CHAPTER XV.

HOVINGHAM SPA.

CHAPTER XVI.

CROFT AND DINSDALE.

CHAPTER XVII.

GUISBOROUGH AND REDCAR.

CHAPTER XVIII.

BUTTERBY SPAS—DURHAM ; HARTLEPOOL.

CHAPTER XIX.

SUNDERLAND—TYNEMOUTH—NEWCASTLE.

CHAPTER XXIV.

ILKLEY ; OR, THE MOUNTAIN SPA.

CHAPTER XXV.

HORLEY GREEN—LOCKWOOD SPA—SLAITHWAITE—ASKERNE—HALIFAX, AND LEEDS.

ERRATA TYPOGRAPHICA.

Page 25, line 32, for *established, be through,* read " be established through."—p. 30, l. 4, for *unwieldly* read " unwieldy."—p. 46, l. 15, for *S. E.* read " N. E."—p. 61, l. 8, for *that the lists,* read " that the number in the lists."—p. 66, l. 29, for *Studely's Royal stately park,* read " Studely Royal, stately park."—p. 130, l. 32, place *and* before " owes its striking."—p. 150, l. 16, for *Olive Mount,* read " Oliver Mount."—p. 184, l. 8, for *Cross,* read " Croft."—p. 290, l. 10, for *Magazine whom,* read " Magazine which."—p. 345, l. 27, for *Geneva,* read " Genera."—p. 378, l. 10, for *impetuous,* read " reckless."—At pages 392, and 394, l. 21, the article *the,* has been omitted before " conveying" and " water."—p. 397, l. 29, the pronoun *its* has been omitted before " re-establishment."

LIST OF ILLUSTRATIONS OF VOL. I.

VIGNETTES.

FIRST TOPOGRAPHICAL GROUP.

NORTHERN SPAS AND PRINCIPAL SEA-BATHING PLACES.

B

NORTHERN SPAS.

CHAPTER I.

CLEARING THE WAY WITH THE PUBLIC.

A Dialogue introductory—Character of a travelling Physician—Pros
and Cons—Remonstrances and Explanations—Ignorance better than
Wit—Silence wiser than Talking—Can a Book on English Spas be
made attractive ? Reader, read.

" So here you are again, just returned from another grand
aquatic tour of some months," observed to me an old and
very intimate friend, on my getting back to my quarters, late
in the autumn of 1839, after having travelled very nearly
3,000 miles in search of information respecting the mineral
springs of England.

I assented.—" The necessity of such a tour," I observed,
in reply to my friend, " seemed to have been made manifest
by the success of my account of a previous tour to the
German Spas; by the eagerness with which the better classes
of people in England availed themselves of the information
contained in that account; and lastly, by the anxiety evinced

B 2

by thousands of invalids to try on themselves the efficacy of those health-giving springs."

" Truly," rejoined my friend ; " but you seem not to have contemplated, while planning and executing this second task, how far your own personal interest might be injuriously affected by the variety of observations and opinions which the completion of that task and the publication of its result would inevitably give rise to."

My looks betrayed the difficulty I experienced in comprehending the precise meaning of my friend's allusions.

" You require an explanation, I perceive, and I will give it to you candidly. First then let me assure you, that in the great world here, this frequent appearance of a physician before the public, in the character of a traveller, must damage his success as a settled London practitioner. On assuming the latter character you spontaneously entered into a compact, to be at the beck and service of those who are disposed to place confidence in you. The first return they expect from you for that confidence is, that you shall always be at your post. But how is that compact fulfilled by you, if when most needed, the suffering patient or his friends learn that you are at some hundreds of miles off, gone heaven knows where, to Russia or to Italy perchance ; to Germany or to France ; or perhaps only to the fens of Lincoln and the moors of Yorkshire ? If the world finds it is so once, twice, or thrice, they set you down at last as a mere *travelling* physician, pleasant enough to peruse in writing, yet inconvenient to have to consult personally. In good truth such is the actual opinion entertained by many in regard to yourself, as I have repeatedly heard to my sorrow ; and your brethren have not taken any especial care to enlighten those many on the subject of their misconception. I put no hypothetical case, but a real one for your consideration."

It was impossible to mistake the zeal and friendly intention which dictated these remarks. Still it was in my power, if not to doubt the consequences with which I was menaced, at all events to contradict the facts from which it was supposed that those consequences would flow.

" I admit," was my answer, " that the impression gone abroad may be such as you have hinted at. I have myself found it already formed among patients, in more than one provincial town, during my recent tour; and it must certainly prevail to some extent among my provincial brethren also, or I should not have remarked that previously to their addressing patients to me for consultation in London, no matter at what period of the year, they write to ascertain ' whether I am likely to be in town.' And yet how incorrect such an impression would appear were the real facts better known! and if incorrect, how unjust to encourage it, and suffer it to produce such consequences as you threaten me with! I am therefore glad you have afforded me an opportunity for an explanation.

" What are the real facts? It is now three-and-twenty years since I regularly settled in the metropolis as a candidate for practice. In the course of that long period I have absented myself from town on five different occasions. Twice on account of my own health, seriously damaged by the exercise of one of the most arduous branches of the medical art, which I practised for eighteen years incessantly, and to an extent that few have exceeded while it lasted ; and thrice besides on professional engagements. The entire period of absence, taken collectively, has extended to twenty months; making hardly one month in each year of my service to the public. Why there is hardly any one of the London physicians in extensive practice who does not take a longer holiday every year."

" Still from the manner in which you occupied your time during your absence," replied my friend, " and from having told the reading public how you were employed, even in their service, when not at your post, by the production of octavo volumes of travels—people have come to the conclusion that you must be better pleased to be away than at home ; and even your uninterrupted residence of nine and ten years at one time, without ever leaving the metropolis for more than one day (which I happen to know to have been the case), goes for nothing, or is forgotten."

" So then, had I held my peace after my return from my occasional peregrinations, and kept to myself the fruit of those peregrinations, or what is still safer perhaps, had I wasted the time of my absences in amusements, and returned to my professional labours at the commencement of the season, without the information I have gathered, I should not have exposed myself, according to your present belief, to the chance of being looked upon as a medical attendant who is here one day and away the next, and consequently not to be relied upon. Well! if such must be the price at which I am to secure the continuous support of the public, I at once renounce it on such terms ; and will proceed in my own way to tell that public what I have endeavoured to accomplish in my absence, for their benefit and information."

" But you will have also to submit to the penalty of such a resolution. I will now proceed to give you my second reason for considering this new task of yours likely to act injuriously to your interest. The great success of the book on the spas of Germany, you say, has made manifest the necessity of another book on the spas of England. The proposition is a *non sequitur*. But grant that the necessity for such another book does really exist, you surely have chosen the time for its publication too precipitately! The curiosity and the interest excited by the work on the German mineral waters are scarcely sufficiently abated for you to hope to supersede it by a second publication on an analogous subject. You therefore damage the value of the latter, and your own reputation as the writer of it, if you cannot secure public attention to its subject."

The reply to this second scruple of an over-anxious friend is as conclusive as that in the first case. " By the former work on German mineral waters, I sought to benefit a class of opulent and aristocratic people, who may amount perhaps to five or six thousand yearly visiters to those waters. A very large proportion of these I have seen and sent thither myself since the publication of that work, and on their return they have testified to the great efficacy of the waters in their own various cases, of which I keep a faithful register. The remainder are directed to those springs by my professional brethren, who have all, at last, found out that their patients, encouraged by the contents of the book in question, are determined to try the effect of the German spas. It being clear that thither they will go ; their professional advisers recommend them to do that which it is not in their power to prevent.

" But what are, after all, five or six, or even ten thousand individuals who may be partial to foreign mineral watering places, and likely to keep to the perusal of my former work, compared with the hundreds of thousands of almost every section of what are denominated the easy classes, who may be expected to require, and to be ready to use if properly recommended to them, the home mineral springs, and consequently to be likely to take considerable interest in a work which shall detail to them every particular connected with those means of cure as well as diversion? The only thing needful to attend to, in order to command attention to another work on spas, is to make it as full and as useful as the first has been considered to be; and the result cannot be doubtful. The consequences, therefore, which you seem to deprecate, my good friend, as likely to arise from this new production of mine, the result of an absence of about three months from my post during the last summer, I hope are not likely to follow its appearance."

" May you prove correct in your conclusions. To the

third ground of objection which I take against your present task, however, I apprehend you will not be in a condition to direct any thing like a satisfactory explanation. With all your experience as a traveller, and a writer of travels, it will hardly be possible for you to invest the subject of mineral waters in England with sufficient interest or importance to secure a proper return for your trouble, labour, and care, in an increase of confidence on the part of the public, either in the treatment by mineral waters in England, seeing that they are notoriously inferior to those of Germany, or in yourself as the practitioner who recommends them. Is it not true that almost all the English mineral waters are inefficient in comparison to those of the Continent?"

It is evident that I could offer to my over-scrupulous interrogator no better answer to his third objection than the perusal of the whole work, the existence of which he so pertinaciously laments, as likely to prove injurious to his friend the author of it. To that perusal, therefore, did I urge him to apply himself with convenient speed, and until completed, "to suspend his judgment;" and I ask the same favour of the reader.

CHAPTER II.

RAILWAY TRAVELLING.

Quick Travelling makes Short Books—PRINCE GEORGE, Arthur Young, and the Railway—Is the latter a blessing, or the reverse to Travelling Invalids ?—Important Question for a Doctor to solve—Supposed grievances and positive Advantages—Author's Experience—Qualifications and Exceptions—THE LONDON AND BIRMINGHAM RAIL-CONCERN—Its Bustle and Bullyism enough to kill a Nervous Patient—Contrasted with other Lines of Railroad—Difference between PROMISES and DEEDS—Imposition and Rapacity—Necessity for a Parliamentary Interference—The London and Birmingham, and the Grand Junction Contrasted—Other Sins of the London and Birmingham Line—Promise kept.

OF the many unexpected results consequent upon the enormous change in the internal communications of the country, brought about by railway travelling, there is one in particular at which writers, as well as readers, of books of travels, ought equally to rejoice. Railway travelling has left the former no excuse for dilly-dallying at the very outset of a journey, on a long, tedious, and uninteresting road, to regale their readers with some exquisite bit of novel information, touching the number of milestones and turnpike-gates ; and it has taken from them the power of filling up the first twenty pages of a book with preliminary *verbiage* about what nobody cares for : it has, in fine, compelled them to plunge immediately *in medias res*—that is, to come to the

purport and burden of their song at once, and leave all preparatory notes, of difficulties to be overcome, and fatigues to
be undergone, out of the question. This is no trifling boon
to the reader, who thus finds his curiosity likely to be speedily
gratified without previous tantalization.

Nothing is so tedious as the narrative of preliminary steps
in a book of travels. The *locomotive*, thanks to the philosopher of Soho, has at one stroke of a piston, swept all
such prolixities away. When Prince George of Denmark
undertook to visit Petworth, the royal traveller was engaged
for nine hours in toiling down to his destination (a distance of
about fifty miles); and the account given by contemporary
chroniclers of the measures taken to ensure safety and expedition on that occasion, together with the narrative of the
mishaps on the journey, is as irksome to read as the journey
itself must have proved to the royal traveller. Now behold
the difference which a little more than a century has brought
about in these matters! Look at the wonders of a *locomotive* as compared to a state-carriage!

Another royal prince, on his way to this country, to become what George of Denmark was at the time, quits the
station-post of a Belgium railroad at the extremity of a line
of one hundred] miles, to reach the sea that separates him
from his queen; and in half the time of his royal predecessor, accomplishes more than double the distance without a
single event the telling of which could occupy more than
a line in the narrative of his journey.

Arthur Young was a great traveller in his day, and wrote
almost as many books as he had journeyed miles. But look
at his narratives! One-half of the time of his reader is taken
up with the perusal of entire pages of anathemas against
roads and road-makers, and in lamentations at his own slow
progress.

" I know not in the whole range of language," he exclaims
in one of his tours to the North of England, " terms suffi-

ciently expressive to describe this *infernal* road," &c. &c. ; and further on he adds, " Let me most seriously caution all travellers who may propose to travel this terrible country, to avoid it as they would the *devil*—for a thousand to one but they break their necks or their limbs by overthrows or breakings down."

And where do my readers think that such dismal adventures were portended to the traveller in honest Arthur's time, namely, just seventy years ago ? Why, between Preston and Wigan, a nearly direct line of about seventeen miles in length, which I actually rolled over twice last summer, in less time than one occupies in sipping his breakfast—that is to say, in twenty-eight minutes each way !

How delightful it must be to all who feel the *pruritus peregrinandi* to know that from the identical place whence an active traveller dated his lamentations of old against the almost insurmountable difficulties of journeying to his destination, lines of communication, of equal velocity to the one I have just referred to, are shooting out in a northerly direction, one of which will reach Lancaster before the expiration of 1840, thereby affording the means of transport in ten short hours from London, to within twenty miles of the pure atmosphere of *Winander Meer*, and the other lakes in the north. To a person of delicate health and susceptible nerves, such a journey, with comparatively little or no fatigue, and less of adventure, must be a real blessing.

But is it so, in sober earnestnesss, with regard to all invalids or susceptible persons who may attempt or be recommended to avail themselves of these propulsory modes of travelling ? What is the formed opinion of medical men on such a point ? Have we sufficiently studied the operation of railway travelling on our patients, or even only upon such people as are prone, liable to, or threatened with disease ? What, if a person is endowed with such exquisite sensibility of the nervous system, that the clumsy slamming of a door by a careless footman at home, or the tumbling down of a set of fireirons, at once produce a start, a commotion, and a headach for the day? Can such a person trust himself to railway travelling? And if a lady be thrown into a fever and a state of agitation at the sight of mere ordinary bustle—at the incessant grinding of a carriage ploughing a gravelled road—or at the rapid passage of objects before her, — is such an individual fit to travel by railway? Should, in fine, a person of either sex, subject to what is commonly denominated fulness of blood in the head, risk a rapid journey in one of the locomotives of the Western or the South Western trains, to rattle on at the rate of thirty miles an hour?

These are important questions for a physician to treat; especially if, in undertaking a work wherein travelling may form a prominent subject of recommendation, he is likely to point out the convenience and facilities of the new and striking mode of transport, which forms the subject of the present chapter. Such are precisely the reasons which gave rise to the chapter itself, and but for which some of my readers might think it out of place in a work on " The Spas of England!"

I am not aware that the question has been fully considered or discussed in medical works. Incidentally there have been opinions mentioned as emanating from medical authorities, which are, however, as yet unsupported by sufficient experience and undoubted facts. Some one or two awkward or unfortunate events that have occurred on a railroad, to travellers supposed to have been in infirm health, have been explained in an off-hand manner, and upon very feeble evidence, as the effect of railway travelling on such constitutions—nay, some of my brethren have gone so far as to analyze with mathematical and nosological precision the different degrees of mischief, which the various incidents, inseparable from railway travelling, are likely to produce.

It has been alleged, that the being wafted through the air at the rate of twenty or thirty miles an hour, must affect delicate lungs and asthmatic people; that to such as are of a sanguineous constitution, and labour under fulness of blood in the head, the movement of rail-trains will produce apoplexy; that the sudden plunging into the darkness of a tunnel, and the emerging out of it as suddenly, cannot fail to make work for the oculists; and finally, it has never been doubted, but that the air in such tunnels is of a vitiated kind and must give rise to the worst effects; while that at the bottom of deep cuttings or excavations, being necessarily damp, will occasion catarrhs, and multiply agues!

Such is the list of alleged grievances said to have been started by medical men, against railway travelling.

I have availed myself of that mode of conveyance as often as possible upon all rail-roads, good, bad, or indifferent, in all directions and in all classes of carriages; from the superb mail chariot with its spring cushions and well-stuffed back and sides, to the open platform in which passengers of the humblest description, as on the Manchester and Leeds rail-roads, are penned-in like sheep. I have tried a journey of nine hours consecutively in one of the close carriages, and again, in the second or open class of vehicles. In the course of all these goings and comings, I have studied not only myself but my neighbours, and purposely entered into conversation with them as to the effect of railway travelling, on themselves and their friends or acquaintances.

It is in this manner alone, that positive information on such topics can be obtained. Well, the result of all my observations is, that there is not much of truth in the alleged medical grievances against railway travelling, and that, *per se*, such a mode of conveyance is not more likely to do mischief to people's health than any other hitherto adopted.

I am bound, however, to qualify this declaratory opinion by stating, that constituted as rail-roads are at present, without proper and responsible control, or uniform legislative regulation ; and varying, as almost all of them do, in their mode of construction, management, and condition, so that while one is smooth, joltless, and almost noiseless, another is the very antipodes of all these ; it is not impossible that some easily affrighted dame, some highly nervous old gentleman, or a readily excitable person prone to fulness, may suffer from railway travelling or from some of its concomitants.

But these are the exceptions and not the rule. I admit, that if the first of those morbidly disposed individuals, on presenting herself at the station of the London and Birmingham line in Euston-square, in order to procure a ticket for any one of the classes of carriages on the rail-road, is made to go through the necessary process in the most hurried manner possible, and without the smallest chance of gathering a syllable of information, or a civil answer to a question, from one of the spruce clerks busily employed in slicing and distributing pink, blue, and yellow slips, for pounds, shillings, and pence, which keep flowing in from every quarter : I admit, that if, at the beckoning of a policeman, the same easily affrighted lady be squeezed through a funnel-like passage, as if she were forcing her way with the rabble at half-price into the pit of old Drury, in order that she may afterwards find her way, *tant bien que mal*, to the platform from whence she is to embark on her venture : I admit, that if, having once reached the platform, dragging her own portmanteau and *sac-de-nuit*, she finds the former suddenly snatched from her by some lusty porter, and thrown upon a new-fangled pair of scales at the bidding of a young fop, who at the same time peremptorily demands some additional ten or twelve shillings, for an alleged excess of weight in her luggage : I admit, that if, marvelling at so exorbitant a demand while questioning its justice, the first signal-bell for the passengers to take their seats is heard to sound, and the servants of the company, running to and fro, hardly offer to relieve her of her burden, or place her and it in the carriage she is to occupy, but leave her to do all that in the best way she can : I admit, that if, while perplexed as to what she ought next to do, she hears the last signal-bell ring, and a second policeman addresses her with "Now, ma'am; you'll be too late, ... in with you, ma'am, quick, quick, or you'll be left behind ;" lifting her at the same time from the platform on to the step of the nearest carriage (probably not the one she ought to take for her destination), and the train all the while moving forward : I admit at once, that if all these things are to take place, if an easily affrighted dame is to be thus jostled, hurried, and bullied, then the railway journey which is to follow is likely to prove of serious injury to her.

But reverse the picture : see the same person going through the quiet, easy, civil, and reasonable proceedings which accompany railway travelling on any other line, the South Western for example, and our easily affrighted lady will find no inconvenience whatever, but on the contrary every comfort from that mode of conveyance.

The rail-road, from London to Birmingham, is in fact an ill-managed concern. Present yourself in any garb you please to the counter of their offices, assume the most affable or beseeching tone of inquiry you can, still you will either get no answer at all, or one which you would hardly give to your own menial servant. The difference in that respect between the two ends of the line, the London and the Liverpool lines, is quite striking; as compared to London, all the officers and servants at the Liverpool terminus are perfection, and their arrangements incomparably superior.

The rapacity, too, of the persons managing the concern has no end. I have before me their soft-lipped, alluring prospectus of 1833. Not only was *safety* and *expedition* promised, but *economy* also. The latter was illustrated by comparison to the then inside fares of stage coaches, of which the charge for the first class of carriages on the railroad was to be less than the half. This forbearance did not last long. The price was soon raised to the full amount of the inside of an ordinary stage coach ; and within the last few months, with as much reason for any further increase in the fares of the principal classes of carriages as there was for any addition before,—namely none, but the good will and pleasure of the directors, and the despotic uncontrollable power granted to them by a loosely and vaguely defined act of Parliament,—they have raised the principal carriage fare by an additional half-a-crown, and have visited with a still heavier demand the traveller who prefers the second class of carriages, by increasing his fare five shillings more, that is, double the increase upon the first class carriages, by way of penalty, it must be supposed, for presuming to prefer the second to the first class of vehicles !

This is hardly honest towards the public ; and done too in the face of many successive favourable reports from the Board of Directors, upon the progressive gains of the company, and the declaration of high dividends.

Where is this eagerness after lucre, unvisited by any usury laws, to stop, if Parliament does not interfere in behalf of the public, which the legislature has hitherto left unprotected, and at the mercy of any set of rail-road monopolizers ?

It is really worth while, as we are on the subject of railroad travelling, and as I am disposed on the whole to recommend the use of it to certain classes of invalids, not only as a convenient but as a salutary mode of transport from one place to another—it is worth while, I say, to reduce to a few formulæ of numbers the iniquity of this mode of proceeding on the part of the London and Birmingham Railway Company. For this purpose we have only to contrast what is done in regard to charges upon the two extreme lines, between London and Liverpool, which meet at Birmingham as a centre.

The distance between the last-mentioned city and Liverpool by railway is ninety-seven miles and a quarter. The charge for the first class carriages is and has invariably been one guinea. That it is a remunerating charge, we may conclude, first, from its never having been raised; and, secondly, from the recent declaration of a very high dividend to the shareholders. Between London and Birmingham the distance by railway is 112 miles (so laid down in all their maps and sections); the charge, therefore, if that of one guinea for ninety-seven miles and a half be an equitable and remunerating charge, ought to be twenty-four shillings and fourpence. But it is, in reality, thirty-two shillings and sixpence; *ergo* there is, in this case, a positive extortion of eight shillings and a fraction above what is *equitable*.

Such an extortion, however, becomes even more glaring when we take into consideration the London and Birmingham fare for the second class of carriages, which, as before stated, has been lately raised without notice or reason to twenty-five shillings. On the Grand Junction the distance of 97¼ miles is charged 14s. 8d. for that class of carriages. The proportionate charge, therefore, for the same class of carriages on the London line should be 16s. 3d. Instead of which it is 1l. 5s.; *ergo*, there is here an excess of nearly nine shillings above what is just and equitable! And the legislature, in granting acts for this new mode of conveying passengers, never provided against the possibility of such extortions being practised on the public!

But these are not the only sins against the London and Birmingham management. Their behaviour with regard to the charge for luggage is even more reprehensible. In all their printed documents it was stated that all excess of weight of luggage above 100lb. would be charged one penny per pound. Even to this day it is so printed on some of the luggage tickets. It is the charge still demanded on the Junction or Liverpool line, and I may add on many other lines; though several of them make no charge whatever for luggage. But one penny is not so good as double that sum : so thought some able financier at the board, on some unlucky day for the public ;—and his compeers assenting, the printed *one* is forthwith changed into a written *two* on the luggage ticket.

In that guise the charge stands on my own ticket of the 18th of July, 1839, now before me (8 P.M. o'clock train), by which an excess of luggage weighing 72 lb. above what is allowed, and which, according to the declaration of the chairman of their board to a committee of the House of Commons, made two or three months before, would have been charged six shillings, now cost me twelve ! What Chancellor of the Exchequer would, by the stroke of a clerk's pen, venture upon doubling the amount of any tax on the public, in the truly off-hand manner of these executives?

The said luggage consisted of a leathern portmanteau *only*. It was rather bulky to be sure ; still it was but a portmanteau, and I could carry it with one hand. I ventured, almost tremblingly, to put in one word of remonstrance against the unexpected transmutation of one into two, which I saw juggled before me by the clerk's quill, and also against the amazing ponderosity discovered in a *clin d'oeil* in my portmanteau, which had been thrown carelessly on a newfangled weighing machine that left no leisure or means to verify its operation ; but I was instantly abused.

As I am not of the most pacific temper in such sudden emergencies, I, too, raised my voice and plucked up courage to demand for myself, and others (who by this time had entered the office with similar protestations), some explanation. But lo ! I might as well have tried to out-whistle the steam which just then was rushing with a violent hissing noise out of our locomotive. " Pay, or your luggage *shan't* go !" I did pay, and told them they should hear from me,—and thus I keep my promise.

CHAPTER III.

RAILWAY TRAVELLING CONCLUDED.

ABUSES Abroad and Abuses at Home—Reform necessary—Every other Species of Conveyance under Legislative Control except Railroad—DANGERS and Inconveniences of Rail Travelling—Author's Experience —FIRST START—Darwin's Prophecy—Progress—Impediments—Accidents—Delays—RESULT—Sum total of the Benefit to Mankind, and Invalids in particular, from Railways.

I DARE say that when these pages see the light, some one will stand up to defend the Company in the proceedings described in the last chapter. But then I know, that the whole voice of the public is with me on the subject. Some reviewers, too, will be retained, to show up the Author for introducing questions of this nature in a work professing to treat of mineral waters.

When on a former occasion, treating of the mineral waters of Germany, I exposed the impositions practised at the frontiers and custom-houses of some of the continental ptaces on those who travelled to and from the several spas, no one found fault with my proceedings, but rather applauded the act. Is it only when abuses are met with in foreign countries by a traveller, that their exposure is proper? and if the same individual travels at home upon a like errand, and discovers equal, if not worse abuses, does he not render the same service to the public by exposing them likewise?

That a corrective reform must take place of all such abuses connected with railroad travelling, and at the hands, too,

c 2

of that very legislature which allowed the creation of many fruitful sources of these abuses,—every thing around us seems to indicate; and that reform cannot come too soon. Railroads, to be a blessing to this country, must be placed under wholesome and distinct parliamentary regulations, and watched over by authorities *wholly independent* of the speculative part of the undertaking. Not the pecuniary part of that undertaking alone, should be regulated and put under control, with a view to the protection of the public; but the safety of the latter also should be considered—a point of the most vital importance, for which, as yet, no provision whatever, of an official character, has been made or thought of.

If a smack, or the smallest bark, is to be licensed to trade from London to any port of Great Britain, certain precise and definite regulations to ensure its safety and that of the crew are strictly enforced, by a Trinity board or some such authority. Some of these vessels, placed under the command and management of a master, may be manned, perhaps, by three seamen and a cabin boy only. Yet that master has certain strict orders to observe, for the protection of the four lives temporarily placed under his care.

The legislature has in such cases, and from time almost immemorial, interposed to save human life. Among the many public carriages that convey a dozen passengers to and from the various cities of England, not one is permitted to ply without strict rules being laid down, established by acts of Parliament, by which its management and progress on the king's highways are strictly defined; so that the limbs of the traveller therein and thereon, may be, as far as possible, protected. In this second case again has the legislature interposed to save life.

But how differently stands the case with the new mode of railway travelling authorized by the very same legislature! Why, instead of three or thirteen, three hundred, or three thousand lives have often been committed in one day, on the several railways of England, to the sole direction of one man, an engineer, so called, or engineman, whose skill, prudence, sobriety, alertness, presence of mind, strength of nerves, promptitude in action, and knowledge of the Leviathan power he has to control, have never been preliminarily examined or ascertained ; neither have they been acquired by regular scientific training or education ! And yet on the failure of all or any of these requisites, in a man having the momentary charge of so many human lives, may the whole or most of those lives be suddenly extinguished, or as many limbs maimed and disfigured.

I would advise those who have feeble nerves, and especially travellers of the weaker sex, when once embarked in one of the well-stuffed coaches of the Great Western, or of any other railroad, after having surveyed the superb display of closed and open vehicles arranged on rails under a splendid colonnade, in one almost interminable line, teeming with live beings,—not to suffer their thoughts to revert for an instant to the consideration of how and by what mighty power, and under whose sagacious and provident direction, all these creatures, beaming with life and spirits, are to be transported to their remote destinations. Such a reflection, at such a moment, would deter them from the prosecution of their journey, or make them miserable throughout it if they proceeded. It is in such cases as these that I admit the possibility of railway travelling being likely to prove detrimental to health.

To glance at all the possible dangers to which the traveller on a railroad is at present liable, from the mere want of a uniform and intelligible legislative enactment to regulate that new and prodigious invention, which seems destined to annihilate space,—is a task to be shrunk from, were it not thrust upon us by the very nature of the subject and intention of the present chapter. In fact, no other mode of travelling is encompassed by so many dangers.

In the course of the professional tour which the following

pages are meant to describe, the author purposely availed himself of every species of conveyance along a circuitous route of nearly three thousand miles, ranging through almost every county in England ; in order that he might be prepared to give his best advice, founded on personal experience, to those who are likely (as in the case of the Spas of Germany) to apply for that advice, respecting the most eligible mineral spring to be resorted to, or the most desirable mode of conveyance thither to be adopted.

Railway travelling formed the larger proportion of the various modes adopted by the author. Carriages drawn or pushed by locomotive as well as by stationary engines; carriages sliding down an inclined or dragged up an ascending plane; carriages moved along by a trotting horse on iron rails; all these were employed in turn. The inside and outside of mail and stage coaches were also put in requisition, and so were postchaises, gigs, and errand-carts. Finally, a saddle-horse, a canal-boat, and a coasting-steamer, were not forgotten. All these means of conveyance were purposely had recourse to by way of experiment; but none suggests to the mind so large a category of perils almost inherent in it (so long as it shall remain in its present state) as that one marvellous species of conveyance on which we have been descanting.

We will imagine that we are about to start on a railroad, from the terminus or first station. A long line of carriages charged with their live lumber awaits the signal. Hitherto the huge locomotive, which had been brought out of the engine-house like an impatient warhorse, and placed at the head of the line,—had only given tokens of its presence to the passengers by the continuous hissing of its steaming breath issuing through a narrow opening. But now the bell has sounded—the carriage-doors are all secured—the farewell and the good-by have been given to the travellers by the friends who remain behind and who retreat back on the platform—

" All's right," cries the inspector at the end of five minutes. The monster-engine, roused by fresh fuel and loosened by the swarthy engineer, first changes the hissing into a hoarse yet shrill whistle, throwing up a shower of misty water into the air like a huge Leviathan of the Greenland seas; and then panting loudly, and in measured beatings, sets off on its rapid journey, dragging along with it (chained to each other) the fifty vehicles to which it has been harnessed, " and outstripping," as a recent writer has said, " the fleetest race-horse and antelope in its speed."

How clearly did the illustrious Darwin, in his Cruscean distich, predict this wonderful consummation of man's industry, many years before it had even been dreamt of by the world !

> Soon shall thine arm, unconquered steam, afar
> Drag the slow barge and drive the rapid car.

Once launched on its errand, the train is at the mercy of one man's skill and carefulness; and all that are committed to it have suddenly and voluntarily changed their individual chances of the worldly perils likely to affect their existence. The train in its rapid course has come into collision with another, or with a ballast train which did not get out of the line into the siding at its proper time; or it has overtaken a long train of goods which had set off before, but had been detained. In each of such *rencontres* the effects have been tremendous.

Presently the train has found the moving rails, or switches, which are to direct its course, turned the wrong way, by the neglect of a policeman deputed to set them properly ; and the engine, with the string of carriages, by being suddenly thrown off the straight line upon a sharp curve, have been fatally overturned. Such switches, upon a lofty embankment, turned the wrong way, have precipitated the whole train down its sloping sides.

In some places the train of one railway and that of another have to cross each other on a level at certain angles ; as in the case of the Great North of England and Clarence Railroads, for example:—who can contemplate the effect of a collision, should the two trains meet by miscalculation of time or accident? Yet such a collision has taken place on the Darlington and Stockton railways.

Farther on the train is to change the line, in order to enter upon another at right angles. The time appointed for this is arranged, so that no other train may be at the point of confluence of the two roads at the same time; but some accidental occurrence has baffled this pre-arrangement, and two trains have reached, from two different lines, the point of confluence at the same moment of time, and the contact has been terrific and fatal. Newton station can testify to that fact.

Similar, though not equally dangerous rencounters, the trains may fall into, from the railroad crossing in places, and on the same level, ordinary highways.

Presently the train reaches an embankment, the soil of which, loosened by the effect of heavy and continued rains, and incapable of supporting any weight, is unsteady and gives way, just as the rumbling engine advances over it, and is suddenly imbedded in the quaking mass of earth.

In another part of the line, a long train of carriages has entered a very deep cutting, the banks of which are not sufficiently inclined away from the railroad. Incessant rains for two or three days have loosened the earth of these banks, which the vibration caused by the train has afterwards shaken down, overturning the engine and half burying several of the carriages. The Grand Junction can bear witness to the possibility of both these occurrences, and November 1839 is not too far remote a period for recollection.

Lastly, a bridge or a viaduct has broken down at the very instant of the string of vehicles passing over it, and some of them have been precipitated into the chasm. The Greenwich, the Birmingham, and the St. Germain's railroad in France, have, each in turn, furnished an example of this species of danger, inherent in railroad travelling.

Next to such danger come inconveniences ever inseparable from a mode of travelling of this description. Of these,
that of delay on the road is, perhaps, the most lamentable;
in as much as the causes of it have hitherto been as frequent
as they have proved disastrous. At one time it is a stray
cow or a sheep lying athwart the rail, which the engine's
scuper tosses into the air, being itself checked in its progress by that act.

At another time, a deaf railway-labourer is knocked down,
or a drunken policeman falls just as the engine approaches
him, and the rapid machine passes over their bodies, being
thrown out of the line at the same moment.

A supply of water to feed the boiler is required; the train
reaches the pump at one of the stations, but the pump is
frozen or refuses to work. The stoker, who ought to be like
Argus, ever vigilant, falls asleep now and then; the fire
goes out; and the locomotive, which was to have conveyed
the night-mail at twenty-five miles per hour, is standing
stock-still.

Here and there the rails will be covered with snow, or be
excessively wet; and the wheels refuse to *bite*, wasting their
power in useless girations. All these *contretemps* will cause
delay, though not so much so as when, upon some unlucky
occasion, a grand explosion takes place, and all power of
locomotion is suddenly annihilated.

These inconveniences and dangers are not imaginary or
merely possible; they have actually all occurred upon some
one railroad or another; they have all been recorded in the
public journals, and been admitted in evidence before a parliamentary committee; neither will they be averted until superior arrangements shall be made, and a general supervision
of all the railroads established, be through the agency of a
general Board.

The immense advantages, however, of this stupendous invention still remain; and although, as in the case of almost

every one of the more surprising discoveries of man, practically applied by his ingenuity to the curtailment of labour, the increase of wealth, and the multiplication of luxuries,—the result has been obtained at the expense of new dangers, with an increased liability to the loss of life ; nevertheless, the great, the enormous sum of benefit that must accrue to mankind from the establishment of a means of conveyance which seems to level all topographical distinctions, and not only brings distant cities, but remote countries nearer to each other, and annihilates time and distance,—is not to be questioned, and becomes every day more manifest.

Railway travelling is a fruitful theme of many important reflections, besides those which I have deemed sufficiently akin to the general objects of my present work to introduce into this and the preceding chapter. Its reference to political results—to agricultural considerations—to statistical conclusions—and to the possible amelioration of the condition of the people, form so many points of interest, which it is not my province to touch upon in this place, yet to some of which I may perchance have to allude in the course of this work, with certain illustrations drawn from personal experience. At all events they are points well worthy of the consideration of statesmen, as involving questions of the first importance,— whether in regard to the immediate interests of enterprising persons, and the convenience and intercourse of the community at large, or in reference to the safety and protection of human life.

CHAPTER IV.

ROAD TO HARROGATE.

The Euston Station—Philip Hardwick—The departure Parade—
Arrival of Passengers—The train—Vagabond Post-office and flying
bags—Suggested Improvement—Off-we-go—No sooner gone than
arrived—Theatrical Effect—Railroad Suppers; cheap, plentiful,
and quickly swallowed—Irish M.P.'s—Facility of travelling makes
Travellers—Sundry Illustrations—Where will it end?—Arrival at
Liverpool—The Adelphi—Farther Progress—Arrival at Harrogate.

Having now done my duty by pointing out the many
glaring defects in the management of the Grand Junction,—
not without hope that it may mend in consequence,—I hesitate not in asserting that, but for it, I should probably not
have undertaken my present laborious task.

To know that—thanks to the grand junction rail—I should
find myself, in the course of a few hours only (those hours
snatched from sleep, and consequently of no great value)
within a short distance of one of the most central, and at the
same time one of the most interesting spas of this country,
to begin with,—was certainly an inducement for me to make
that beginning; and I therefore set out with a light heart and
good cheer, on my instructive and professional excursion to
visit all those important localities.

To a traveller who is in a hurry, and desires to enjoy as
many of the comforts of a railroad as he can procure, the
night train is unquestionably to be preferred. The very sight

of its preparation for departure is inspiriting, and there is hardly a more dramatic or soul-stirring scene enacted by gas-light any where in London, than that which may be witnessed every evening under the colonnade of the Euston-square station.

The arrival of the mail train from the country at an early hour in the morning at the same station, is tame in compari-son. One only advantage does the stranger enjoy who arrives by that conveyance on a fine morning, which those who depart late at night have not: it is the sight of that imposing and massive entrance erected by Philip Hardwick, on the purest principles of a Grecian Doric elevation, which rises to the height of seventy feet, and imparts to the locality a grandeur commensurate and in character with the gigantic nature of the entire road, considered as *one* line of communication be-tween two extremes—the first and the second commercial cities in England.

The departure parade, as it is called, at the hour of eight o'clock, p.m., is swarming with bustle. The experienced tra-veller in this species of conveyance reaches the spot in full time to see his luggage safely lodged on the top of the coach he is to travel in; and within that coach he afterwards secures his seat, by the number marked on the ticket he received in the office. He then has leisure to survey the throng, and examine the long string of vehicles prepared to carry to their respective destinations an almost incredible number of tra-vellers like himself, whom he sees arriving in groups and shoals, pouring in upon the departure parade from all the outlets of the various offices; some panting and fearful lest they should be "too late;" others coolly sauntering, *cigar en bouche*, like old hands at this sort of work; and many frightened at the mere idea of losing both property and passage.

First come the carriages of the second class, which slowly move on, like automatons, to take up their station at the outer end of the parade, where the headmost is yoked to the locomotive. These carriages are closed with glass windows, and are sufficiently snug in winter, but have not the luxury of cushions, stuffing, &c. An experienced traveller, however, will bring his own cushions and plenty of great-coats, and make himself as comfortable in this particular class of vehicles as if he had selected the better class, and at an expense, which, until it was unexpectedly and unjustly raised last year, amounted only to two-thirds of the expense of the higher class of carriages.

Then follow next in succession the carriages destined for Manchester, forming the first division, and consisting of four, five, or more, according to the number of passengers who require them. After these comes what is emphatically styled the royal mail-coach, followed by the several carriages destined for Liverpool, which constitute the second division, composed like that of Manchester, of several first-class carriages and the mail-coach. The latter, in both divisions, is a smart dashing vehicle, within and without, most luxuriously fitted up inside, like the new chariot of a young baronet going to court on succeeding to his title. The former, also, are decked within with every comfort. They are well stuffed, have soft cushions, and a most convenient upright, with resting-places for the elbows, and a pillow-like swelling on each side of the traveller, who can hardly resist from applying his cheek to either, and committing himself to the god of slumber. Should he be sleepless, however, or by nature vigilant, a friendly lamp hangs suspended from the centre of the ceiling, bright enough to allow him to strain his eye over a guide-book, or the " unstamped," which are sold at the station *pour tuer le temps.*

But one of the most interesting portions of this long chain of vehicles, is the huge caravan-looking machine which follows in the rear of all the carriages, and which reminds one of the old days of Cross and Exeter Change. On peeping into it, an oblong square, well lighted and fitted up with pigeon-holes on every side, shelves and tables, presents itself, the direct purport of which is very soon made manifest, by the introduction of unwieldly and foul leathern bags, crammed full of letters, which are being dragged in by men in the post-office liveries; while the operation of sorting the said letters is going on within. During the progress of the train, smaller letter bags are formed out of the larger ones, which, being afterwards hung outside the caravan in some opportune place, protected by a net-work, are, upon arrival at certain points on the road, snatched off without any detention, by a simple machine, whose alertness is never at fault; and thence they are conveyed to the respective offices in the neighbourhood for distribution.

The sight of this bee-like industry within a confined hutch, while the train is swiftly sliding on to his destination at 25 miles an hour, suggests the idea of a different and preferable arrangement, for the conveyance of passengers in trains travelling to greater distances, like the one from London to Liverpool for instance, or the other (that is to be) from the metropolis to Exeter, and a third from the capital of England to the capital of Scotland. I mean the adoption of long omnibusses instead of coaches, fitted up with a long central table, around which the passengers may sit, and either write, read, play at cards, converse together, or take refreshments, as in the state cabin of a steamer, and as I understand it to be the case on some of the long railroads in the United States, where people value their time too much, and are too busy, to afford to go to sleep, or be idle for so many hours even in a railway carriage.

The line of vehicles along the departure parade is terminated by the tender, the luggage-van, and the truck for private carriages.

At twenty minutes before nine, P.M., this long procession started. In one hour and twenty minutes it had reached

Tring; at a quarter before one, Coventry lamps hove in sight; and with a continuous movement, vibratory at times, and a noise generally drumming, but occasionally clashing, we reached Birmingham as the illuminated clock, under a much more stupendous colonnade than that of the terminal station in London, marked twenty-five minutes to two, A.M.

One hundred and eleven miles of ground had thus been passed over in five hours (no prodigy for a railroad to be sure), before one could get *ennuyé* or fatigued. I am thus minute and particular, on behalf of such of my readers as are invalids, or of a trepidating nature, who will not be sorry to peruse what may appear trite, worthless, and common-place to others. I shall not easily forget the flattering re-mark made to me by a patient returning cured from one of the German Spas, Gastein,—who asserted that the very minute description I had given of the difficult road to that romantic and elevated spring of health, had, by putting him on his guard, been the means of saving himself and party from many difficulties and a perilous rencounter.

If the starting from Euston station be dramatic in effect, the arrival at the Birmingham-station is no less theatrical. The sudden entering under the cover of a vast area, brilliantly lighted up like a fairy region, with the whole train, which pushes its course home to the very furthest verge of the plat-form, facing a grand building destined to give asylum and refreshment to the hundreds of passengers who arrive by the Liverpool train—is accompanied by sensations not experienced under any other circumstance. Neither are these sensations rendered tamer by the next spectacle that, in the vast tea-room, offers itself during the halting-time, of three-quarters of an hour duration, allowed to such as have to proceed to Liverpool or Manchester; although the room in question is not so elegant and ostentatious as the great morning or re-freshment saloon just alluded to, designed and erected by the same eminent architect to whose imagination is due the Doric arch of Euston-place.

The strange effect of suddenly beholding, upon emerging from the slumbering and dark monotony of a night journey, three hundred people of both sexes, arranged as if by magic, and in an instant within a spacious and well lighted room, around several cross lines of parallel tables, who, but five minutes before, were variously distributed and apart from one another in thirty different carriages—is in itself amusing. But its entertaining character is considerably enhanced if we follow these people in their operations, attacking and demolishing tea, coffee, chickens, tough ham and stale bread—beef, pork, and stuffed pies—and all in ten minutes and for two shillings.

On this occasion I recognised, among the hungered, many Irish M.P.'s returning to their home after a laborious parliamentary session, and not, as one may easily suppose, among the least eager in the work of demolition.

I used to think the sight of a mail-coach supper or a long journey to Edinburgh, a marvellous odd sight. But this swarm of human mouths suddenly put in motion—these two hundred pair of hands, setting-to at once with forks and teaspoons, to sweep clean off from a set of long tables many pounds of sugar, and gallons of tea, and dishes innumerable of various food, under which they were before groaning—but the faces and grimaces, the chattering and the jargon, the approbation and disapprobation, expressed in loud tones, of so many minds, mouths, and stomachs, that accompany the scene,—these I say are features of the moment, far more exciting than all, and may prove a moral lesson into the bargain.

Surely the facility of travelling has given people a new propensity to locomotion. For at what time were there ever congregated together in any one night, so many as 150 to

200 passengers in this halfway-house city, when long coaches only, and short mails plied on the road, to convey people, either for pleasure or business, from one point on the line to another ? What other proof need we have of the truth of the proposition with which I set out than the fact, for example, that between two insignificant towns in Yorkshire, Darlington and Stockton, where hardly enough travellers could be found formerly to support a coach three times a week on a road of about twelve miles, the subsequent establishment of a railroad has induced upwards of two hundred persons daily to travel that distance ?—or the other fact, that between Manchester and Liverpool, a similar railroad facility of communication being once established, about thirteen hundred passengers have been *daily* availing themselves of it every year ; whereas twelve or fifteen coaches sufficed before, for the number of travellers who plied between those two cities?

It is, therefore, unquestionable, that to afford cheap and speedy means of travelling for the people, is to induce people to travel who would otherwise have staid quietly at home ; and if this process is to go much further, the whole nation, at length, will be on the move; no one will ever be at his post ; restlessness will be the order of the day ; and we shall be on the go, so much and so often, that we must go *au diable* at last, railroads and all. This is the moral lesson, and mark the issue of it !

As the rosy-cheeked milkmaids of Liverpool were plying their shining pails from house to house, calling the half-slumbering inmates to their doors; the passengers in the London train reached the terminus in Lime-street, whence many of them proceeded to that most showy and bustling of all hotels in England, the Adelphi. It was, unluckily, the second day of the Liverpool Races, and all the black and white legs from the metropolis had congregated in the house, and secured all the habitable parts of it; leaving me the alternative of either proceeding elsewhere, or putting up with a dark bath-room seven feet by three and a-half, to dress in, as the best accommodation the house could afford to a new comer.

This was no great grievance to one who only wished to *débarbouiller* himself, eat a hearty breakfast (and no coffee-room in England supplies a better one than that of the Adelphi), and after making two or three inquiries, on account of which he had taken Liverpool in his way, instantly to depart for Manchester,—where, in fact, I arrived in an hour and a quarter, after finishing that most delightful repast.

The object of my next movements being to reach Harrogate with as little delay as possible, I staid not, this time, to inquire after old friends in Manchester; but leaving the Royal Hotel (a house which, for its situation, I can well recommend to my travelling invalids), immediately after my arrival, I committed myself to the top of " the Earl of Harewood ;" on the slow wings of which, after a flight of seven hours and a half through all the densely-populated and manufacturing cities of this district of Yorkshire (Rochdale, to wit, Halifax, Bradford, Shipley, Otley, &c.), I made good my journey from the metropolis to Harrogate Spa, in the course of one night and a few hours of the following day, and took possession of a small neat back bedroom, at the end of an interminable narrow corridor *au troisième*, in the Crown Inn.

Now, to the physician who undertakes to visit Harrogate for information only, such rapidity of motion from the metropolis may not be objectionable, nor the miscellaneous mode of proceeding thither fatiguing. But to an invalid whom the doctor may have to send to that Spa, a less hurried and heating manner of reaching his destination would be more convenient and desirable.

For this there is every facility and appurtenance imaginable. The railroad from Manchester to Leeds, about to be completed, will expedite, without increasing its fatigue, the journey to that Spa; to which from the last-mentioned city, the distance left to be performed by ordinary coach or post-chaise conveyance, is only sixteen miles.

But until the railroad in question be completed (and none promises better), the traveller in delicate health proceeding to Harrogate, may rest at Birmingham a night, having left London by one of the afternoon trains; reach Manchester the following day by a similar train; advance with baggage and carriage in the morning by the railroad again, as far as Littleborough; and thence with post-horses, go forward to his destination, with hardly any fatigue.

CHAPTER V.

HARROGATE.

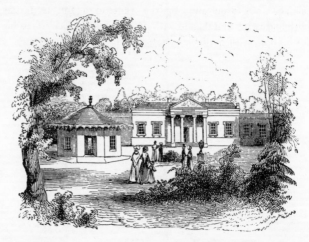

Doings at Harrogate—First Intelligence—Early Season and Late Season—
Cockneys and Aristocrats—Short History of Harrogate—Genuineness
of its Waters—Its Situation,—Low HARROGATE and HIGH HARROGATE
—Discovery of Saline Waters—The OLD WELL—The MONTPELLIER—
"Stinking Waters"—A Legal Squabble—The Lawyers always best off—
Expense of Quarrelling—Boon obtained worth nothing—Sulphur Water
Plentiful at Harrogate—The Cheltenham Saline—ROYAL PROMENADE
ROOMS—Discovery of other Saline Waters—Recapitulation—Analysis
of all the Waters at Harrogate—Dr. HUNTER of Leeds—Sir CHARLES
SCUDAMORE.

HARROGATE has the very air of a watering-place. A
stranger traversing its elevated common as he comes in from
the south, by the Leeds or Manchester road, could not mis-

take it for any thing else. But if the first and rapid survey upon arrival should leave him in a state of doubt, conviction of the fact will force itself on him through eyes and nostrils, " at early morn."

Well acquainted from former visits with the localities, and knowing that I should find more than one of my patients and friends in the place, I proceeded soon after my arrival to visit one of them, whom I expected to be my cicerone for the week, and kind remembrancer.

" It is yet early for you to see this unsophisticated place to advantage (so my friend had written to me early in July), for it is, as yet, full of clothiers from Leeds, and cutlers from Sheffield, besides all the red noses and faces in England collected together. There is not a livery-hat in the place but our own, and ours, at present, is the only 1*l.* 1*s.* subscriber on the books at the sulphur well; showing the caliber of the company, who cannot afford more than five or ten shillings, and most of them the half of the smaller sum. But Sheffield and Leeds will soon loom homewards, and then, they say, better company will come."

My correspondent was right. The cold which prevails yet,—particularly at night—in the month of July, and the frequent showers of rain, render Harrogate ineligible as a mere summer residence, at that period, and would scare away the more exquisitely susceptible among those of "gentle blood." At the close of that month the Spa season properly speaking begins, and this lasts till Doncaster races. Before that time, carts and gigs empty their gatherings daily. Coroneted chariots, britzschkas, and postchaises, ply about in abundance, after that, bringing their more noble cargoes of aristocratic visiters.

It suited my purpose to be betwixt and between, like Mahomet's coffin. I wished to see the tail of the "unwashed," and the head of the "exclusives," and I just hit my right time for that purpose.

Like most of the really celebrated Spas in England, Harrogate was, at the first discovery of the springs, a mere village ; but unlike most of them, Harrogate remains a village to this day, though upwards of two hundred and seventy years have elapsed since the first mineral water was tapped on its bleak heath, by a Captain William Slingsby. While Cheltenham and Leamington have converted themselves, in the course of a few years, from mere villages that they were, into smart and pert towns, Harrogate has remained a village still. It has been brushed up a little to be sure, and extended somewhat, both below and above ; but so wildly and irregularly—so without any design and consistency, and at such distant periods of time—that pretension to any thing above a village it has none.

This is precisely the circumstance that has saved the reputation of Harrogate. Who can cavil at the nature, genuineness, and efficacy of the Harrogate waters ! On the other hand, who has not cavilled, and cavils to this day, at the waters of both Leamington and Cheltenham ? Those of Harrogate are unsophisticated, because the place itself remains as it was ! You dip your cup into the fountain-head, and get your *strong* waters. There is no shuffling, and the mind is convinced at once. Elsewhere you have the complicated machinery of pumps, the ends of whose pipes may terminate heaven knows where, and you drink in faith, but not in conviction. Harrogate is, in fact, a true and genuine Spa.

Its situation is delightful. For elevation, above the Irish and German oceans, midway between which it is nearly placed ; for position, at about equal distances from the three capitals of the United Kingdom (about two hundred miles) ; and for geological formation, favourable to human life—Harrogate stands almost pre-eminent.

That such a place must enjoy a salubrious air it is hardly necessary for me to add. The extensive heaths which, with

immense tracts of finely-cultivated country, surround this
favoured spot, allow full play to the sweeping breezes, and
render the air remarkably pure and bracing.

Upon this point we may readily confide in the assertion of an
enlightened physician, Dr. Hunter of Leeds, who has studied
well the climate of Harrogate, and the powers of its waters,
touching which he has written an able treatise, that has gone
through several editions. That writer declares that " no case
of pestilential cholera had been known to have occurred in
Harrogate—neither have infectious diseases of any kind ever
been prevalent."

There is a Low Harrogate and there is a High Harrogate.
In point of antiquity, as a place worthy to be marked on the
map, Low Harrogate bears away the palm. Yet mineral
water was first discovered at High Harrogate. But High
Harrogate has only chalybeate springs, very excellent in
their way, still only chalybeate, and there are hundreds such
in the north. Low Harrogate, on the contrary, has the
" true, genuine, stinking wells," and they were only discovered, or at least used for the first time, one hundred and
thirty years after the former.

The latter wells, nevertheless, are those which gave and
give its reputation to Harrogate ; so that when we send
patients to drink the Harrogate waters, or to bathe in them, we
send them to Low Harrogate, though they choose to live in
the upper village, which is what almost every body tries
to do.

After all, the local distinction consists merely in having to
walk about half a mile on foot, ascending all the while a
pretty stiff acclivity, crossing two or three streets of the lower
village, which lies in a cup or narrow vale—then a field or
two, and so reach the wider expanse or area with its " green"
and " race-course;" hotels *à prétention*, a new church, two
libraries and the post-office, constituting the only important
points of the Upper Region or High Harrogate.

The communications between the two places are free and commodious, there being no fewer than four, namely, two for carriages, and two, much shorter, for pedestrians, as already described.   The two villages stand in the relation of east and west to each other.

Low Harrogate has, within the lest few years, gained additional importance as a mineral watering-place, by the discovery of purely saline waters untainted by any sulphur.   This circumstance has added a new feature to Harrogate as a Spa, and has given occasion for the erection of a noble building, a representation of which stands in front of the chapter.

Of these saline springs there are several; and I have noticed by the compass that *they* are found in what is called in Yorkshire a *beck* or trough (the bed of a rivulet) to the northward of a line running S. E. and S. W., and that southerly of that line no saline, but on the contrary, all the sulphur springs are to be found.   Of the latter, two principally deserve our attention.   On the morning after my arrival I betook myself early to the examination of all the springs.

Between half-after six and eight o'clock, A. M., all the world was up and stirring.   I could from my window survey the various throngs, as they formed and moved to the different points of their destination.   Some directed their steps to the original or OLD WELL, as it is called, a few yards from the Crown Hotel, in which I was staying; and there, under a squatty and ugly dome, supported by rudely-carved stone pillars, they found a gratuitous beverage of fetid water.

Others passing a little to the left of the said hotel, entered the garden, formerly known as the Crown Gardens, but now designated as the Montpellier Pleasure-grounds, in which they found the Crown Sulphur-well, so formerly called, but now styled the MONTPELLIER SULPHUR-WELL, which its new proprietor assures us furnishes a larger proportion of the stinking gas than the original well.

These, then, are the TWO principal sulphur-springs at Harrogate, and their analysis will be found in the general Table at the end of this work—a plan I have adopted, as in my former publication on the Spas of Germany, for the sake of convenience, as well as with a view to avoid any interruption in my narrative, by the introduction of chemical numbers and chemical names, which can interest only a few readers scientifically or medically inclined. The plan was much approved of in the former publication, and I shall adopt it in reference to *all* the mineral waters I may have to mention in the present one.

Besides the two principal sulphur wells I have enumerated, there are two other wells with sulphureted water, one of which has changed its denomination even since Dr. Hunter's late edition, and has been converted from the CRESCENT into the VICTORIA New Pump-room and Baths; while the other, known as Thackwray spring, or No. 5, has acquired a *notoriety* far superior to its celebrity, from the circumstance of its having been the subject of legal contention between certain proprietors of hotels at Harrogate, and the person who claimed to be sole owner of it.

That contention, for which great preparations had been made in the way of scientific evidence on both sides (never used, and lightly paid for), and a still more formidable array of legal talent brought up (too much used and too heavily paid for), terminated, as such causes generally terminate, in the men at law gaining every thing, and the litigants nothing.

The question was, who was to have the sole command of the well—the inhabitants or Thackwray? The judges proposed to split the difference. Thackwray was declared to be the owner, but was bound to erect a room over the well, with a pump in it, which however was not to be maintained at his expense. From " noon till eve" the said pump-room was to be kept open for any body to use the water of the well, as they list, and both plaintiffs and defendants were at liberty to put a lock on the said pump, to prevent its being used out of season.

Now mark the result of the quarrel. The plaintiffs, who gained the cause, had to disburse 1,352*l*. 7*s*. 3*d*., for their victory, towards which sum the visiters, who, the lawyers contended, must feel the deepest interest in the cause, contributed the magnificent quota of 14*l*. 2*s*. ! And the defendant, who secured the nominal ownership of the well, died (probably of broken heart) a few months after the assizes !

And after all, what think my readers has become of the well, the pump-room, and the pump ? Why, the latter has got so fast locked in rust, from never having been used at all by the visiters, or plaintiffs, that upon my trying to work it, in order that I might taste the water, I got a strain at my shoulder, and was grinned at by a gaping clown or two with red hair for my useless efforts ;—and thus almost all these pretended patriotic displays generally end " *in fumo et caligine*."

Not so with the men of law, however ; for they always take care of themselves too well, to permit any such result : and accordingly we find that on that memorable occasion (March, 1837) they shared among themselves a picking of 789*l*. 9*s*. 3*d*. leaving a sum of 341*l*. 7*s*., to be divided in various proportions among the late Dr. Smith, the father of English Geology, the illustrious Dalton, Professors Phillips and Daniel, and the late Dr. Turner.

Both the disputed well, and the one which supplies the Victoria baths, are within a few yards of the spot in which surges the original OLD WELL, the glory and pride of Harrogate, from which almost all the water exported thence is bottled—and may be bottled by any body.

This proximity induced people to fancy that the *disputed* and the *old* well might be only one and the same spring. But there are strong reasons to dissent from such an opinion ; and I for one feel convinced that more than one other spring might be discovered, by tapping the lowest level of the vale on one

side of the bank before alluded to, without interfering with
any of those already in existence. Indeed, within the memory
of the youngest inhabitant, not fewer than three other springs,
with waters charged more or less with the sulphurous gas,
were known to be used, all in the same line of stratification,
and within one, two, or three yards of the old well.

These springs were mentioned and much noticed by Dr.
Sprat and Bishop Watson; but they can hardly be said to
form part of the present arrangement of useful springs at
Harrogate. The curious and the whimsical excepted,
almost all invalids and visiters are satisfied with the Old Well
water, and that at the Montpellier Garden, for drinking; and
with that of the latter, and of the Victoria, for bathing.

I have already alluded to the additional reputation which
Harrogate has acquired of late years from the discovery of
purely saline springs. Within a Doric temple, measuring
one hundred feet in length and thirty-three feet wide, lighted
on one side by a series of lofty windows, we find the first
spring of this class; the discovery of which dates only since
1819. From a supposed resemblance in composition to the
famed Cheltenham waters, this spring has been denominated
the Cheltenham Saline, having dropped its two aliases—of
Oddy, and Williams—by which it was at first designated.

The discovery of a water of a medicated nature, free from
sulphur, and endowed with purgative properties, was hailed
with enthusiasm. Forthwith a pump-room, worthy of its
importance, was planned, and under the care of Mr. Clark,
of Leeds, the structure just mentioned was raised, to which
the name of Royal Promenade and Cheltenham Pump-room
was affixed.

The building is in every respect worthy of praise; but it
lacks space for the many other conveniences required to
enable its present occupier to complete it in all parts, as a
regular Cur-saal, in imitation of those on the continent. Mr.
Gordon, who rents the place, is willing and spirited enough

to undertake all that is necessary, and much of that he has indeed effected already. But he lacks support and encouragement. Much as Harrogate is frequented ; and cheap—unusually cheap—though the subscription to the room be, Gordon would be a considerable loser by the concern, were it not for the benefit he derives from a stated number of balls given during the season in this grand saloon—one of the best of its kind in England.

A band, engaged purposely for the season, from London, enlivens the hours during which the promenaders frequent the pump-room. The architect has for this purpose erected a small gallery within a recess in the wall, opposite the windows immediately above the pump which supplies the Cheltenham saline, about the centre of the room. The affable Mrs. Gordon superintends a small and select library of volumes of light reading, placed behind a glazed screen at one end of the room ; while on several of the tables are laid the more popular periodical publications, and most of the metropolitan and provincial newspapers.

Concerts *à la Musard* serve to quicken the steps of the promenaders in the evening; and nothing in fact has been spared to render the establishment attractive.

It was not likely that a discovery, leading to such important consequences to Harrogate, being once made, should not induce spirited individuals to seek for similar springs on their own grounds. Accordingly we find, in the recent history of that Spa, that the master of the Crown Hotel, who had already, in 1822, found a sulphur spring in his garden, (to which I have alluded under the denomination of the Montpellier Spa, where the sulphureted water is both drunk and used for baths,) did, in 1836, discover a saline mineral spring, analogous to the one in the Great Promenade-room, which he immediately added to his establishment in the same gardens, thereby rendering that establishment complete. This new saline spring, like the other, lies in the same direction from the *beck* which divides the Vale of Low Harrogate.

By way of recapitulation, then, before we conclude the chapter, it will be useful to repeat, 1st, that at Harrogate—that is, on the common above Low Harrogate—there are two purely chalybeate springs, without sulphur, and with few saline ingredients besides; which springs bear the names of the *Old* or *Sweet Spa*, and *Tewit Well*. 2dly, that in Low Harrogate we have two principal sulphureted springs, the *Old Well*, and the Crown or Montpellier Spa, besides the sulphur spring which supplies the Victoria room and baths. 3dly, that two principal saline springs, called Gordon's Cheltenham, and Thackwray's Cheltenham, have been added to the number of late years; besides minor ones of both classes, which will be alluded to hereafter.

All these waters have been analyzed at various epochs, and by different individuals of merit and authority; some of them very recently indeed; as for example, that of Thackwray's Cheltenham saline, which has undergone within the last two months a fresh analysis by Mr. West, of Leeds, who was instructed to forward me the result of his inquiry. Of that result I have availed myself in the general Table of analyses.

I have already mentioned the valuable work of Dr. Hunter amongst the most recent productions touching Harrogate. With that physician I had the good fortune to form a personal acquaintance during my tour, which has tended to increase the confidence I already felt disposed to place in all his statements respecting Harrogate. He resided on the spot, and watched the effect of the several waters for some years, and in his researches he was aided by the scientific as well as practical skill of Mr. West, whom I found upon many occasions, both personally and through correspondence, to be a minute, painstaking, and accurate chemist.

Did I address myself solely to the profession (which heaven

forbid !) I should hardly have deemed it necessary to add in this place, that the " Treatise on Mineral Waters," published by Sir Charles Scudamore, the second edition of which is now lying before me, contains a short account of the waters at Harrogate, with analyses undertaken by himself and Mr. Garden, the well-known and justly-esteemed operative chemist of London.

Of these also I have availed myself in drawing up my general Table. Sir Charles's work unfortunately is almost too strictly scientific and professional to find its way among the general reading public; and I only lament that my excellent friend had not given to it a more popular garb on its second appearance. It might perchance have spared me my present task.

CHAPTER VI.

HARROGATE CONTINUED.

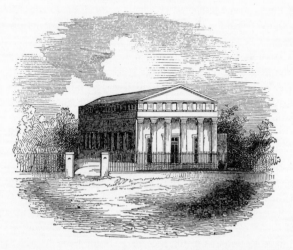

An Impromptu Ball at the Promenade Room—The Company—Introduction—A few Characters—The *Elegantes*—Mutual Invitations—
Dancing the Order of the Day at Harrogate—The Place not well provided with other Amusements—The Montpellier—Appearance, Taste,
and Effect of its Water—Effect of too large a Quantity being
taken—To be Drank Warm—Proper Doses of it—Grimaces—The Old
Well—Character of its Water—Effect of both Waters—Author's
Experience in them—What is wanting in Harrogate Water—Mistakes
respecting the Saline Water—No Analogy between it and the Cheltenham or Leamington—Its Effects—Montpellier Baths—Building
and Internal Arrangement—The Victoria Baths—The Victoria Promenade Room—The Crescent Old Well—Walker's Carbonated Water
—Its value requires confirmation by a fresh analysis.

" Come, come," quoth my friend and quondam patient,
Colonel ——, now for three weeks enjoying the benefit of

Harrogate water and Harrogate air, " you must, for once, unbend, stiffen your cravat, and substitute light pumps for Wellingtons, and ' *honor*' us with your presence at the first ball of the season in the Royal Promenade-room, of which I am the principal steward and M. C. *pro tem*. It is an *improvisé*, done to serve a worthy man, the present *entrepreneur* of the promenade-room, who rents it for 300*l*. for the season, besides paying a band from London at twelve guineas a week.

Tired as I was, I yet could not resist joining in a work of kindness. Moreover, as I had come to see and learn, it struck me that an *improvisé* ball was as likely to teach me the humours of such an assembly at Harrogate as one more deliberately got up.

The Doric temple shows off to great advantage by night, like many of the ladies who figured in it; and with a superior company, such as we meet here at a more advanced period of the season, a ball, in it, must be a mighty fine thing for killing time at Harrogate.

The place was not crowded ; but a good sprinkling of people of almost every sort was scattered over the floor, or occupied the different ottomans in the recesses. Some were dressed as for an evening party, for there had been sufficient notice given in the afternoon of this impromptu. Others had not thought it worth while to go home to dress, and the ladies appeared *sans façon*, in morning bonnets, with their partners *en frac*. Amidst these heterogeneous groups, the six or eight stewards, with their white rosettes and smart coats, appeared like so many turkey-cocks strutting among the motley inhabitants of *la basse cour*.

My first introduction was to Colonel Sir ———, a gay cosmopolitan Scotch baronet of 62, once a dragoon, who hardly ever opens his lips but to spout distichs, either in praise of Harrogate water, which had cured him of a liver complaint, or on his birthday, and on his having been forsaken *so young* (poor thing !) by the fair sex !

My next acquaintance was a young man of property, fashionably attired, who had also derived great benefit from his visit to this Spa. He is one of the *sommités* in Cheshire, with whom I felt much pleasure in conversing at some length, on his intended journey through Greece and Turkey, for which he was preparing himself, by laying in an additional stock of health.

With the history of a few more of the young men present, with whom I had thus suddenly contracted that sort of acquaintance which one is not loth to form under circumstances like the present, I became sufficiently versed in the course of the evening, as they whisked by me, with their fair partners in the mazy rounds of a waltz. There was Mr. ——, the son of Sir Thomas ——, a Cheshire man also, a marriageable youth, much ogled by the ladies' mothers ; and also a penniless *ci-devant roué*, a wreck in health and fortune, though allied to high noble blood, who could now not boast of as many pence as he once had pounds.

Wales, as well as Cheshire and Lancashire, had supplied its humorous contributions to the *soirée's* entertainment, and I was much amused with the minute details of important warlike matters from an old militia colonel, a short punchy man, who had changed his name for a fortune, and acknowledged St. David for his patron.

The fair exhibited rather to advantage, though almost all of them *inconnues*. Three or four were decidedly pretty, and a couple of them perhaps might have been called *élégantes*. Indeed all seemed surprised that so goodly a display should have been brought together at such short notice, considering how few names of any importance there were on the Spa books.

The thing is done somewhat more splendidly, and certainly more gaily, further on in the season—when the regular balls at the Crown, on every Wednesday evening, and at the other principal hotels, on other days in the week, take place by mutual agreement ; or whenever, by some sudden frisk or inspiration, "The ladies and gentlemen at the Granby or Dragon present their compliments and request the favour of the company of the ladies and gentlemen at the Crown," or *vice versâ*. But on the whole what I saw may be taken as a fair specimen of all the rest.

Dancing is the principal amusement for the company at Harrogate; and it is one that greatly conduces to aid the mineral waters in their effect. There is scarcely any other occupation for the invalid and visiter, except excursions to the neighbourhood, and a promenade, *de long en-large*, from one well to another.

The lords of the creation have also the billiard-table, and the cigar; the weaker sex a circulating library; and occasionally a concert is concocted, or an itinerant lecturer comes amongst them to unravel the wonders of the heavens, or display the beauties of nature.

These are so many godsends to shorten *ennui*, for the preventing of which Harrogate is but ill provided. And yet no watering-place in England ought to have more sources of amusement; for Harrogate is " a genuine Spa."

To the Montpellier Gardens I repaired the following morning, anxious to become personally acquainted with a spring which had apparently worked such wonders as I beheld the preceding evening in the persons of our dancers. I followed the throng, who took the direction of a small and neat octagonal building, covered with a projecting Chinese roof, and surrounded with flower-beds and grassy banks, between and over which undulating footpaths afford a limited and circuitous promenade to the water-drinkers.

Within the building two pumps, side by side, supply the sulphur and the saline waters; the latter of which, as I before observed, has been but very recently discovered. This system of pumping mineral waters is decidedly bad, and need never be had recourse to. Why it was adopted in the present istance I know not; but unquestionably the water at the

Old Well will always be drunk with greater confidence, for the
very reason that there are no leaden pipes to draw it. That
few people, *comme il faut*, avail themselves of that well is
simply because what costs nothing is, in their estimation, not
worth having; whereas here, at the Montpellier, the large
sum of two shillings per week is charged, for each person subscribing to drink the waters and to have the right of parading
up and down the grounds.

I shall have occasion to say something more on this system
of pumping mineral waters out of the bowels of the earth—a
system not adopted in a single instance in Germany, and
greatly to be deprecated. At present, I applied myself with
a serene countenance and an empty stomach to the quaffing
of a large tumbler of the fetid stream, previously warmed by
mixing with it some of the same which is kept constantly
heated in stone jars placed on the top of a fireplace.

The water is perfectly colourless and transparent, and
almost brisk from the escape of gas. The first impression on
the tongue is intensely salt, followed by the peculiar bitter
taste of salt water, but leaving an *après-goût* like that which
remains after chewing bitter almonds. It goes down oily, and
at the temperature at which I drank it (115°) the sulphureted
gas is scarcely perceptible. I repeated the same quantity
four times, diminishing each time the artificial temperature
until I drank it cold, thermometer then marking 52°, while
the external atmosphere was at 60°, and the nauseous taste
had increased with the descending temperature.

The whole quantity I took in four times, I noticed people
to drink at twice only, and quite cold. Writers on this
water have recommended the latter practice. This is an
error which I was sorry to see committed at all the English
Spas. There are few stomachs which can bear with impunity
the weight of two doses of three-quarters of a pint each of a
cold, salt, and sulphureted water, drunk with a short interval
between. Few stomachs can stand the slow extrication of

the imprisoned gas, which, once ingested with the cold water, is gradually disengaged by the warmth of that organ. It then mounts into the head, and produces a confused, heavy, and unpleasant feeling.

This I have put to the test of my own personal experience. Drunk quite cold, I found the water particularly heavy on the stomach, and in an hour's time my head ached not a little. Some of my younger patients in this place experienced similar effects ; and, indeed, upon inquiries among strangers, who were religiously following the recommended practice, I ascertained the case to be precisely the same. At all events the first glass or two should be warmed, but not so much so as to drive off the whole of the sulphur gas.

With respect to quantity, that point has been determined by long experience, and by very competent authorities. It did not appear to me that people on whom devolved the management of the water, at the several Spas I visited in this county, were sufficiently aware of the importance of this consideration. The quantity drunk, at one time, should be such that during the fifteen minutes' walk, which is to elapse between one dose and the next, the stomach may nearly have got rid of the first before it receives the second. Four ounces of liquid ingested will nearly disappear from the stomach in the course of twenty minutes, particularly when assisted by walking exercise.

Such is the opinion and practice at the Spas in Germany, where beakers holding hardly as much as four ounces are used by every invalid, and not the half-pint and *whole pint* tumblers which we see employed here, at Cheltenham, Leamington, and elsewhere.

I have entered into the consideration of this subject in this place once for all, and I wish to be understood, that I adhere to the German mode of administering mineral water, in opposition to that adopted in this country.

It is yet early morning. A group of young children of

various ages, from five to nine years, are just brought in.
The maid immediately doles out to them their prescribed
modicum of the " nasty" water, and in such large tumblers,
full and so cold, that I am not surprised at the children
drinking it with reluctance, and making sad grimaces at their
nauseous dose. How half a pint of such a liquid is to be
swallowed otherwise than with disgust by the babes, at this
chilly hour of the morning, when the governess herself takes
care to spit out two-thirds of what she drinks, it is not easy
to conjecture. Seriously, this is a very objectionable mode
of administering the Harrogate water to children.

Day by day I noticed that the physiognomy of the several
groups which wandered about the grounds of the Montpellier,
was improving in the scale of civilization. Every day has its
fresh arrivals. Young ladies are particularly numerous. Old
people too are not scanty—many scorbutic, some herpetic,
and not a few with pustular noses. These are seen wandering to and from the sulphur spring, not unfrequently extending their walk to the OLD WELL for a last sip, a *bonne bouche*,
as it were, before they return home to breakfast.

To that well I next extended my trial of the water upon
another morning. Sallying out for that purpose at 8 A. M.,
I found that " holy temple of Hygeia" thickly surrounded
by people of the middle class. No contrast can be stronger
than that which exists between the sort of people seen to
quaff large goblets of the water here, and at the subscription-
rooms; and the old women, nearly in tatters, placed in a
row behind a species of stone parapet, over the top of which,
as upon a counter, the salutary fluid from the well is delivered to every applicant, formed a curious sight to one who
had been accustomed to behold the neat, pretty, and alert
handmaidens of the Sprudel.

These noisy creatures (who look like so many fishwomen)
administer the water either cold, or mixed with some
previously heated, and in tumblers, in size nearly a pint.

The well is behind them, and there is no lack of the water, which is squandered profusely at no charge whatever, save perhaps a solitary copper-piece, which some one, more generously disposed than the rest, throws with an air of protection on the stone counter.

I quaffed twice of this second sort of sulphur water, about six ounces each time, and warm. It goes down as oily as the Montpellier, is not quite so intensely salt to the taste, and is decidedly without that *après-goût* of bitter almond which I think is a pleasant feature of the sulphur-water at the Montpellier; and which, in the latter case, remains adhering to the tongue for some hours after drinking it.

Like the Montpellier, the water of the old well, especially if taken cold, troubles the head, and some days gives the headach; it produces eructation of sulphureted gas, as when one has been eating half a dozen eggs boiled hard, or in a *worse* state; it acts promptly on the kidneys, and seems to promote the action of the intestines, as well as to influence the character of its secretions in the course of the morning. When neither of these effects are produced, the water is not properly digested, and the head is the more affected.

To render the water at Harrogate perfect of its kind, it should have held in solution about thirty grains of sulphate of soda in each pint. It unfortunately holds none, and therefore it only derives the little of purgative qualities it possesses from the large proportion of common sea-salt it contains, which amounts to one hundred and eight grains in the pint.

If the so-called Cheltenham saline at Harrogate (both the one in the promenade-room, and the other found by the side of the sulphur well in the Montpellier grounds,) had been in reality endowed with the peculiar ingredients known to enter into the composition of the real Cheltenham water, one of which is sulphate of soda or Glauber salt, we might then, by

mixing the saline with the sulphur water, render the latter
aperient, and consequently more useful and effective. Unfortunately, not only is there no sulphate of soda at all in
the *soi-disant* Cheltenham saline at the Royal Promenade-
room, and only two grains and a half of it in the Cheltenham
saline of the Montpellier Gardens, according to the very recent
analysis supplied me by Mr. West; but there is in both a
largish proportion of oxyde of iron,* which at once renders
the mixing of the two waters perfectly impracticable.

That the two waters are incompatible, the good lady at
the pump-room in the Montpellier occasionally does show,
by pumping half a tumblerful of the water from one pipe,
and the remainder from the other closely adjoining,—when the
mixture is instantly converted into something like ink, much
to the amusement of the old and young.

With deference to Dr. Hunter, who, I think, first suggested the notion that these so-called saline waters at Harrogate, of recent discovery, " held a middle rank between the
waters of Leamington Priors and the saline chalybeate wells
at Cheltenham," I must avow my surprise, that he should
himself have adopted, and justified in others, the assumption of
the name of " Cheltenham saline " or spring, in regard to the
water found in the Royal Promenade-room, — when, in
reality, there is no similarity between the two. For a very
potent ingredient (iron) is largely present in the saline at
Harrogate, and totally absent in the Leamington waters, or
exists only in a very minute portion in the Cheltenham
wells; while another equally effective (and in mineral
waters strongly characteristic) ingredient (Glauber salt) is
found in sufficiently large proportions, both in the Leaming-

---

* I can only afford a note, to mention that in the grounds of the
Royal Promenade-rooms, and close to the saline spring, there is a well
of pure steel water, which is not used at present, but of which a proper
use might be made by serving baths with it, as I suggested to the proprietor, Mr. Gordon.

ton and the Cheltenham waters, but not in the saline waters of Harrogate. The very minute quantity found since in one of them was unknown to Dr. Hunter.

Sir Charles Scudamore, by simply calling the said modern waters of Harrogate " Saline Chalybeates," has avoided falling into the error of viewing them as at all like the waters at Cheltenham. The fact is, that the waters in question are chalybeate springs, holding in solution an unusual quantity of common salt, with some muriates of lime and magnesia; and, as such, they are most valuable combinations, and fully entitled to the commendation bestowed on them, both by Dr. Hunter, and Sir Charles Scudamore.

I partook of both waters in their turn, and in sufficient quantities. The temperature at both wells, after repeated trials, I found to be 60°, external air being 65°. In appearance it is opalescent, and slightly turbid, having a vestige of an ochry tinge. The taste, when drunk cold, is saltish, hardly bitter, and it is soft. The saltish taste continues some time in the mouth.

As I happen to require any thing but steel water, I felt, as I expected, very ill on both the days on which I drank of those saline chalybeates. In the head in particular I suffered greatly, and the state of uneasiness generally produced by this tightening fluid pervading the system, was one of great discomfort, until I betook myself to the *soulagement* of half a bottle of Pullna, which I always carry with me when travelling.

Both these saline waters and the sulphureted waters are used as baths, with wonderful success at Harrogate. The practice, of course, is as old as the place; but baths were formerly administered at the different hotels and lodging-houses, in the most inconvenient and unsatisfactory manner. The bath-tubs were placed any where, and the water fetched from the adjoining bog-springs was used for two or three baths without being changed. At present, on the contrary, two superb establishments for bathing exist in the place, equal to any thing of the kind at other Spas.

The Montpellier Baths, formerly called the Crown Baths, come first in point of appearance, though not in priority of existence. The Victoria Baths come next. The building is five or six years old. Hence it is evident that Harrogate, though slow and late, has nevertheless improved in some respects; its baths in particular.

There are six bath-rooms on each side of the building, to which access is had through separate waiting-rooms—the one side being for the ladies, the other for gentlemen. In the hall, or under the portico, in warm weather, a band plays in the morning. The bathing-tanks are exceedingly neat, being of stone of an elegant form, partly sunk into the floor. Inside they are lined with white tiles; externally they are painted and varnished; while the ledge is of polished black marble. They are very deep, and of good length, and admit of the flow of either hot or cold water, by the simple turning of one handle. At the widest end of the bath a band, made of canvas, is hooked across, and serves to support the head, and keep the shoulders away from the cold tiles; a great improvement in all warm bathing.

In two of the rooms on each side of the building the baths are deeper, and are called the upright or sitting baths. In them the bather may sit in such a manner as to be almost standing; a contrivance likely to be of use to certain invalids or elderly people, or to those who, when lying down, may feel the weight of the water on the chest too oppressive.

The water for these baths is drawn from six different springs, by aspiring pumps. A small steam-engine pumps the water through them into a reservoir, where it is heated by steam from the boiler of the engine. The supply of water, both of the sulphur and saline kind, is amply sufficient; nor is the former much deteriorated in its quality by the application of heat, as we might naturally expect; for it is found, when admitted into the bath-tanks, that it retains much of the sulphureted gas.

As if Harrogate had been destined to exemplify publicly the marring influence of legal quibbles, besides what has already been detailed respecting Thackwray's fifth spring, we find a very pleasing and creditable small building of the Ionic order, containing thirteen bath-rooms, sunken below the level of the ground, as if erected at the bottom of a quarry, to which you have access by descending steps, and separate entrances for the ladies and gentlemen. These are now called the *Victoria Baths*, the first establishment of the sort formed in Harrogate; now the property of a Company, who have spared no expense to render them worthy rivals of the Montpellier Baths.

The reason why these baths were built *in*, and not *above* the ground is, that the proprietor, Mr. Williams, was precluded by a clause in the surrender of the plot of ground, from raising any building on the surface of it, and so he dug and erected the baths below it!

This building, however, is perfectly dry, and the arrangement of the baths themselves is very creditable. Although there is not a separate dressing-room to each bath-room, the latter is so large that it admits of a curtain being drawn across, to separate and conceal the bathing-tanks, which are oblong, and ample, and altogether sunken into the floor, and tiled.

They are narrower than those at the Montpellier, and not so smart, yet very comfortable and clean. The terms are three shillings for each warm bath in both establishments. About 4000 are used during the season at the Victoria, and 6000 at the Montpellier.

Almost adjoining to the Victoria Baths is a large promenade-room, with an organ at one end of it, used for public meetings and lectures, and also open to subscribers. It was formerly called the old promenade-room, and was erected in 1805, at the suggestion of Dr. Caley. It now bears the name of the " Victoria Reading-rooms and Library." It is nearly opposite the Old Well, and is frequented principally by the company who make use of the water of that well.

In order to clear the ground of all I have to say in reference to the mineral springs at Low Harrogate, it is right that I should mention in this place the existence of two mineral waters, totally distinct from the rest, which have been noticed in Dr. Hunter's, and Sir Charles Scudamore's works, as the *Crescent Old Well*, and the Crescent Hotel Saline Spring.

The former, which, if it ever was really endowed with the properties ascribed to it by Dr. Garnett of old, must have been a most important spring, is now in a state of utter dilapidation and neglect. I could not procure a single drop of the water ; but I have induced the proprietor to undertake its cautious restoration. The second is now called Walker's Strong Saline Spring, or Leamington Spa Water. It is obtained by a pump, in a small room adjoining Mr. Walker's extensive wine premises; and as it neither contains sulphur, nor a single trace of iron, with the largest proportion of carbonated soda of any of the springs at Harrogate, the water is, in my opinion, a most valuable one, and might be rendered useful in a variety of complaints in which no other of the Harrogate waters is suitable.

I find the analysis of this spring on Walker's card, and he assures me that West is the author of it. The same analysis appears in Dr. Hunter's work; it *is* therefore to be relied upon. Still a fresh analysis is desirable, and I recommended it. Should the composition of the water be as here predicated, I could point out applications of it of the utmost consequence for invalids visiting Harrogate, even supposing them to require the baths of the peculiar water of that Spa.

Walker's saline spring was formerly in the garden of the Crescent Hotel, which hotel has now changed its name for that of Northumberland House.

Harrogate's fetid water is sent to all parts of the kingdom, and every body here professes or undertakes to export it. The Old Well principally supplies the necessary quantity; but the bottling process I there witnessed is imperfect and objectionable. Still, enough of the fetid gas remains to last for some months.

The water, however, does not keep well. Mr. Fryer, assistant at the Montpellier Baths, sends the water of that stronger sulphureted spring in glass bottles, of a pint and a half each, at seven shillings per dozen, bottles included, to all parts of the kingdom.

CHAPTER VII.

HARROGATE CONTINUED.

Influx of Visiters at Harrogate—Larger Number than at any other English Spa —Best Time for Attending it—Scarborough a proper Conclusion of the Course of Mineral-water Accommodations—HOUSEROOM—Situation and Aspect of the principal Lodging-houses—Comparison between Low, High, and Middle Harrogate — YORK HOUSE — THE QUEEN—HOTELS: THE CROWN AND DRAGON—THE GRANBY—BELLEVUE, the crack Mansion of the Place—Panoramic View from it—The Promenade PLEASURE-GROUND — Groups of Invalids — The Interesting Widow—The Lame Boy—CHANGEABLE FACE—The Newcastle Alderman—Distinguishing Marks of Society—Is there any thing in Blood?

SUCH a profusion of important mineral springs collected in one place, renders Harrogate what I styled it—a " genuine Spa," to which thousands must flock annually to seek health —some under proper advice and management, others at random. Accordingly I find, from inspecting that very ably conducted periodical, called the " Harrogate Advertiser," established in 1836, by Mr. Palliser, the intelligent bookseller and postmaster at High Harrogate, that the lists, weekly published, of the strangers or visiters actually in Harrogate on each day of publication, has seldom been less than a thousand, and frequently several hundreds above that number.

Beginning in the first week of June of last year, when there were about five hundred visiters, and ending in the last week in October, up to which latter *cold* date even, there were still about three hundred visiters in Harrogate—twenty thousand five hundred and eighty-six appear to have been registered. But as most of these remain two or three weeks, during each of which their names appear on the list, it will be necessary to deduct something like two-thirds of that large total, in order to come near the true number of arrivals. Hence if we assume that between seven and eight thousand visiters had arrived, and resided three weeks at Harrogate, during the season of 1839, we shall be within, rather than without the mark.

Now this is a considerable number, and one which bespeaks the favour in which Harrogate is held; for even in Germany, hardly any of the most popular Spas, Baden-Baden, Wisbaden, and perhaps Carlsbad excepted, can boast of having had, during any one year, a much larger assemblage of water-bibbers.

By far the largest number of strangers at Harrogate arrive about the 10th of August, and continue to pour in largely until the 15th or 20th of September. To those who at that season are quitting Harrogate, I should strenuously recommend a sojourn of six weeks or two months at Scarborough, to complete their cure.

Now let us see what sort of accommodation and house-room Harrogate can offer to this crowd of pilgrims hastening to its shrine. This one feature of a Spa I hold to be of such paramount interest to invalids, that in all the mineral watering-places in this country which I visited last summer, I invariably followed the plan adopted regarding the German Spas; namely, that of procuring personally every possible information respecting hotels and lodging-houses, and of ascertaining by ocular inspection, that the information was correct.

Houseroom, independently of that which is to be found in the principal hotels, is plentiful at Harrogate, and of every description, from 10l. per week (which a very wealthy and amiable heiress first set the fashion of paying during the last season but one) down to two guineas. Bellevue is the dwelling which has produced the former sum. Two other houses nearer to the Montpellier let for five and six guineas a week. They are convenient, and look westerly. One of them, at the time of my visit, held a family of thirteen children, and their respective progenitors. Other detached houses are to be hired in what is called middle Harrogate, which boasts of a *Parliament-street*, and a *Waterloo-place*.

Ascending higher along this line towards the Common, one meets with a range of stone buildings, having a certain degree of *pretension* to something like architectural design. They are enriched in front with very neat flower-gardens, and look down over the esplanade of Low Harrogate, on one side of which is a public library; and the Crown hotel and terrace on the other side, with the Church on the right hand.

Beyond this " Prospect-place," the road, as it keeps still ascending towards the Common or " Muir," as they call it here, insensibly winds by several other buildings or rows of houses; among which are conspicuous the range called the QUEEN, with its pretty gardens and beds of roses in front, and a showy private house, standing back by itself on a plot of grass within a railing, belonging to Mr. Sheepshanks, a wealthy, good, and benevolent gentleman of Leeds.

But all these buildings, and many of the rest which follow, have the drawback of an objectionable aspect, looking either northward or north-eastward. An invalid will find amongst this great variety of edifices wherewithal to suit his taste and wants, either for a small or a large family. All of them have lying before them the extensive Common, which is intersected by the Leeds, the York, the Ripon, and the Otley roads.

Although the air is purer and lighter at this elevation,—the prospect which the houses of Middle Harrogate have to the south and west, is far more cheerful than that which a vast plain indifferently cultivated, or wholly barren, can offer. In the latter situation it is the keenest eye only (that which can compass an horizon at a distance of ten and fifteen miles) which can find an agreeable or pleasing object before his dwelling. At Harrogate, for an invalid, these are not trifling considerations, and I think I am doing no mean service to those among my readers who may have to spend a season at that place for the benefit of their health, in informing them beforehand as to the most eligible situation for their temporary dwelling.

One great inconvenience attaches besides to the houses in Upper Harrogate, which is the greater distance an invalid has to go over, in order to reach the sulphur springs, all of which, as already mentioned, are in Low Harrogate. Yet with all these disadvantages, many more neat-looking buildings are now starting into existence on the margin of the elevated common.

Of the boarding-houses on this table-land, YORK HOUSE has the most favourable aspect, being direct south, and sheltered from the prevailing blasts of north-north-westerly and westerly gales. The Queen, and other houses, I have already mentioned. They form a continuous line, which extends to the left of the common, as far as the insulated and showy hotel of the Dragon, by which the line is terminated.

The church of High Harrogate, a neat stone edifice, stands in front of this line, on the right of the road, at some distance on the common ; and some distance past this, with a western and the best aspect on this wide expanse of ground, is seen the GRANBY, the truly aristocratic hotel of the Spa.

In this direction is one of the purely chalybeate springs, called the *Old* or *Sweet Spa*, enclosed within a small circular building, erected by Lord Loughborough, and open to the public. To the water of this spring I attach more importance than I am inclined to do from experience to that of the second chalybeate spring, called Tewit well, situated in a little hollow, or swampy piece of ground, at the east corner of the common. The water of the *old* chalybeate having reached its stone border, overflows into a channel, and passes out of the covered well into the open air, in a basin that is accessible at all hours. A slight deposition of red oxide may be seen on the border stone, but hardly any at the bottom of the well. The water looks perfectly clear and transparent, and is delightfully cool, the outside of the glass becoming instantly dimmed as it comes out of the spring, into which it is dipped by the attendant girl, by means of a stick, terminated by a cup-holder, as at the German Spas. The water tastes very pleasant, and agreeably sapid, with a slight *goût* of iron, as if the tongue had been applied to the blade of a steel knife. It sits very lightly on the stomach, and does not affect the head. It is most certainly a valuable auxiliary in curing weak stomachs and dyspepsia, with acidity.

Nearly opposite to the church just mentioned, upon crossing the road from the common to the line of houses before described, and not far from the house of the resident surgeon, Mr. Richardson, and from Langdale's circulating library, that convenient footpath leads to Low Harrogate which I before mentioned, shortening the way thither from the common by more than half the distance.

BELLEVUE, the crack house of the place, twice alluded to, in which I spent many agreeable hours in the society of some of my patients, is an excellent square stone building, with several bedrooms on the first floor, of very good size, and well furnished, of which those at the back look over a pretty long slip of garden, full southward. On the ground floor the drawing and dining-rooms are made *en suite*, and a smaller parlour by the side of them has been converted into an ordinary dining-room. Altogether the conveniences of the house are such as one could desire.

From this house a full view is obtained of the principal objects in Low Harrogate. It stands midway between the latter and High Harrogate, near the Salem chapel, and not a great way from the spot where begins the footpath, already alluded to, which leads across the fields to the upper town.

Two acclivities, running N.N.E., and W.S.W., beautifully wooded, are seen ascending insensibly from the flat level of Low Harrogate to the plateau of the upper town, separated by a narrow dell, at the bottom of which meanders the *beck*, or rivulet, previously noticed, running eastwardly. At the entrance of this dell, and on the left, standing rather high, we find the wide-spreading *Swan* hotel, with its modernized face turned to the south-east; while on the right, the ground is occupied by the Old Sulphur Well, the Crown hotel, and the Victoria rooms and baths.

Following the line of this hollow in an easterly direction, the eye meets with the Montpellier Spa, and, still further on, the handsome temple-like edifice which shelters the Cheltenham saline spring. It is from the back of this last building that the remainder of the wooded dell, forming the beautiful pleasure grounds of that establishment, extends upward to the level eminence of High Harrogate. This line serves also to mark the two regions of sulphur and saline springs, the former being all situated to the south, and the latter to the north of that line.

It is this picturesque arrangement of nature and art which the front of Bellevue and other lodging-houses a little higher up the acclivity, and in the same line, overlook. In the farthest ground, the landscape is bounded by the segment of a horizontal circle, on the waving line of which Studely's royal-stately park rears its ancient clumps, and splendid groves of oaks and columnar beech trees, forming a pleasing and interesting object, constantly under the eye of the inmates of these dwellings.

I have just named the pleasure-grounds of the Cheltenham Spa. To invalids the advantage of such an addition to that handsome Cur-saal, for a mere weekly subscription of

three shillings and sixpence, is immense. It is decidedly
the prettiest spot in Harrogate, and may be made quite
a *bijou*—a very Tivoli—by means of a few improvements and
alterations, which I ventured to suggest to Mr. Gordon, the
proprietor, and which he is most willing to undertake if properly encouraged. Neither Leamington nor Cheltenham
can boast of such a rural promenade in the immediate vicinity
of their springs.

In these grounds there are two lines of walks ; the upper,
measuring thirteen hundred and eighty feet,—the lower, or
the one nearest to the *beck*, eleven hundred and fifty-two
feet ; so that the visiter may, without going twice over the
same ground (as in that wretched paddock of the imperial
pump-room at Leamington), take a very agreeable walk of
half a mile, mostly very much sheltered by lofty forest trees,
his steps inspirited by the distant musical tones of the band
playing from the top of the terrace, the cadences of which serve,
as it were, to mark his own movements, which are quickened
or retarded by the occasional shrill blast of the trumpet, mingled with the softer notes of the harp and the flageolet.

The grounds are prettily waved and distributed. From
the terrace first alluded to, at the back of the great pump-
room or temple, slopes of grass and winding paths, with
seats and tents, offer a more lively scene than we find farther
on, where the wild forest-like character has been preserved.
The *beck*, or stream, so often mentioned, descending from
the great bogs above Low Harrogate, traversing the latter,
and skirting one side of these grounds, has been restrained in
its course, and swelled into a " lake," or sheet of water, with
a tortuous path on its elongated margin, a thousand feet in
length. A boat waits on its unruffled surface the pleasure of
such visiters as prefer the exercise of rowing to that of walking,
after drinking the saline spring in the morning.

It were to be wished that this water could boast of a more
crystal-like hue. But as the sewage of the village, and the

waste water from the Montpellier and ictoria baths, must be conveyed through it and out of it, the transparency and clearness of the Cumberland lakes will never be imparted to it ; added to which, bog water is never colourless. The idea of adding boat exercise, and the aspect of a large sheet of water, to a spa, is excellent ; and we must regret that the materials for carrying it into effect are not better.

Seated on a bench fronting the principal path, from whence I am sketching the present description, the company, which has collected in pretty large numbers at the Royal promenade room, attracted by the fineness of the early morning, now spreads in groups over the grounds, and exhibits to the keen observer their several characteristic peculiarities and infirmities. A lovely widow has just passed before me, whose weeds seem recent ; she accompanies an only son, whose left leg has been cut off to arrest the ravaging inroad of scrofula, which seems to have seared also his pale and sunken face with scars and swellings. Perhaps the father, whose loss the sable of both mother and son plainly tells, has been swept away by the same fatal disorder ; the poisonous lymph of which, creeping along with the paternal blood, has propagated itself to the unhappy offspring.

Another boy has just been led along to the margin of the lake, for a ride in the boat. His appearance marks the presence of a hip-disease. He is lame, weak, and walks not without sufferings. He has drank, I am told, of the sulphur well for some time past, and is now using the saline chalybeate. His progress towards recovery, of late, is said to be wonderfully great.

Faces still bearing the marks of previous illness, but which my kind cicerone the colonel, who had watched them from the first, assured me had been before saffronized and resembled tallow, —now pass in review, in walking lines, or appear, here and there, dotting the lawns, and exhibiting daily a notable progress towards a better complexion.

Anon, and I recognised among the invalids a good hospitable gentleman, an Alderman of Newcastle, at whose house I had been kindly entertained during my sojourn in that city, at the meeting of the British Association in the year preceding. I had known him in excellent health. He appeared now as if rising from the grave, accompanied by a young and interesting guardian angel—a most affectionate niece—ever watchful over the safety of her uncle. He had been recommended by Doctor Hedlam, the eminent physician of Newcastle, to come hither after a severe and dangerous bilious fever. On his arrival he seemed so ill that the surgeon, Mr. Richardson, would hardly venture to sanction the use of the waters. He had all the symptoms of a confirmed hepatic disease. He drank the sulphur water and bathed in it, and he was now quite restored.

After all, these panoramic glances at the congregated numbers of invalids who apply to the mineral springs for health, are the most instructive. Here the merest superficial observer will detect with ease, from among the mere imaginary valetudinarians, those that are really ill; he will trace the daily changes for the better which the latter exhibit; and he cannot fail to be struck, particularly at Harrogate, with the wide distinction of classes among the large number of visiters who frequent the Spa. Here the difference in the company, month by month, as the season advances, is remarkable. The visiters seem to rise in importance and quantity of blood, as the thermometer rises with the increasing heat of the summer sun.

Surely there must be something more than mere fancy in that peculiarity observed in the mould of countenance of certain people in each distinct class of society. But besides " blood," which is always sure of showing itself, and is different in different castes—the distinction of faces must have been implanted on the physiognomy of certain individuals, by the respective daily occupations—the habitual state of their mind—their diet—and, above all, their associations.

CHAPTER VIII.

HARROGATE CONCLUDED.

The Substantials at Harrogate—TABLE D'HÔTE at the Crown and other
Hotels—Living not cheaper than in London—Sorts and Prices of
Provisions—Public and private Ménage—HOTEL-KEEPERS Lords of the
Place, as at Baden—Hotels for the Lords and Hotels for the Gentry—
Associations and Gaieties—MEDICAL NOTES on the Harrogate Waters—
Importance of not taking them without Advice—Best Mode of using
them—Drinking and Bathing—Complaints benefited by them—Imme-
diate Effects of the Water—SCEPTICISM of English Physicians, as to Mi-
neral Waters, on the decline—STRIKING CURES by those at Harrogate—
Author's long Experience — Mr. RICHARDSON's Opinions valuable—
Rules as to Quantity and Mode of administering the Waters—Mud
Baths first suggested by the Author as a means of Cure, entirely overlooked at Harrogate—The BOG-district—The Hospital—The Observatory — CLIMATE—Inhabitants— Uniqueness of Harrogate— Public
Spirit wanted—CONCLUSION.

DIET and associations ! These, next to the mineral waters,
are the most important points to attend to in estimating the
value and merits of a Spa.

At Harrogate all who live at the Hotels, have the convenience of a table d'hôte. From experience I can recommend
that at the Crown ; and from what I have heard visiters of
consequence say respecting them, those at the other hotels
are equally entitled to praise.

At all the principal hotels, whether of Low or High Harrogate, the banqueting-rooms or saloons in which the dinner
takes place, are large, well appointed, and admit of the

enjoyment of a band at dinner-time. There are also with-drawing and separate sitting-rooms for the company, the former of which are common to all who sit at the table d'hôte, whether resident in the hotels, or simply accidental visiters.

The living is not much more reasonable at Harrogate than in London. Bread tolerably white and well flavoured, and butter indifferently good, sell at precisely the same high prices. The milk, owing to the meagre pasturage in the neighbourhood, is poor and thin, and the cream scanty. Mutton is excellent, and eightpence per pound. Fruit, par-ticularly strawberries, is plentiful, but at no lower price than in London.

In fact, though a *rural* Spa, Harrogate has all the domestic inconvenience of a *town* one. The reason is plain enough. In the first place, all the supplies, indifferent as they are, come principally from Knaresborough; and in the second place, about six or seven large hotels, four of which, as I before ob-served, are first-rate ones, have to provide at a weekly charge (which, individually, is very reasonable) board for at least one hundred guests each day. They, therefore, absorb all the provisions that can be gathered in the neighbourhood. Mutton and poultry, and the most preferable or choice vege-tables, are quickly snapped up by them ; and even the fish, as it makes its rare appearance in the market from Scarborough, is instantly appropriated : so that the dwellers in private houses or in lodgings stand a poor chance of getting any thing good or cheap, or enough of it even to satisfy the pretension of cookery.

Hence families who propose to live in separate houses, and to " keep house," must not expect to live at *Harrog*ate for much less than at *High*gate, had their doctors sent them thither from the metropolis for a change of air.

And yet of the two, a private family, if at all numerous, had better have their *ménage* in a separate house, than live at an hotel, even at the risk of being looked upon as stingy, and

of the common herd ; a stigma they are very likely to have cast upon them.

At an hotel the ordinary charge for lodging and board at the public-table, is two guineas and a half a week, with half a guinea more for the servants of the house, whom you are *censé* to employ.   If you have a servant of your own in livery, then the charge is three shillings and sixpence per day extra ; besides which there is a tax of three shillings a week for wax lights.

All this together, making a total of either three pounds six shillings without a servant, or five pounds per week with one, is bearable for one or two persons ; but let a *Chef* and his lady, like some friends I knew in one of the principal private houses, with three young ladies and three servants, take up his residence at the Granby for example, and a sum of not less than twenty guineas a week would have been required, even though using the public-rooms, without being either so comfortable or so independent as in a private house ; a great consideration, by the by, where four ladies, three of them young and one an invalid, are concerned.

Still fashion, for the higher classes of people, wills it that they shall live at the principal hotels, and to them accordingly they proceed ; though few of these illustrious remain the usual period of time necessary for a successful treatment by mineral waters.

This state of things has given immense importance to the hotel-keepers, and in that respect Harrogate is something like Baden-Baden. These gentry are, in good troth, the lords of the place at present.   What does not suit them, that must not be ; and in the pursuit of this object, each pulls his own way, and cares not what becomes of the rest.   They go so far as to command (for it's a threat in the shape of a request) the closing of the hospital, as before stated , during the season, lest the sight of the poor lepers, and still more so, the use they make of the sulphur water out of the upper or *bog*-wells, as they are called, should interfere with their own establishment of baths and invalids.

The hotels are of two classes; but this division, which was a well-marked one a few years back, is now dwindled away, from the force and change of circumstances. At one time your opulent Leeds, and Sheffield, and Manchester factors, whose ideas of supreme happiness at a Spa were limited to a moderately dear hotel or boarding-house, no more dreamt of stopping at the gates of the Dragon, still less at those of the Granby, for admission, than they would at the palace of my Lord Harewood, by the way, for that purpose. No; they sneaked into the Swan, the White Hart, or the Wellington, or, as the *summum bonum*, into the Crown, to occupy some one of its hundred little bedrooms, low-roofed and without bells, arranged on each side of narrow corridors, which crossing each other at right angles, and in all directions, would puzzle the most expert topographer. The Dragon and the Granby were sacred places. The lords only graced the latter, while the wealthy commoner pleased himself in the former.

Now, *nous avons changé, &c.* Pretty little *gauche* misses and their snuff-coloured coated papas boldly stalk into both houses without being "called;" cutlers and cotton-spinners aspire to great assembly rooms and gigantic banqueting-saloons; and nothing pleases the wealthy townsman of Bradford and Huddersfield, Halifax and Rochdale, but the *lambris dorés*, the well-stuffed sofas of red damask, and the *cuisine par excellence* of those two crack hotels.

The season, however, presently arrives, when the smoke of their native places recalls them to their duties, and when the complexion of the previously pimpled damsels being well polished by the sulphur bath, and the lining of their papa's stomach altered into a fresh manufacturing power by the Cheltenham chalybeate,—they must take their departure and leave London luxury at Harrogate for Lancashire and Yorkshire homeliness. And then the Right Honourables, the

M. P.s,—the baronets, and their ladies, pour into Harrogate, chase away all the vulgar before them, fill the Dragon and the Granby with " Ha—ha-s," and " How do-s," imprisoning the real invalids at the Crown ;—where, by the by, I lived for a week very comfortably, to be near the Montpellier Spa and the Old Well.

Then begin the real *gaieties* of Harrogate, then the money flies, and six weeks of a plentiful harvest enables the respective landlords of those aristocratic establishments to keep them up during the rest of the year, with expenses and taxes upon them that would appal a chicken-hearted Boniface, and which could not be met but for the extravagant charges the landlords themselves make on their customers of " gentle blood."

The well-ascertained existence of four distinct classes of mineral waters at Harrogate, namely, the pure chalybeates, the saline chalybeates, the saline without any chalybeate, and lastly and principally, the sulphur water, will render it necessary for medical men, when they recommend the water of Harrogate to their patients, accurately to specify of which class the patient should partake.

Nor is this all. According to the analyses, the springs of the same class seem to differ among themselves. Thus we have the strongest sulphur at the Montpellier, the middle degree of strength in sulphur at the Old Well, and a minimum degree of strength of sulphur at the Knaresborough or the Starbeck well. These distinctions should be attended to in prescribing.

Judging from my own experience, and the effect the several wells have had on me, I should feel disposed to begin the full course of sulphur water-drinking, with the Knaresborough, and end with the Montpellier. For warm baths the strongest is perhaps the best to be used at once.

Hitherto the sulphur waters alone have been used for bathing purposes. But there is no reason why the saline chalybeates, especially those which have a less quantity of the muriate of soda, and are therefore less likely to irritate the skin, should not hereafter be employed for baths. On the contrary, there is every reason why they should be so; since amongst many hundred cases of invalids who visit this Spa, a large proportion of them cannot bear, and some do not require, the application of sulphur to the skin; whereas they would be benefited by, and many positively require, a chalybeate bath.

Mr. Richardson, with whom I visited a patient or two at Harrogate, and had long conversations touching the virtues of the sulphur waters, entertains a general sweeping view respecting them and their effect in disease, derived from long experience. In all sluggish constitutions inclined to glandular disease, in scrofulous tendency, in obstruction of the mesenteric glands; in all cases of biliary derangements, of light dyspepsia, in constipation; but above all in the squamous, defedating, slow-acting diseases of the skin, he has found great benefit from the sulphur water, accompanied by sulphur baths. On the other hand, if there be fever, great irritability of the nervous system, or of the skin; if the tongue be furred, or white and dry,—the skin parched, hot, and feverish; if there be any palpitation of the heart present, not symptomatic merely of indigestion but idiopathic; or if any degree of active inflammation of the lungs is going on,—the sulphur water will do mischief.

Where the sulphur water is suitable, it purges when taken in the quantity of a pint and a half in the morning. A smaller dose will hardly do it. Mr. Richardson orders it to be drank in two tumblers of three-quarters of a pint each, with an interval of twenty minutes between; and he considers the course to last from three to six weeks; sometimes inter-rupting the course by a short excursion between. He seldom recommends more than twelve baths.

Mr. Richardson admits that where it does not purge, or in those cases in which it disagrees even when it purges, the

sulphur water will affect the head, and produce confusion
and distress. He has been in the habit of recommending
often a little blue-pill or some aperient medicine to assist the
water when the latter does not operate unless drank in large
quantities; as in such cases he looks upon the harm that
might arise from the mercury as a lesser evil, than what
would inevitably be produced by the ingestion of a very
large quantity of the water.

When after drinking the water for a period of two or three
weeks he finds that the patients nauseate the dose, he invariably directs them to desist from it altogether. That the
sulphureted water is an agent of great power, he is quite
convinced, although Mr. Richardson (like myself in the case
of the Spas in Germany), found most of his brother practitioners of eminence in the north of England sceptical, and
inclined to laugh at his faith in the waters. " And yet,"
says he, " they will send me patients very often to be treated
and cured by the very waters they seem to despise." " You
have yourself noticed," continued Mr. Richardson, " the
success operated on Mr. ——, of Newcastle. He was despatched hither by our common acquaintance and brother
practitioner, Dr. ——, a leading man in that city, despair-
ing of his recovery almost, and sceptical as to the power of
our sulphureted waters. He will be much and agreeably
surprised when he beholds him come back next week. At
his arrival in Harrogate, I assure you I hardly knew whether
I should mislead him with any hope of success from these
waters, so ill was he; but we tried, and the conclusion is
most gratifying."

I attach more importance to these general and practical
remarks and precepts of a man of good sense and respectability, with that degree of professional acuteness which is
sufficient to enable a medical man to turn to account his
long experience in the treatment of diseases by means of the
Harrogate waters, than I do to many a learned treatise based

on presumed analogies, supposed philosophical inductions, or wirespun scientific theories.

With most of Mr. Richardson's views and ideas, my experience of some years in witnessing the effects of the Harrogate waters on several of my patients, coincides. But having had a much wider field of practice in the general application of mineral waters for the treatment of disease, than he can have had in the single locality of Harrogate, I differ somewhat from him in all that relates to the quantity of water to be taken, the manner of taking it, and the effects to be produced.

I differ first in point of quantity. A pint and a half of the strong sulphureted water is an exorbitant dose, because a pint of it contains 108 grains of common salt, and the whole dose 162 grains, being fully a third of an ounce of common or kitchen salt; by far too large a quantity of that stimulating condiment for any stomach.

Had there been in combination with it any sulphate of soda, or even of magnesia, to qualify the physiological effects of so large a proportion of sea-salt, and thus add to its solvent and purgative power, my objection would be considerably weakened, perhaps removed. But as the analysis shows no such saline ingredient to be present in the water, the objectionable properties of an excessive dose of sea-salt swallowed in the course of less than an hour and a half before breakfast, are left to act unmodified upon the coats of the stomach; and accordingly we find that people taking it, are liable to feel uncomfortable and heated about the pit of the stomach, and to experience a peculiar headach, under which I have myself suffered to a considerable degree from that cause.

This headach differs from every other species of headach, and is much more severe and alarming, in as much as it seems to occupy the centre and basis of the brain, and is accompanied by a sensation of distension in the blood-vessels, together with a feeling, that if you were to move the head quickly, one of the gorged blood-vessels must give way. This species of headach, however, is principally to be ascribed to the large quantity of sulphureted hydrogen gas, which in each prescribed dose of one half-pint of water, amounts to 60 per cent. in the strongest well. An effect equally unsatisfactory, occasioned by the latter cause, may be noticed in respect to the abdominal secretions, which appear dry and burnt up, denoting clearly a feverish and irritated state of the mucous lining of the intestines.

As to the mode of administering the water, I must object, with all those who are well versed in the practice of a mineral water treatment, to its being drunk, at one time, in such a quantity as I find it recommended in this country. The Harrogate water, like many other mineral waters endowed with energetic properties, is an agent of mischief when inconsiderately prescribed. To order more as a dose than the stomach can digest in the course of twenty minutes, is to inflict injury on the patient; and the Germans, who limit the quantity of each draught of their waters to four ounces, with an interval of twenty minutes between, act wisely and from good experience.

I also think that the first dose of the fetid water should be taken diluted with hot water of the ordinary sort, and the rest warmed by a mixture of the same water previously heated. Rather than rely on quantity for the aperient effect of this water, I would add to it, according to each individual case, that which it lacks, namely a small proportion of Glauber salts in the first glass.

It is the same with respect to bathing in the Harrogate water. I have found the baths too stimulating when the water has been used undiluted ; and in proportion as the stimulation has been great, so has the reaction been after it, when the blood seems to flee from the surface, to congregate in the centre, and to produce, at one and the same time, a great sensation of heat internally, and thirst; while the surface, particularly of the face and extremities, is miserably chilly, and almost blue.

A young lady, a patient of mine, using the baths by my direction at Harrogate, had found them to produce the two distinct effects just mentioned, up to the time of my arrival; whereas by explaining to her the cause, and avoiding it by proper dilution, as well as by exciting a gentle glow immediately after coming out of the bath, through the usual means, I soon released her from all unpleasant effects.

Mr. Richardson, on being questioned on the subject, assured me that the sulphur waters are excellent in verminous disorders; and that gout, or a tendency to it, is often effectually checked by the same means, as well as rheumatism, in its various chronic forms, and not otherwise.

Against complaints like these, however, and for inveterate and the most difficult cases of cutaneous disease, Harrogate possesses, in my opinion, a much more powerful agent, which has hitherto entirely escaped the attention of the profession, and to which I desire most emphatically to direct it—namely, the MUD-BATHS.

The material well calculated for that purpose is near at hand. Upon a high ground, a short distance from Low Harrogate, in a westerly direction, is a piece of moss or bog earth, which has commonly but erroneously been supposed to be " the mother of the Harrogate waters." The whole surface there, to a considerable extent, presents an extraordinary phenomenon in the physical history of the place. Deep sulphur wells, two or three pools of water impregnated with tannin and more than one saline chalybeate, as I ascertained on the spot by tests, dot an area of some acres, which altogether has the appearance of a great chemical laboratory of nature. Cuttings in the quaking surface at various distances, and natural denudations, have discovered the character of bog-earth, with its redundancy of free sulphuric acid.

On the margin of this curious district, a Hospital for both male and female patients requiring the use of the Harrogate waters has been erected, through the exertions of Mr. Richardson and a few benevolent individuals, aided by the liberality of the Earl of Harewood, lord of the manor, who has secured to the miserable objects requiring such a boon, in the best manner that his tenure would allow, the possession of the grant of the land he made to them, and on which the hospital stands.

"I have, on my part, done my best," said his lordship at the foundation of the hospital, "(next to alienating altogether the land—which I cannot do,) to make it a permanent possession to the poor; and I hope I may answer for the benevolence and philanthropy of my descendants."

The establishment is small, but useful, and has done much good. It is well managed ; but during the season it is kept closed, by reasons to which I have alluded, and which are not creditable to the parties who impose such a condition. The patients supply themselves with the necessary sulphur water from the springs of the bog tract close at hand, which springs being open also to all the inhabitants, supply many of them and their baths with water, fetched away in appropriate vessels.

Well then, it is this very tract of land which should supply the material for the mud-baths ; and an intelligent, enterprising person, acting under the direction of an able physician well versed in the theory and practice of mud-baths, as now greatly and most successfully used in Germany, would confer great benefit to society, and secure immense advantage to himself, by the establishment at Harrogate of sulphureted mud-baths, like those of St. Amand in the department of the North in France.

If the pedestrian from this current tract of land, extends his excursion further westerly, about two miles and a half, either along the high-road, or across an extensive boggy moor (which I nearly had reason to repent I had ever attempted), he will reach the foot of a lofty tower, standing isolated, like a great beacon, rising one hundred feet, upon an extensive waste. To the interior of this he will be admitted through a curiously-wrought-iron gate, which marks the number of visiters as they are admitted,—and so ascend to the top; where by the help of twelve telescopes, there placed in the direction of radii to a circle, he will sweep every part of the horizon, but will look in vain for the two seas—the German and the Irish—the expectation of beholding which originally induced Mr. Thomson to erect this " Observatory."

As proprietor of it, that gentleman has turned the building to account, making at least ten per cent. for his money, which he has taken good care to protect against any possible desire of appropriation on the part of the keeper (an odd character), by the contrivance before alluded to.

One improvement Mr. Thomson might adopt at the summit of his observatory—one adopted at the Belvidere of Neufchatel, in Switzerland, where glasses are placed to survey an extensive horizon of Alpine country—and which consists in having the names of the remarkable places to which the glasses are directed, and their distances, engraved on a brass plate fixed to the parapet beneath the glass.

I will conclude what I have to say on the subject of the treatment of disease by the Harrogate waters, by stating that during the last season, patients afflicted with hepatic disorders, glandular affection, rheumatism dependent on sluggish secretions, frequent eruption of boils and other disorders, whom I had recommended to proceed to Harrogate, returned thence completely restored.

While speaking of the treatment of diseases by the minera waters of Harrogate, our mind is naturally directed to the consideration of its climate and territorial aspect. Nothing can be purer than the air at Harrogate. Its elasticity is felt by every new visiter immediately on his arrival; but the situation is exposed to high winds, and the temperature is generally low—lower by two degrees than in the town of Knaresborough, placed in a lower part of the valley.

Judging from my own experience and the affirmation of the oldest inhabitant, or assiduous frequenters of the Spa, it rains, on an average, four days in the week during the summer months; and it is seldom that the sky is perfectly free from lowering clouds or gloom. But as the soil is of that light porous limestone, which absorbs all moisture with great rapidity, the rain sinks speedily into the earth ; and a few minutes after the heaviest shower, one can walk out on the paths and in the streets without inconvenience.

This very quality of the soil is averse to the success of agriculture. There is generally a character of poverty about the land of the immediately surrounding districts, and there is no large timber. Green crops are the principal occupants of the land, and these do not seem to be farmed so well as in Northumberland and other northern counties. The characteristics of prosperity are not visible around Harrogate ; and there is an appearance of dilapidation, more or less marked, even in the hedges and gates that divide the fields.

As to the native inhabitants of this particular district of Yorkshire, whether of the industrious or of the consuming classes, they are not, as in many other parts of that county, particularly well favoured by nature. It is seldom that one meets with a handsome adult woman, or a very good-looking man. This is not the district for tall life-guardsmen ; yet in children the character of their physiognomy is pleasing.

I have dwelt more largely, perhaps, than is consistent with the nature of the present work, on the Spas of Harrogate. But among the few really important Spas of which England can boast, in comparison to other countries, I hold Harrogate to be of such manifest superiority—indeed, I was almost going to say, *uniqueness*—on account of the peculiar nature of its waters (if properly managed), its sulphur mud, now first recommended, and its situation, that I felt anxious to bring all its merits before the general readers more fully than any medical treatise had done before. It is for this reason that I have entered into details which the medical treatises I allude to could not embrace, but which, to a non-medical reader, are of paramount interest.

Harrogate has the elements within itself of becoming a Spa of the first magnitude, even to the extent of attracting foreign travellers; but there is much to be done to bring it to that state. At present the condition of Harrogate is quite primitive, and as such, liable to all those impediments to progress which appertain to the *petits pays*. Hence one hears without surprise of the bickerings, piques, and feuds, between Low and High Harrogate. They of the latter envy those of Lower Harrogate their springs and Well, at the same time that they boast of their superb hotels and large establishments. But these are sneered at by the Low Harrogate people, who, in their turn, point to their noble pump-room, and promenades, their Crown, and their Swan.

In Harrogate no vestige of any form of government obtrudes itself on the notice of the stranger; and not a single representative of the smallest civic authority is to be found here, not even a guardian of the night, or a day-policeman. Hence encroachments on public privileges and rights not unfrequently are attempted; and, but for the watchfulness of the threatened victim, would be carried into effect. Thus, last year, in order to annoy the low Harrogatians, a determination was expressed by somebody to cut down a tolerably fine row of beech-trees, which, at this moment, form the only shaded walk for visiters who are returning from the baths at Low Harrogate in very hot weather. The thing would have been done, though the timber could not have fetched at a sale more than a few hundred pence, and though it grows on crown land; when a spirited remonstrance from the Low Harrogate people to the board, stopped the intended act of vandalism.

If true public spirit existed between the two places, Harrogate would soon rise in the scale of Spas. At present, I fear, from all I have gathered from the very best authority, such is far from being the case. Nay, it has been remarked, that if the dwellers of Low Harrogate project any improvement for the general good, in order to increase the attraction of the place, those of High Harrogate will not join to defray the expenses.

With the exception of one or two individuals with whom I conversed on the subject, and who are connected with the bathing establishments, I have found very little disposition in the proprietors of the springs, or the permanent inhabitants, to effect any thing to promote the advancement of the place, or to make known the value of its water, together with the gradual though slow ameliorations that are taking place from year to year. They are all apathetic, and prefer to leave things to take their course.

I hope they may be roused by what I have here stated, and by the very favourable opinion I have given of the Spa in general, to a more enterprising conduct. A spirited capitalist would find an unexplored mine of wealth in Harrogate; which is not one of your ephemeral Spas, dependent on fashion. Its almost peculiar waters are lasting, and so must and will be their reputation.

CHAPTER IX.

KNARESBOROUGH AND ALDFIELD.—ENVIRONS OF HARROGATE.

Best Mode of Killing Time at a Spa—Excursions from Harrogate—
Vehicles—*Martyr et Souffrance*—Knaresborough, or Starbeck Spa—
Its Sulphur Water preferable in some Cases to that of Harrogate—
Baths not so Irritating—Recent Restitution of the Starbeck Spring—
Conduct of Physicians at the English Spas, with reference to Mineral
Waters—Objectionable, and why—Not pursued at Harrogate—Knares-
borough Castle—St. Robert's Chapel—Mother Shipton and the Drop-
ping Well—Geological Features—The Cave!—Rómantic Situation—
Banks of the Nidd—A prating Old Dame—Tombs of the Recluses—
Eugene Aram—His Skull—A Bone to Pick with the Phrenologists—
Brimham Crags—Superstitious and Practical Explanations—Imposing
Scene—Gay Group of Visiters—Richard Weatherhead and the Merry
Widow—Magnificent Prospect—The Bees' Villa—A brilliant Equi-
page — A Farce, and a Fracas of Crokery — Aldfield Sulphur
Spring—Character, Taste, and Virtue of its Water—Its Situation.

What are the most prominent features observable among
the temporary inhabitants of a Spa? Idleness and want of
occupation. This *dolce far niente* is among the very best
auxiliaries to the mineral water, in the cure of disease. To
cast over your shoulders all care, and turn your back on
business, is to be half cured of your disease. But for the
same reason *ennui* would soon take hold of the visiters at a
Spa, if the twelve or fourteen waking hours daily passed at it
were wholly unemployed.

One of the most effectual and satisfactory, as it is also the
easiest mode of occupying some of those hours, is by making
excursions in the neighbourhood of the Spa. Harrogate, in

that respect, offers an almost endless variety of resources; and the means of conveyance to some of the nearest, as well as the more remote objects of attraction in the country around, are to be found with sufficient readiness, and at a moderate charge. Carriages by the day or by the month, post-horses, saddle-horses, flies, gigs, and phætons, are all to be had either at the principal hotels, or from some of the tradesmen in the place, who turn livery-stable men *pro tem.*

Public vehicles standing out for hire, are few and miserably equipped. Nothing can equal the wretched appearance, for example, of the donkey-phæton. Those all-enduring animals, with their hairless hides broken to the bone, drag a miserable-looking carriage for one shilling per hour, and are seen wincing, yet still proceeding, whenever a buckle, or a knot in the harness, or the sharp edge of a tight trace (as the poor animal pulls up a hill), has eaten away the flesh! The " *Souffrance*" and " *Martyr*" of the poor French *voiturier* are not more applicable appellations of his two miserable nags, than they would be to the ill-treated twin asses of Harrogate.

Yet with these, or something analogous, though in general with more pretending means of conveyance, do the numerous dwellers for the time being at the Spa of Harrogate, spread themselves almost daily on all points within a circle of twenty miles; some beginning their excursions soon after breakfast, and extending the same to the utmost limit of a long day's duration; while others, unwilling to lose any of the " prepaid" repasts at their hotels, are satisfied with an expedition which can be compassed between luncheon and dinner.

KNARESBOROUGH

Is an auxiliary Spa to Harrogate, a species of suffragan watering-place, which the visiters at the latter more frequently proceed to,—not because the mineral springs are *at* Knaresborough,—for they lie midway between that town and Harrogate,—but rather with a view to look at the castle, visit the shaded banks of the Nidd, and inspect the cave rendered so famous by the most popular novel-writer of the present day.

Thither accordingly, like every body else, I proceeded in goodly company on a fine day, stopping by the way at the " Knaresborough Spau," as it is now denominated, or the *Starbeck* Spau, as designated upon the map of the Forest-award.

This spring, known since the beginning of the 17th century, had been suffered to fall into a state of dilapidation, and, some time after the passing of the act of inclosure of Knaresborough forest, was ploughed over and destroyed. Yet to judge by the very many publications that had appeared from the pen of not fewer than fourteen physicians and one learned prelate, its virtues and importance must have been considered as great during its existence. The same impression has probably incited the inhabitants of Knaresborough to recover the well since; and accordingly we find that, in 1822, a subscription having been entered into for that purpose, the necessary operations were began, and the Spa was duly opened with a grand masonic ceremony soon after.

The Spa consists of two distinct springs; that, the water of which contains sulphureted hydrogen gas, being the principal one. The other by the side of it, and at the distance of about fifteen yards to the right, is a chalybeate, and of secondary importance.

The sulphur water springs from a triangular space in a rock, in the quantity of about one gallon in a minute, without any considerable variation, except during the prevalence of rainy or very dry weather. I found its temperature, as in the sulphur spring at Harrogate, to be 52°, but in very frosty weather, I was told, it gets as low as 48°. It however never freezes.

The water is clear and beautifully colourless, and not by any means unpleasant to the taste. Being slightly impregnated with sulphureted gas, its odour is not so disagreeable as that of the Harrogate water, nor is the excessive taste of common salt of the latter, perceptible in the former. For both these reasons I should recommend it as the most proper sulphur water to begin with. I have prescribed it with success in many cases in which the stronger sulphur water of Harrogate had decidedly disagreed. In addition to which there are in the Knaresborough sulphur water larger proportions of magnesian salt, according to Dr. Murray's analysis, than in the water at Harrogate; a circumstance which would induce me to view the water as a more effectual alterative and depurative of the blood. The advantage also of drinking it without the aid of leaden-piped pumps, and in its genuine state, is not a trifling addition to its value.

In order to secure this valuable spring a little stone building was erected over it, whence the water flows into a stone bason in the centre of a square space sunken some steps all round, and paved. A cottage was built also near it, and a poor family placed in it, to wait upon the visiters who frequent the spring.

But the most important step taken in regard to this Spa, has been the erection of some baths adjoining the cottage,—forming, with the latter, a very pleasing object externally, and constituting a very essential part of the establishment.

The arrangement of these baths is creditable, though the space is contracted to the utmost limits of economy, and their number too small to satisfy the demands for them.

My experience of these baths coincides with that expressed by Dr. Murray. We hold the water of this spring to be far preferable, in many cases of irritable diseases of the skin, to those of Harrogate, owing to the smaller quantity of common salt present in them, and the greater proportions of muriates

and carbonate of magnesia and lime, which give to the water
an extreme softness and a peculiar smoothness.

At my second visit to this Spa, for the purpose of trying
the baths, I met the father of three lovely little girls who were
covered with pustular eruptions, and had been for a month
bathing at Low Harrogate, with a manifest increase of the
irritation of the skin and its disease.   Here, on the contrary,
as the mother expressed it to me, in the course of only eight
baths at the sulphur Spa, they were recovering *à vue d'œil*.
A dashing equipage was in waiting to receive them, and I could
not help envying the parents, as they darted up the lane
planted with beds of flowers, which leads into the Harrogate
and Knaresborough road, at a very short distance, the gratification they must daily experience, at the beneficial effect of
this mineral water on their cherished children.

In another case under my immediate care, finding the
Montpellier baths too exciting, and the sulphur water at Low
Harrogate too heating, I ordered my young and fair patient to
trip it along to the Knaresborough fountain on a donkey every
morning, and there drink of the salutary stream as well as
bathe in it; all of which had the most beneficial result.

Of the chalybeate water found in the same locality and
forming part of the Spa, I know nothing; nor do I think that
much is recorded, or indeed that anything is done with it,
judging from the state and appearance of the well.   As a
chalybeate nothing in the neighbourhood of Harrogate is
better than its *old Spa*, already described.

For all the measures adopted in restoring Knaresborough
Spa to its present state of usefulness, and for having roused
the inhabitants of that town from their previous apathy
respecting it, the public are indebted to Mr. Calvert, of
Knaresborough, who published, in 1836, a small historical
and descriptive account of the Spa.   Dr. Murray, also, by
analyzing the water, contributed to give it publicity.   He

was long resident at Knaresborough, and enjoyed the character of an amiable, as well as of a charitable man :

" A friend to the poor, and medical guide,"—

as the macaronic poet, author of " A Week at Harrogate,"
has said of that excellent person, whom we shall presently
meet again in another place, and whose testimony in favour
of the Knaresborough sulphureted water, obtained personally from himself, has confirmed me in my opinion of its
efficacy.

It was supposed, at one time, by the Knaresborough
people, that the Faculty, at Harrogate, had, from motives the
reverse of amiable or just, spoken with derision of the *Starbeck* well ; lest its reputation should endanger that of their
own place of residence. What is meant by *the Faculty*
at Harrogate I know not. At present I am acquainted with
only one influential medical man at that Spa, whose opinion
of its waters is generally sought for by the visiters ; and he,
I will take on myself to say, is not likely to experience any
feelings of jealousy against Knaresborough. Even supposing *self* to be (which heaven forbid it should) the ruling
consideration of a medical man in the position of Mr. Richardson, the surgeon generally consulted at Harrogate, his
recommending visiters at that place to drink and use the
waters of the *Starbeck* Spa, cannot clash with his interest or
that of Harrogate ; since the patients, even in that case,
would reside at the latter place, as being equally handy to
the *Starbeck* spring, and far preferable, as a *séjour*, to
Knaresborough.

But such a personal consideration, I am convinced, would
never enter into the mind of my medical brother just mentioned ; inasmuch as I found him to be precisely what a
medical man at a Spa should be, namely, acquainted with
the nature of the water, directing his patients how and when

to take it, and obtruding as little as possible of his own physic, or prescriptions upon them besides, in the same manner that medical men act at the Spas in Germany.

It is this becoming forbearance, on his part,—far different from the conduct pursued at other principal Spas in England, where patients are besieged and surrounded with all the array of medicine, and where the action of the waters is impeded or interfered with, so that at last people are disgusted with both the place and the waters;—it is, I say, this forbearance from all such intermeddling on the part of Mr. Richardson, that induces the large number of visiters I have quoted elsewhere to resort to Harrogate with confidence in its salutary springs. And they will continue so to resort, so long as no physician sets himself up in the place, to insist upon the frequenters of the Spa undergoing a " preparatory treatment," an " accompanying treatment," and a " concluding treatment;" consisting of *physic, physic, physic.* Indeed those frequenters seem to have settled the question for themselves; since it appears, that of late years hardly a single physician has settled at Harrogate who was not glad to leave it again for want of occupation. When cases occur at that Spa which require better medical advice than is to be procured there, the talented physicians of York and Leeds, Belcombe, Simpson, or Hunter, and from some other places also, are summoned for that purpose.

The tourist who is on his way from Leeds to Ripon, passing through Knaresborough, or the temporary dweller in Harrogate visiting the same place, would probably, in days of yore, have halted for an hour to view the scattered fragments of its fortress, its towers, and semi-round buttresses, or its square keep, whose extraordinary walls of twelve and fourteen feet thickness now serve for purposes far different from those of their original destination.

From its highly elevated site upon the loftiest rock that hangs over the deeply-embosomed Nidd, the traveller would for a moment enjoy the splendid panorama that offers itself to him on that spot. Or he might be satisfied with simply sketching an east view of the dismantled tower and dilapidated arches, now falling fast into decay, but presenting a very picturesque group for the pencil.

If local tradition interested him, he would penetrate into and examine that chapel cut out of the solid rock, exhibiting fantastic figures, pilasters, and niches, the patient handiwork of some recluse, which has been supposed to have sheltered St. Robert; who, by the by, must have been an ubiquist, as caves equally cut out of the hard rock by the same saint, on the brink of precipices, are to be seen in many parts of Germany, Salzburgh to wit.

Or the observer would mount the steep cliffs near the picturesque low bridge over the Nidd, to admire the many dwellings excavated out of rocky sides, stopping at that particular one to which the name of *Fort Montacute* has been given, and which a poor weaver and his son were sixteen years in completing. Or, lastly, he might proceed to the house beneath the cliffs, which boasts of having been the birth-place of that celebrated character, Mother Shipton, whose knowledge of futurity puzzled even the poor prelate of Beverley.

All these objects of interest would the ordinary tourist to Knaresborough in former days stop to examine, and then pass on ; or if he had a smattering of a naturalist about him, he might have extended his inquiries to, and indulged his curiosity in contemplating, the far-famed dropping well, which exhibits the paltry farce of water, highly impregnated with earthly particles, being transmitted, by means of concealed pipes, across a chasm left by the detaching of a bulky rock from the cliff; from the upper surface of which rock it is suffered to trickle down in an expanded sheet of perpendicular drops— depositing, in its fall, on various objects exposed to its action, calcareous sediments, which have been called petrifications.

Or, as a geologist, he would rather have been looking at that magnificent section of the new red sandstone supporting the yellow magnesian limestone, which is to be seen under the castle-rock near the cotton-mill, and which sandstone shortly after, towards the high bridge, disappears when the limestone descends to the bed of the Nidd, exhibiting, in its structure, at a place just beneath the ancient encampment, veins of *celestine*, both blue and white, occasionally finely crystallized.

At present, however, one object alone gives an all-absorbing interest to Knaresborough, and attracts thither, at some time or other, all the visiters at Harrogate, who care little or nothing for all the natural and artificial wonders just enumerated. A common occurrence, culled out of the Knaresborough Newgate Calendar, has, of late years, given a degree of celebrity to that place, which it hardly enjoyed before the fervid imagination of the author of " Eugene Aram" clothed the life and death of a scamp, better educated than the commonalty of rogues are in this country, with the charms of his inventive pen. The cave, the cave, " St. Robert's Cave," is the watchword of the idle visiters at Harrogate, as they sit devising the operations for the following day, over the last bowl of punch at the supper-table in the long-room of the Crown or the Dragon. And to Knaresborough all the disposable conveyances of Harrogate are ordered for the morrow.

Thither my merry friends, who had patiently witnessed my operations and inquiries at the Starbeck Spa, and whose company would have given interest to the intended expedition, had none belonged to it, drove me in their carriage. In this we followed the example of the many; but not, I trust, without being duly impressed with the wholesome reflections which a visit to the scene of a deliberate, artfully managed, yet, after all, detected homicide, is apt to suggest; especially when that foul act has been perpetrated by an individual who, if knowledge made men virtuous, ought to have been the last person in the world to have committed such a deed.

Crossing the bridge over the Nidd, which, for a minor river, narrow and not over limpid, presents some characters of beauty as you look down upon it, and follow its tortuous stream until it is lost round the castle cliff; a short carriage drive brought us to a small wicker-gate, kept by an old dame, who readily extended her palms to receive whatever contribution the visiters felt disposed to drop into them.

She has her story quite pat. A few ruinous steps, without a railing or a parapet, lead down to a platform or small terrace in front of the famous Cave, which is small, not deep, and hollowed out of the rock. The river runs a little way below the terrace, on the margin of which a dwarf stone-wall, supported by the sloping green bank, has been erected. By this contrivance, no access can now be had to the Cave by the river side; nor is the spot liable to the inundations to which it was previously subject.

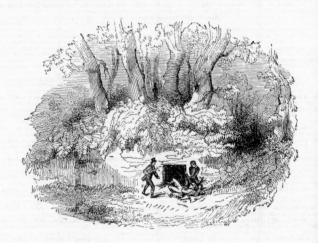

About the middle of this terrace, chance, a short time back, brought to light an excavation two feet deep, and in shape like the inside of a stone coffin, made in the solid rock, with hollows at the bottom to receive certain projecting parts of a human body—such a one having been found in it in a state of decay at the time of the discovery. In tossing up the earth, by which this tomb was encumbered, a small silver coin was brought to light, which the good old dame exhibited, but which none of our party could decipher, as the inscription is not very legible. The coin would probably have informed us respecting the age of this sepulture, and the name of its inmate.

Had such mortal remains been discovered at the period when Eugene stood arraigned of murder,—no doubt he would have made good use of the circumstance in his extraordinary and very clever defence, by practically exemplifying his line of argument, that the bones found in St. Robert's Cave need not have been those of the murdered Clark, but rather might have been those of some recluse anchoret who there perished in due course. But " blood will have blood;" and Providence willed it that the discovery which would have supplied an argument to the arraigned schoolmaster too strong even for the law to withstand (when circumstantial evidence alone directed the jury), and which would have snatched guilt from condign punishment, should not have taken place until long after that punishment had been inflicted, and, it is hoped, after it had time to operate salutarily by its example.

Ever since the appearance of Bulwer's interesting novel bearing the name of the culprit, public sympathy has been attempted to be excited in behalf of his memory. The most successful, clever, and highly interesting effort made to that effect, is that of Norrison Scatcherd, Esq., who in two well-written little works, full of curious details, the one entitled, " Memoirs of the celebrated Eugene Aram," and the other " Gleanings after Eugene Aram," has endeavoured to place the history of that extraordinary character (for extraordinary he certainly was in many respects) in its proper light, and to enlist the kindly feelings of his readers in behalf of his hero.

His remarks on that interesting girl "Sally Aram," the favourite and only affectionate child of Eugene, who followed him to Lynn, and clung to him in York Castle, whither, with a devotion and fidelity, characteristic of her sex where a beloved object is concerned, Sally had attended her father, are replete with pathetic feelings. The composition does great credit, not only to the author's head, but to his heart; for he concludes with a "moral" deduced from the sad lesson he has composed, and does not, like a certain learned physician at one of the meetings of the medical section of the British Association, exclaim against the injustice of a sentence contended, by the latter, to have been little short of a legal murder.

And why so? because upon a skull deemed to be that of Eugene Aram, upon no *direct* evidence whatever*—upon evidence, indeed, which Dr. Fife, of Newcastle, said to be an able supporter of phrenology, considered to be "neither moral nor legal"— certain particular manifestations were found present and others wanting! The latter reasons, which I perfectly well recollect being adduced emphatically at the time, it is but justice to add, the learned author has disclaimed in his subsequent publication. But assuming even that the skull is genuine, and taking its phrenological developments to be as there stated, no ruffian was ever more deservedly hung than Eugene Aram.

---

* Dr. James Inglis, who so ingeniously brought forward the subject of Eugene Aram at the meeting in question, has since published a small pamphlet in corroboration of his previous statements; in which, however, he only reiterates the same indirect (and certainly in a court of law insufficient) evidence, to prove the identity of the skull exhibited at the meeting.

On our return to our respective quarters at Harrogate, we beheld a long cavalcade, a line of vehicles just come in from an excursion to that extraordinary region near Brimham, ten miles north-west of Harrogate, which induced the topographer Pennant, in 1773, to call it " the seat of wonders," capable of exciting astonishment unspeakable.

This far famed region, which is only inferior to that curious and extraordinary district near Dresden, called *Saxon Switzerland*, so fully described in my work on " St. Petersburg," and which leaves far behind in interest the much talked of druidical circles of Stonehenge, on Salisbury Plain, forms a never failing object of attraction for the Spa-drinkers, as well as for strangers visiting the interesting part of Yorkshire in which it is situated.

On approaching Brimham by the Harrogate road, a scene presents itself, which to an unprepared traveller would appear almost as fantastic or of another world. Twice have I visited the celebrated crags on Brimham Hill, and yet the impression of something supernatural in the whole scene—an impression I have scarcely received in any of the many romantic regions of the continent I lately visited—an impression too, against which as a mere geologist I ought to have been proof—continues fresh and vivid on my mind.

For the first acquaintance with this locality I am indebted to one of those rapid rides of twelve miles and back, intended to digest a luncheon and prepare for dinner, which a certain great judge of the land, remarkable for amenity of manners and a good heart, strong health, and a still stronger mind, proposes as a sport to his fellow visiters enjoying the hospitality of Studely. It is some years ago that after a ride from the latter domain—a ride rendered most agreeable by his powers of conversation—that excellent person first plunged me, totally unprepared by reading or verbal information, into the very centre of what I thought looked like a dilapidated city, of Babylonian origin. A second and a recent visit of two

weeks to the same hospitable mansion, affording me an opportunity of again beholding that region, I rode thither at
leisure, on one of those brilliant days which seem appropriated
purposely to enjoy the beauties of Yorkshire.

My direction from Studely was south-west, on the Pately-
bridge road. Having reached Grantley lodge, within which a
broad canal, with a sweep of lofty trees on one of its gently
curved banks, marks the avenue to the hall of the Nortons,
the road creeps over a very steep hill, from the summit of
which a picturesque peep of Grantley Park is obtained.
From Studely to this point, the country exhibits a most beautiful and varied prospect of undulating grounds all the way.
A mile farther, however, after ascending another hill, the
first sight is caught of the great " Muir," north-by-east;
and for a wide circle thence, eastwards, all seems desolate
and barren.

Anon, some pretty patches of well cultivated ground in the
lowlands come to relieve the scene of sameness. But all
traces of the rich, luxuriant, and cultivated part of the country,
is left behind, on progressing towards the seventh mile-
stone, being shut out by the high ground I had been descending to reach the Fellbech houses. In all directions, around
these insulated humble dwellings, naught is seen but bleak
plateaux of the same great moor, one placed lower than the
other, to an almost interminable extent northwards. The
bright yellow and sandy carriage-road alone, shining across the
bleak and brown surface, in a descending and waiving line,
breaks the monotony of the scene, and is observed tapering in
breadth as it proceeds farthest, until it fades in the horizon
formed by ranges of blue hills. A finger-post at this mile-
stone points to the road on the left, leading to the crags, or
nooks, as they are called by the country people.

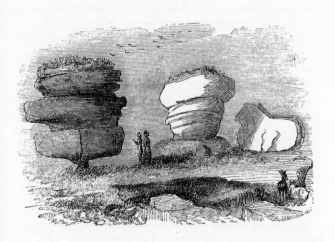

There they stand before me, those mighty stones, of forms the most singular, to which various appellations have been given, as they were supposed to resemble natural or artificial objects, and many of them of most stupendous size. A mile yet divides them from the summit of a steep hill, in the carriage-road (lately widened and much improved), on which I halted to hail their first appearance ; and yet they seem to be within reach of the out-stretched arm.

On the top, and on its margins, and down its sides, the Brimham hill bristles with huge projecting masses of rocks. It looks like the seat of an ancient castle of giants ; one (the Idol) rock prominently conspicuous ; the others planted here and there around, like watchful deities of minor rank, to guard their chief.

The western sun, which was darting its horizontal rays on many parts visible from where I stood, darkened by contrast those whose aspect did not admit of being lighted up by the glorious planet. A gale portending the approaching equinox, (it was September,) had just set in, and whistling dismally through the crags, swept along the bleak and dark surface all around, like the waves of the dead sea.

The carriage-road winds round the base of the hill, and during fine weather, I should say, may be very passable : and horse-bridle paths on the acclivities are innumerable. After many windings, the carriage-road reaches and stops in front of a house erected about a half century ago by the late Lord Grantley, for the accommodation of visiters. Its aspect is turned to the south, and being also placed on the most elevated pinnacle of the hill, it looks surrounded by the mighty masses of gritstone that are scattered in all directions, but more extensively in that of the east. From its upper windows a magnificent view of an extensive and rich country is seen.

To one who follows and listens to the guides in exploring this curious region, the whole scene is puzzling ; but when we examine it minutely we can easily discern that the hill on which the scattered masses appear, is an elevated stratum of sandrock, the composition of which varies, from a fine sand, yellow and grey, to a coarse gravel intermixed with rounded and crystalline pebbles. In some parts the material seems of a looser and more friable texture. The most prevailing line of stratification is with a dip south-south-east on the one side, and north-north-west, and even west-north-west, on the other side of the hill. In this respect whole lines of consistent strata may be traced, separated here and there by vertical fissures more or less important, splitting the general mass into so many insulated pillars. These having subsequently by the action of air and water, and more especially by frost and the frequent exposure to storms of wind that visit them, been worn down at their edges, bases, and summits, but most commonly parallel to their stratification, have gradually assumed shapes the most fantastical.

In some parts large masses of the grit having been deprived of their support, by the wearing away of their bases, formed by some horizontal fracture at considerable elevation from the ground, became ill-balanced, and were hurled-down to an inclined, an upright, or a prostrate position. The rocking-stones found on this hill are certainly nothing but the fortuitous result of such operations as these; while the same agents scooped out those mystical wells and hollows on the top surface of some two or three of the rocks, to which the guide ascribes so much importance.

Balderstones, so produced, are to be seen spread on the east declivity to a great distance, as well as among the variously shaped and figured remains. These remains are not like those of the pillars of carbonated lime on the banks of Saxon Elbe, but more grotesque and various, from the more easily destructive action of air and water on these less compact materials.

The scene altogether is grand and imposing ; and invested as it has been with a religious origin and supposed superstitious rites, it becomes doubly interesting. That druidical priests should have taken advantage of such mighty remains and geological accidents is no wonder. In the various shapes of the rocks they saw the figures of their Gods. In the trembling condition of some of the masses, not yet precipitated from their nicely balanced position, they found a reason for ascribing miracles to their idols. In the perforations made through the coarse masses by natural causes, and in the fissures due to the same, when the gale whistled through them at particular times of the month, and at particular hours of the day, they might pretend to behold the sacred organs by which their deities communed with them.

But that these priests should have fashioned this gigantic theatre for religious purposes, no one will venture to assert. In no part whatever of the entire scene did I see the hand of man ; neither does it seem necessary that, for all the objects of superstition, those crafty religionists should have required any effort of their own to shape these mighty and

singular wonders of the spot into more supernatural performances.

From these silent tokens of primitive ages, turn we our
looks towards the gay and noisy groups just landed on the
little platform in front and a little below the One-house, from
every species of vehicles, and from the back of every riding
quadruped. They come hither from Harrogate, and instantly
place themselves, with submissive discipline, under the guidance of Richard Weatherhead, the happy successor of the late
husband of our buxom and pert landlady, who, with her
hand, bestowed on Richard the right of conducting the company through the mazes of Brimham hill. The late lord had
been an inhabitant and *custos rotulorum* of this desolate
scene for nearly seventy years ; inhabiting, at first, a miserable
hut, and next, the present house of refuge, as it would be
called on the alps summit, during the rest of his life, in
winter as well as summer.

As I stood watching on the threshold of this asylum, I beheld the numerous wanderers, threading in long lines of
variegated dresses, with black, brown, and white hats, and
yellow bonnets, the intricate ways of the hill's declivities;
meandering among the rocks ; now suddenly lost to view as a
black mass of gritstone intervened between us, or as they
sunk into a lower path ; and again appearing, all at once,
as they mounted a rising bank, or climbed over a rock. Some
seemed boisterous and inspired by the scene ; others looked
agast, and listened to the explanations of the guide with
amazement ; while most of them, *mouton*-like, followed in the
wake of the rest, merely because they had come to see " the
Nooks." In this number it was easily to discern some young
couples, who instinctively went along with the general procession, without caring for the objects of it, more occupied with themselves, and with improving their casual
acquaintance, made at the last night's ball at the Crown.

In this diorama of moving figures, Richard, like a magician

with his short wand, was seen to skip from rock to rock, addressing from his elevated stations the company, by explaining to them the miracles of druidicalf anatics; " the lover's leap," and " the rocking stone;" and then scampering, like a mountain hind, from one raised platform to the next, he seemed to be glibly repeating the same long list of names and appellations given to the single stones, or groups of stones, for the edification of his hearers.

Here he points his finger upwards to the round head of a rock, the celebrated " Idol Rock," nineteen feet in height, and forty-six in circumference, which stands on so small a pedestal, that, at first view, the beholder is inclined to consider the whole a deception. Anon, and he is mounted on " the Pulpit rock," resting his hand on " the Parson's head ;" and presently applying the whole weight of his person to the edge of a table rock, suspended on a nearly pointed pivot, and over which he strides, Richard sets the whole mass in motion ; concluding with " Now ladies and gents, I have shown you all that is worth seeing, and you may now take your pleasure, for nothing all over the place."

And sure enough the company take their pleasure, some of them picknicking under the " Oyster-shell rock," or between " the Baboon's and the Serpent's head rocks ;" while others, returning to the house, set about finishing their frugal repast, and drain to the very dregs their ginger beer bottles, the only liquor allowed in these regions.

The prospect I beheld in various directions from my station, and the contrast between the fine country north-east and south-east of the hill, and the bleak moors, around the crags and down the slopes, are singular and striking.

I did not ascend any of the rocking-stones, from whence the view is said to be of the most extensive description, comprising the lofty towers of York Cathedral, the dusky outline of the Yorkshire Wolds, with the Hambleton Hills to the east, and far away to the north, Hackfall (another of the objects of attraction within reach of the Harrogate visiters), Marsham, and an extent of country stretching to the foot of Roseberry Topping, in Cleveland.

This centre of a vast moor-land, covered with a fragrant hether, had often, it seems, been converted into a " house of recovery " for all the industrious bees from the neighbouring towns and villages.   Dining, some months after my visit to Brimham hill, with the Reverend Dr. ———, a prebendary of Peterborough Cathedral, he informed me that many years before, while visiting the crags, he had noticed a great number of bee-hives, which the old guide assured him were annually sent to him from all parts, to pass the two summer months of July and August, during which he lodged and boarded the industrious insects, giving them house-room and the full range of his moorish possessions.   From their marauding expeditions his busy winged protégés returned with their honey charged with the aroma and fragrance of the heath.

Richard at length having saddled my horse, which had been browsing in the rear of the house, I was preparing to quit, when the front steps were suddenly obstructed by a group of four smart *belles* and a beau, just landed with a pa and a ma, (owners of B—— hall, a few miles distant,) from a brilliant landau drawn by four bays in silver harness. This startling equipage for such a region, with its outriders and postillions in sky-blue and jocky-caps of the same, had been seen for some time winding up the rugged way, and finally halting in the flat below.

As the party rushed past me, with looks and the air of protection, to reach the book of arrivals, on which one of the fair white gloved hands inscribed the title and appellation of the two elders, together with the euphonous names of Miss and the Misses Jemima, Wilhelmina, and Dorothea—they happened to disturb the equilibrium of an enormously fat person, " a very Lambert," who was at the time filling the whole entrance door with his bulk, tottering like a rocking-stone, from the effects of frequent application of his wife's bottle of comfort to his lips. The slight concussion was too much for him, and down he went, barrel fashion, rolling again and again over the inclined slope, till his ulterior revolutions were checked by the thick stump of a friendly shrub, against which he pitched with a jerk that made his paunch resound like the belly of the Trojan horse when struck by the spear of Laocoon.

His dear rib, a most worthy *pendant*, who had shortly before cautiously descended the steep brow of the hill, to stow the remnants of their pic-nic into the *sociable* (or " sousable," as I heard an old lady once call these leather-curtained cars for four) in which they had come hither; hearing the well-known voice uttering a cry of distress, turned suddenly round to whence it came, knocked the heavy bundle of *fragiles* out of her own hands by coming in contact with the tattered carcase of the little driver of their vehicle, and he in his turn fell sprawling on the ground, cutting his nose against the newly-made fragments of smashed crockery. In the midst of the general merriment excited by this scene, I spurred on my hack, and was presently lost among the mazes of the *Stony Forest*.

ALDFIELD SPA.

Returning to whence I came, Studely-park, Aldfield Spa lay in my way, and thither I directed my steps, to examine more minutely that sulphur-spring, which I had visited on a former occasion with less attention. As I rode along a private road in an eastward direction towards Aldfield, when about a mile north of Brimham-hill, and while following the edge of a rising ground, which appeared to be an offshoot from it, I noticed a strong illustration of the correctness of my view respecting the geological origin of the crags, in some denuded strata of the same grit of which those crags are formed, having the same dip, and exhibiting in certain parts above the surface of what is now cultivated ground, portions of the rock as fantastically carved out by time and weather as any among the Nooks. Indeed on looking into several of the working quarries which I passed on the road, I saw a confirmation of that view, in the existence of the selfsame grit in them, with a precisely similar inclination of the visible strata of that rock of which the entire district seems formed.

Aldfield Spa is found in a sequestered part of the valley of the Skell, called the "Spa Gill," about a mile and a half westward of Fountain's Abbey; from which there is a pretty footpath to the spring; the latter being accessible also by a high road through the village of Aldfield. By the kind permission of my Lord de Grey, on whose property the well is, people from all parts are allowed to have access to the spring at all times, and to make use of the water. He has also permitted a room in an adjoining cottage to be fitted up with the necessary conveniences for either a warm or a cold bath of the mineral water; and has appointed a goodly dame at the cottage, to attend and perform all such services as the use of the water may require.

The well in every way resembles the principal one found on the bog lands above Low Harrogate, being rudely-covered over, and sheltered, except in front, by upright and horizontal flagstones. The water remains constantly level with the upper part of the well, at a depth of four or five inches, above which it is allowed to flow out by a discharging-pipe, which conveys it down a stream-way, close by. A stone hollowed out in the centre, and the hollow bored with a round aperture about eight inches in diameter, permits the water to surge from the rock underneath, accompanied by a succession of little air-bubbles every two or three minutes.

The water is transparent and colourless. It has a temperature of 52° Fahr., a temperature I found to appertain to all the *rocky*-sulphur springs in Yorkshire. No air-bubbles rise from the bottom of the glass, nor do any appear adhering to its inner surface after the water has been suffered to rest awhile. The taste is one of pleasing freshness, though rather soft. It is almost wholly free from the peculiar flavour of strong saline waters, and the smell and taste of the sulphuretted gas present are akin to those of the mildest of the Harrogate waters.

I drank several glasses of the water on more than one occasion, and applied the ordinary tests at the spring, to ascertain the principal components of it, and which seem to be somewhat analogous to those of Harrogate; holding a middle rank between the sulphuretted water of that place and Knaresborough. The water is not aperient without the addition of a quarter of an ounce of some neutral salt. Epsom salts is what is added here, in which the people are wrong. The cases of recovery from disease by the Aldfield Spa, which the good woman of the cottage remembers, among the many patients who have applied to the well since she has been in charge of it, are very numerous, and one cannot but believe her.

The situation of the spring is pleasing, but not of a romantic character. It is a purely sequestered and rural spot, the valley of the Skell being here smiling, and not imposing as at Makershaw, another part of the same dale. To the neighbouring countrymen and their families, the facility of procuring a natural medicinal agent of this desciption is a boon for which they cannot be sufficiently thankful.

CHAPTER X.

ENVIRONS OF HARROGATE CONTINUED.

The French tourist who observed that, " *C'est à la campagne qu'on voit les Anglais,*" said truly. He alluded to the upper classes of society, and meant to contrast the comparatively insignificant mode in which they display their own importance and wealth in the capital, with the pomp and splendour they exhibit at their seats and ancestral mansions in the country.

The aristocrat of the English commonwealth, and the opulent commoner who is descended from a long line of ancestors, take a pride in maintaining intact, as transmitted to them, the species of *seigneurie* or independent domain, with its manorial dwelling—be it magnificent or unpretending—by which their individual rank and station in society seems marked and distinguished, and through which they can attract and command in their immediate neighbourhood, an obsequiousness bordering almost on vassalage.

This keeping up of a certain *prestige* in the particular district which, from long location of the family in it, has become almost patrimonial, has, moreover, certain solid and real advantages, such as an Englishman alone can appreciate, and knows how to turn to account in forwarding his own or his family's worldly interest. Hence, the maintenance of all those splendid country residences which dot the fair surface of England, and which so much struck the French traveller, as well as the pompous style of living displayed in them, are both necessary, to satisfy family pride and family interest ; and as those two motives are not likely ever to fade, so are the means by which they are gratified likely to remain for ever.

In the vast capital of this empire the vortex of society is so wide-mouthed and rapid, that whoever approaches it must submit to be dragged within its all-absorbing eddy, nor hope to be able to keep aloof and on its margin, conspicuously grand, and exempt from the all-extinguishing effect of the whirlpool. People are conscious of this striking characteristic of London ; and hence no attempt is made, even by the wealthiest individuals, or the more noble in society, to set up, by the same means which serve in the provinces, any claim to seignorial importance. We find therefore in London (few exceptions indeed being made) no palaces and imposing mansions standing out of the common rows, terraces, and squares—no great train of domestics—no extraordinary equipages, reminding one of a princely retinue—no greater display of banquets and brilliant assemblies in one particular house than in five hundred others—finally, no exercise of that splendid and extensive hospitality among the great which is especially conspicuous among them in the country, even to ostentation. Nothing of this will the stranger who has just witnessed it all, and probably partaken of it in the provinces, notice in the capital. London is only a temporary *pied à terre* for the great—a spot to transact business in—including that *keeping before the public*—a place to watch and be watched in, for particular purposes during a certain definite period—a locality in fine suited to recruit faded influences and shore up the tottering interest of dynasties.

The country is the genuine theatre for the display of grandeur for the support of privileges, for the upholding of family importance ; and hence it is that, " *l'Anglais doit être vu en sa maison de campagne.*"

The upper classes in England may be said to stand in the same relation between town and country, that the real Russian noblemen stand between Moscow and the Imperial Residence, as St. Petersburgh is called.   Whoever desires to form an adequate idea of the wealth, pomp, and power of a Russian Boyard, must view him at Moscow, not at St. Petersburgh.

In this respect France differs from England as the poles differ.   Paris is France, and *les provinces,* nothing.   The illustrious who lives *en prince* in the capital — even the pompous " *ministre d'Etat,*" who temporarily dwells in the gilded and almost royal saloons of the *hôtel du ministère*—displays therein all that " *les grands*" of France can display in this world.   You must not visit them at their " *châteaux*" in the country.   There, all *prestige* has vanished, and Mons. Thiers even is no more than one of the *Tiers-etat.*

My return to Studely Royal from the little expedition mentioned in my last chapter, and my residence of many days, on that as well as on a former occasion, under its hospitable roof, suggested the preceding train of reflections. But even the sight of that domain, truly denominated royal, would not alone have warranted the remarks just made on the condition of high English society in the country. Good fortune has furnished me with many more striking examples of the general application and truth of my remarks.   Whether as a simple stranger, permitted to view those very mansions and country seats to which I refer, or as a guest invited to some of them to witness and partake of their inward and domestic comforts and splendour,—I have had opportunities sufficient to enable me to subscribe to the opinion expressed by my French traveller, repeated by myself, and entertained by so many people, that it has at last become almost trite.

The hundreds who daily flock from Harrogate to the extensive and magnificent grounds of Studely, and are suffered by the kind permission of the amiable mistress to wander through every part of them, and who hardly expect the amazement they will experience at the sight of Fountain's Abbey, forming part of these grounds—such visiters, I say, will partake in the opinion in question, and admit that private individuals need not, in this country, envy the sovereign his royal domain, his parks, or his pleasure grounds.

Often have I bent my way to the great entrance into the grounds of Studely from the mansion, by the door of its most superb banquetting-hall, through the dressed flower-garden divided into innumerable beds of gaudy and showy plants, following an avenue of venerable oak trees, the youngest of which reckons a century, and still further on a stately aisle of lofty pillar-like beech trees, which seemed to direct the steps of the pedestrian, until at last I reached the principal lodge, where twenty or more carriages of every form and colour stood waiting, unhorsed, for the return of those parties they had deposited from Harrogate in the morning, and which were now rambling within the *grille* in all directions.

I have seen many of the groups, lost in ecstasy and admiration, admit that of all the excursions which their temporary séjour at the "genuine spa" had enabled them to make, this was the most "surpassing strange" and imposing. They would often linger with unsated curiosity before the temples —the cascades—the canal—the statues—the splendid banks of laurel—the lakes—the river—and lastly the holy shrine of our Lady of Fountains; they would cling to the latter and its glorious accessories and appurtenances; nor could the approaching feeling of hunger, after a ramble of many hours, recal them to the appointed time of the projected pic-nic in one of the pavillions placed on the border of the outer lake, wherein such repasts are permitted to the visiters, by the kind proprietess.

Of such parties I have met in one day, when the fineness of the weather tempted people abroad, as many as ten and twelve and they each of them were numerous. Every party had a conductor, who, taking charge of them from the very threshold within the great iron-gate, escorts them all the time, explaining every thing as he goes along the many and varied walks, and through labyrinths, journeying between walls of yew trees, luxuriant laurels, hollies and evergreens of every kind, and passing by many plantations that cover the hills as well as the plain, until they arrive at the Italian division of the gardens, and so on to the celebrated ruins of Fountain's Abbey, the Mecca of every pilgrim who is attracted to the spot, and one suited to attract even those from a greater distance who have not the excuse of being at Harrogate.

This is the gigantic feature and the pride of Studely. Where is the spot in Europe, be it fashioned by unbounded power or incalculable wealth—by taste, the handmaid of the arts, or by mere seignorial pride, destined to serve as the country residence of a sovereign—on which we shall find, *as part of the pleasure-grounds*, the most magnificent remains of a most magnificent abbey, left standing for centuries, in the picturesque condition of ruinous integrity? Let Bolton, Kirkstall, Rivaulx, Glastonbury, and Tintern Abbeys claim each their individual superiority; but never shall the palm be wrested from Fountains'; which, equal in architectural beauty, pictorial preservation, and in extent also to some of them, and superior to others—outstrips them all

in being surrounded by an extent of park and pleasure-
grounds in character, which none of the other abbatial remains can boast of—Bolton excepted.

But it is not merely as a vast extent of pleasure-grounds,
equal, if not superior to Windsor Park and gardens, to the
Giardini Boboli, to the *Lustgarten* of Schweitzinger, or to
the groves of Nymphenburg near Munich, that Studely is
to be viewed. In many of those princely domains, art has
done more than nature. The earth has been tortured into
many fantastic ways; hillocks have been raised on plains, to
give undulation to the ground; rocks have been manufactured, and covered with every possible vegetable production; dales have been dug out, and water made to run at the
bottom of them. But here is Studely: it is hills as ancient
as the universe that we behold, springing up into the air
some hundreds of feet, clad to their summits with forests
coeval with William of Normandy; it is the precipitous
descents into dells, bathed by a classic river sang by Spen-
ser; it is ravines cleft by diluvial torrents, and a succession
of valleys, of which that of *Makershaw* alone measures
some miles in extent. It is such features as these, in fine,
placed within a ring-fenced area, that would occupy a traveller on a goodly horse in exploring it, from sunrise to
noon, and thence to the hour of declining day, which
entitle Studely to be considered " an unrivalled territory."

Coming to sober prose,—what a magnificent sight does not
the endless variety of forest trees, indigenous as well as
exotic, offer, which are to be found in all directions in
Studely grounds? A few years back Mrs. Lawrence employed an artist of merit in designing fac-similes of the principal trees in the park and pleasure-grounds. The trees
were measured at the same time, and represented in pencil-
drawings of the folio size, and are true portraits. Mr.
Jukes, the artist, was engaged five months in his work, and
as it was during the winter principally that he designed the

trees, they are of course leafless, except the firs and spruce.*

Fountain's Abbey has engaged the pen as well as the pencil of many eminent persons, and needs not my poor description in this place. Yet as a noble monument of gothic art, and as a remembrancer of times singularly romantic in the history of England, every visiter possessing a soul will be apt to view it with feelings such as no description or drawing can do justice to. The time of day, too, at which these noble ruins are seen, invest them with different interest. The early morn, just as the sun darts its first rays from over the summit of the lofty wooded hill that faces the abbey, where the deep and straight valley, in which the ruins lay imbosomed, prepares to bend, and the river expands into a semicircular lake, gives to the scene a mellowness which gradually vanishes as the meridian sun covers the whole of the ruins with a flood of light.

At eve, seen from the banks of the Skell, seated under a clump of trees on one of the benches purposely placed there to enjoy it, at the distance of about the eighth of a mile in a straight line, the spectacle is of a more sombre cast. The sun, setting behind the ruins, throws out in dark shadows against the

---

* It will not be altogether uninteresting to enumerate a few of the most remarkable trees in question, as a matter of curiosity and comparison with other places. A Spanish chesnut 112 feet high and 22 feet in girth. Another 89 feet high, 12 feet in girth. A Lime-tree, 101 feet high, 17 feet 3 inches in girth. Beech, 114 feet 6 inches high, 22 feet in girth. Ash, 104 feet high, 20 feet in girth. Three oaks nearly 90 feet high, and 24 feet in girth. Another (oak sessiliflora) *one hundred and eighteen* feet high, and 33 feet in girth, divided into five principal upright stems ! Alpine fir, 130 feet high, and 20 in girth. A black American spruce, 121 feet high, 9 feet 11 inches in girth. A silver fir, 96 feet high, with a girth of nearly 11 feet, and a spread near the ground of 50 feet. A sycamore, 100 feet high. A Dutch elm, 95 feet, and an English elm 108 feet high, with 26 feet 8 inches in girth, and fifteen principal upright stems;—and *sic de cæteris.*

firmament, the outlines of this massive structure, and serves to carve, like a fine embroidery on the gilded sky seen through them, the open traceries of the upper casements in the tower. Thrice have I seen with enchantment this touching scene, which is rendered still more impressive by the surrounding forested hills, the noisy rippling of the Skell, and the warbling of many birds bidding adieu to departing day.

Still the most imposing view of these ruins, I must contend, is by the light of a full moon. During a sojourn of two weeks at Studely last summer, the facility of a *passe partout*-key given to her guests by the amiable hostess, tempted me to frequent rambles through that enchanted region. An expedition even at midnight to the Shrine of Fountains is by no means of rare occurrence with the company staying in the house. It is one, at all events, which many would compound to travel some hundreds of miles to partake in, and of which I myself partook more than once.

" Never can the solemnity of the scene (as I once before stated in another publication), be effaced from my memory. There lay the towering and multi-shaped pile, swelled into larger dimensions by the illumined atmosphere of night, quietly reposing in a vast lake of moonlight. Now and anon some of its noble parts would be suddenly snatched from our view, by a solitary black cloud scudding before the westerly gale, and passing between the moon and this grand theatre of wonders. But the cloud disappeared quickly over the top of the surrounding hill, and all was brilliancy again. The stillness too of such a night-scene had its peculiar effect on the beholder, different from what we experience at the calm silence which pervades this secluded spot even at midday. Of such stirring nature is the sun's light, that it can hardly be associated with silence. It is a clamorous, it is a life-giving light. That which the moon sheds, on the contrary, seems to command stillness : it is, in fact, silence itself—it is the grave. Its tranquillity is catching, and the soothing influence that attends it, steals upon us unawares, and seems to lull, for a time at least, every passion within our troubled bosoms.

The breeze that moved the occasional cloud before it on that night, kept playing with the top branches of the tall cedars planted on the highest pinnacles of the adjoining hills, and shook, with a hissing moan, the dark boughs of "the Seven Sisters"—yew-trees said to have been planted by the founders of the abbey. These murmurs, mingled with the babbling noise of the Skell, that sparkled in the moonshine,

"Like woven sounds of stream and breezes,"

scarcely interrupted the general harmony of these silent regions, where

"The dead are sleeping in their sepulchres,
And mouldering as they sleep."

Their voices we evoked from their tombs, within the lengthened and gloomy cloisters, as one moonlight night, accompanied by two or three fellow guests at Studely, whose acquaintance one remembers with pleasure,—we all stood surveying the mysterious pile. Ensconced within an elliptical niche, scooped out of a huge jutting gritstone-rock, that forms part of a high hill near the left margin of the river, and at the distance of a few hundred yards, with our faces turned to the ruins, we roused the sleeping genii of the place with our loud interrogatories, and every word of ours was heard most distinctly repeated *within* the ruins, though in an altered and generally a louder echo. When two of us sang first and second, and followed each other as in a canon, the effect was both singular and pleasing.

The question of selecting proper building materials for the new Houses of Parliament, was just then under consideration; and a commission was travelling over the country to inspect quarries, examine churches, and other old public buildings, and make a choice of a proper stone for the required object. I know not whether the said commissioners did or did not take pains with Fountain's Abbey. Its structure merited attention, which must have been but superficially bestowed, if it be true that they have reported Fountain's Abbey as one of the sandstone edifices " in an advanced state of decomposition."

On examining it, I find that several varieties of sandstone have been employed : some having fine crystals, and very minute sand in their composition; while others, on the contrary, have large grains of quartz and nodules. Here and there a regular bit of compact flint-stone is to be met with. The calcareous stone is chiefly of the magnesian kind, and a calciferous grit has been employed likewise. Fragments of each of these, as if they had been the rubble left in the quarries after the working of the stones, have been used to fill up large spaces between the inner and outer faces of many of the walls in the less important parts of the building.

In the neighbouring valley, strata of all these modifications of calcareous grits are to be seen, which have evidently been worked for the building; and to judge by the state of integrity of surface in most of its parts, one cannot deny that the choice of materials made by the monks was highly judicious.

We often wonder where Prout and Stanfield could have found the many glaring tints with which they colour their buildings. In these remains of the abbey the truth of their selection is beautifully and most picturesquely illustrated, and every tint of the most gaudy description may be seen here. The surface of an inside wall of a square department adjoining the long cloisters, and to the east of them, open to the heavens above, and hardly protected by small arches springing from corbels, exhibited at my visit almost every colour on

a painter's pallette, the pure effect of lichens. The lilac, the
chrome-yellow, the iron-red, the deep orange, and the greenish and bluish tints, were all strongly visible on this multi-
tinted wall, and contrasted pleasingly with the natural
colour of the stone, which is of a creamy yellow. In some
few places a lichen nearly of a pearly white came in, in
patches, to harmonize with the rest.

It is not otherwise with the south side of the great quadrangle, a most exquisite piece of gothic structure, with a noble
arched door in the centre leading to the Refectory. The
upper or first story of the latter, particularly the wide and
centre pier supported by the arched door is tinted by similar
causes in the manner just described, and produces a most
beautiful effect. None is a more skilful painter than Nature.

The visiter at Harrogate, whose curiosity is not already
satisfied with the various objects I have enumerated,—placed,
as it were, within reach of his head quarters, purposely to
aid the salutary effects of the Spa, by furnishing him with
agreeable and instructive recreation,—will find many more
besides to occupy his attention.   That romantic region,
Hackfall, to which so many equestrian parties direct their
steps,—Ripley Castle, with Sir William Ingilby's extensive
gardens, greenhouses, and a pinery excelled nowhere in
the north of England,—also *Almais* Cliff,—and the Armida
gardens of Swinton, presided over by the amiable heiress of that
domain ; and perhaps even Bolton Priory ;—those will furnish
occupation for many a day.   And after all, the visiter may
feel that something yet remains undone, if he performs not his
devotion within the great sanctuary of Ripon, its massive and
unostentatious Minster.   The recent elevation to episcopal
rank of that cathedral, has invested it with an importance
which it probably possesses not intrinsically.

The first thing that strikes the beholder on entering Ripon
Cathedral, is the unusual shortness of its nave, as compared
with those of Lincoln and York.   The distance between the

central west door, to between the pillars which support the
west arch of the square transept, or St. Wilfrid's Tower, facing
the screen, is only sixty-four paces. The effect of this arch,
which has on the right, or south side, a heavy gothic pillar
instead of an Anglo-Norman, like the one opposite, is very
curious. It brings the said pillar forward, so that neither the
screen nor the door in it is in the centre, under the arch,
when viewed from the bottom of the church, but both are as
much as three feet and a half nearer to the south than to the
north side of the transept.

This deformity was occasioned by the rebuilding of two of
the old Saxon arches supporting the lantern, which were
broken down by the fall of the spire about two centuries ago.

The interior of the church is not remarkably imposing, from
the presence of any conspicuous monument or decoration. It
has received many and recent ameliorations under the direction of an able architect, by means of subscriptions, as well
as subventions from the coffers of the Dean and Chapter.
But the covering of the walls and pillars with a yellow distem-
per wash, which contrasts violently with the flat and rather low
roof of reddish wood over the nave, was a sin against sound
taste which must be attributed to inferior hands.

It is refreshing, while shocked by this incongruity, to peer
over the ancient stone screen that divides the choir from the
nave. Attracted by the magnificent east window, which has
at different and recent epochs been repaired, the eye loves to
pass over the new and beautifully groined arched roof of that
part of the church, substituted, under the direction of the
same able artist, for the old ceiling, which previously hid the
apex of the fine gothic arch now advantageously seen over
the new organ. Many of the oak-carvings in the choir deserve attention; but they are surpassed in exquisiteness of
workmanship by other cathedrals in England, and still more
so by many of the churches in Flanders.

As I was stepping across the sacred temple for the purpose

of ascertaining some of the preceding facts, the great western door was suddenly thrown open, and a solemn procession entered and advanced along the great nave, pacing the hallowed ground at the sound of a mournful dirge-tune, sung with organ accompaniment by six or eight boys and as many adult chaunters, all in white surplices. They were marshalled by a verger in his black gown, carrying a silver mace.

> " Who is this they follow ? ————
> It doth betoken the corse."

The great bell had been previously tolling for half an hour those dismal quarter-minute strokes, which in Christian lands announce the departure of our fellow-men from this world of strife, and prepared me for the affecting scene that followed.

Behind the surpliced chaunters came the lifeless being to whose memory and for whose soul-sake this *requiem* and *motet* was raised, in touching and harmonious accents, to the vaults above in this House of God. It laid unconscious of these devotional honours in its narrow coffin, carried to its last dwelling—its last resting-place—by mourning bearers, not on the shoulders, but at arms' length downwards, and only a foot from the ground. The principal mourner touched with his right hand all the while the head of the coffin, which went forward first. Mourning relatives mostly clad in deep sable followed, principally aged people, who must have reflected at the time, on how near their own hour must be when a similar ceremony would be performed for them.

Like Hamlet upon a similar occasion, " I crouched awhile and marked," behind the shadow of one of the side pillars. What a subject for reflection at such a moment! Many friends of the deceased and his family were there, together with some that had been attracted with mere curiosity. There was no appearance, or even the affectation, of a tear or of desponding grief. The deceased had lived his full term of life, and had died of nature's decay. He had outlived the keenest feelings of attachment on the part of his kindred. But a modest gloom was spread over the countenance of some of the nearest relatives, which contrasted sadly with the levity of the strangers, and the yawning of such as had attended to oblige the family, or to be civil, or to avoid offence.

Alas! how little any of them cared for the departed! He had been a tanner, and in that humble calling had realized a fortune, when he retired, and became a *gentleman*. All this had secured to him the present cathedral honours, at his exit from a world which he had entered under the thatched roof of a miserable hut wherein had dwelt his mother, a poor labourer's wife!

How impressive, how thrilling, is the ceremony of consigning' the mortal spoils of our fellow-creatures to the grave, accompanied by the sound of solemn music and solemn rites! This is a remain of the Romish mode, wanting only the sprinkling of holy water, the lighted tapers, and the gorgeous dresses of the priests, instead of the coarse linen surplices of the chaunters (as in this instance of protestant worship) whose ordinary dress is ill concealed by the temporary investiture of a sacerdotal habit. The ceremony is the same, the intention identical, but the pageant somewhat different. We all look for and aspire to a future state of happiness, and pray that those who are gone from us, and before us, being "delivered from the burden of the flesh, may be with the Lord in joy and felicity." But the Romish churchman views an intermediate state, one of probation and of expiation, after which there is final judgment and redemption; and, therefore doth he pray, that the final adjudication may be favourable to the departed. The separatist from the church of Rome, on the contrary, believes not in an intermediate state of expiation, and views the final adjudication of the dead on the glorious day of resurrection as decided, or at all events, not to be modified by prayer, at and after the demise of a Christian. No praying therefore will avail for him;

since, according to the impressive and simple liturgy of the
burial service, " the spirits of them that depart in the Lord
and the souls of the faithful, after they are delivered from the
burden of the flesh, live with Almighty God and are in joy
and felicity." Their fate then is determined, and prayers can
avail not. And yet we have here, in the ceremony I was a
witness to, the semblance of something like an intercession,
through prayer, in behalf of him who is released from " *and
no longer present in the flesh over which we pray.*"

I repent me of having hastily declared that no sincere or
really grieved mourner accompanied the deceased to his grave.
When his remains had been committed to the ground, " earth
to earth," and the several parties had dispersed,—a group
of persons in the deepest mourning did pass me along the
south aisle, on their return from the churchyard, from one of
whom heavy sighs and groans proceeded, as from anguish,
and who would have fallen but for the support of a venerable
elderly man. I withdrew to let the afflicted go by. It was
the surviving partner, as I afterwards learned, of the deceased,
who had struggled with him in his difficulties, and rejoiced in
his success; who, in life, had been his happiness, and, in
death, was now his only and sincerest mourner.

That I might lose not a single vestige of this impressive
moral lesson, thus unexpectedly read to me, I stepped
into the churchyard, to behold the new-made grave, and
reached it just as the two grave diggers, as waggish as the pert
interlocutor of the Prince of Denmark, were shovelling the
last handful of loose earth over the sepulture, to level with
the rest of that field of death the last habitation of " the
rich tanner of Ripon."

This melancholy operation took place within a few feet of
that nearly subterranean recess of death, called the *Bone-house.*
The massive door was open, and I descended into the crypt,
the three vaulted arches of which are filled with skulls and
detached jawbones, with leg and thigh bones, in some parts
piled twelve feet deep inwardly, and seven feet in height, in

careful tiers one at the top of the other. The crypt is thus
internally virtually walled in all round with dead men's
bones ; and the floor likewise is composed of them to the
depth of three feet. These bones were found, and some of
them piled up in these vaults, about twenty-five years ago,
and the rest, amounting to about four thousand complete
remains, were at first heaped up like a great wall against the
outside of the church, between two east-end buttresses. There
they remained until eight years ago, when a great pit, ten
feet square, was dug in the churchyard, and the whole heap
of skulls and bones were thrown into it *pêle-mêle*, the
ground being afterwards planted with trees.

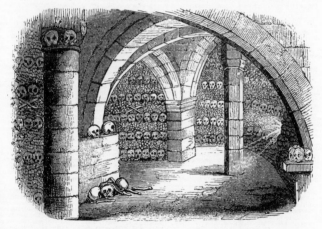

The floor on which the visiter to the bone-house (or
skullery, as Theodore would call it) unconsciously treads, is
strewed with skulls, lightly covered over with a thin coating
of yellow sand. This, in some places, may be brushed off
with the feet, when suddenly the eyeless sockets of some
unknown genius, destined to perish in obscurity in life as well
as in death, stares you in the face ; or the gaping jaws of a
decrepit lawyer, yawn like the portal of death, to remind us
how that grim deity, like the art which the owner of those

jaw-bones professed in life, swallows up all without mercy or distinction.

To behold here repeated in untold numbers the outer case of that material substance which is said to think, and which in the lapse of centuries has distilled itself into nothing— while its external covering, on the contrary, remains as before, unchanged and unaltered, one would doubt if man have really any other allotted duty to perform beyond the grave. The spirit once flown, must either return defined in quantity from eternity to the general mass of the *aura mundi* from whence it came, and with it mingle as one of its integral parts, until refashioned into some other modification of matter; or it will lie still. At all events it could neither suffer nor enjoy, grieve, nor rejoice, without fresh materialization ; since it lacks that which it has left behind, and which even death cannot take away, for here we see it before us ages after spirit and matter have severed partnership. So reasons the half-witted materialist.

Had we no greater, had we no loftier, and far nobler reasons for believing in the existence of another and an active life hereafter, than what is to be deduced from material feelings—then what will explain to us the dream—ah ! the dream which tells us that we may act, suffer, or enjoy keenly, acutely, and earnestly through a something that is within us, and is not the body, since the body in dream lies prostrate, immovable, and unmoving, and often appears as dead to the bystanders. Is not this a fair picture of what our life may be in another world ? But therein shall we behold and recognise those who were once so dear to us, and whom we have lost.

Before bidding adieu to the Minster, where I had now spent some hours, the present condition of its interior building engaged my attention. This is a point of great interest at this moment, when extensive public buildings are meditated or in progress.

Two distinct materials enter conspicuously into the structure of the Minster;—a compact sandstone of a yellowish cast and fine quartzose grain, occasionally varied with streaks of red, or of an iron-ochry tinge; and secondly, a firm limestone, also yellowish, not scaly nor friable, compact after exposure to the air, and free from shells or any other fossil remains. The earliest portion of the building yet left standing, and said to have been erected by Wilifred, at the east-end, is of sandstone. It has now withstood the east, south-east, and north-east winds for nearly a thousand years, and is by no means in a damaged state; although, as a useless portion of the building, it is not much attended to.

The second erection, by Thurstan, Archbishop of York, its west front, its window, and the two square towers, are of sandstone also, the surface of which is almost intact. In the remainder of the additions made successively under Henry the Second, Henry the Third, and Stephen, both sandstone and limestone were employed; and were I to give an impartial opinion of the state of integrity of the two stones, comparatively speaking, I should unhesitatingly declare that the sandstone is the least affected by age or exposure. The side of the buttresses sustaining the eastern wall and sides of the eastern window, which are exposed to the direct north wind, are much and roughly handled over their surfaces. The sandstone employed is supposed to have been found at no great distance from Ripon.

Having had the honour, at Studely, of being introduced to the Bishop of that newly created diocese, with whom I afterwards partook of one of those splendid banquets which daily distinguished Mrs. Lawrence's most hospitable establishment, we discoursed on the state of the Minster, and by a natural transition on the episcopal palace also, which was then erecting upon an eminence a little way out of town, commanding a view of Ripon, but altogether devoid of trees, and in the midst of arable land. "A palace!" I said, "why, with ten thousand pounds or thereabout, and no more, which it has been proposed to expend for that purpose under the control of certain commissioners, what palace can be erected? A moderately-sized dwelling-house, in what his lordship called *a collegiate style* of gothic structure, is even now rising, and probably, by this time, has been completed. It will shelter the prelate of Ripon, but it will not be a palace. Its front porch and narrow doorway bespeak no palace; neither is the elevation or height palatial, notwithstanding the contrivance of cutting down, around the base of the building, part of the hill on which the gothic structure stands, so as to impart to it the appearance of being upon a terraced sub-basement. The architect is the same who successfully competed for the Nelson pillar.

The diocesans of Ripon, who have not been long in discovering the great worth and excellent qualities of their first Bishop, like most of those who have the honour of knowing his lordship, regret that an edifice more in character with his high dignity and personal attainments, had not been raised by the government for his residence. They can hardly help reverting to the splendid palace erected by the Catholics for their own district prelate, near Bath, as a contrast to the *mesquinerie* allotted to the protestant Bishop of Ripon.

As in almost every thing else that evinces public spirit, patriotism, and goodness of heart, whenever the welfare of Ripon is concerned, so in the very transactions of finding a site for the Bishop's house, of ceding additional land for a domain around it, (which, after all, will extend only to very little more than one hundred acres,) and of building the house itself, for which she furnishes the stone out of her own quarries, the mistress of Studely has acted a generous and conspicuous part. Wealth that is so applied cannot be grudged to the possessor, whose days, it is hoped will be spared for a long period to come, that the poor may continue to reap the benefit of them, and bless her.

Preparations were now making for taking my leave, that I might proceed with my intended inquiry into the mineral springs and principal sea-bathing places of this county, when the Earl of ————, also a visiter at Studely, proposed a ride to Newby Hall, and a visit to its noble proprietor. Although acquainted with that manor from a former visit, the temptation of once more viewing its statue gallery was too great to be resisted. We accordingly proceeded thither, were courteously entertained, and every facility was afforded me to inspect the many valuable objects of art which the mansion contains, including the unique gobelin tapestry of the drawing-room, the several pictures hung in divers apartments, the prettily painted ceilings, by Zucchi, and the bijoux morning-room, or boudoir, of the Countess de Grey, in which, among many other beautiful objects, arranged with peculiar taste, there are two exquisitely finished portraits by Lawrence.

The gallery of statues is an additional building connected with the older edifice. It communicates with the library, and is divided into three compartments, the centre of which rises into a cupola. The gallery is about seventy feet long, and the library fifty feet. They constitute one apartment as it were, facing the south, having the river Ure running in front of it, though too low to be seen from the rooms. A cheerful lawn, skilfully planted, stretches between it and the house, with a distant view beyond it of a pretty country.

The glory of the gallery is the statue of Venus, formerly known as the *Barberini Venus.* It was purchased through the Abbate Jenkins, at Rome. The statue is larger than that of the Medici Venus; it has been restored in several parts; but the torso is magnificent, and equal to the best works of art handed down to us by the ancients. It is highly finished, and the restorations are very creditable. I was struck also with a head of Caracalla in the collection, and with a *statuette* of Cicero sitting in his consular robe, and very like the ancient bust of that great orator. This performance is set down in the catalogue as the figure of a senator.

Newby Hall and its various treasures of art are, by the liberality of the Earl De Grey, open to the visiters at Harrogate daily.

CHAPTER XI.

MASTER DANIEL, who dwells in a shop not far from the Bellevue, at Harrogate, is a useful person in his way. He lets out a gig at a fair charge, and drives his *fare* himself; and being very intelligent, to boot, he answers the purpose of a cicerone mighty well.

Under his guidance I placed myself on quitting Harrogate on my way to the spring of Thorpe Arch ; intending afterwards to halt at York for the night and two following days, as an excellent starting-post for a public conveyance to Scarborough.

Our tract lay direct south, with the Almais Cliffs on the right at some distance, and on the left Kirkby Overblow, a small but picturesque town, whose rich and fertile valley is traversed by the high-road.

"They are rather sparing of their *metal* in these parts," observed Daniel, " in mending the road, and my nag feels it. See how she ploughs, instead of rolling, as she did nearer home, on a smooth and hard surface. The fact is," continued the shrewd rate-payer, " as the people here are obliged to fetch their stone for road mending from the limestone quarries at Harrogate, for which they pay tenpence per square yard, and as much more for carriage and breaking, road mending becomes an expensive job, and so *they* are left to mend themselves."

Kirkby is most favourably placed. It looks, westwardly, on a lovely plain entirely surrounded by hills, covered with the finest verdure, and thickly wooded. The most striking object in this mass is York, whose elevated buildings appear so near, to one who looks eastward from the ridge of Kirkby, that you would fancy the city lay at your feet.

We came at last to Harewood Bridge over the Warfe, where the clear stream offers to the idler from Harrogate the sport of trout fishing. Parties adjourn here from the Spa for fish dinners after the sport ; and on the same occasion, visit the noble mansion and grounds of the Earl of Harewood, which are liberally open to them every Saturday.

There is a nearer approach to the former through the plantations, over a great and steep hill projecting in the road, and round which the carriage must wind its way for three quarters of a mile, after coasting the great wall of Harewood Park over the bridge. To avoid this the pedestrian uses the right of way along a winding and ascending path, through a small gate placed on the right of the road, at the foot of the hill. Many follow this path, in order to enjoy the magnificent panorama which successively unrols itself at their feet as they ascend and now and then turn to view the extensive and fertile dale to which the Warfe, conspicuously sparkling in the sun, has given its name.

The ruins of Harewood Castle, with its two remaining square towers, mantled with ivy, are close at hand, and a tunnel-gate through the summit of the ridge, leads to a farther point in the high-road, where, at a few hundred yards distance, is the great entrance into Harewood Park, through a lofty and grand Italian arch, with a handsome lodge at each side. The position of this entrance, at the confluence of three wide and straight avenue roads, with the neat and uniform stone dwellings of the village at their points of union, is one of the most seignorial-looking I have seen in England. Beyond it the expanding grounds are seen through the large iron *grille* to great advantage.

A casual passer-by, evidently of the place, whom I accosted whilst Daniel proceeded to take care of his nag, informed me that the noble proprietor was "at home;" and began to descant eloquently on the personal worth and merits of that nobleman. "O, yes, we all rejoice that my lord be come back from London. Every body in the village gladdens whenever their kind master and mistress return to the hall. My lord and my lady are so good!"

Is not this the best eulogium a good and wealthy man can desire, who is placed by rank and fortune over the destiny of many of his fellow-creatures? Alas! one of the eulogized parties has since departed " from the hall " for ever!

Though the day was not that of ordinary admission to the mansion and grounds, my card procured me that privilege, accompanied by a flattering message. To describe the interior of the house, the whole front of which, divided into a centre and two wings, measures nearly three-hundred feet, owes its striking and rich corinthian design to Adams, of London, and Carr, of York, would be to occupy more space in these volumes than I can spare—considering what yet

remains before me to accomplish. Agreeably to the usual
routine on all such occasions, I passed, accompanied by the
portly housekeeper, who had been summoned for that purpose by an officious powdered lacquey, from the hall, of excellent dimensions, into the library ; thence through the state
bedrooms, the saloon, the yellow and white drawing-rooms ;
the lengthened and striking gallery, lighted by seven windows,
over each of which hang festoons of mock curtains in carved
wood, ready to let down, executed in so masterly a manner
by Chippendale, that the sharpest eye might be deceived in
them ; and lastly, the dining and music rooms, with the circular room, and so to the great staircase, painted by Zucchi.

All the ceilings are most beautifully decorated, particularly
that of the gallery, which forms the extreme end of the west
or right wing, from the windows of which there is a view
full of charms. But different far is the more extended and
delightful prospect before the centre portico, which covers
the grand terrace outside of the room called the saloon, at
the back of the house fronting the south. Here the edifice
seems as if perched upon a hill springing up from a valley, at
the bottom of which the produce of a single spring has been
skilfully spread out into a magnificent sheet of water, towards
whose margin the verdant sides of the hill have been made to
slope with great taste and judgment.

Some walks in various directions, and the use of a portable
telescope, enabled me to take in at various points the many
beauties of the general pleasure-grounds, which, I understand, comprise about a hundred and fifty acres, and were
laid out by Brown, at an expense of sixteen thousand pounds.
At the end of one of these walks, the ivy-mantled church,
placed within a thick grove of trees, which gives it an air
of solemnity, becoming the last resting-place of the lords
of this domain, arrests the steps of the visiter. Historical
recollections tempts him to enter the small and sacred temple,

which, for the number and perfect preservation of its tombs, is said to surpass every parish church in the county.

On the threshold of the churchyard stood my former honest interlocutor:—" I thought you would be coming to see our parish church. Most people do come hither from Harrogate; but only to satisfy curiosity, not to attend divine service. For they say as how there is no comfort to be had in the high-Calvinistic exhortations that are thundered from this pulpit—no profit to the soul to hear constantly the hard doctrines of Calvin. God surely cannot be so hard-hearted as they represent him. And to hear too, as I have heard, those discouraging doctrines preached when the heart is broken—at the burial of a beloved parent—detaining for that purpose the grieved relatives on the brink of the grave, that they might hear of nought but the speaking of hell,— oh, that is the hardest of all. However, the archbishop, they say, has put a stop to that at last, and we hope for better things."

Daniel had, by this time, wheeled round his gig to the great entrance-gate, and without any farther loss of time we hastened to the Spa of

THORPE ARCH.

Most of my readers are probably strangers to the existence of such a mineral watering-place. Yet, in its immediate vicinity, and even to a great distance in the neighbourhood, its reputation is considerable. From a most insignificant village, Thorpe Arch has risen into a place of importance, owing to its chalybeate spring, which holds in solution a large quantity of muriate of soda, and has been well described and analyzed by Dr. Hunter of Leeds, who, at two different interviews I had with him, gave me every information respecting it.

The water tastes something like the one at Knaresborough; but I could not detect any sulphur-smell in it, not even so feeble as that of the Starbeck well. I fancy that if there be any present (as the people of the Spa stoutly assert) it must quickly evaporate; and as the water is now pumped out of the spring,—which they have been obliged lately to cover, in order to prevent its further inundations from the rising of the Warfe, to which it was subject,—into a pump-room, built on a rocky bank of the river, at about fifty feet elevation from it—sulphuretted gas can hardly be expected to be present in the water when used for baths. Yet, the opinion on which the water is drunk and used for bathing is, that it is " like Harrogate ;" and so they say of every spring in Yorkshire, that has the slenderest claim to the smell of rotten eggs.

In the case of Thorpe Arch, however, I was determined to put the question at rest, by inducing Mr. West of Leeds, to go down to the Spa, and on the spot test the water for sulphur. His reply, after complying with my suggestion, within the last four months, is conclusive as to the absence of all traces of sulphuretted hydrogen from the Thorpe Arch spring. Besides testing the water with acetate of lead, nitrate of silver, and sulphate of copper, Mr. West subjected a quantity of this water taken immediately from the well, to a severer trial, by boiling it in a flask, the mouth of which was covered with paper moistened with acetate of lead. No change whatever took place.

The situation of the Spa is charming. The lofty bank of the Warfe behind it, whose limestone aspect here assumes the most picturesque shapes—and the rich verdure of the opposite bank, contrasting with the more waved and broken surface of that from the bottom of which the spring issues, are features of perpetual interest, which must work their wholesome effect on the water-drinkers.

" Jutting points of gray or creamy rock," observes Dr. Whitaker, " appear immediately above the right and left of the spring ; and the sides are covered with ash, hazel, and whitebeam to their summits, so as to give the whole the appearance of primeval nature."

The stream of the Warfe darts past with great rapidity; yet both salmon and trout are caught by the Spa-drinkers, after they have quaffed their morning draughts of the chalybeate.

Baths, both warm and cold, and shower-baths, are given in a very humble-looking building, and still humbler bathrooms, which ought to have been better, considering that they are erected as a speculation by a company of shareholders. This facility of having baths recently added to the Spa, has made it much more frequented.

As you drive through the village, which at present consists of a long series of modern and neat-built lodging-houses, many of them extremely elegant, favourably placed and with gardens in front, you are surprised to find them all occupied. Upwards of a hundred such houses have been built within the last twenty-five years.

On turning out of the village to the left, towards the Spa, a beautiful reach of the Warfe is immediately seen above and beyond the Spa-house; just behind which a very lofty square building rises, generally filled with company at the proper season of the year.

Dr. Hunter states, that the Thorpe Arch water is diuretic, and operates mildly, and with considerable certainty. It must be taken in the morning for that purpose, and in large quantities. The disorders of the human constitution successfully treated by it, are said by Dr. Hunter to coincide very nearly with those treated by the Harrogate waters; but Dr. Walker, who wrote many years before, and whose book is carefully preserved in the little waiting-room at the Spa, insists that the Thorpe Arch water is superior to the sulphur-water of Harrogate, in cases of general relaxation, bilious disorders, glandular obstructions, and stomach complaints.

Dr. Hunter upon this observes, that the truth of such remarks, as far as he himself had witnessed or learned from others, appeared unquestionable; and he adds, that the water of Thorpe Arch had acquired considerable reputation also in some complaints of the sex—in headachs and habitual jaundice.

It has already been stated, that numerous as the visiters have of late years been at this Spa, the accommodations provided for them have been ample and very comfortable. Among these I may mention in particular, and from my own knowledge, Farrer's hotel, a very neat, well-looking, and commodious house. Coaches arrive to and depart from it at convenient hours every day, to and from many parts in Yorkshire; and a light omnibus conveys visiters hither from the railway-station at Tadcaster, at the distance of only a mile and a half; whereby, Thorpe Arch is placed in direct and quick communication with York on the one side, and Leeds on the other, and consequently with every important city or town in the north.

Situated near the ancient town of Wetherby, and the immediate neighbourhood of several extensive parks, one of which, Bramham Park, is very well known as a most beautiful domain extending over a space of eleven miles, the situation of Thorpe Arch is, as may be supposed, charming. Nature has been almost lavish of her rural beauties upon this favourite spot, which is considered also one of the healthiest in Yorkshire. The facilities afforded to invalids for taking every species of exercise over excellent roads, or on fine smooth and elevated downs, with many delightful prospects from them or for visiting spots, not far distant, of antiquarian or historical interest, have been an inducement to many among them to make this desired village their home, in which to spend the evening of their days.

As we proceeded nearer to the capital of the county, and left behind us the many enchanting beauties of the West Riding, I could perceive the great, though insensible, change for the worse which became visible in the aspect of the county, in its agricultural condition, and its soil. Lighted by the huge and brilliant gas-lamps of York, hung about in profusion, Daniel at length deposited me at the door of the Old George, in "Pavement," and we parted, excellent friends, after a day's companionship in travelling, and the payment of *one guinea*.

To judge by its central situation, I should have considered this hotel to be one of the best in the place, had I not detected my error afterwards. It certainly fell far short of what I expected in such a city as York. The Black Swan and Winn's Hotel have a better aspect, and are larger; but the constant noise of coaches that traverse, at every hour of the day and night, this central city of England, and pass along Coney-street, render those establishments rather objectionable. Here I had a decent though small bedroom, with an excellent bed, scanty and old furniture against the walls, a single towel, and the foulest-looking water to wash in that I have seen out of London.

In a spacious and old fashioned sitting-room, a breakfast, worthy of the gastronomic reputation of the county, was spread out ready for my use on the following morning. Two large bay-windows stood open before me, as I sat at the table, and showed me the busy stream of people coming down "Pavement." "Saint Crux" was close upon me, so as nearly to shut up one of my windows, and "All Saints" stared me in the face. Indeed churches are as plentiful as houses; and in that respect York may be said to resemble Cologne; a resemblance, by the by, which many of the streets, and contracted thoroughfares, and short cuts to get at the sacred temples, and far-famed Minster, with the bustle on the quays of the Ouse, its steamers and passage-boats, serve to strengthen.

York certainly lacks the mud, or rather the filth of the streets of Cologne ; for here, as in London, the inhabitants prefer drinking that miscellaneous amalgam of all abominations (diluted in their ordinary beverage and culinary solvents) which the Colognists studiously keep away from the water they drink, and reserve for their noses.

York, moreover, boasts of *trottoirs*, albeit they be narrow ; and its atmosphere is not so scented as that of the archiepiscopal see on the Rhine. But *per contra*, York has only water of the dirtiest description that of London excepted, either for drink or cosmetic purposes, to set off against that never-to-be-too-much-lauded compound, the " Eau de Cologne."

York is a city of a hundred gates. There is no end of them. Having passed the outer toll-bar, and come in through Mickle-*gate*, along Lower Ouse-*gate* and High Ouse-*gate*, the stranger has a right to expect that he is fairly *within* the gates of this " second city of the British Empire," as the Eboraceans are pleased to style it. *Pas du tout ;* for as we advance a few steps farther to the right and to the left, or straight forward, we find ourselves out in our reckoning,— for Collier-*gate*, and Foss-*gate*, and Stone-*gate*, and Castle-*gate* and Goodram-*gate*, and Walin-*gate*, and Peter-*gate*, and Davy-*gate*, meet us in, though they bar not, our progress.

A wag, who evidently had not the fear of the archbishop before him, observed, in reference to the two latter gates, that they were properly placed in the vicinity of the great church, to remind us that, according as we stick to *it* or not, Peter's *gate* will be opened unto us, or old Davy's, whenever our allotted time comes, for going to " Davy's Locker."

As we parade through the intricate streets of York, and meet at every corner some relics of olden times, and a church in most of them, with two or even three such in some others (greatly dilapidated or verging on final decay though they be), it is impossible not to feel that we tread on ground rendered classical in the history of England, and that of the Reformation. At the latter epoch there were not fewer than forty-two parish churches, seventeen chapels, eighteen hospitals, three abbeys, two priories, three monasteries, and a religious college. " Of these," says honest Drake, who was any thing but a papist, " there was not so much left in the depredations committed at the Reformation, as to sustain and keep up little more than half the number of parish churches, two or three of the hospitals, and a chapelry or two at most. . . . . " No sooner was the word given, *Sic volo sic jubeo*, but down fell the monasteries, the hospitals, the chapels, and the priories in the city, and with these the eighteen parish churches, the materials, and revenues of all being converted to secular uses." . . . " It is shocking," continues the same writer, " to think how far these depredations were carried ; for, not content with what they could find above ground, they dug open vaults and graves in search for imaginary treasure ; tossed the bones out of stone coffins and made use of them for hog-troughs,—a piece of inhumanity as, I believe, the most savage nation in this world would not have been guilty of."

Contemporary historians are agreed in detailing all these and many more abominations, by means of which the Reformation was carried on in the north of England, and bitterly lament that " our most excellent Church should have its origin deduced, or its restoration take date from, such execrable times." " The Reformation (observes a zealous and learned historian of that era) put a stop to all religion."

And in good truth we find, from the records of those times, that those who had undertaken to reform the dominant religion of the country, were little prepared to supply its place

with another; for it is manifest, judging by the preamble of
an act in the first year of Edward the Sixth, that instead of
a superstitious yet learned religion which they had pulled
down, no other means of religious rites could they substitute,
or supply more than a few churches with service, and those
even by ignorant and worthless persons. " And no person
(so recites the said Act) will take the cure but of necessity, as
some chaunting priests—which for the most part are unlearned and very ignorant persons, not able to do any part
of their duty. By reason whereof the said city (of York) is
not only replete with blind guides and pastors, but also the
people much kept in ignorance, as well of their duties towards
God, as also towards the king's majesty and commonwealth
of this realm, and to the great danger of their souls."

Three centuries have worked wondrous changes in these
matters. Instead of no cure we have too many *cures* in " our
city of York," and for " the unlearned and very ignorant
persons not able to do any part of their duty," we find a clergy,
who like most of their brethren in protestant England, are
remarkable for being the best educated and most erudite servants of God in Christendom—save always a few monks and
recluses and protestant pastors to be met with in many parts
of the continent.

And a noble and a magnificent temple have that clergy to
perform their holy service in ! The present was my first visit
to York cathedral. Need I say that at the view of that colossal pile, lately cleared of all incumbrances from around it
—and standing (though in a contracted space) a pure model
of symmetrical beauty in Gothic structure, particularly in its
unrivalled front, and towers unequalled—I was much and
impressively struck, as must all be who contemplate that far-
famed Minster ?

Its interior excites feelings akin to these impressions ; and
the recollection of the eventful fire which on a particular day
in February, 1829, levelled into a mass of mouldering ruins

the choir of this beautiful temple, and was nigh proving destructive to the whole fabric, mingles now irresistibly in every beholder, and makes him offer up thanks that so wonderful a structure, the work of two centuries, raised by means of *indulgences, bulls,* and *relaxations,* and other of the very abuses which it was the object of the Reformation to abolish, should not only have been spared during the depredations of that revolution, but have escaped, even now, the ravages of an incendiary fire.*

It is a great drawback to the enjoyment of scenes like these if the beholder be gifted with too keen an eye; else I should not have felt fastidiously unhappy, while wrapt up in ecstasy at every thing I saw around me, on observing that the beautiful modern doorway, with its iron gates in the stone screen, (itself a most gorgeous piece of tracery,) is not placed in the centre. It is, on the contrary, considerably nearer to the left; and as the middle of the organ, placed over this doorway, corresponds exactly with the apex of its arch, it follows that neither the door nor the organ is in the centre of the nave,—a defect very striking and singularly obnoxious to those who enter the church through the great western door.

It is curious that the writer of that able work called ".The New Guide," recently published by Hargrave, one of the principal booksellers of York, should not have noticed a deformity so glaring, in a structure otherwise so perfect. Indeed the effect of this want of symmetry is visible in another incongruity resulting from it—namely, that when viewed from the centre of the great western door, the screen shows only four and a portion of a fifth of the statues of the kings placed in the niches of the north side of the entrance

* This was written a few months only before the recent purely acci
dental calamity, from the same destructive element, had rendered the
paragraph almost inapplicable.

whereas, on the south or right side, as many as six are fully seen.

On leaving the cathedral one is tempted to make the tour of its exterior, by the free circulation which has been established all round the edifice, from the Minster-yard to the new deanery; as well as by the showy appearance of the latter building, which was completed about the year 1831, in the Tudor style, by order of the present dean, a gentleman of refined taste, under whose direction, I believe, another house of less pretensions, equally Tudorian, called the New Residence, was erected.

The old monks are said to have taken care invariably to set themselves down in snug and comfortable places. Much to the credit and taste of the present representatives of those by-gone recluses, they also have taken care (in this place at least) to suit themselves with a fine and delightful spot for their residence. Nothing can be more enchanting than the Minster-green, from the centre of which I could survey the various parts of the cathedral around me, the chapter and vestry also, with the library, some remains of gothic arches, the new residence and the deanery, as well as the pleasure-grounds which are interspersed among these various buildings, all breathing the favourite and hallowed spirit of Gothic architecture.

To a medical man, travelling too in search of professional information, York offers one or two attractions which may well be alleged by me as an excuse to my readers for lingering in this city, on my way to another of the Spas I have undertaken to describe. These halts, made for self-instruction' sake, may not turn out altogether unprofitable to my readers; although I have felt throughout my present work, that, in introducing matter somewhat extraneous to its main purport, I not only labour under the great difficulty of endeavouring to offer new matter on home, familiar, and beaten topics, but also incur the imputation of presuming to bring in matter *à-propos de bottes*, into the more legitimate delineation of the objects to which I ought in strictness to confine myself. In this respect, I do not stand on the same vantage-ground I stood upon while writing on the Spas of Germany; for then I was certain of being able to submit to my readers what, to a large majority of them, must have been quite new, and being *foreign*, good *of course*. I trust, nevertheless, that by the plan I have adopted, it will not be altogether impossible to impart to a work on "the Spas of England," sufficient interest to secure the attention of English readers.

The objects which principally attracted my attention in this city, besides those already enumerated, were the New Museum, and the celebrated "Retreat." A friendly intercourse with the two principal physicians, who divide between them the best part of the medical practice in York, and, with Dr. Wake, for many years physician to the York Lunatic Asylum, enabled me to accomplish much in a short time.

I was not equally fortunate in meeting the chairman of the directing committee, Samuel Tuke, the descendant of the philanthropist William Tuke, founder of the "Retreat"—an establishment that has acquired an European renown. But with the ready assistance of Thomas Allis, its able superintendent,—who, with a straightforwardness and candour highly creditable to himself and the institution, laid open every chink and corner of it, during the unexpected visit I paid him,—I was able to make myself master of the condition, management, and prospect of an establishment for the treatment of mental disorders, which is inferior to none in existence, and superior to many having the reputation of being models.

It is not to be denied that much of the gratifying results obtained in the York "Retreat," is due to the singular combination in one individual—the very superintendent I have just named—of every requisite that can constitute excellence

in such an officer.   Friend Allis has, from the earliest period
of his life, been brought in contact with the "afflicted of
craziness," and seen their ways and the effect produced on
them by various sorts of treatment.   His experience on this
point, therefore, at his present mature period of life, must be
unquestionable.   He has undertaken to exercise in his station
functions in which he delights, because of the good they
tend to; and he, therefore, exercises them not reluctantly
as a mere matter of duty, but *con amore*.

No one is fonder of natural sciences than Friend Allis, few
more expert or learned in the practical departments of them.
Hence the hours not devoted to the discharge of his official
duty, are wholly consecrated to preparing, classing, and describing objects of natural history; and this very disposition of his
mind has he turned to account in forwarding the intention
of the institution; inasmuch as he sometimes brings to the
consideration of those attractive and interesting works of
nature, the intellect of the afflicted under his *surveillance*,
so soon as he perceives that mighty engine struggling to
recover from its fall.   He at the same time, by pursuits like
these, of so tranquil and contemplative a nature, renders more
intense his already strong sense of " adhesiveness " to the
field of his operations.   Lastly, nature has endowed him with
an imposing figure, tall and of a robust make, the very aspect
of which has often been found to command, even without the
utterance of a syllable, respect and obedience in refractory or
irritable patients.   And yet no superintendent of a lunatic
asylum possesses more conciliatory manners, or a milder tone
of voice.

In going round every part of the establishment with him—
in listening to his conversation with the patients of both sexes
and of all ranks—in witnessing the manner in which they all
addressed him, looked at him, or smiled kindly as he passed
—in reflecting on the many illustrations of his peculiar views
with which he supplied me as we went along, and on the

replies I obtained from him to the various inquiries my visit suggested,—I could easily perceive that Friend Allis was the very man William Tuke needed, to carry into effect his own judicious and philanthropic views on the management and cure of lunatic patients.

The " Retreat " was one of the first establishments for the treatment of insanity founded in England, on the principle of employing more humane and wiser measures than those heretofore resorted to in the management of the unfortunate beings afflicted with that disease. It has now been in operation forty-four years, and the statistical details connected with it, open to the inspection of every visiter, are full of interest. Its original destination was for patients belonging to the Society of Friends; but that destination has been enlarged, and other patients are equally admitted. At the time of my visit there were nine among the whole number who were unconnected with that Society.

The several buildings forming the establishment, which presents, from the summit of the hill, about two miles distant from York, an attractive front, have very recently been enlarged, and rendered infinitely more comfortable for the hundred patients they are intended to accommodate. A considerable sum of money has also been laid out for the purchase of excellent land, twenty-seven acres of which now surround the building. These two expensive improvements have enabled the committee to provide for the better classification of the patients, as well as to increase their accommodations.

The latter are of the very best description, especially in the apartments of both the male and female patients of the better class, who pay the highest weekly charge for their maintenance. I could not desire for the most beloved friend deprived of his nobler faculties a better asylum or a superior treatment. There is nothing grand, nothing ostentatious, but every thing for use and for comfort ; and matters appeared to me to be managed with so much effect, and so little fuss, that I could hardly have imagined myself in a lunatic asylum from aught I beheld around me ; but that " the vacant eye, the stare, the unmeaning grin" told their own story quite plainly. The Society of Friends need well be proud of having been the originators and of being the warm supporters of such an establishment. As much as this, or to that effect, I inscribed with pleasure in its album, on taking leave of the " Retreat" and of Friend Allis.

Dr. Wake was my next conductor through an establishment of a similar nature to the " Retreat," but of a more general and public description. The report of its committee for the year ending June, 1839, gives a satisfactory view of the general state of the York Lunatic Asylum ; and from what I saw in the course of my visit, as well as from the information readily communicated to me by Dr. Wake, at the time, I should conclude that the asylum has made many steps in advance, and is likely to improve farther. As yet the system of coercion is in existence at this County Asylum. We shall see, elsewhere, that one of the next and greatest improvements in its management will be to abandon that system.

I have already made honourable mention of Dr. Belcombe. As I knew that he was well connected with Scarborough, through his late father, and his present brother-in-law, the much-respected vicar of that place, I gladly availed myself of his kind invitation to dine and spend one evening with him, during which I derived much profitable information on points of my immediate and intended inquiries.

The doctor is a true man of the world, with that sort of open and affable manner which is calculated to win the confidence of his patients. I found him conversant with every novel or important fact, of the most recent date, in his profession, and stored with much general information—the result of extensive reading.

From all that I learned in my conversation with Dr. Belcombe, I was induced to prolong my stay in York for one

additional day, in order to visit the Museum; and I have reason
to rejoice at the delay, as it procured me also the advantage
of an interview with another able colleague, Dr. Simpson, to
whom I have already alluded, and who gave me many interesting details of a Spa (Hovingham) of which I had never
even so much as heard the name mentioned; but which I
determined upon visiting in consequence.

Dr. Simpson, like his colleague, lives in the vicinity of the
cathedral, and occupies, though a bachelor, a large and
palacelike-looking house in Grey's-court, which was originally
made a freehold by Henry the Eighth, who took possession of
it in person, at the Reformation, and sequestration of church
property. Charles, also, once held his court where Dr.
Simpson now sees his patients. The presence of two such
physicians in York is a fortunate circumstance for the inhabitants.

It was a happy idea of the architect of the new Museum
in this city, standing in an enclosure of about three acres of
land, surrounded by about six more of other pleasure-ground,
to set up in beautiful contrast with the lovely remains of St.
Mary's Abbey (one of the many gems of Gothic and sacred
structures in England) a Grecian Doric Temple, appropriated
solely to the scientific and learned objects of the " York
Philosophical Society."

The venerable ruins just mentioned occupy the north-west
side of the enclosure. The Roman multangular tower
separates it from the city to the east. On an eminence in the
centre stands the Museum, with its noble front of a hundred
and two feet in length, designed by Wilkins, looking down
upon the river and the extensive landscape beyond it.

The entrance to the grounds from the city is by a Doric
gate. On either side of the wide path which leads thence to
the Museum, the ground is appropriated to a botanic garden;
the remainder of the enclosure is laid out and planted, so as
to produce a picturesque effect, as well as with particular

reference to the favourable display of the exquisite remains of antiquity which adorn, and consecrate, as it were, the ground.

The front of the Museum is decorated with a central portico of four columns, 3 feet 6 inches in diameter, and 21 feet 6 inches high, extending 35 feet, and projecting 10, with bold steps all round. The space on each side of the portico, which is terminated by a pilaster, has three windows, ornamented with suitable architraves. A bold and massive pediment rests upon the columns, and the entablature is continued the whole length of the front, and returns round the ends of the building, which is of Hackness stone, and about 24 feet deep.

Within it, besides a theatre for lectures, a small library, and a committee room, we find a museum of antiquities and natural history, divided into several apartments, with a collection of Saxon, Roman, and Gothic sculpture and architecture in the underground floor. Scattered on this, many exquisite specimens of knots and groins, which had formed part of St. Mary's Abbey, are to be seen as they were brought to light by recent excavations; and well would it have harmonized with certain beautiful remains of former times, still left in the Minster, had the architect, while engaged in restoring that class of ornaments in that part of the cathedral which the fire of 1829 had destroyed, directed these beautiful specimens of St. Mary's to be taken as models, instead of carving those now *in situ*, exhibiting a meager invention, or rather a sameness not to be found in any of the Gothic cathedrals in this country.

It will be sufficient to name John Phillips, as the curator of the Museum, to be quite certain that its geological portion (and in that respect the collection is very valuable) is scientifically and skilfully arranged, agreeably to his own geological map of England, and the nomenclature he has adopted. The curator at the time of my visit was engaged in restoring a neat Gothic building, placed immediately beyond the ruins of St. Mary, which he was to hold on that condition of the proprietor of the Museum, and which would become his private dwelling.

I heard of another threatened restoration of ancient remains in these grounds, which it is to be hoped may never be carried into effect; although a few individuals who are favourable to that restoration have already subscribed the sum of five hundred pounds towards it. The building to be restored is a miserable-looking barn, to which some middle-age recollections are attached, and upon its being restored, the said barn will be converted into a ball-room. The connexion between a restoration of an old hut and the establishment of a public ball-room, is not, methinks, very manifest.

But I must close my note-book, or I shall never reach my next destination, Scarborough, whither I proceeded by the Scarborough mail, a conveyance which leaves York every day early in the morning, immediately upon the arrival of the mail from London.

I should have halted in my way at New Malton, where a kind and pressing invitation from Dr. Travers, the principal physician resident in that large market-town, would have secured me a hearty welcome. Besides the temptation of making the personal acquaintance of a young and intelligent physician, active in the pursuit of science, which might have induced me to stop, there was also that of examining a mineral spring, formerly much in vogue, and well known as "the New Malton Spa." But the importance of any immediate inquiry by myself into its character and properties not being very manifest, I passed through Malton without stopping, and rely entirely on Dr. Travers's report, which I here transcribe.

" The saline-chalybeate spring at this place was celebrated nearly two centuries ago. Attention was first directed to it by Mr. Simpson's 'Treatise on the Malton Spa' in 1669, and afterwards by the general work on mineral waters in 1734, by Dr. Short, of Sheffield.

" The present handsome pagoda over the well was erected by the late Earl Fitzwilliam, about five-and-twenty years ago, and stands prettily in the gardens adjoining the hotel.

" The water flows in a very copious stream, is quite clear as it issues from its source, but on standing a little time, leaves a ferruginous deposit. Its specific gravity is very little greater than that of distilled water, and its temperature is not affected by the season of the year. It has a strong saline-chalybeate, but not unpleasant taste, and possesses considerable purging and diuretic qualities.

" There has been no very recent analysis. An imperial gallon of the water yields three drachms and forty-five grains of residuum, consisting of sulphate of magnesia, sulphate of lime, common salt, and a portion of protoxide of iron.

" The water has been found highly efficacious in many chronic diseases; particularly affections of the liver, indigestion under its various forms, and general languor of the system. It is taken in doses of from one to four half pints, at short intervals; the early morning being considered the most favourable time for that purpose.

"This Spa, however, has ceased to be a resort to persons from a distance; which is rather a matter of surprise when (apart from the valuable properties of the well) we take into account the very superior and extensive accommodation at the hotel, and the attractive character of the surrounding country.

" The district abounds in picturesque rides and drives, and is one of no ordinary interest to the botanist, the practical farmer, and the geologist. The hill above the well-house is of the oolite formation."

CHAPTER XII.

"The QUEEN" of Sea-bathing Places—First Impressions on seeing Scarborough—Substantial Breakfasts—Prominent Features of Scarborough—Natural Phenomena—Geological Attractions—FLAMBOROUGH Head—Filey Bay—Robin Hood Bay—Striking Improvements—Mr. Dunn, the principal Surgeon—Other Medical Practitioners—THE NEW SPA—View from the " Cliff"—The CLIFF BRIDGE and Menay Bridge—Scarborough Races and the Roman Arena—Paths leading to the Spa—The New Building—Sea Wall—The Terrace—The Promenade, or Saloon—Gothic Architecture on a Sea-shore—Mr. WYATT and a gallant M.P.—Lively interest taken by the latter in the welfare of Scarborough—The Two SPRINGS—Taste, Appearance, and Quantity of the Water from each—Former Analysis—A new one necessary—Performed successfully by Professor R. Phillips.

I AM enchanted with Scarborough. And who would not be who has sojourned but a single day at this " Queen" of English sea-bathing places, at the close of the summer months, or in the early days of a bright autumn ? To me Scarborough was a surprise, to the full extent of the word. I was not prepared to find a bay of Naples on the north-east coast of England; nor so picturesque a place perched on lofty cliffs, reminding an old and experienced traveller of some of those romantic sea views which he beheld abroad, particularly in Adriatic and Grecian seas.

" And can the people of this county," I involuntarily asked to myself, after only a few hours' residence in Scarborough, on the day of my arrival, which was a glowing and a brilliant one—" can they, if money and time can bring them to such a sea-berth as this, voluntarily prefer to it their Margate, their Brighton, and their Hastings? O for more taste, and better judgment!"

Scarborough, an hundred years ago, was what the last-mentioned places have become since. Then the Earls, the Marquesses, and the Dukes were as thick at that Spa as berries are on hedges. This I collect from a list of visiters for the season of 1733, referred to in a curious book, bearing the title of " A Journey from London to Scarborough," in a series of letters from the author to his friends.

To be sure, travelling with hired horses was not quite so expensive then as now, and " a trip to Scarborough " was an easy journey, which one could perform with four horses at a shilling a mile; albeit days were employed in it, where hours would now suffice! Inns, indeed, were but passing indifferent at that time, and lodging-houses worse still; a circumstance which the waggish author in question considered as a great convenience, inasmuch as " it made people rise early." Notwithstanding this, Scarborough was then what Brighton has since been during its palmy days of Royal countenance. And what, I ask, has made Scarborough less than Brighton? Can the reader solve that problem?

I know not whether to attribute the feeling I experienced on my first arrival at Scarborough to the exciting nature of the air into which I found myself suddenly plunged, when the mail pulled up at that most intricate turn in front of " the Bell "—or to the sight of the glorious ocean—or to the appearance of sundry eatables spread on the well-decked table of that inn. But to whichever of these causes it may be owing, that feeling was one of inward contentment, accompanied by a buoyancy of spirits such as I had not lately enjoyed.

Unquestionably, the being admitted to the privilege of

sitting down at once with three or four merry persons, and a lady or two to boot, at a table where I was presently helped with all the good things of this world, after an early morning drive of three or four hours, with " an unfreighted stomach," was likely to put in good humour even the crossest-tempered fellow alive; and, perhaps, that had its influence in the present instance. Bread good, and good looking; excellent tea, tea-cakes, muffins, and new-laid eggs, would satisfy any reasonable bachelor at a London club-house. But what if he found within his reach at the same table a *piéce de resistance* of cold beef, and raised pies, and shrimps, and potted and marinaded fish of many kinds, to satisfy wherewith either his hunger or his whim !

And yet such things, and such a breakfast, are to be found at Scarborough, not only at the Bell Inn, but at many other hotels; and they constitute one only of the four daily repasts which honest and civil Master Webb (and I heard that other landlords do the same) gives you at nine, twelve, four, and eight o'clock p.m., at his ordinary on Bland's Cliff, for the sum of six shillings per diem, including lodging !

These *substantial* breakfasts, by the by, seem to be the order of the day at all the English Spas. At the Crown at Harrogate, I noticed a similar practice; but there, instead of sitting all round the same table, its company is divided into groups, or solitary individuals, sipping their bohea at their own separate little tables, and calling as they require them for all the side-board et ceteras, which an obsequious waiter is ready to hand over to them.

This arrangement has its advantages; but it also proves a most effectual damper to all sociability at a Spa. Breakfast is a repast they hardly know how to enjoy at the Spas in Germany. In England, on the other hand, the thing is overdone, and the rules of diet, for such as have just quaffed four or six tumblers of mineral water, are set at defiance. The mingling together of tea and coffee, eggs and ham, mustard and cream, chicken and veal, with two half-pint tumblers of the " stinking water," at the Montpellier at Harrogate, or indeed of any mineral water, whether there, here, or elsewhere, at Cheltenham or Leamington, is a practice I have witnessed at all those places. How, then, is mineral water to produce its *salutary* effect ?

Scarborough is, perhaps, one of the most interesting marine Spas in England. It combines the advantages of mineral springs with those of a convenient and luxurious sea-bathing shore. It is surrounded on the land side by numerous objects of attraction, to which either roads or footpaths, over moors and dales, like radii from a centre, offer a ready access to the visiters. Some of those objects, indeed, have acquired well-merited reputation.

In modern architecture, enriched and heightened by extensive gardens, plantations, and arcadian groves, there is Castle Howard, which the visiter will perceive on the right of the high road, immediately beyond Malton.

In ancient structure Rivaulx Abbey, which is supposed to have been the first Cistercian monastery founded in Yorkshire, presents ruins of considerable extent, more perfect than those of most of the same class of monastic buildings in the county, Fountain Abbey excepted.

In natural phenomena we have the strongly marked geological formation of the coast, right and left of Scarborough, with its cavern and promontories—its clefts, its dislocations, and its elevation—all sufficiently denuded to exhibit a very museum to the lover of geology. From Robin Hood's Bay northward, to the Flamborough Head southward, a distance of thirty-three miles of coast, every inch of the land which may be inspected at low water, over a course of the finest sands in England, is pregnant with interest.

Indeed, Flamborough Head of itself would be a sufficient

feature to stamp any sea-bathing place with importance and attraction. Its lofty cliffs of nearly five hundred feet elevation, of the purest limestone, remind one of the " White Cliffs of Albion," at Dover. But here the circumstances of the cliffs teeming, during the spring and summer months, with thousands of birds of every species and plumage; and, above all, the stupendous caverns that penetrate into the very bowels of the cliff shore, particularly that which is called " Robin Lyth Hole;" invest this mighty promontory—one of the many frontal guardians of the Seagirt Island—with indescribable interest.

The deposit of fossil plants in the shale and sandstone of the oolitic series at Gristhorp Bay, five miles south, and also at Haiburn Wyke, seven miles north of Scarborough, must also prove very interesting to the geologist, as well as to the botanist, as it offers specimens of the ferns and lycopodium orders in greater variety and preservation than any other known locality can offer. Many of them closely approach to existing species, and not a few of them are most distinct in fructification. Occasionally, as in the *solenites,* named after Dr. Murray of Scarborough (the gentleman to whom I am indebted for the present geological memorandum), the process of fossilization has been so imperfect, that the plants retain elasticity and combustibility, and even traces can be found in them of the vegetable principles of tannin and resin. These fossil ferns of Gristhorp, being usually of a perfectly black colour, displayed upon a gray ground, resemble drawings in India ink, and are, consequently, more precious than those of the coal formation, which merely present black upon black.

But, independently of these geological attractions, the lover of romantic landscape will be highly gratified with the wild and beautiful scenery of Gristhorp Bay, perhaps the most striking and pleasing of the numerous little bays which indent the rocky coast from Scarborough to Filey.

And what a lovely and curiously seated fishing village this very Filey is, with its beautiful and ample bay, displaying at low water the finest sands on this coast, to the extent of nearly three miles! Even here a mineral spring is found, and there is one also at Bridlington, four miles south of Flamborough, besides a good sea-bathing place at Bridlington Quay, of late years much frequented. Both springs are chalybeates.

Similar in general character, but infinitely more romantic in appearance, is another bay, a little more distant from Scarborough than Filey is, but in an opposite direction, namely, northward. The freebooter Robin Hood, who seems to have sought refuge in every romantic spot in the north, has stamped this bay with his own name.

Far more interesting than the association excited by such ballad heroes is the contemplation at Whitby, six miles farther off, of the venerable ruins of its once renowned abbey, and of a rich collection of fossil remains, including probably the most splendid specimens of ichtyolites in the world.

Such are a few of the many attractions near and around Scarborough, towards which a visiter would naturally hasten soon after his arrival; and which, therefore, I have at once enumerated to my readers, without attempting any elaborate description of them ; a description, indeed, rendered unnecessary by the existence of the able and learned works of Phillips, Young, Smith, and others, to which I must refer my readers for more extended information.

Of another publication I must not omit to make honourable mention also, which will prove to the visiter at Scarborough a fund of amusement and instruction, namely, "The History and Antiquities of Scarborough," by Thomas Hindewell, who was bred to the sea, and all his life a sailor. The first edition of this work appeared in 1798, and a revised one with a memoir of the author, a native of Scarborough, in 1837.

To such as love to scan doggrel verses, and laugh over a

few caricature sketches by an " H. B." of Scarborough, the work published by Green and Rowlandson, in 1812, will be a source of fun and amusement. Glorious days those of 1812 must have been for Scarborough! *Revien-dront-ils?* I think so.

Every thing has been done, and is doing, to verify my prediction. It will not be the fault of those more immediately connected with the place, neither will it be from any lack of zeal and love of truth on my part, if the prophecy be not in a short time fulfilled. We will now proceed to examine in what that " every thing" consists.

The reader (generally attracted by the illustrations of a book) ere he peruses this chapter will have glanced at the cuts, in which three of the most striking objects at Scarborough are faithfully represented. Two of them are connected with recent improvements; indeed of these one, "The Spa," is but just completed in all its parts. To it I proceeded in company with Mr. Dunn, the highly and justly popular surgeon at Scarborough. This gentleman, to the qualifications of a first-rate surgeon, ready and able to undertake any thing that a hospital surgeon in London would venture to undertake for the relief of suffering humanity, joins the rarer attribute of being a sincere friend to science, especially geology, with the practical part of which he is quite conversant.

Aware of the object of my visit, and prepared for the manner in which I was likely to conduct my inquiry into Scarborough, and Scarborough Spa, Mr. Dunn took every pains imaginable to facilitate my object, and render it complete, and with equal readiness and candour supplied me with all the particulars I desired.

It is evident that industry alone, or even the best experience in the conducting of such investigations as I had undertaken, would not have enabled me to obtain all that information which I deemed requisite in matters of this kind.

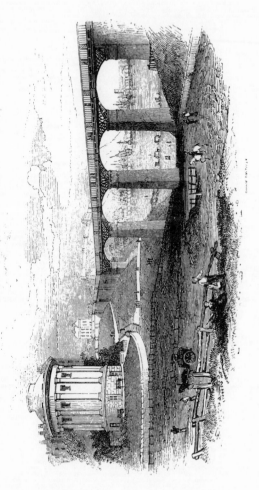

SCARBOROUGH CLIFF BRIDGE, AND MUSEUM.

How, for example, could I have learned aught respecting many points of my inquiry,—such as, for instance, the climate and salubriousness of Scarborough—its ordinary or average temperature, and its barometrical variations,—except through the verbal communications of some intelligent and old inhabitant, or from an erudite medical man?

I gladly, therefore, availed myself of the kind assistance afforded me, not only by the active medical person just named, but by his associate also, Mr. Travis, and likewise by Dr. Murray, whom I have twice already introduced to my readers, and who enjoys now at Scarborough the fruit of his former professional exertions.

" What structure is that," inquired I of my kind conductor, " which, like a turreted castle, is strongly seated on a sea wall nigh the shore, at the foot of that high bank covered with green, beneath Olive Mount—for such I heard you call that lofty hill on our right, bearing all the features of an oolitic formation?"

" That is our NEW SPA," replied my guide; " within that striking edifice, which has sprung up in the last few months, to serve as a new landmark to the mariner approaching our coast, are placed the two mineral springs, of which, doubtless, you have read, as being celebrated in the olden days for their healing qualities. They were formerly very insufficiently protected by a mean-looking building, from the inroads of the sea. Now the art of Wyatt, directed by the taste of one of our worthy representatives in parliament, has secured those valuable springs to the invalid, while it has also afforded the latter an accommodation of a superior class during the hours of drinking the water, which they enjoyed not before. They have now a saloon of good proportions to assemble and walk in, with other smaller rooms and contrivances, such as are found at some of the Spas in Germany, so familiar to you. We look for your approbation of our waters, when you shall have examined them; and of the building likewise, which has added unquestionably a striking feature to our landscape. The idea was happily conceived, as we trust it has been executed, though not without difficulty, owing to the great proximity of the sea to the springs, which had washed away a former edifice."

We were standing in the centre of a circular platform with its convex brow (formerly the projecting ledge of what is emphatically called "the cliff") turned to, and connected with the magnificent bridge, of which I have introduced a correct view in the present volume, and which bears from its connexion the name of "Cliff Bridge." Its existence dates only from 1827, and is due to private subscriptions, amounting to 9,000*l*.

The view which offered itself to us from this favourite spot with the visiters to Scarborough, is, perhaps, the one best calculated to produce in the beholder that impression of amazement which I experienced on my first arrival. At our feet the wide strand encircled the margin of the ocean, the more distant expanse of which, lost to view on the left hand, seemed bounded on the right by a succession of beautiful bays and concave shores, which extend between Scarborough and Filey to the utmost verge of the horizon. Nearer to us the shore, bold in some parts, and almost *a-pic*, looked gracefully green, rounded, or tabular in proportion as it retreated from the water in a series of oolitic cliffs backed by Oliver Mount, loftiest of the range, and 490 feet high.

Between this spot, and another nearly equally high ground opposite, beyond which stand the two springs just alluded to, a chasm four hundred feet wide yawns with a depth of nearly eighty feet, which in former days must have rendered all communication between the town and the Spa difficult, and even painful to invalids. Across this chasm a bridge has been thrown, resting upon light iron arches, and supported by three square stone insulated piers seventy feet high, besides the two end piers or bridge walls that connect the structure

with the two opposite cliffs. The floor of the bridge, which
is fourteen feet wide, is formed of transverse planks, and a
lofty, open, iron railing serves as a protecting parapet along
each of its sides.

A moderate toll of half-a-crown a month is charged for
each person desirous of enjoying the convenience of this
bridge. As I paced cautiously at first this airy structure, I
could hardly look down to the far-removed strand below,
through the slender plank pavement, perforated with apertures
for the escape of rain water, without a recoil of the blood,
a dizziness, and a feeling of horror. Yet a bold charioteer
with four well-trained steeds in hand, undertook, at the
opening of the bridge in July 1827, to drive a coach over it
amidst the acclamations of the myriads who covered the
adjoining buildings and surrounding hills, which, on that
eventful day for Scarborough, were swarming with human
faces, all eagerly intent on that single object.

The looking down upon the road below, which, descending
rapidly in a slightly curved line from a neighbouring hill,
sweeps between the two centre piers, and goes to join the
strand, reminded me of a somewhat analogous position I had
trod in some years before when crossing that magnificent and
imposing structure the Menai Bridge. There, vessels in full
sail glide under the suspended arches, and look like coasting
boats on a deep blue lake. Here vehicles of all sorts, and
animals, and people, rendered dwarfish by the depths at
which they are seen, wind their way to and from the sea-
shore.

On the broad sands of that very shore the Scarborough
races are held, and what, at one hour, was the estuary of
living waters, murmuring in successive bow-like waves towards
the foot of the cliffs, becomes in the next hour, upon that
occasion, the course-ground and the theatre of the equestrian
as well as pedestrian display of man's skill and animal agility :
thus reversing the destination of the Roman arena, which,

after the course of the quadrigæ and the fights of the gladiators, was presently inundated to afford scope for the representation of mimic naumachia or sea-fights.

The view of the horse-races from a place suspended almost in the air, at such an immense height over them as this, is enjoyed perhaps uniquely in this country, by the people of Scarborough and the visiters at the Spa, from the CLIFF BRIDGE,—which may indeed be said to be, on such an occasions, the grandest *stand* of any race-ground in the world.

Beyond the straight line of the bridge a wide path has been made along the brow of the cliff, leading now in a straight and now in a zig-zag direction to the building of the new Spa already mentioned, and which, at my visit, was just completed in every respect, except as to its interior decoration. The whole structure will cost from nine to ten thousand pounds; defrayed by subscription.

Mr. Leslie, the engineer, first raised a species of sea-wall, or break-water, at low-water mark, and built it up to above high-water mark, with baulder stones, in appearance strong and gigantic, and resembling a mighty bastion. How far such a defence will resist the repeated shocks of the thundering waves from the German Ocean, by which it is almost daily assailed, or the wearing action of high-tide, and the dilapidating effect of the south-eastern gales, which blow directly over the coast, it is not for me to decide : its stability is not doubted, else the great terrace spread on the top of it, on which is seated the whole range of the new Spa buildings, would not have been so placed.

At one end of that terrace the springs of mineral waters, two in number, are to be found, to which you descend by a few steps, much in the way that the visiters at Kissingen descend to drink the Ragozi. Adjoining is the saloon already alluded to, or promenade-room, suitable, from its length, for walking in rainy weather. It is lighted by several windows facing the sea. From the small casements of the upper portion of the turrets, as well as from the flat roof of the building, the visiter has an opportunity of enjoying a variety of views of the sea and coast.

The style of architecture adopted in this edifice, as will be observed in the plate, is the Castellated Gothic, with embattled walls and towers, from one of which a smaller turret rises to bear the standard of Scarborough. The stone used in the building is of a brown, ochry colour.

Mr. Wyatt imagines that this is the only style of architecture suited to English scenery, and to the broken and wild slopes of the shore; although, by the by, the cliff which rises immediately behind and above the new Spa, to the height of one hundred and fifty feet, consists of alluvial rubble, loose, and without any compact adhesiveness,—and not of wild and broken features.

Originally that cliff was almost perpendicular, and upon the slightest interference with it, or after heavy rains, threw down destructive avalanches. It was consequently cut down, and made to decline with a gentle acclivity, from the terrace of the new Spa upwards. But this remedy has not yet been applied to all the parts of the cliff which overhang the new buildings of the Spa. Nor has the newly-created surface of the slopes been planted with shrubs, so as to give it a pleasing and soft aspect, instead of its present unsightly and rubbish-like appearance.

The gravel walks also are sloppy in wet weather, and too loose and unconnected on their surface in exceedingly dry weather. The fact is, that the new-made soil is not sufficiently compact and adhesive, and requires, as I ventured to suggest, the application of a thick layer of chalk under the gravel bed, to render the surface perfect. This is no trifling consideration for the visiters at Scarborough, who have to walk once if not twice a day in all weathers, to and from the new Spa, for the purpose of drinking the waters, and who, even at other hours of the day, are disposed to make use of their privilege of meandering along the various paths on this cliff, which, when more thickly planted, will be a great resource to the invalids.

The author of that magnificent idea of an architectural embankment of the Thames,—which will always be considered as the origin of whatever improvement may hereafter take place on the banks of that filthiest of all the metropolitan rivers in Europe, whether it be after Rennie's, Martin's, or Walker's plan,—suggested and watched over (so I understand) most of these recent improvements at Scarborough ; indeed the designs for the building of the New Spa were supplied by him. The gallant member for Scarborough, accustomed, from living in one of the prettiest places of his own in Ireland, to the contemplation and enjoyment of what is beautiful,—conversant, moreover, from travels, and the society of the skilled in fine arts, with whatever constitutes genuine taste,—was likely to suggest nothing which the most fastidious could not approve. We may conclude, therefore, that by adopting his ideas, and following the impetus he has given to those measures which are to resuscitate from its long lethargy one of the Spas best favoured by nature in England,—Scarborough will secure to itself a full share of popularity and success.

In a small, sunken court of the castellated building, paved with flagstones and surrounded by stone walls, are the lion-mouthed spouts, placed at some little distance from each other, from which the mineral water is continually pouring,— the excess passing away through a small stone basin, and by discharge-pipes, down to the strand below. From their respective positions these two springs have received the names of North and South Wells or Spas.

I tried the waters of both several times. That of the south well is colourless, and very limpid ; two qualities which it shares in common with the north well. The former does not taste like a saline water, though it is supposed to hold more ingredients of a purgative nature than the other, and has, in consequence, been called hitherto the saline or salt well, in contradistinction from the north spring, which has always been considered as a purely chalybeate water; yet the taste of iron is not much more marked in the one than in the other spring. In the south well that particular taste is not elicited until after drinking two or three glasses of the water. In the north well the same taste may be said to be more immediate, though it approaches more to what would be called *goût apre* than to the *goût* of rust of iron.

The flow of water is different in the two wells. That in the south spring is at the rate of half-a-pint in twenty seconds; whereas, in the north spring the same quantity of water is obtained in seven seconds. I repeated the experiments often with Mr. Dunn's assistance. The north well, therefore, supplies seven hundred and sixty-five gallons of water in twenty-four hours.

Most of my readers are probably aware that for a long succession of years, Scarborough mineral water enjoyed universal reputation in England. That reputation diminished in proportion as fashion brought other mineral springs into notice, and attracted the higher classes of visiters, who formerly used to flock to Scarborough. That the efficacy of its mineral waters depended on something substantial in them, and not on capricious imagination, no one can doubt who is at all conversant with the medical history of the place. But even the well-tested effect of such waters will not prove sufficient to fix permanently the opinion and favour of the public in their behalf, if medical men of influence and character, practising on the spot, publish, from time to time, an account or analysis of their component parts, each of which differs from that of its predecessor.

That such has been the case with regard to the very mineral waters we are now considering, I collect from a statement made by Mr. Dunn at a public meeting held last summer at

Scarborough, in which I find it laid down that of five successive analyses which had appeared in the course of perhaps
two-thirds of a century, there was not one that did not differ
from the rest in every essential particular. They all disagreed,
for example, as to the total weight of saline matter in a given
measure. They disagreed in the quantity of iron present,
and still more so in that of carbonic acid gas. Some too
admitted ingredients as present in the waters, which others
had not even mentioned. Thus insensibly was the confidence of the public shaken in the real composition of the
waters, and by a natural consequence, the confidence also in
their medical virtues.

In this state I found the knowledge respecting the composition of the Scarborough water at my visit to that Spa,
and the personal observations I had occasion to make at that
time, though merely cursory, served only to add to my former
state of doubt, as to the real chemical nature of the two
springs. Accustomed as I have been for some years to examine mineral waters with a professional eye, I was not long
in perceiving that in one or two points the analyses hitherto
published could not be correct. I saw no trace of free carbonic acid ; I could not distinguish any greater quantity
of iron in the well emphatically called the Chalybeate, than
in the one called the Salt, or Saline Well; and as regards
the latter, the great difference stated to exist between its
proportion of common salt, and that of the same salt in
the chalybeate spring, I could hardly detect.

The probable origin, as well as composition, of the water
of these two springs may be anticipated from a study of the
nature of the geological formation of the cliffs from which
they surge. According to J. Philipps, that formation exhibits calcareous, and iron stone* strata, with their long,

* Iron nodules and stone are to be seen even on the strand, and I
understand are carried away in boats, and sold by the Corporation to
people from Newcastle.

straight and intersecting fissures, often lined with double lamina of oxyde of iron, between which, sometimes, there occurs a white, compact, soft, smooth substance, said by the Rev. W. V. Vernon to be a compound of alumina, silica, and perhaps magnesia.

We should, therefore, expect to find in the Spa water— Carbonate and sulphate of lime, Alumina, Magnesia, Silica, Oxyde of iron ; and, probably, the alkaline muriates.

But a fresh analysis of both waters ought to be made by a professed chemist, a man of undoubted eminence, whose name and well-known experience in the difficult art of properly analyzing mineral waters shall stamp ever after the analysis of the Scarborough wells, to be given to the world, with an authority and authenticity never to be questioned.

All this I took the liberty to represent to my intelligent cicerone, adding that, "Although I respected, and indeed applauded, every preceding effort made by the several individuals who had published an analysis of their own of these waters; yet the discrepances that existed among them called for a fresh investigation. Perhaps for medical purposes, the approximating analysis of the probable ingredients at present received may be deemed sufficient, especially when we add the taste, temperature, specific gravity, and physical impression made by the water on the organs of digestion. Still a precise knowledge of the real composition of the waters was in my opinion a desideratum, which it was unquestionably to the interest of the leading inhabitants of Scarborough to procure. I for one would not undertake to speak positively of the nature and efficacy of those waters without possessing such an analysis.

To the credit of all those concerned in the affair, it is gratifying to have to record that the suggestion was soon after my departure taken into consideration at a general meeting; when it was resolved to apply in turn to the several eminent chemists, whose names I had supplied, for the purpose of securing the services of one of them on the occasion. The choice fell on professor Richard Phillips, who has produced, with his accustomed ability and philosophical precision, a report of his chemical inquiry into the composition of the Scarborough waters, which has stamped them at once with a sufficient degree of value to warrant my previous recommendation of them; a recommendation which, having been made publicly known soon after I left the place, occasioned in the course of that very season the demand for the water to be threefold what it had been.

Professor Phillips's report has very properly been printed, by order of the Cliff Bridge Company, and a copy of it sent to every subscriber. The analysis it contains of the north and south well I have, as usual, placed in my general tables. In this place it will be sufficient simply to mention, that the result of Mr. Phillips's analysis affords a practical verification of those chemical characters of the water which I had deduced from geological data, and upon the strength of which, as well as upon the effect of the waters upon myself and others, I ventured to speak in commendation of their use.

CHAPTER XIII.

SCARBOROUGH CONTINUED.

MEDICINAL Virtues of the Scarborough Springs—Quick Remedy for Heartburn—How to cure a Fermenting Digestion—SCARBOROUGH after Harrogate—Principal Complaints cured by the Mineral Waters of the Former—Effect of the work, "The Spas of Germany," on English Practice—SCEPTICISM quickly changed into Faith—Self-interest works Miracles on Doctors—Indiscriminate and injurious recommendation of Foreign Baths—THE RESULT—Lamentable Cases—Author's Practice and Method—Opinion of able Medical Men respecting it—A Dishonest Reviewer—A VIEW of Scarborough.

THE mere consideration of the ingredients now distinctly ascertained to enter into the composition of the two mineral springs at Scarborough, suffices to explain, and accounts for the several cures said to have been effected by them during many years past, and points out at the same time to the experienced physician the particular complaints in which the waters in question may be successfully employed.

Supposing a visiter to be directed to drink a half-pint tumbler of the water of the South well, he will then take into the system about half a drachm of soluble salts, principally of the alterative and laxative kind, which is a very agreeable and fit dose for daily use. Combined with this he takes also a little more than the tenth part of a grain of a preparation of iron, different from those we are in the habit of prescribing, namely, iron in the first degree of oxydation, combined with double the usual quantity of carbonic acid found in the ordinary medicinal preparations of that metal.

The latter circumstance is of immense importance, as it renders steel admissible in many complaints of the stomach, even when accompanied by morbid irritability, in which the more usual preparations of steel—such, for example, as those generally prescribed by a very popular physician at another of the English Spas—would prove injurious.

Of this fact, which I originally assumed from mere inference when I tasted the water at the spring, long before Phillips's analysis had been instituted, I felt convinced on personal experience. Being, at the time of my visit to Scarborough, subject to severe attacks of acidity and pain at the pit of the stomach soon after every repast, no matter how light in kind and quantity (an inconvenience which I attributed, first to the state of morbid irritability produced in my stomach by the repeated trials I had made of the strong sulphurous waters at Harrogate; and secondly, to the frequent change in my food, arising out of my then erratic life from place to place)—it struck me that a small tumbler of the South well water, taken soon after meals, would prevent the unpleasant effect before alluded to. In this I was not disappointed. Further experience taught me also, that if I drank the same quantity of that water, while actually smarting under that most disagreeable sensation, to which the name of *heartburn* has been given, in less than half-an-hour after, the symptom would disappear.

It is pleasant at all times to drink, while suffering from the effects of dyspepsia or laborious digestion, a small quantity of cold limpid mineral water taken at the very source; but I can hardly express the luxurious feeling with which I used to quaff two or three moderately-sized tumblers of the South spring at Scarborough, after a substantial dinner of mine honest host Webb, of the Bell, which had set the biting vipers at work within the recipient of all his good things. In a few minutes after the ingestion of the water, the disturbance in the last-named receptacle was effectually quelled.

And here I must, before I proceed farther with the consideration of the virtues of the Scarborough waters, express my great approbation of the arrangement made in the new building, for retaining the old mode of procuring the water from the spring, by means of a simple spout through which the water is seen constantly flowing, instead of introducing the very objectionable, unscientific, and often nasty process of pumping for the water when required. There is a freshness in the very look of the old mode, which is not a little influential in favouring the effect of the water.

Even from the little I have said, an inference may be drawn, that after a course of the Harrogate waters, the daily use of the south spring water of Scarborough would form the most appropriate and beneficial appendix to the treatment of a vast number of disorders, for the cure of which the powerful and exciting effect of the sulphuretted waters had been deemed necessary; as that remedy may have set up a morbid sensibility of the nerves of the stomach, and an irritability of its lining membrane, which a feeble solution of bi-carbonate of the protoxyde of iron, combined with half a drachm or a drachm of Epsom salts, would be calculated entirely to remove. I must, therefore, invite the attention of medical men who may have to send invalids to Harrogate, and that of invalids themselves who may happen to go to Harrogate without advice, and feel grieved, after a course of the waters, to find that their stomach is in an irritable condition,—to the fact that by going afterwards to Scarborough they will find means to counteract that unpleasant result.

In the same manner, with reference to some of the Spas in Germany, we find it necessary, after exciting the system by the Carlsbad waters, to send the invalids to be cooled and tranquillized by the Kreutzbrunnen, or Ferdinandbrunnen at Marienbad.

But in the case of Scarborough, that place offers two other important reasons for recommending to the Harrogate invalids a conclusion of their course of treatment with a sojourn at the former place. The one is that the air at Scarborough in the months following the termination of the Harrogate season, is more genial and elastic, and purer than that of the moors, which are then charged with moisture. And the second is, that an opportunity there offers for sea-bathing of the very first description.

On the subject of the medicinal virtues of the Scarborough waters, referring principally to that of the south spring, I held a long converse with Mr. Dunn, who had seen me take on the spot two or three doses of the water, followed by the good effect I have already described.

" We find," observed my interlocutor, " that this water exerts considerable action on 'the kidneys, and will prove likewise sufficiently aperient if the invalid, before he begins the use of it, takes care to prepare the way by one or two brisk purgatives, and afterwards drinks daily and regularly in divided doses from a pint and a half to two pints of the water. In this manner I have known even chronic cases of constipation, to be effectually and permanently cured."

" I have noticed in some of the works written on the Scarborough Waters," I then said to Mr. Dunn, " that they have been found serviceable in cases of debility, relaxation of the coat of the stomach, and sickness ; also in pains of the loins attendant on gravel, and in some distempers of the skin. The water from the north well in 'particular, which, from containing a smaller proportion of the aperient salts, tastes more inky, and is more heating, has been recommended to those of the fair sex who are very delicate or relaxed : as it has been found to brace them up, and add

strength to their limbs as well as colour to their blanched
cheeks."

" Just so," was the reply; " we have had, every season,
instances of the most satisfactory kind, to prove the correctness of those assertions. They were made by their authors
upon grounds of positive experience, and our own subsequent
observations have tended to confirm those of our predecessors.
This remark will not surprise one who has, like yourself,
studied so extensively the effect of mineral waters on the
human system; and has, by his work on the Spas of Germany, effected a revolution in the system of scepticism prevailing among us English practitioners. We look to you, therefore,
for carrying out this fortunate change to its utmost extent; and
gladly do we see you engaged in studying the mineral waters
of this country, which you will, no doubt, make known to
the world with the same success you did those of the
continent."

" A period of three years," said I, " since the publication
of the book you have alluded to, has worked marvellous changes
in the mind of my professional brethren in London. From
being sceptical, they have now become universal admirers of
mineral water treatment abroad; so much so that as the proper
season comes round for proceeding to the foreign Spas, the
London physicians are now for sending thither all their
patients;—with what discrimination as to places—with what
positive acquaintance with the peculiarities of the spring and
localities they select—with what personal experience with
regard to the effects of the water they recommend—I must leave
you to guess, who have read my exposition of the state of know-
edge of foreign mineral waters existing in this country, when
' the Spas of Germany " first made their appearance in 1837.
These indiscriminate recommendations, as I must in
consequence call them, have led to disastrous as well as
ridiculous mistakes, many of which have fallen under my
notice, and I have had to rectify them. Patients have

returned to England made considerably worse by being sent to a distant Spa, upon no other apparent ground than because it bore a popular name, or had been very flatteringly described in the work you have mentioned. Of this a most lamentable instance has occurred this very summer, in the case of an amiable and most interesting noble lady whose end was manifestly hastened by, to say the least, a useless journey to one of the Bohemian Spas. In one or two instances patients have come to me, on their return from abroad, complaining that they had not derived the peculiarly soothing and delightful effects I had promised them in my book, under the head of Wildbad, whither they asserted they had proceeded at the recommendation of their own medical man. But upon inquiring further into the matter it turned out that ' their own medical man,' who probably had never condescended to peruse the " Spas of Germany," in which the peculiar baths of Wildbad were first made known in England, had sent the patient to *Wisbaden*, a name more familiar to their ears, and which they considered to be probably one and the same Spa with Wildbad. In fact, there is no end to the mistakes that have occurred ; and many of them have been serious."

" It passes my comprehension ; it certainly does not agree with the principles of common honesty towards their patients," observed Mr. Dunn, " that medical men should undertake to recommend any particular bath, being themselves unacquainted with its real nature, rather than direct the patients at once for advice to the individual who has given public proofs of having studied the subject of mineral waters most maturely."

" I have kept," so ran our dialogue, " a digested register of those patients who have consulted me on the propriety of using the German waters, either abroad or at that useful establishment at Brighton, ever since the publication of my work. They amount to upwards of seven hundred regularly indexed—

exhibiting many very extraordinary cases of disease wholly eradicated by mineral waters, and others materially benefited by them although of many years standing. I have not got the return of all the registered cases, so as to be able to speak confidently of the success in all; for some of the patients do not think it worth their while to report the result of their case after coming back from Germany. But I have every reason to be satisfied with the total result of all the cases that have come to my knowledge; nor have I had a single instance in which either the patient or myself had to regret the choice I had made of the particular Spa for their recovery. Methinks that a similar precision, and with it a similar success, may be ensured in the case of the English mineral waters, to the study of which, as means to cure disease, I am now applying myself in the same manner that I did in Germany. My unbounded confidence in the efficacy of mineral waters as agents calculated to combat disease with immense effect is such, that I have extended and introduced their use in the treatment of ordinary complaints, even such as occur every day—namely, acute diseases and fevers. In the two latter classes, instead of draughts, and mixtures, and powders, and pills, without end, intended to produce but two effects— namely, purging and perspiration—I administer an appropriate mineral water, in divided doses, diluted with warm water, which accomplishes all the indications of the case in the most satisfactory manner, and certainly with less disgust and worry to the patient."

" I thank you for the hint," rejoined my scientific guide. " I am already indebted to you for a valuable mode of expediting the cure of certain diseases requiring counter-irritation, and I shall be too happy to add this other mode of treating general disorders by the employment of such admirable compounds of nature—instead of the many more complicated drugs we generally employ. It is but due to you, and a mere act of justice on my part, to state that the counter-irritating lotion you first recommended in your work upon the means of expeditiously curing disease by external application, has, in my hands and those of my respected and experienced partner, produced all the effects you predicted, and that neither of us ever go out now without being provided with that powerful and most valuable agent. The day will yet come when the profession will render justice to the inventor of a preparation the effects of which are as certain as they are immediate ; and the rationale of which is based on the soundest principles of physiology."

I purposely report, even at the risk of being taxed with vanity, the preceding honest and candid opinion on this all-important subject, (spontaneously given) of a fellow member of the profession, who enjoys the largest share of practice in a populous place, and who spoke from his own knowledge and experience. A similar opinion had been expressed before by the able physicians whom I named when describing my visit to the city of York ; and analogous sentiments have been conveyed to me by others whom I shall have occasion to allude to in the sequel of the present work, as well as by letters from total strangers in various parts of England and the continent.*

Our conversation ended, we slowly retraced our steps, taking the direction towards the Cliff Bridge, on the thresh-

* Such disinterested testimonials, founded on a real knowledge of facts, from so many able individuals in the same profession,—together with the singular unanimity of commendation from more than twenty reviewers, regarding one of my recent medical publications † referred to by Mr. Dunn,—may well be considered as more than sufficient to neutralize that single example of nefarious condemnation of the same work, which appeared, without one word said of the contents of the book, not in one but in *two* successive numbers of a quarterly medical publication, conducted by Dr. Forbes, of Colchester, who is hired to " do " that journal by a medical bookseller in London.

In this new capacity, the disappointed physician and unsuccessful
† *Counter-irritation, its Principles and Practice ; with one hundred cases, &c. &c.*—1 vol. 8vo, 1838.

hold of which a very striking panoramic view of Scarborough presented itself, inferior only to the one represented in the engraving, taken from a boat at a small distance from the harbour, and given in the title-page of the present volume.

The back being turned to the sea and its sweeping bays,— the two straight and prolonged lines of the lofty iron-rail parapet serve to direct the eye to a converging point, where the toll-gate stands, at the furthest extremity of the bridge. Here the circular platform of " the Cliff " expands, backed by its oblong square, formed of neat dwelling-houses, which are generally well filled during the season, as they enjoy an open prospect of the bay.

On the left, the long side and square tower of Christ-church, a modern sacred edifice, raised by a subscription of three thousand pounds among the inhabitants, arrests our attention.

Following the direction of that object still further to the left, Beavor-terrace appears; so named in honour of the Duke of Rutland, who, although he has ceased to be the absolute patron of the borough, is still as much revered as ever by its inhabitants.

translator, delights to vent his impotent spleen against every thing that is either beneficial to the world, or above his feeble comprehension.

My recent extended tour through the country has proved to me the sort of estimation in which such a journalist is [held by the profession: inasmuch as, in a great many instances, I found that, disgusted with the uncouth and unlettered style and general bearing, as well as with the frequent and gross inaccuracies of the British and Foreign Medical Quarterly performance, medical men had discarded it for another which possesses far greater and prior claims to their support, as being infinitely superior to its rival in information ; and for honesty, without a competitor.

Such a performance is not likely ever to fall into the hands of any of my readers ; but should it by chance meet their eye, I caution them against supposing that it contains even the semblance of truth respecting the works of many of his superiors, which the editor incapable of under-standing or appreciating them, slashes in the most scurrilous jargon, under pretence of reviewing them.

Separated from this terrace by a wide opening intended to be the site of a new street, the beginning of a projected grand crescent is seen, half-a-dozen of the houses of which are already finished. These houses are much in the same style of architecture as those commonly seen at most of the fashionable watering-places, St. Leonard's especially. One or two among them are distinguished by size and greater pretensions, and are the residence of the Woodwards, a family of great consequence, and much respected among the permanent inhabitants of Scarborough.

There are but two or three of these superior dwellings (by far the best in the place for situation and comfort) which are let as lodgings.* When this crescent shall have reached the farthest end of its projected line, it will mask an unsightly range of stables erected on the same ridge, which, at present, obtrude, and offend the eyes.

Descending towards the sloping ravine at the bottom of which runs the road that passes under the bridge, to reach the Strand,—the ridge in question terminates in a green knoll, on whose summit stands an insulated and smart house (the best situated in this locality) the residence of G. Knowles,' Esq., who laid out the various paths and walks on the hill above and beyond the new Spa.

Of the semicircular line of land-views just described on our left, the centre point (about midway on the lofty embankment) is occupied by the Scarborough Museum—a rotunda of Roman-Doric structure, thirty-seven feet and a half in its external diameter, and fifty feet in elevation.

If the eye now returns to the centre of the Cliff Bridge, and tracks the outline of the landscape to the right or north side, far different objects present themselves. A bold line of cliffs, the summit of which is variously shaped and figured

---

* An excellent opportunity offers here to a spirited speculator in houses; as land for building contiguous to Beavor-terrace, is to be purchased for five shillings per square yard.

by natural accidents, as well as by many buildings placed thereon, is seen to emerge from within the opening of Scarborough harbour, and to project into the sea. It rises higher the farther it stands out, until upon its loftiest point, which measures more than three hundred feet above the highest tide, it exhibits the once famed but now ruinous castle, within the surrounding walls of which lie concealed nineteen acres of smiling green land. The ancient and conventual-looking church of St. Mary,* with its square tower, seems placed on purpose in this direction, though farther inland, to add to the effect of this picture by its contrast with the remains of the embattled walls of the castle; beyond which, the outline, gradually descending to the horizon, terminates at some distance with the piers of Scarborough harbour.

Here the small craft form picturesque groups; while the many and heavy clusters of red brick dwellings of the humbler classes, which are thickly huddled together right and left of the opening of the harbour, spread some way inland, and form the primitive or old town of Scarborough, canopied over by hovering clouds of blue smoke which rise in light and curling columns.

* This is the parish church of which the Rev. Michael H. Miller is vicar, and in which public worship is performed five times a week. I have already alluded to the exemplary character of this most worthy churchman.

CHAPTER XIV.

SUCH is the sea view of the new, as well as of the old
town of Scarborough—the fashionable and the unfashionable
end of this celebrated watering-place. A scene cannot be
imagined of greater contrast in its two composing elements,
or of greater interest in its *ensemble*. Whatever progress
modern structure may be destined to make southward,
whether inland, or upon the various points of the great amphitheatre which faces the ocean, it is heartily to be wished that the
sacrilegious hand of improvement may never dare to touch a
single vestige of the primeval huts and cottages of the fisherman
and the mariner. The picture is now complete. The like is
not often beheld in other parts of this island ; and its existence is, to my mind, one of the many merits peculiar to
Scarborough, as a temporary residence for invalid strangers.

That improvements will take place, and building be carried on to some extent, no one can doubt who is aware, as I am, of what Scarborough is still susceptible. Every facility in the mean while is afforded for such an enterprise. Land for building, contiguous to Beavor-terrace, is to be purchased (as I have said) for five shillings per square yard; and the Kelloway Rock, a ferruginous sandstone with fossil shells, abounds on this part of the coast, particularly under the Castle hill, where it is seen above the pier. The new Museum, to the architecture of which I have already alluded, is constructed of this stone (the gift of Sir J. V. B. Johnstone, Bart.), which is alone worked for building purposes at Hackness, and hence often called *Hackness Stone*. It is a beautiful building-stone, as well as a valuable one. While in the quarry it is very soft, easily chiseled, and readily fashioned into architectural decoration; but it soon becomes hard on exposure to the air, and then possesses much durability.

Having reached the threshold of the scientific temple just named, belonging to the Scarborough Philosophical Society, it was not likely that my kind cicerone, one of its most indefatigable officers, should suffer me to pass by without entering its precincts. And well does the establishment deserve a visit from every stranger who may chance to be at Scarborough. To those who make that place their residence for a month or two, such a museum must prove a most delightful source of amusement and intellectual gratification. Every temptation, even upon the score of economy, has been offered to the scientifically inclined, or even to the merely curious, to visit frequently that institution, for the admission to which only two-and-sixpence is charged for a month to a single individual, or five shillings for the same length of time to a whole family, no matter how numerous.

Considering the extent of its collection—its methodical and novel arrangement, due to the late Dr. Smith, the geologist (who suggested also the circular form of the

building for the display of British geological specimens), and
the short period that has elapsed since Scarborough was
without this additional and attractive feature,—the Museum
offers a remarkable instance of what may be effected for
science, by perseverance, great activity, and an earnest desire
to support it. In 1828 no vestige of a scientific collection
was in existence at Scarborough, yet its Philosophical Society
was formed. At one of its meetings a desire was expressed
that a Museum to contain the many rich specimens found on
the adjoining coast, and other objects of natural history,
should be constructed. Instantly a liberal-minded and
wealthy Baronet who presided over the Society, takes up the
subject, subscribes liberally himself towards its attainment,
and gets others to do the same. Having procured from that able
architect, Mr. R. H. Sharp, of York, the design of a chaste and
classical edifice, the worthy president presents all the necessary
building-stone from his estate at Hackness, and with an energy
and promptitude seldom equalled, seconded by the unremit-
ting co-operation of Mr. Dunn, then Secretary to the Society,
succeeds in adding to Scarborough, in less than two years,
one of its present most prominent and attractive features, at
an expense of 1893l. for the building, fitting up, and
decoration altogether.

On entering the principal room, which is thirty-five feet
high, and lighted from an aperture in the dome, around me I
beheld arranged on sloping shelves, and in the order of their
strata, very numerous fossils, showing at one view the whole
series of this kingdom. Among these specimens, which are,
perhaps, some of the most perfect in England, one cannot
overlook two admirable collections of fossil corals—the one
purchased of Mr. Williamson, the Curator—the other
presented to the Society by Mr. Duesbery, being the valuable
collection of the late Mr. Hindewell, the historiographer of
Scarborough.

Below these sloping shelves an horizontal one is placed,

sustaining the general arrangement of fossil, and recent shells; while the birds and animals are placed above the geological arrangement; so that every part of the Museum can be seen at once.

Among so many objects deserving admiration, it is not easy to specify those that attracted most my attention; yet it isimpossible not to single out the magnificent saurians of the Scarborough collection, the fragment of one of which, alone, is nine feet long, and that only half the length of the animal. Neither is it likely that, on quitting the Museum, the visiter should fail to notice the skeleton of an ancient Briton and his oak-tree coffin, placed just outside of the building, recently brought to light, and supposed to be 2000 years old. The teeth are all perfect, and the skeleton would appear to have been preserved by the tannin found dissolved in the water, which had penetrated into the coffin.

All these various objects are ably explained to the visiters by the keeper, Mr. Williamson, who is himself no inconsiderable object of attraction. Originally a working gardener, and fellow-labourer with another equally-distinguished naturalist of Scarborough, whom I shall presently introduce to my readers, Mr. Williamson has by his own industry educated himself to be an excellent naturalist, has made nearly the whole of the collection of pebbles and fossil remains in this museum, and is bringing up to the medical profession a son who bids fair to prove a worthy scion of of his sire.

The sight that presented itself below us as we emerged from this repository of science was of the most cheerful description. The sun, long past its meridian hour, was lighting up the magnificent scenery around, and inviting people abroad. Long lines of pedestrians were approaching from the cliff to the bridge, and passing through the tollbar, deployed themselves over the whole length of that stupendous structure, making it their afternoon promenade.

Many groups and parties extended as far as the tortuous paths on the opposite hills. Amongst them, I recognised many and was accosted by some whom I had the honour of being known to professionally, and all of whom spoke in praise of the place.

The bearing of many of these visiters bespoke the rank in life to which they appertained. Lady R——, the relict of the opulent Yorkshire baronet, near Ferrybridge, whose great wealth has descended to a minor grandson ; Colonel M——, and his lovely family, nearly allied in blood to a recently deceased earl ; Sir L. O— ; the Rev. Dr. F——, a distinguished divine and dignitary of the church ; the Honourable Lady and Miss W—— ; the Ladies H—— ; the Earl of T—— and his Countess ; were a few of the *distingués* I could discern in the moving crowd. Others my kind guide named to me, and the presence of all showed that, with a very large number of the superior classes, Scarborough retains still its natural attraction. And well will it be for them and all of the kindred class, if, while debating whither to go during the summer and autumn in search of health, and the enjoyment of nature's beauties, they do not forget that Scarborough offers both gifts, to an extent not easily equalled on other parts of the British coast.

I mixed not in the gay scene, but parting with my friend, whose professional avocations called him away, I threaded a tortuous and descending path down the side of the hill on which stands the Museum, and then reached the broad strand, from which the waves had but lately retired. To my right the soft yet firm and level sands extended as far as the distant sea-wall of the new Spa, which is accessible at low water from the strand, by means of steps practised in the great sub-basement of the Spa-terrace. On my left an equally level and wide zone of the purest sands I had ever beheld, stretched as far as the piers of the little harbour, skirting the foot of the Castle-hills.

Straggling groups of people are seen basking in the sun, or leisurely pacing the strand in this part, at the earliest hour of day. Early equestrians too I have beheld taking possession of the level expanse, and pirouetting their chargers on the soft sands—the best riding-ground in the world ; while led horses go through their morning exercise, sniffing the gentle sea-breeze that has just set in.

Fronting the sea here, some neat houses appear, which are let as lodgings, and are called the marine houses. They have a small adjoining building for cold and warm baths,—the sea, at spring tides reaching nearly to the threshold of its garden front. A lofty and sloping bank, from a hundred and fifty to two hundred feet high, thickly covered with shrubs and trees, rises from hence, and in a southern direction, like a species of crescent bower, goes to join the cliff bridge. On the brow of this green embankment, at various elevations, between one hundred and one hundred and forty feet, stand many of the best houses, with a south or south-eastern aspect. On the sands below, a file of thirty or forty bathing-machines is ranged on their broad wheels, ready for use. Those belonging to Chapman, twenty in number, appeared to me to be the largest and the best.

The arrangements for bathing in the open sea by means of these machines are of the most satisfactory kind, particularly for ladies. The almost insensible descent into deeper water, with the softest bed imaginable for the feet to tread upon when immersed in the water, and the peculiar transparency and purity of the returning tide upon these open bays, render the operation of sea-bathing in this place not only perfectly safe, but one accompanied with almost luxurious feelings. If sea-bathing is to impart vigour to an infirm constitution, or restore a morbid frame, surely the having it in great perfection must be one of the first and most desirable of its recommendations.

Sea-bathing, judiciously prescribed, and properly employed, I hold to be, next to the use of mineral waters, one of the most powerful means a medical man can wield for the restoration of his patients. Even where the complaint requires to be treated with mineral waters, I have known a great many cases which could not be completely and permanently restored without sea-bathing, as a concluding measure. In this respect, Scarborough offers, for those who judiciously use Harrogate, or Cross, or Dinsdale, or Shotley Bridge water for their ailments, not only the advantage of great proximity as a sea-bathing place, but also that of being one of the very best places of that description.

I hold it to be an unfortunate circumstance for the Germans, that their country affords them not the means of having recourse to sea-bathing, after having been at their own delightful and very efficient Spas. Those among them who can afford time and money to procure the luxury of sea-bathing, have but one place to fly to, and that is in consequence much frequented by them : I mean Scheveningen, near the Hague —a spot perfectly desolate and insulated, below a range of sand-hills, and affording only the accommodation of a single large building perched upon those hills. Here, in 1836, I beheld invalids who had come from distant parts of Germany for the benefit of sea-water, and who were dying of *ennui*. Had they' stretched across the German ocean and landed at Scarborough, how different their situation and the ultimate result would have been !

Of the advantages of sea-bathing in a professional point of view I have spoken in another part of the present volumes, and I have only to add in this place, that in addition to the great sea-water bath afforded by the incomparable sands at Scarborough, that place offers the convenience and accommodation of some of the neatest and most elegant baths, within special buildings placed on different parts of the cliffs, that I have seen any where. Travis's baths are on the " cliff." They are of marble, and fitted up with much taste and every convenience, and supplied, as I ascertained by in-spection, with the purest sea-water. Every form of baths, whether warm or cold, is administered when required, including shower, pumping, drenching, and vapour baths.

The above are, I believe, the oldest baths in the place. But the very *ne plus ultra* of a coquettish bathing-establishment is attained in the comparatively modern baths of Dr. Harland, and those of Champney. The former are placed in a neat modern building very favourably situated not far from Beavor-terrace. The reader can hardly form an idea of the boudoir-like and costly manner in which these baths and their dressing-rooms are fitted up. The expense for a single bath at all these establishments is moderate—being half-a-crown, with a trifle to the attendant.

By this time my readers will readily believe that I must have been weary with my researches and peregrinations. I returned to my hotel to arrange and collect my flying notes taken on the spot, and found a merry party assembled at dinner; at which some of the finest fish was served up. Scarborough is noted for that delicate article of the table; and it is to be procured at very reasonable prices. The fine turbot laid on our board had cost only five shillings ; and for sixpence one can get three large haddocks.

Living on the whole is somewhat cheaper at Scarborough than in London, and certainly not so extravagant as at Harro-gate. From inquiry of an excellent manager, the mother of a large family, I learned that the prime pieces of meat, with all bones removed, cost but eightpence per pound ; that poul-try, eggs, and butter, are one-fourth cheaper than in London ; and that a fair-sized codfish may be had for one shilling, or a pair of the largest soles for that sum. Bread and milk are tolerable, and water is excellent—rather hard but well-flavoured and limpid.*

* This, which is called the Falsgrave water, is obtained from land-springs and collected into reservoirs where it deposits its mud. The cistern is

Water and bread! These are no trifling comforts at a Spa—and though they may appear trite in their nature to some people, yet the enumeration of them will have its value with a large majority of my readers.

House-room, whether in the form of lodgings or of separate houses, is not to be procured good at a very cheap rate. The average rent for the latter is ten guineas a week. A large house near the cliff bridge lets for thirteen guineas during the season, which is reckoned to begin on the 1st of July, and to terminate on the 12th of October. After the latter date, house-rent falls to one-half its former amount. Lodging and boarding-houses are of three classes, and at all of them four meals are allowed. The respective prices are 4s. 6d., 5s. 6d., and 6s. 6d. per day, including a bedroom.

I have already mentioned the charges made at the Bell. I occupied in it a bedroom facing the south side of the castle, and under it the two piers of Scarborough harbour were visible. Below I looked upon the clustered streets of the marine portion of the town, and on turning my head to the right, I beheld the beautiful bays down to Filey point. The house stands on a shelf of " Bland's Cliff," and the view from its apartments is not interfered with by any of the rows of neat lodging-houses which are arranged in front of it, for they are below its level.

covered, and thence the water takes its course through iron pipes to four conduits, where women fetch it and carry it to private houses at a penny a pail. One of the reservoirs is a natural one, connected with which there is a curious anecdote of old Smith, the father of English geology, who by giving the name of *Corn-brash* to one of the rocks of the series on this coast, identified himself with the geology of most parts of the country. Scarcity of potable water during one summer, induced many persons to consult Smith, who having found a natural fissure from which the scanty supply of water was obtained, desired them to bore in that place, when the water surged with a profusion that both pleased and alarmed the people. Old father Smith upon this uttered an exclamation of joy at the result of his own sagacity, and declared that the water was what had been pent up since the deluge !

A visit I paid to Captain S—— (a former acquaintance), at Reed's Hotel, enabled me to examine with attention that crack establishment of the place. For situation, interior arrangement, and fitting up, it appeared to me to be the best of its class. The charge is 6s. 6d. per diem, and half-a-guinea a week for the bedroom. The *sommités* who visit this Spa generally alight at this well-conducted establishment. Among other conveniences Reed's Hotel boasts of a spacious ball-room.

But, alas! of what use to the place is such an accommodation, except for some mediocre concern now and then? Of all the auxiliaries so much required at, and generally forming the boast of, other Spas, Scarborough repudiates the two principal and most cheering ones—dancing and sociability. The Scarborough visiters have hitherto been the greatest separatists in England, and would as soon think of returning a bow to some " small unknown" to whom they had never been regularly introduced, as they would to dance with any one not belonging to their own set. This should be reformed, and the sooner the better.

Nor is the theatre better supported during the season. It made one's heart ache, almost, to see the bewitching widow of a late gallant life-guard officer, whose histrionic efforts, aided by a very handsome person, and eyes that are

Stars, stars, and all eyes else dead coals,

London audiences know so well how to appreciate, struggle to perform with spirit and frolicsome gaiety the task she had undertaken for her own benefit, before nineteen spectators!

No—excursions inland, or a walk to the summit of Mount Oliver, where, upon a terrace six hundred feet above the ocean a most superb panorama of land and water is enjoyed; and parties on the water, especially for the purpose of exploring the interesting coast right and left of the town, which offers a very museum of geology,—these seem to be the principal amusements peculiar to Scarborough.

Numerous boats are always in readiness to take parties out to sea at the moderate charge of one shilling per hour; while from thirty to forty horses, and donkey-carts and other carriages, may be seen at the end of the road under the Cliff Bridge, at one shilling and sixpence per hour the single, and three shillings the double harnessed vehicles.

To those who are fond of angling I would recommend a walk to the banks of a noted trout-stream in the Forge Valley, not far from Scarborough, where visiters have hitherto been permitted to fish. But a club is about to be formed for the preservation of the fish, which is, however, intended to be on very liberal terms.

Scarborough has its Gazette of fashion and arrivals during the season, in which the aristocracy of the farmers from the East and West Ridings figure away in long lists at the hotels and boarding-houses. As the season advances, and the two days of the races, held on the sands, in August, pass away, the great mass of visiters of ignoble birth gradually retire and make way for those of a superior class. The number of visiters of every description who have of late years frequented this watering-place during the season has amounted to about two thousand. It ought to increase to four times that number.

Their presence, in one respect, has been so far beneficial to Scarborough that it will have occasioned the erection of two additional churches. Hitherto, hardly any provision existed in the place for affording to the poorer people, especially sailors and fishermen, an opportunity of attending divine worship. St. Mary's, besides being too far removed from the shore, was found insufficient, and the want of room in that parish church probably gave rise to the many meeting-houses for dissenters which are to be seen about the town. A new church (the *Christ-church* before mentioned) was consequently erected a few years back, to the south of the Castle Cliff, not far from the principal street; and a certain number of free seats were reserved in it for the sole use of those classes of people whom it was desirable to induce to attend the national form of worship.

But here again the number of strangers, who from the different hotels flocked to the new church, took possession of the free seats, and the more humble worshippers saw themselves deprived of every accommodation in the house of God, unless they submitted to the inconvenience of attending church at a much earlier hour than the usual time for divine service.

This was greatly felt by the excellent vicar, whom I have already introduced to my readers. In his heart was he sorely grieved to find, on the one hand, that the class of persons who stood most in need of true religious instruction were without the means of obtaining it; and on the other hand, that the absence of such means was the main cause of the daily advances made among the population, by the spirit of separatism from the church of England.

The consideration of these two important facts induced the worthy pastor to solicit contributions from the faithful towards erecting a new and modest temple to God, down upon the Strand, and he has every reason to rejoice at the prospect that his most anxious wishes on this point will be fully realized at no distant period. To this end he has strained every nerve, and exerted himself zealously for a long time past; making frequent appeals to that effect from the pulpit of the parish church. Within that church I once attended divine service, when I was much edified by his discourse and mode of delivery, which are such as to have given him a great hold on the esteem and veneration of his flock, among whom he enjoys the well-merited reputation of being an excellent preacher.

The few hours I spent in the society of this gentleman at

his house in the evening tended to confirm the favourable impression I had received in the morning, of the conscientious manner in which, even at the expense of his private fortune, this worthy minister discharges his duty.

In point of intellectual amusement Scarborough offers many more resources than are to be found at other Spas. Besides the Museum and the Library of the Philosophical Society, there are the Agricultural Library, and Mrs. Theakstone's News-room and Circulating Library.

But one of the most intellectual treats besides, is a visit to Mr. Bean's unparalleled collection of shells, both recent and fossil, including complete series of corallines and British shells, decidedly superior to any other in the country. The latter are scientifically arranged according to the most approved modern authorities, in two large cabinets, containing from sixty to seventy thousand specimens, among which Mr. Bean showed me almost every recorded variety in this useful and most delightful branch of science.

I noticed among them three recent specimens of a shell (*Panopœa Glycymeris*) which, until Mr. Bean had discovered these specimens, was considered to be an extinct animal, every naturalist having the fossil specimen, but not any of them a recent one. On the other hand, Mr. Bean has a fossil *Pholas*, which is a recent species supposed never to have been found in a fossilized state. Professor Grant saw it. Lyall and Sowerby were expected to visit it.

A great number of Mr. Bean's corallines have lately been figured in "Johnstone's British Zoophytes;" yet many new and rare species remain undescribed in his cabinets.

As for the geological specimens from the Yorkshire coast in this collection, they are on a par with the rest of this superb museum, being as perfect and complete as human research has yet been able to make them. In the *Cornbrash* limestone alone Mr. Bean has found one hundred and fifty species of fossil remains, most of which he has described in the

Magazine of Natural History. His fossil plants vie with those of the Scarborough Museum; many of them are as yet undescribed, and deserve the close inspection of the fossil botanist.

It is impossible, in the present work, to speak otherwise than generally of this scientific and matchless collection, or rather I should say, this series of collections, which Mr. Bean began and completed in the course of twenty years, during which period he discovered and named many new species and varieties. He at first began to look for fossils, but finding he did not know how to class them without being previously acquainted with the recent shells, he set about forming the present collection of them, by walking twenty miles for five or six hours every day backwards and forwards; and unquestionably he appears to have made the most splendid collection of British shells in the country. The genus *Helix* (snail), in particular, presents a most splendid arrangement.

But it would much exceed my limits to attempt any thing like a specific enumeration of such treasures. Those who visit Scarborough and can have access to the museum of Mr. Bean, whose urbanity and communicativeness are the theme of praise, will find it an honour to the place, and a lasting monument of the genius and skill of its possessor.

The produce of geological research in the vicinity of Scarborough is not altogether applied to scientific purposes; some of it has a more pleasing destination—that of forming ornaments for the fair sex. I would single out in particular the beautiful manufactory of jet—for which both Scarborough and Whitby are celebrated. At the latter place jet is found in large blocks, which are cut afterwards, at Scarborough, by an Italian artist and jeweller, named Vassalli, into every species of ornaments, such as necklaces, chains of every variety of pattern, crosses, waist-buckles, paper-folders, and rings. There is much taste displayed at times in the choice of the form given to these several objects, and their high finish renders them still more acceptable. Their price is about one-fourth of what would be asked for them in London; and it is curious enough that some of the lady visiters informed me, in regard to other objects appertaining especially to their toilet and comforts, that they found at "Crawford's shop," in Scarborough, the metropolitan fashions, from Ludgate-hill and Regent's-street, at a lower price than in the capital. Indeed the Everingtons, and the Merringtons, and the Swan and Edgars have their district depots for the season in Scarborough, as they have at Harrogate.

The climate of a place such as I have described, which recommends itself by so many advantages to the attention of all who require to recruit their health, is a point that deserves particular notice in a work like the present. I have already alluded to the purity of the atmosphere, its elasticity, and bracing quality. From its exposure on the east coast, a mistaken notion is entertained by many, that winds in an easterly direction (which are universally feared) must be of longer continuance at Scarborough than elsewhere. The inspection of a table of prevailing winds, given me by Mr. Dunn, exhibits as the mean of seven years (from 1832 to 1838 both inclusive), the number of ninety-eight days only, during which, winds blew in the course of each year from the east, north-east, and south-east quarters. The mean number of days in which the north wind blew during the same period of years was forty-five days and a half.

On surveying the bay, I noticed how it is sheltered by hills from the north and east winds, except the south-east; while it is also open to the whole day's sun. These local circumstances necessarily render the winters remarkably mild; it having often happened to strangers who had prolonged their stay at Scarborough as late as Christmas, and on whose veracity I can rely, to be able to dress in the morning with the windows open, through which a genial breeze blew in from the sea.

The opportunities afforded me at Scarborough and since, to examine the meteorological tables kept by Mr. Williamson and Mr. Hawkridge at the museum, and those of the registrar of births, marriages, and deaths, by Messrs. Donner and Woodall, have convinced me of these important facts: First, that the mean average temperature in the month of January 1838 and 1839, at Scarborough, was higher by six degrees than at York, and by nearly four degrees than in London, and only one degree less than that at Torquay. Secondly, that for many years past the mean temperature of the autumnal quarter has ranged between forty-four and forty-nine degrees, while for the whole year it has been as high as $52\frac{3}{4}$ degrees. Thirdly, that the average number of days of rain throughout the year has been somewhat more than one-third of the year; August, September, October, and November being the months, generally speaking, of less rain. Lastly, that the claims to a superior longevity in favour of the inhabitants of Scarborough, over that of other parts of Yorkshire, is fully established: it appearing, besides, that the period of the visitation of strangers is at the most healthy time of the year.

On these several points Mr. Dunn has drawn up a series of tables and memoranda, which he was kind enough to send me, and to which I trust he will be induced to give publicity. I much regret, that the nature of the present volumes precludes me from making a more extended use of their valuable information.*

I now bid farewell to Scarborough—of all the English Spas I have visited, the one which has left the most pleasing impressions on my mind, probably in consequence of its combining the luxury of sea-bathing in perfection, with the more solid advantage of efficient mineral springs.

* My wish, in this respect, has been since accomplished. Mr. Dunn presented his Tabular Vital Statistics of Scarborough to the Medical Section of the British Association, at Glasgow, and has since published them.

CHAPTER XV.

HOVINGHAM SPA.

The VALE OF PICKERING—Railroad to Whitby—The German and Irish Sea, almost one—A strong and a strange Case in proof—Road to Kirby Moorside—The BUCKLAND CAVE—Antediluvian Relics—Desolation—DUNCOMBE Park—The Dog of Alcibiades—RIVAULX ABBEY—The Village of HOVINGHAM—The Spring no Spa—Properties of the Water—Cures performed with it—Proposition to establish Sulphur MUD-BATHS—A Tour—Botany and Agriculture—Sowing wheat *versus* planting Trees—" My Son Edward's Children"—Who is the greatest Benefactor ? Surgeon WILCOCKS—Parish Work and Commissioners' Pay.

WITHIN the last twelve years much has been said, and much more has been done, to impart notoriety to a sulphuretted spring brought to light in the immediate vicinity of a small village, called Hovingham, in the vale of Pickering. Printed papers and circulars of all sorts were sent round, proclaiming the virtues of the recently discovered spa ; and invitations, as well as many hints, were thrown out to capitalists and hotel-keepers, to come and settle at Hovingham, which it was expected would become a favourite resort for invalids. No quantitative analysis of the water was ever made, or published, however ; but a general account of its ingredients, ascertained by simple tests, was placed in my hands, with the respectable name of Dr. Travis. of New Malton, attached to it; and this was a sufficient inducement for me to journey from Scarborough to Hovingham.

Anxious to see the country, I engaged an open carriage, with a conductor who had been well recommended as one capable of giving me much local information. Posting in a gig is not only a very convenient, but also a by no means unfrequent mode of travelling in Yorkshire; and during summer weather, a most delightful mode of conveyance it is. A succession of very brilliant days enabled me to enjoy it in perfection, and use it to advantage.

It is impossible to leave Scarborough, and not to cast a last look towards it as we reach the summit of that great hill distant about two miles, which, when once we have descended westwardly, will stand, like a mighty screen, between us and that town. It is from that very summit, that the first view of Scarborough and its south bays, and the great promontory on which the castle rears its dismantled towers, bursts on the traveller who journeys thither from Malton. Seen from thence that ancient citadel seems to stand apart and away from the mainland. The dark mass, contrasting with the yellow sunshine that covered the waste to the right and to the left, appeared as if unconnected with the general outline of the shore.

Looking westward soon after, I caught a glimpse of the remains of Wykeham Abbey, and a general view of the rich vale of Seamer, the latter once a flourishing town, and now a mere village, yet a village magnificent in appearance.

After an excellent breakfast at a neat inn at Snainton, I changed my vehicle and driver, and set off for Pickering, along an enchanting by-road; though the road itself is neither smooth nor in good condition, from the friable materials, the calcareous grit of the county, employed in making it, as well as in keeping it in repair.

The smart lad who sat by my side first pointed out to me Mr. Osbaldeston's villa on our right, passing which and before reaching Allerston, I beheld on my left, from the crest of a hill, the rich champaign country, still called the Marshes, with New Malton in the distance, and Castle Howard at the foot of the Howardian hills; the whole bounded by the Wolds, south of the York road.

Next he introduced to my notice Thornton Dale, placed in a hollow, with its trout-stream crossing the road and Mr. Hill's park, in the vicinity of which we chanced to meet a fair country lass travelling unattended, on horseback, in the fashion of the county. One cannot speak satisfactorily of the appearance of the several villages through which we passed. The houses of the yeomanry, built of the yellow-coloured stone so general throughout this oolitic district, did not give one the idea of comforts within. My quick-tongued companion alleged as a reason for it that the inmates were not in easy circumstances, owing to low wages and hard work. Being himself the son of poor farming people at Brompton in the neighbourhood, he admitted that he had been kept at the school in that village, at Sir George Cayley's expense, for nearly six years, where he had learned but little reading and writing, and was just able at the end of that time to manage his bible and no more. I inquired if people drank much in these parts, " Yes, a goodish little," was the answer. " And what is it they do drink ?"— " Why all sort, ale and rum, and brandy, and gin, and sometimes three or four young farmers, who can afford it, will club together for a bottle of wine, and drink that instead, to be thought gentlemen like."

To the north of the market-place at Pickering, an ancient broad carriage-way with the remains of a line of lofty elms, which once formed part of a great avenue, leads to one of those undulations or swells in the limestone formation, which like so many ribs, descend from north to south, down the lofty moorland into the vale of Pickering. On the summit, of one of these, the remains of Pickering Castle are still visible, though in a very dilapidated state; the walls of circumvallation, in some places lofty, and in others depressed, following the undulation of the ground, mark still the extent of 'the castellated territory. The view from the hill into the vale of Pickering would be exceedingly beautiful were it not for the unsightly stone fences and boundaries, which, with straight and right angular deformity, offend the eye, and have considerably spoiled in this, as in most parts of Yorkshire, the picturesque appearance of the country.

Pickering owes its present prosperity to the railroad which placed it in immediate communication with Whitby. Its inexhaustible quarries of limestone would have been useless but for the new facility thus acquired of disposing of that produce. By bringing York, too, in nearer communication than before with the Port of Whitby, there being but twenty-five miles of coach-road between the terminus at Pickering and the metropolitan city of the county, the German ocean has been, as it were, approximated to the Irish sea.

Of the reality of this fact, I met with an illustration in the person of an American skipper, who having put into the Port of Whitby from the Baltic, had there found letters summoning him instantly to return to his native land, with or without his vessel. He had consequently left the latter in charge of his mate, and mounting one of the carriages on the single line of horse-rail to Pickering at five o'clock in the morning, reached that place in time for the coach to York, where I saw him get out and immediately enter the carriage train on the railroad to Leeds, on which I was myself preparing to travel at the time. It was then about noon. Leeds we reached in a little more than an hour, and here my hurried skipper, who had allowed himself scarcely a moment's breathing-time, took coach again as far as Littleborough, where he would arrive at four o'clock, quite in time for one of the afternoon trains on the new railroad, which from that place conveys the traveller in three-quarters of an hour to Manchester. Thence, I need not say that our transatlantic traveller intended to proceed by one of the numerous trains which leave for Liverpool, so as to reach that seaport at the expiration of an hour and a half, quite soon enough to enjoy a hearty repast, the first refreshment on that day, and ship himself off in one of the steamers, which, at the close of a long day in July, drop down the Mersey with the evening tide, ready to take advantage of the land-breeze that is to waft them into the Atlantic.

Thus a man who rose in the morning, on the eastern coast of England, his face turned towards Russia, would, ere the sun of the same day had set, be seen quitting the western coast of England, his face turned towards America. Such is one of the miracles of railroad travelling!

The drive from Pickering to Kirby Moorside, is through a succession of the richest and most extensively-cultivated lands I had yet seen. The road happily undulates with the dips and risings caused by the many dales and ridges descending from the north in almost parallel lines, and affords many an opportunity of casting a bird's-eye glance at the subjacent plain. The entire surface is teeming with tokens of social life. The villages are here neater,—few of the dwellings being thatched, but generally tiled and built of stone. They trail the rose and the honeysuckle up to their chamber casements, and the population seems numerous, healthy-looking, and well clad.

Our course ran so tortuous, that it afforded all the accidents of an ever-varying landscape. Some of the ridges that divide the nearly parallel dales to which I have just alluded, are thickly clothed with wood ; while others, which the eye could track to their highest and most distant point, though green, were bare of forest-trees, and terminated abruptly and nearly perpendicular in the vale; divulging by their denuded faces the characters of their geological structure.

I had thus far committed my notes to my tablets, whilst my vehicle was driving through Kirby, where it presently halted in front of the great quarry at *Kirkdale*, on the western side of which I perceived the fissure in the rock that marks the celebrated Buckland Cave, or repository of antediluvian relics. A desolate hole, truly — the whole quarry, and opening of the cavern seemed ! As if the terrified beasts of a former world, in quest of shelter from the one universal devastating flood which threatened their existence, had by instinct purposely selected a spot too frightful to entice any persecuting enemy of their race to follow them.

The steep descent of the road to reach this scene, the hanging wood overhead, and the rocky-shallow *beck* that you must cross to reach the neighbouring kirk from the dale—are all sombre objects, quite in character with the overpowering recollection of the vast dissolution of living creatures which once took place in this sequestered spot; but the hand of man is already at work upon this hallowed ground of science, and a few more months of pickaxe and gunpowder-blasting will have swept away all vestiges of a scene rendered so interesting by the able and enthusiastic professor of Oxford.

From sombre to gay the transit is often rapid. Nature and art afforded me a strange example of this trueism, at the present conjuncture. Scarcely emerged from the gloomy recess I have just described, a valley of surpassing beauty received us, presenting many interesting objects upon a large extent of champaign country, defined on many points by the line of the Hambleton hills. Upon the summit of one of the lesser and subsiding eminences of this lofty range I beheld the manor-house of Duncombe Park, presenting one of its imposing porticoes to the west, and commanding an extensive view over one of the richest valleys in Yorkshire. The brow of the hill before the house has been converted into a lengthened terrace, the two ends of which are marked by an Ionic and a Tuscan temple.

This is by far the most favourable view of Duncombe House, and surpasses that which is obtained on approaching it from the York road, through a Tuscan archway of indifferent design, bearing on the top of it, in the inside, an inscription to Nelson. The noble host, by whom I had many years before been consulted in conjunction with Sir Henry Halford, on account of one of his sons, was out in the grounds, and I was prevented from paying my respects to him. But the dog of Alcibiades, which guards the vast hall adorned with Corinthian pillars, tempted me to trespass, and I examined that imposing entrance with feelings of the highest gratification. I required no further indulgence, and being moreover, pressed for time, instead of loitering through the various apartments, I hastened to another part of the demesne, where pacing a velvet lawn of exquisite beauty, shaped in the form of a grand terrace, many times larger and more grand than Windsor terrace, and terminated, like the terrace in front of the mansion, by a temple at each end, I beheld at my feet the gray and weather-stained remains of Rivaulx Abbey, to me less interesting and less picturesque than those of Fountains Abbey.

These deviations, and a short visit paid to Mr. Dawson, —the resident surgeon of Helmsley, a very quiet and intelligent person, well read in his profession, who received me hospitably, and gave me much valuable information, especially on the subject of the mineral spring I was about to visit,—retarded my progress; but I was amply repaid at the sight of the fertile and rich vale into which the road insensibly descended, after quitting Duncombe Park, and which is, beyond conception, grand. All I have seen to-day (so I find it noted in my diary) of the North Riding south of the eastern moorlands, has impressed me with a most favourable idea of the wealth and high condition of the county, fertilized no doubt by the *débris* swept down from the great north ridge that stands at an elevation of twelve hundred feet, by the numerous *becks* which accompany the several ridges that pass down southwards from that high crest into the vale of Pickering. Many of these very *becks*, or little rivers, by the by, according to Mr. Dawson's statement, who had ascertained the fact in more cases than one by personal examination, suddenly dip it seems, and disappear into the earth at certain places, and again come to light at some more distant spot; an ingulfment noticed also by Buckland.

Mr. Wilcocks, medical practitioner at Hovingham, who has resided in that sad-looking village for nearly thirteen years, received me with kindness late in the day, and after an evening entertainment at his own house, procured for me a most luxurious bed at one of the three principal inns in the place, facing Hovingham Hall, for which the charge of *sixpence* was made the following morning by the good-natured landlord.

Mr. Wilcocks, who has from their very first discovery (1829) taken great pains to study and properly to appreciate the Hovingham mineral water, accompanied me that same morning to the spring, respecting which I may say at once, in order to save time, that neither from its locality, nor from its quality, nor indeed from its quantity, is it ever likely to become a favourite.

After walking nearly a mile and a half from the village, by an indifferent road and along a path through several fields in a low situation, which after every rain are generally in a complete state of irrigation,—I was surprised to find myself in the midst of a regular, quaking, and elastic boggy ground, threatening at every moment to sink under my weight, and in one part of which the sulphuretted spring (for it is of that nature) is found.

I examined attentively the whole of the ground adjacent, and felt convinced, on the spot, that the little square well containing water, charged with a very distinct though faint portion of sulphuretted hydrogen gas, which it parts with very rapidly by deposition, is nothing else than the collected draining of the water distilling through the strata of inflammable bituminous shale, and the fetid, compact, oolitic beds, into the vale of Pickering, to the south or inclined part of which Hovingham is situated.   From the well in question the water is allowed to flow, through an iron pipe, into a species of reservoir; the surplus being conducted to a miserable-looking wooden hut, in which there are two baths, much resorted to by the common people, and used quite cold.

Such is Hovingham Spa, with no accommodation for a safe and easy approach to the well to drink the water, and no provision made for the better classes of visiters for using it either as a warm or a cold bath.   Visiters, however, Hovingham has none; and notwithstanding all the various notes of preparation sounded to entice them thither, the Spa, as yet, can boast of no more than a limited local reputation. All that is known of the composition of its water is that it smells and tastes like all mild sulphuretted water, and that it contains, according to Dr. Travis, of Malton, five grains of solid matter in every sixteen ounces of the water, consisting of sulphate of magnesia and muriate of soda.

That such a water, notwithstanding the simplicity of its composition, possesses properties which recommend it to the attention of medical men, I have the authority of Dr Simpson of York, of Mr. Dawson of Hemsley, and of Mr. Wilcocks himself, for asserting; and indeed it is a fact to be deduced physically from its constituent principles.   As a diuretic, and in calculous disorders, it has been found beneficial.   An elderly woman, after having been afflicted with pain in the loins for several years, accompanied by inability to move, and supposed to be suffering from lumbago, having drank largely of this Spa, passed a calculus, which Mr. Wilcocks showed me, and was cured.

As was to be expected, the water is much used in cutaneous complaints, for which the place was at one time so much frequented by the neighbouring people, that the farmer who rents the land, used to collect from them, in sixpences, a sum of about thirty pounds per annum. These people used also the water as a cold bath, descending into it at its natural temperature of 48° Far., remaining three minutes up to their chins, and never complaining of chilliness, but rather of an excessive glow on coming out of the water. These baths, however, which are in their rudest form, are very little frequented now, and the utmost use made of the water is by the inhabitants of Hovingham, who drink it as their common beverage.

One mode, which suggests itself, of fertilizing the peaty earth, impregnated throughout its extent with sulphuretted hydrogen, and probably with some free sulphuric acid, as in the case of the land near Egra, in Bohemia, would be to apply it to the purposes of mud-baths. The materials might be quarried, as at Egra, and conveyed to the village, where a suitable building should be erected, with bath-rooms; and the mud being previously heated by steam, might be employed to fill appropriate tubs into which the patients might be immersed.

The beneficial effects of such baths I have already fully descanted upon in another part of the present, and likewise in a former publication. In this respect Hovingham might perchance vie with Harrogate, provided handsome and convenient accommodations for the patients were established; for the materials are equally proper at both places. But as a Spa to supply sulphuretted water for internal use to any patient above the lower classes, Hovingham will try in vain to supplant Harrogate. The worthy baronet, Sir William Wolsey, lord of this extensive manor, who has been doing all in his power to give Hovingham the benefit of a Spa, might, and I trust will, turn to account this professional suggestion.

My kind brother practitioner insisted upon escorting me from his place of residence to one of the principal market-

towns on the great north road, on my way to examine other
sulphuretted springs in this part of Yorkshire.   After travelling through a large part of the grounds of Wolsey Park, which
afforded me a partial view of Hovingham Hall, we took a circuitous route along by-roads and private drives, purposely to
become acquainted with this interesting part of the country,
which offers at this moment one or two important facts on
agriculture, besides an ample harvest of botanical curiosities.

Among the latter, one cannot help distinguishing the very
many exceedingly beautiful varieties of heath which are to
be met with at every step in Lord Carlisle and Lord Feversham
woods, or on the moors belonging to the Fairfax of Castlegil-
ling, the descendants of the great parliamentary general, and
those of Mr. Garforth of Wiganthorpe.   A large collection of
these heaths was made some time ago and deposited in the
York Museum.

But to a traveller much attached to agriculture, as I profess to be, a far more interesting sight was that of large tracks
of moorland, redeemed only since the previous Christmas,
by the last-named gentleman who had added them to his
other cultivated lands, with every prospect of success, as to
the crops I observed on his new enclosures.

The mode adopted here of converting moor or waste land
into tilled or arable land is by burning off the surface of the
heath; then paring the ground, and piling the heath in large
blocks, which are set fire to again.   The earth underneath is
necessarily scorched ; and, over it are scattered the ashes from
the burnt heaps, which are ploughed in, when a crop of tur-
nips is taken, and the land very soon after converted into
corn land.   The soil thus turned to good account looks favourable, is adhesive, free from stones, and of a rich brown
or black colour ; not unlike that of the recently recovered
tracks of land in the Lincolnshire fens, near the Witham.

The view of a very extensive district of waste land just
brought into cultivation, is calculated to suggest more than

one important consideration. That which claims attention first, is the question of preference between that process and the much vaunted one of *putting money out at interest*, by planting trees. " I am sowing my son Edward's children's fortune," observed to me many years ago a thrifty M.P. in the west of England, to whose seat I had been summoned on the occasion of that very son's (a mere child) serious illness. The senator was then engaged in planting nearly half a million of trees upon some hillocky and sandy tract of waste land, which in my opinion required nothing but a proper supply of *Flemish* manure from the neighbouring town to be made into most excellent corn land. Edward grew up and his children have since come into the world, and a large proportion of the trees (their intended fortune) have been growing up at the same time ; the growth and height of their stems being duly and regularly measured and noted down from year to year. But the children are growing faster than the trees, and the square feet of timber in the latter are not yet such as to realize the expected fortune.

Now had my friend, instead of his own speculation, adopted the scheme of the Yorkshire squire of Wiganthorpe, the vast tract of land he has condemned to nearly half a century of unprofitable returns, would have yielded not only an ample fortune to Edward's children, but one also to their *father* and *grandfather*, inasmuch as both the latter, as well as his son after him would have derived an immediate and yearly profit from the conversion of waste into arable land.

If, while driving along one of the newly-made moor roads on the Garforth property, we contrast the smooth newly-turned-up surface, oily, black, and lumpy, covered with turnip-plants, which is seen on the one side, with, on the other side, the rough and hillocky surface of the primitive moor, covered with unproductive heath, chequered by water-pools (with only a scanty portion of short pasture here and there) ; besides the large tracts on which, after rain, your horse sinks to his knees ; the conclusion to which we must instantly come is, that the man who converts most of the latter into the former sort of land, is the greatest benefactor to his neighbour, to his country, and to the world at large—for he adds at once to the general mass of food for God's creatures.

After passing through the Garforth property, our way led us to the brow of a hill, whence, upon clearing a wood on our left, a most magnificent panorama burst upon us, York Minster forming its central point. Straight before us rose, upon a hill, that curious *enclavé* of the Bishop of Durham called Crake, marked by a solitary short square tower, the remains of a castle renowned in baronial times. Between it and the foot of the hill on which we stood, Brandsby Hall, the seat of Francis Cholmondeley, Esq., lay imbedded in a wood, with the rectory just behind it.

The vast plain, now stretched like a great map before us, appeared rich, and highly cultivated, containing large tracts of the finest grazing county in England, on which the short-horn and the Leicester sheep are bred to a very great extent; as I had occasion to ascertain in part while going through the farms of Mr. Wiley, the celebrated and largest gentleman-grazier and breeder in these parts. Easingwold is the market-town immediately adjoining.

At Thirsk, the next post-town, I bade adieu to my kind and intelligent guide and brother practitioner, and heartily wished him better luck in his laborious and ill-requited office, of surgeon to a Union of sixteen parishes, for which he receives the paltry sum of twenty pounds a year! Mr. Wilcocks is the son of the Rev. James Wilcocks, who, while trout-fishing one day, discovered the Spa near Guisborough; of the grammar-school of which place he has been master for many years.

CHAPTER XVI.

CROFT AND DINSDALE.

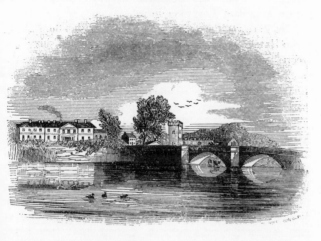

Arrival at CROFT—The Spa Hotel—The "OLD SPA"—Its properties and physical characters—The CANNIWELL—Surgeon Walker and his pet Spa—His extensive practice, and Analysis of the Waters—The "NEW WELL"—Pump-room and Baths—A *tremendous* Water—Its Appearance, Taste, and Immediate Effect—Marvellous Error!—Effect of the Water on the Author—Interior of the SPA HOTEL—Efficacy of the Croft and Dinsdale Waters in the Cure of Diseases—Consumption and Prussic Acid—The Author's claims—Dinsdale Hotel—View from the Hill—Eligible Residence in Summer for any body—DINSDALE SPRING —Taste of the Water—Its Virtues—Danger of divulging your Name —Middleton One Row—The principal Inns—Fashionable GAZETTE —Spelling-book—A Circulating Library—BURY *versus* BULWER—A Project—A Failure—Sad Misfortune—The Hen and the Eggs.

WITHOUT any further delay I hastened towards CROFT, keeping always in sight, on my right, Black Hambleton Hills until I passed Northallerton, and alighted at the " Spa Hotel," in full time to examine, leisurely and with care, the various parts of this comparatively modern watering-place. The road, before reaching Croft, passes under one of the arches of the great railroad now constructing from York to Darlington, which is projected across the valley, and forms part of the great north of England railroad.

John Emerson, the very civil and obliging landlord of the " Spa Hotel," in manners far superior to persons of his class, escorted me to the springs, at about a quarter of a mile from the hotel, in a field near the road-side, where the "Old Spa " is situated.   Nothing can be more primitive or of ruder aspect than the whole concern.   At a very short distance from a very humble-looking cottage is the spring or head of the well, which is generally kept covered with a flagstone.   Here the mineral water is collected, and travels thence, by a short pipe, to a little cistern by the side of the porch of a cottage or Spahouse, for public use ; as well as to the interior of the same building, where it fills up to a constant level a cold plunging-bath, six feet and a half long and four feet wide, sunk four feet into the ground.   Five stone steps lead down to the bottom, which is paved with large flagstones.

The water keeps incessantly running, coming in from the head well at the rate of about twenty-four pints to the minute, according to my experiments.   It is beautifully clear and transparent, and smells of its peculiar gas, though not so strongly as Harrogate water.   I should compare it to the Aldfield water, near Ripon, already described, and it must be looked upon as the draining of the north-east side of the great Richmond Hills, in the same manner that Hovingham spring derives its origin from the draining of the south-west shale and limestone strata of the eastern moorlands.

The temperature is 51°, and never varies.   A deposit of sulphur, as at Aldfield and Hovingham, is observed in the head well, and on the stone troughs through which the water runs, as well as upon the grass twigs near them.   Its taste is precisely like that at Hovingham—saponaceous and alkaline. People drink from three to seven half-pint tumblers of it, and find it strongly diuretic.   They, however, prefer bathing in the water, which operation is always performed at its natural low temperature of 51°.   They take three or four dips overhead in the plunging-bath without complaining of chilliness, and assert that they experience, on coming out of the bath, a most genial glow of the skin, which feels quite soft after the immersion.   This bath, however, is only resorted to by the common and working people—principally on Sundays.

The " Old Spa " was closed upon the opening of the new bathing-establishment ; but in consequence of the water of the former being preferred, and people coming to it from many distant parts, it was again put into operation ; and one or two nice lodging-houses were built near the spot.

Entering a wood at a short distance from the " Old Spa " we find, after walking a quarter of a mile, a small hillock by the side of a narrow but rapid *beck* or brook, within which is a well of sulphur-water, lined with red sandstone taken from the Tees.   The water smells and tastes more strongly of sulphur than that of the " Old Spa."   It is conveyed by *tile*-pipes to the building of the new baths, to be described presently ; and its waste runs into the beck at the rate of fifty pints in a minute, and from thence into the Tees.   The poor people prefer drinking this water on the spot, thinking it more genuine.   The name it bears is *Canniwell.*

Thomas Dixon Walker, surgeon at Harworth (a small place between Croft and Dinsdale), a gentleman so much engaged in practice that he is never to be seen except either mounting or alighting from a horse, and always equipped in top-boots and spurred, has published some " Facts relative to the medicinal properties of the Croft and Dinsdale waters."   The work has gone through three editions, and must consequently have been read ; yet, oddly enough, the little volume in question contains not the slightest description of the local arrangements of the Spa, with the exception of a ground-plan and elevation of the new baths. It is to supply that deficiency that I have entered into so many particulars.

In speaking of the Canniwell spring, that work states that it rises in the middle of a brook. We have seen that this is an error.

I collect from Mr. Walker's analysis of the "Old Spa," that my notion of its similarity to the Hovingham water is borne out by its slight impregnation with sulphuretted gas, of which he reckons but one cubic inch and three-quarters in a gallon. And I am also pleased to find myself confirmed in the idea I formed of the origin of the old sulphur springs at Croft, by what Mr. Walker relates relative to the history of the discovery of the "New Well." This was done by boring to the depth of twenty-six fathoms, when a much more strongly-impregnated sulphur-water than that of the Old Well rose to the surface.

Over this "New Well," so discovered in August, 1827, or rather in front of it, Sir William Chaytor, of Witton Castle, upon whose property the Spa is situated, caused to be erected a suite of baths, with a pump-room fifty feet by seventeen, with the principal elevation in the cottage style (decorated with a veranda or covered walk) facing the east.

The pump-room is a modern oblong room, plain and unadorned. In it the sulphur-water of the new spring is distributed, as well as that of another or third spring, the *Canniwell*, before mentioned, by means of the objectionable mode of pumping. The first of these waters is generally drunk warmed, and with a tea-spoonful of common salt, as the water is totally deficient in that ingredient. Ladies I have seen promenading at two o'clock in the afternoon under the veranda, who now and then applied to the pump-room woman for a small tumbler of the stronger kind of water, mingling the said quantity of kitchen salt in it. With what appetite they sat down to dinner afterwards I could not learn, as I did not join the gay throng at the table d'hôte in the New Hotel. But it seemed an odd time of day to quaff sulphur-water of no ordinary intensity.

The bath-rooms, with their respective dressing-rooms, are neatly arranged behind and on each side of the pump-room. Among them is a large plunging-bath and a vapour-bath, and convenience for shower-baths; all of which are to be had at prices much the same as at all other Spas—perhaps cheaper. The baths are lined with stone flags, and paved with slate. During the season of 1837 there had been as many as eight hundred bathers; but at the present and last season the number has been sadly inferior to that—a circumstance for which the unlucky author of " The Spas of Germany " was considered responsible.

The water supplied to the cold plunging-bath is derived from the "Canniwell Spring;" that for the warm baths is pumped by hand from the " New Well," adjoining, into a cistern and boiler above the bathing-rooms; and such is the strength of the sulphuretted effluvia of this water that all the doors painted with white lead-colour have acquired a jet black coating. This is not to be marvelled at, considering that Mr. Walker detected no less than twenty-two and a quarter cubic inches of sulphuretted hydrogen in the gallon; a quantity larger than that of any sulphur spring in England.

The source of this *tremendous* water—for such I must designate it—I afterwards proceeded to examine. It consists of a wide shaft or sunken well, kept always covered; upon the inspection of which I found the mineral water reaching to within two feet of the margin, and looking on the surface like thick frothy soap-lees, of an opake bluish-white colour, but appearing very clear when pumped out of the shaft into the cistern, through a large leaden pipe which dips considerably into the water.

When the latter is received into a glass a great many air-

bubbles are seen to ascend from the bottom of it, and to adhere
to the inside of the glass. Its taste I can hardly describe.
It is at first sweetish and astringent, corrugating the inside
skin of the lips; but it soon becomes bitterish and metallic,
as if Epsom salts were mixed with a preparation of lead.
It is a discouraging taste, and I question not but it is owing
to the presence of the leaden pipes plunged into the water—
producing sulphuret of lead, which falls in scales from the
surface of the pipe into the water, contaminating the latter.

How such an arrangement could ever have been permitted
for a moment, it is not easy to conjecture. I stated its fatal
objection to the persons around me, and urged it afterwards
to Mr. Walker himself, who admitted its justice, and con-
fessed (as indeed he had previously done in his little work)
that the water required great caution in its internal use, having often produced hypercatharsis, and even vomiting—at
which I marvel not. I shall not easily forget the momentary
effect which the small quantity of the water I drank in the
pump-room had on my head, my palate, and my stomach ; and
I should be sorry indeed to prescribe any such water internally, under ordinary circumstances, without great and
minute precaution ; but under the circumstance of a large
body of lead being constantly present in it—I should prescribe it never. There appears also to be in this water a
natural oily substance, which Mr. Walker has called *petro-
leum*, and which is not less objectionable than the lead.

On my return from the " New Well" to the Spa Hotel, I
passed Croft Hall, formerly the seat of Sir William Chaytor,
now converted into a school for young ladies, which enjoys
high reputation. The hotel is well situated at the entrance
of Croft, near the bridge, and contains, besides numerous
apartments, a grand ball-room and billiard-room, as well as
a news-room for subscribers. The terms for boarding at the
public table are a guinea and a half a week, with half a
guinea more for a bedroom. A private sitting-room may be

obtained for half a guinea extra; and servants are boarded and lodged at three shillings a day.

I am rather inclined to think that the pet Spa of Mr. Walker, who is lucky enough to live *entre deux*, is Dinsdale; the water of which he considers equally efficacious as Croft's water in hepatic disorders, and cutaneous complaints, in Dyspepsia, Hypochondriasis, Diabetes, and even poisoning by lead. Of all these complaints Mr. Walker has published many cases of recovery effected by these waters. A very recent instance of the lastmentioned accident, the ill effects of which were checked and ultimately removed by the Dinsdale waters, Mr. Walker mentioned to me. It was that of a man employed in some neighbouring lead-works, who had his upper extremities completely paralyzed, and who was sent home quite re-established, after drinking the Dinsdale water, and bathing in it six times.

The same medical practitioner has a long article in his book, on pulmonary consumption, which he considers curable in its earliest stages by the Dinsdale waters—combined with prussic acid. Of the efficacy of the latter medicine in diseases of the chest Mr. Walker, like most of the medical practitioners in this county, has had ample and satisfactory evidence.

It is now twenty-one years since I first introduced to the notice of the profession and first prescribed, in this country, prussic acid in pulmonic and other diseases, with the most complete success. I continued to do so almost single-handed for two or three years—meeting with every species of opposition and unfair hostility from my medical brethren—as I have since met on the occasion of my first making public my peculiar system of counter-irritation—or the mode of curing diseases by external applications. Truth prevailed at length in the case of the first medicine, as it is beginning to prevail in that of the second; and both practices are becoming general :' to such a

degree indeed that some people have appropriated to themselves the merit of the suggestion in regard to the first practice, as well as of my subsequent recommendation of the
second ; sinking my name, all the while, as if " I had never
been." But even with such drawbacks I accept and enjoy
thankfully the satisfaction of finding, from the testimony of
medical men in all parts of the kingdom, published from year
to year, in favour of the use of prussic acid, and of the am-
moniated lotions, that the value of my therapeutical recommendations, instead of diminishing has gathered strength with
the progress of time.*

The traveller who wishes to see the twin Spa of this border
land of Durham, DINSDALE, has only to cross the bridge
over the Tees, here rapid and shallow ; pass through Harworth, the birthplace, as every one knows, of the celebrated self-taught mathematician Emmerson, whose eccentricities gained him the reputation of a necromancer, and
whose biography is one of the most amusing in English literature ; and after a short drive along the north bank of the
river, upon reaching the village of Nesham, turn into the
left road which leads to the " Dinsdale Hotel."

* From a recent statement in the *Penny Magazine,* a publication which
circulates, it is said, to the extent of 150,000 copies, I learn that the college of Physicians, in Edinburgh, have admitted, in the new edition of
their Pharmacopœia, lately published, my formula for the counter-irritation, or stimulating lotion, which I first inserted in the *Lancet* of October, 1838. Whether they have done so with the name of the inventor
attached to it or not, that journal does not mention, nor can I learn, as
I have not the Pharmacopiœa in question at hand. But even without such acknowledgment, I am thankful for the honourable station
that has been assigned to a preparation which will be found more and
more valuable the better it is known to the public and the profession.
The able writer of the article on stimulating applications, in the *Penny
Magazine* alluded to, is entitled to my thanks for giving so wide a circulation, through his pages, to the process for preparing my counter-irritating lotion.

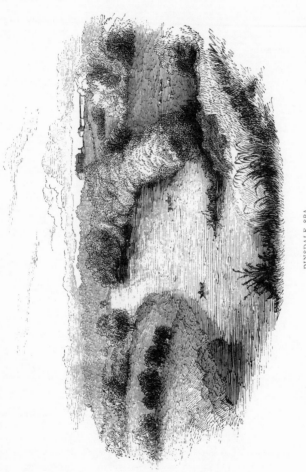

DINSDALE SPA.

The Spa itself is variously denominated Dinsdale, and Middleton One Row ; and some people have imagined (my-self among the rest) that they were two distinct springs. But the double denomination arises from the fact, that the mineral spring is in the parish of Dinsdale, there being no village of that name, but only an hotel ; while Middleton One Row is the village nearest to the well, on the opposite side of the little dale descending at a right angle upon the Tees.

The road to the " hotel" winds up a very steep hill, from the summit of which a fine and extensive view is obtained of the vale of the Tees, and the distant hills both of the North and West Riding. This hotel, which is the offspring of a bright idea of the noble earl who inherits his title from a bordering county, is a large brick building placed within a court planted all round, and having its longest side turned to the south, with ground in front of it tastefully laid out. From its windows, in this direction, the sparkling Tees is seen meandering in serpentine girations through the broad mass of a highly-cultivated champaign country, called the Vale of Cleveland, or " Garden of Yorkshire." The Hambleton hills on the farthest south-east horizon, close the picture.

The hill upon which the hotel stands, as a conspicuous object, slopes gently and park-like to the east, as far as the spring, which is placed in a hollow near the margin of the Tees ; and on the ridge of a corresponding hill on the left, is the row of red brick and tiled houses which originates the name before mentioned, of Middleton One Row. There are pretty paths and walks through the plantations, and beds of flowers grace the nearer portion of the pleasure-grounds, open to the inmates of the hotel.

The interior of this establishment affords first-rate accommodation. There is a large dining-room at one end, and at the east end the great drawing-room. In the centre of the ground-floor there are three private sitting-rooms ; up stairs three other sitting-rooms, and one other room higher still, with a bay-window enjoying the finest prospect from the house. The internal arrangement is commodious and symmetrical, and the furniture, though plain, is good and selected with taste. Dinsdale Hotel, in fine, is one of those places so happily situated, and by nature as well as art so well favoured, that, as a summer residence for invalids, even without the resource of any mineral water at hand, a medical man consulted by the wealthy of the neighbouring counties can recommend it with perfect confidence and pleasure. Of course the situation is lonely and retired, as far as society is in question; there being only that which is to be found in the house. But where the enjoyment of the purest air, with an enchanting scene, accompanied by general tranquillity, is an object, Dinsdale Hotel will be found to afford it most successfully.

It is to be regretted that, of late years, the intrusion of the noise of the approaching and passing railroad-trains between Darlington and Stockton, in the rear of Middleton One Row, has somewhat interrupted the tranquillity of this charming retreat.

I had but a slight glimpse of the landlord of the Dinsdale, Mr. Forsyth, and a still slighter one of the landlady; yet I saw enough of both to make me think that the inmates of their establishment are not likely to complain either of their inefficiency, or the exorbitance of their charges.*

I have dwelt more at length upon this Spa-Hotel than I do in general, and even before treating of the "Spa" itself, because, in reality, I cannot help looking upon it as a most excellent "Maison de Santé" of itself, during summer weather. The sportsman, too, when the invalids have vacated their comfortable apartments, might find this hotel a desirable head-quarter later in the year, being situated in the very centre of the Lambton, Harworth, and Cleveland hunts.

---

* They are a trifle higher than those at Croft.

From the hotel, a pretty winding road, with a plantation on each side, leads down to the spring immediately upon the bank of the Tees. It was discovered by labourers in the service of the Lambton family, whilst engaged in searching for coals. They had just reached, by boring, to the depth of 72 feet, chiefly through red sandstone and whinstone, when the spring burst forth.

The first object I beheld was a plunging bath, in which the water on its surface looked yellow and creamy. The other bath-rooms are commodious, and, like every other part of the Spa, useful, though neither handsome nor pretending. The water comes up through pipes from nearly the level of the river, to a large cistern, and is thence conveyed again by pipes to the pump-room. The latter is a very plain and unpretending apartment, something like a servants' hall; having, however, an arrangement for the distribution of the water, which is very ingenious, and worthy of being placed in a better lodging. Three marble slabs placed against the walls have each two small spouts projecting from them, through which, by pressing inwardly a button placed over them, the water instantly issues in a free stream. Two or three of the spouts are of glass, and from one of these, at one end of the room, the water is obtained, warmed to 90 degrees. This attention paid to the proper choice of materials in using sulphuretted waters, and to the administering of the said water at a uniform degree of warmth, is worthy of being imitated at other Spas of greater pretension.

I could not see the spring or well itself, so as to taste its water at the source; neither could I learn with what material the cistern holding the sulphur-water was lined, and what pipes were used. All seemed behind the scenes, and the attendant pump-room woman could not tell me any thing respecting these points. I asked the same question of one of the visiters; but he had never seen the spring, nor inquired for it!

The taste of the water at the pump-room when cold, and at its ordinary temperature of 52 degrees, is at first sweetish, then slightly pungent, and *âpre*—neither did it go down so saponaceous as the water of the "Old Spa" at Croft. When drunk warm, the taste is at first smooth to the tongue, more saponaceous than when cold, not so pungent, yet still a little so ; and, after a few seconds, some sensation of saltishness is manifested. The charges for bathing and drinking the water are the same as at Croft.

Mr. Walker has the merit of having analyzed this water also, from whose statement it appears that there are in a gallon of it two hundred and twenty-four grains of solid matter, more than the half of which he considers to be sulphate of lime. This point, as well as the manner by which Mr. Walker ingeniously endeavours to account for the presence of so large a proportion of a salt sparingly soluble in water, requires consideration. The proportion of sulphuretted hydrogen gas, ascribed by him to the water, is two cubic inches less than that in the new well of Croft, and yet equal to the strongest water at Harrogate. The analysis will be found in my table.

This water cannot, from its composition, be either a purgative or a powerful solvent. I have already hinted at the several complaints in which it has been found useful. As it requires long boiling to deprive the water of its sulphuretted hydrogen, when the quantity present is as large as that in Dinsdale water, and that of the new well at Croft, it must be evident that both waters are highly calculated for warm bathing, since a fair proportion of the sulphuretted gas will remain present in the water, after warming it—a circumstance that does not obtain when waters, slightly impregnated with the gas, are long exposed to heat.

As a visiter I was requested, while in the act of looking at the pump-room, and after tasting the water, to enter my name in the visiter's book, kept in the ante-room of the Spa. I did so ; but, with the exception of what happened to me at the gates of Warsaw in 1828,—when, having declared aloud to the officer in command my name und character, I was followed by a swarm of Jew beggars with *plica* and sores, urging me to heal them,—I never recollect the declaration of my name in a public place to have led to the result that followed the one at Dinsdale. As I was sneaking away, after having examined every thing connected with the Spa, I found myself successively stopped first by one invalid, who, after a word of apology, asked me whether the cold or hot bath would be the best; then by another, who desired to know what quantity of the water should be drunk in the morning; and, lastly, by a third, who was anxious to ascertain if drinking the water both morning and afternoon would be injurious.

I delivered my opinion to the best of my judgment; but such interruptions, considering the arduous task I had before me, I voted to be a bore. However, it is better to be taken for what one really is, than to be mistaken for something else. At York the driver of my open vehicle from Harrogate insisted on tumbling me into an old coach-inn, the "Old George;" because, from the wrappers I had on, and my black leathern portmanteau, I probably looked tolerably commercial. As a commercial traveller, therefore, I was thrust by the waiter into the commercial room, where, after the clouds of the Nicotian vapours had subsided, so as to allow my arrival to be noticed, I was greeted with "How is trade with you?" and with "Any luck to-day?"

Taking the footpath through the plantations, along the bank of the river, I was directing my steps towards Middleton One Row, from the Spa, when I was overtaken by the man of the baths, who happened to be absent while I had been making my inquiries of his wife, touching the sources and management of the mineral waters. He informed me that the spring is in a rock behind the bath, from which the water issues at the rate of twelve gallons in a minute, and is conveyed to two cisterns—the one as a reserve for the cold, and the other for keeping the water continually warm, fit for bathing; an object which is accomplished not by steam, but by ordinary fire placed under the cistern. These cisterns, or reservoirs, are cleared out every week, when a crust of hard whitish sulphur is removed from the inside. The pipes used, according to this man's statement, seem to be of lead; so that even here we have the same mistake committed, of exposing lead to the effluvia of sulphuretted hydrogen gas!

Middleton, stretching in a crescent-like form on the top of a lofty and gently-sloping bank of the Tees, consists as I before stated of *one row* of lodging-houses, principally for the accommodation of those who come hither to use the Dinsdale Spa water. The distance from the Spa is about a mile, not *below* the baths, as Dr. Peacock, another writer on Dinsdale waters has stated, but *above* it, on the ridge of the hill.

The principal inn, kept by an honest widow (Mrs. Hanson), is very clean, and contains plenty of excellent accommodation at reasonable charges. It occupies nearly the centre of the row or crescent, with a direct western aspect, and I found it quite full,—as indeed were all the lodging-houses. During the season families of the first respectability from Northumberland, Durham, and Yorkshire come hither, as I perceived indeed on glancing at the " Spa and Sea-side Fashionable Gazette," the luxury of possessing which, Dinsdale and Middleton share in common with Croft and Seaton on the Coast. And a smart thing truly the said Gazette is, with all its appurtenances of a vignette and lacelike pattern of a border to its pages! Oddly enough, there appeared in one of the numbers so many monosyllabic names, as those of some of the visiters who dwelled for the most part in the same house, that I was forcibly reminded of my old spelling-book, " Abbs, Bell, Brown, Dees, Hall, Hog, Last, Laws, Meek, Muff, Ord, Stag, Tate, Winn,"—*cum multis aliis.* Most of these oddities were snugly lodged at the " Woodbine Cottage, at Croft,"—the rest were under the same roof with myself; and I imagine, equally as much pleased as I was with the hotel and the treatment they received from the landlady, who is the most civil person in the world. I must not omit to add, that the beds here are particularly good, and that, in fact, one could hardly expect such accommodations, at so reasonable an expense, in such a place.

Who, at a Spa, consisting of merely twenty one-story-high-lodging-houses, brick and mortar built, overlooking the Tees and the vale of Cleveland, would expect to find, besides an Hotel, a Bazaar, an Omnibus, and a Circulating Library, as well as a due proportion of phaetons and donkeys? Yet so it is. Moreover, the *Bazaar* has its raffles, at which articles from Birmingham and Tonbridge are disposed of at prices four-times their original worth. The *Hotel* has its billiard-table, where a few young Durham students knock the balls about; while the opulent Cleveland farmer and grazier, in *shorts*, with strings dangling from their knees, look over the game and whiff their 'bacco-smoke through the fine white clay. Lastly, the *Circulating Library* has its Bulwers and its Burys.

To the latter establishment (which I should have passed by, from having seen " Grocery" inscribed over its door without reading further, had not my good landlady, who was watching me, set me right) I paid a visit, in hopes of there finding Mr. Walker's account of the Dinsdale waters. A very comely young person stepped in at the same time, and deposited an odd volume of a novel, stating that her mamma had sent it back, for she did not like it, and would call on the morrow for something better. I took up the single volume from the counter. It was the " Disowned." "Bless me, Mr. Winter," said I, " how can you afford the newest publications to your subscribers in so thinly an inhabited colony ?"—" Afford, sir? Why it depends on the sort of works. Look ye, sir. This lady has rejected the ' Disowned,' and so have many others before her, though no one will ' own ' it. Not so with the ' Divorced,' for Lady Charlotte is just now a great favourite with both misses and their mammas; though, of the two, the latter have been my best customers for that work. The mere lending her ladyship's novel to them this season has already produced me the sum of five pounds. Upon this, I had made up my mind to get myself a good silver watch out of my lady's duodecimos, and in honour to her, so soon as the pounds should have become guineas : when in an unlucky moment, a lady subscriber, who was perusing one of the volumes while walking through our shaded groves by the side of the Tees, dropped it into the running stream, in one of those moments of absence which the perusal of that work is said to produce. My dream· of the silver time-measure, from that *minute*, vanished."

" In that case," said I, " the fair lady must pay for her absence, and give you the value of the book."

" Poor recompence that," retorted Master Winter, whom I discovered to be a dry bit of a wag. " She may pay for the hen; but who is to pay for the eggs ?" Now this for an " *épicier* " I vow is not bad.

CHAPTER XVII.

GUISBOROUGH AND REDCAR.

The " Quaker's Railroad," as that is called which from
Darlington conveys coals to the mouth of the Tees, is an exceedingly convenient thing for such as are in a hurry to leave
Dinsdale and Middleton, as I acknowledge myself to have
been, anxious as I was to post on for the purpose of visiting
the many other places connected with my present inquiry.
In less than half an hour the said rail conveyance transferred
me from Widow Hanson's comfortable apartments to the
Vane Arms, in the great market-place at Stockton, where retaining the character that had been lent me at York, of a
commercial traveller, I took possession of a snug corner in
the commercial room, and with a knowing air, rang a peal
for my breakfast.

I am here beginning to tread on delicate ground.   At the

conclusion of my tour through Germany in 1836, I had occasion to go over certain minor districts, and visit three or four lesser German Spas, which had been already traced and described by a popular writer with success. In doing that I followed a " Head." I am now about to follow in the wake of another " Head " whilst engaged in looking after *English* Spas; and although our individual objects in making this " home tour " be widely different, yet as some of the places visited by us both are the same, it is not unlikely that I may appear to trench on other people's ground. I can only say that such is not my intention. It is a curious coincidence no doubt, that in the case of two works, the one upon German, the other upon English mineral waters, I should have had for my immediate predecessors, in treating a small part of those very subjects, two brothers equally and deservedly popular. At this I naturally rejoice; and as it is said that " two *heads* are better than one"—so I trust that to *follow* two Heads will be considered better than to have followed none.

Here at Stockton, the author of the " Home Tour" has preceded me with his valuable remarks on coal-waggons and coal Staiths ; but he has said nothing of the town itself and the condition of the people. In the like manner, Sir George has given a faithful and spirited description of " the salmon-leap ;" an artificial cascade, distant about two miles from Dinsdale Spa, up the river Tees—though he has omitted the details of the Spa itself.

Further on, the same writer has descanted on the wonders of Hartlepool, whither I shall also follow him; but he left matters there in an unsatisfactory state, and I had the gratification of finding them the reverse. In fact, although the " head and the tail" may have followed each other (as they naturally will), it does not follow that the latter should *wag* precisely where the other has nodded ;—and so we go on with Stockton.

This town is losing its old topographical station, and

getting a new character, that of an *entrepôt,* instead of being a
seaport of export.   On the one hand, the railroad from Darlington, and the Clarence railroad from Durham, have
brought inland produce to Stockton; and on the other hand
the new town of Middleburgh—the wonderfully rapid creation of the " Friends"—set down at the very mouth of the Tees,
six miles nearer to the open sea than Stockton—have robbed
the latter place of its station as a sea harbour.   Vessels now
anchor at Middleburgh snug and comfortable, which before
strove to mount the river and reach Stockton, after overcoming the sad surf, tossed over the bar by easterly gales :—so
that Stockton, as a maritime place, is become insignificant.

A visit to the waterside soon convinced me of this; and a
further inspection of the principal streets exhibited to my
view the inevitable effects of such a change.   I found every
part near the water-side in a deplorable state of dirt; and
most of the streets branching off from the long and wide
main street (one of the handsomest in any provincial town
in the north) and leading or descending towards the port,
narrow and filthy.

In the upper part of the town, towards the back of the old
church, many of the houses, still retaining their showy fronts,
were closed—the grass was growing in the middle of the
streets—and some of the latter, which seemed quite new,
were unpaved and steeped in mire.   The people appeared
squalid and ill-dressed,—discontented and not well-looking;
yet, according to the authority of an intelligent bookseller
and stationer in the market-place, with whom I had a long
and interesting conversation, matters at Stockton ought to
appear better; for not only coals are brought down to the
place for transmission to and shipment at Middleburgh, but
also the produce of the mines from the western counties,
such as lead, &c.   Stockton is also becoming a manufacturing town.   Already it has a cotton-mill of considerable
extent, and a flourishing pottery, which is about to be

followed by a second, the materials or clay being brought back by the vessels which carry coals hence to the southern coast.

The people at Stockton must have been inclined to the *dolce far niente* when they turned chartists, shortly before the time of my visit, and set about grumbling in good earnest, wandering in groups, the very picture of indolence and wretchedness; else, if we are to believe my informant, they need not have looked as they did, nor have been starving. At no time (so the said seller of stamps assured me), had the industrious classes had less reason for being dissatisfied with their lot; work might have been had plentifully, and none need have remained idle for an instant. Bricklayers, masons, and mechanics could command from twenty-two to twenty-four shillings a week wages, and ship builders as much as thirty. It is in these very classes of operatives, that Stockton found in former days among its inhabitants, many men who attained in various paths of life a high degree of celebrity.

The new seaport of Middleburgh, the site of which nine years ago was marked by a solitary farm-house, now boasts of a population of four thousand souls, all of them engaged in carrying on a lucrative commerce. The extension of the Darlington railroad to this place from Stockton, by means of a suspension bridge over the Tees, has been the main cause of so rapid an increase. A neat Gothic church was lately erected there, for the accommodation of the many who belong to the church of England. Middleburgh in fact is one, and as yet the most important, of the rival harbours which have successfully wrested much of the trade from Tynemouth and Sunderland. We shall see presently that another more formidable competitor is rising on the same coast.

None but those who have visited the district would probably believe the assertion, that a drive from Stockton to Guisborough affords one of the richest treats in England to the lover of landscapes; yet so it is, and I much regretted when the driver of my humble vehicle halted and told me that our journey was at an end, depositing me at the same time at the house of the physician of the lastmentioned place,— who immediately accompanied me to the mineral spring.

In the course of this short excursion, I purposely directed my conductor to lead me through Marton, an humble village a few miles from Guisborough, which boasts of having given birth to Captain Cook. Even to breathe for a moment within the circle in which a man of imperishable name first drew his breath, is a circumstance of stirring interest to a traveller; still more so to one, who during some years of his early life lived on that same element, and was in that same service which witnessed the achievements of the illustrious navigator.

After a drive of a mile and a half on the south-east road from Guisborough, skirting the lesser Cleveland hills, my friendly companion and I entered a narrow carriage-way, which presently plunged abruptly into a thick and intricate wood. Following here a very tortuous path, hardly wide enough for a two-wheel carriage, and keeping along the brink of a murmuring *beck* on an alum-shale-rock bed, noisy and turbulent, we reached at length a most romantic and rocky nook, enlarged from what nature had made it by former alum-miners, but most solitary and retired.

At a spot where the torrent sweeps along a projecting mass of slaty rock, by the side of which it has scooped out its own shallow channel, and under impending portions of the rocks which hang over from the oposite bank, a stream of the most beautiful and transparent water is seen to spout immediately from the shale strata, and being conducted through a stone pipe, issues conveniently for the use of the drinkers.

The taste is slightly sulphuretted, as is its smell; but this removed (and nothing is so easy) the water tastes as sapid as pure spring water. Perhaps after a little while, and on reflection, one can fancy the presence of a little of the bitterness of muriate of lime; but such a taste is very faint indeed.

The stream flows at the rate of thirty pints in a minute; its temperature was 50°, while that of the air was 63°. It is probable that while the alum-works (now wholly abandoned) were rife in this secluded spot, which can boast of having been the place where alum was first manufactured in England in Elizabeth's time, the workmen may have noticed this water; but its introduction to public attention was due to the Rev. James Wilcocks, as I before observed, and is of as recent a date as 1822. Since then, it has acquired a certain degree of local celebrity. A rude bath-room for using the water, either as a cold or a hot bath, has been erected under the rock, and during fine weather a woman attends from Guisborough to supply the wants of the visiters.

The approach to, and situation of, this spring, are the most romantic I ever beheld in England. Its vicinity, also, to Redcar, as well as Whitby on the coast, besides a multitude of country-seats of great importance by which it is surrounded, invest the place with much additional interest. It will not, however, become very readily a 'fashionable Spa, —there being many difficulties to overcome for that purpose, many wants to be supplied, and improvements to be suggested. Around the spring the fractured shaly-rock is covered with aluminous efflorescence.

I have inserted in my general table the analysis of this mineral water, published in 1823, by Mr. Goodwill, an apothecary at Lofthouse. How far it is to be relied upon, I am not prepared to say ; it seems to have been conducted with great care. A water said to contain only 23¼ grains of solid matter in a gallon, or in other words not quite three grains of saline ingredients in a pint, with only the eighth part of a cubic inch of sulphuretted hydrogen gas, cannot be expected to produce any very wonderful effects on the human constitution, except on homœopathic principles. Acccordingly I did not hear of any very extraordinary cure performed by means of this water; although some cases of indigestion,

relaxed and weak bowels, acidity, loss of blood, and cutaneous disorders, were mentioned to me on good authority, as
having been completely restored. This I can readily con-
ceive, and I have no doubt more cases of disease might be
successfully treated by this very water, from the happy combination it contains of alkaline principles, with the moderate
tonic dose of alum.

In returning from the spring through Guisborough, the
remains of the old Augustine abbey, which present to this
day tracery of perhaps one of the most elegant Gothic windows left to us of the twelfth century, together with the arch
of the priory, still left standing not far from those vestiges of
monastic times,—detained me a short time.

But I felt considerably more interested in a conversation I had
with the reverend discoverer of the mineral spring, who being,
moreover, master of the free grammar-school of Guisborough,
entered fully into the subject of education—a question on
which most of the leading public men of our day have recently cast their venture, and staked their reputation as
statesmen.

My reverend friend's experience, however, in practical education, *long* as it had been, could not be said to be very *great ;*
for it had never extended beyond the teaching of the simple
elements of the latin tongue. He was one of the many hundred examples of the little foresight our great ancestors
evinced, in providing for the instruction of their contemporary
as well as succeeding generations, when they left quite enough
to ill-requite a teacher for striving to cram with the rudiments
of a language never likely to be of service to them, the children of petty tradesmen, shopkeepers, and labourers.

In a desolate-looking room, surrounded by empty forms
and benches, designated as the Free Grammar School of
Guisborough, founded in Elizabeth's reign, there sat at a top
table, opposite the seat of the reverend instructor, three
little dirty and ragged urchins, with slate and pencil,

and a Lilly's grammar, who were spending their afternoon hours of gratuitous instruction, in declining *hic, hæc,* and *hoc felix;* at which *happy* work they had been engaged during several successive days ;—and for the trouble of going through with them this daily farce, from year to year—the pious founder of the school had assigned the stipend of fifty pounds to the pedagogue.

When it is considered that in England, sums large enough to endow a first-rate college in each county for the most complete system of general and useful education, are squandered (for as they are uselessly spent, they are in truth squandered) in obedience to bequests, equally miscalculated and unprofit-able as the one of Guisborough school, made in the olden times with the intention of instructing the people; and when we reflect also that in the largest majority of cases the ful-filment of that intention has been perfectly unattainable, through circumstances totally independent of the teachers ; we shall not wonder at the expression used by a noble mar-quis high in the councils of her Majesty, in a letter addressed to the Bishop of Exeter, that " this country, in the scale of *secular* education, is inferior to the central states of Europe."

And yet to read the hundreds of advertisements under the head of " Education," which appear in the papers of the metropolitan city of York alone, one would expect that country at least to afford a marked exception to the noble lord's sweeping assertion. At all events, it cannot be said that, of establishments meant to promote *secular* education in Yorkshire, there is any deficiency. Neither is any allure-ment or soft persuasion spared by the conductors of those es-tablishments, to induce parents to give their children a proper *secular* education. Indeed, on the score of economy alone, it would appear as if those conductors of educational in-struction offered an actual premium to parents for sending their children to school; since in some of the announcements, out of thirty-five which I have now before me in a single number of the *York Herald*, I read of academies, classical, commercial, and mathematical, where every thing is taught for the mind, and where the body is equally well taken care of in every requisite of life, for the sum of sixteen guineas per annum !

The truth is, that with all these facilities, private as well as public, *secular* education among the masses is as Lord Lansdowne designated it ; and the causes of it are obvious : the total absence of a uniform, large, and liberal system of instruction throughout the country, applicable to the classes to be instructed, and to their future wants is the first reason ; and the self-assumption, unrestrained by any law, of the important character and functions of teachers, by any man or woman who thinks the opening of a school likely to prove a good speculation, is the second reason. Until such time as one and the same scheme of popular instruction shall have been defined and enforced by the state, and none but teachers purposely trained, examined, and approved of, shall be appointed to work out that scheme, secular education in England will continue " inferior to that of the central states of Europe."

Hence the true English philanthropist ought to view with gladness any endeavour, however feeble and ineffective at first, that may be made to attain the second of the two important objects, by means of training schools,—in the hope that the good results that may be expected from them, will enable the legislature hereafter to complete the plan, by prescribing a uniform and universal system of tuition.

We have a most triumphant evidence of the good and successful result of such a plan as has just been hinted at, not only in what is now taking place in Prussia, but at home, even in reference to the classical and mathematical education of the superior ranks of society who frequent the universities. Defective as the plan of studies is admitted in many respects to be at those institutions, yet the mere uniformity of that

plan perseveringly adhered to for centuries, and the well-tried
skill of the teachers, who have given daily and visible proofs
of their capability to teach for many years before their appointment, have sufficed to produce not only a fair average of
well-informed people in the upper ranks of society, but also
some of the brightest examples of classical, mathematical, and
philosophical eminence. The principle then which, applied to
a particular class of the people, and referable to a limited plan
only, succeeds so well, when applied to all the other classes
with reference to a more general and more useful course of
instruction will without doubt work as admirably.

I was now in the vicinity of Redcar, which enjoys a local
reputation as a sea bathing-place, for its singularly beautiful
sands. Thither therefore I proceeded, calling in my way at
Up-Leatham, the seat of the Earl of Zetland, whom, to my
regret, I found absent on the continent.

This tranquil retreat, sheltered from the east by vast plantations, and placed in one of those lovely dales which the
swells and lesser hills of the Cleveland range form in the
neighbourhood of Roseberry Topping, that lofty peak sacred
to minstrelsy and witchery, recalls to memory the days of its
chivalrous and successive lords, the valiant Earl of Northumberland, Robert de Brus, and Lord Falconberge.

Thence I pushed on to Marske. This ancient and insulated Hall, which, from its external appearance bespeaks the
times of Charles the First, and which has often resounded
with the noble name of Dundas, stands near the shore, a
short way south of Redcar, to which there is a drive on
sands as smooth as velvet, yet so firm that neither horse nor
man leave their imprint on them as they tread the strand to
proceed to Redcar. This peculiarity has given Redcar (in
other respects a most insignificant sea-village) a certain
degree of sea-bathing celebrity during the summer. Many
people who either for health or pleasure desire to have good
sea-bathing at that season, repair to Redcar from many parts

in the north, in order to enjoy at the same time the daily walks or rides over the broad floor eight miles long and one mile broad, left by the receding waters. Some intention, however, at present exists of giving more importance to the place, by making it a convenient harbour. For this purpose it is proposed to connect the *Scars* (two projecting lines of rocks near the coast) with breakwaters, and to surmount the latter with walls of enormous length, to serve as piers. But the ultimate utility of the scheme is doubted by many, and the speculation, as yet, meets with little favour.

Returning from this sea bathing-place, a gentleman's seat at Kirk Leatham, was pointed out to me, whose name recalls that of a most worthy and honest Chancellor of the exchequer, now a peer of the realm. With its yellow front and Flemish like elevation, that building seemed purposely placed there to mark the foreign origin of the noble lord's ancestors.

Beyond it, a very curious and large edifice appears, built on three sides of a quadrangle, and of a very imposing exterior,—having a statue upon a suitable pedestal representing justice, in the centre of its open court, which is enclosed in front by a handsome iron palisade. This building, from its denomination of, and destination as an hospital, sufficiently commemorates the pious bequest, and philanthropic name of Sir W. Turner, its founder.

Scarcely had this object been left behind than the eye, as we reapproached at a great speed the lofty wall of the Cleveland hills (here rising like a mighty screen to fourteen hundred feet elevation), rested on Wilton Castle, seated on a small eminence not far from the road. Of the ancient baronial seat nought but the name remains. In its stead the plain Elizabethan windows of Sir Robert Smirke's modern elevation, are seen distributed through a great many walls of red sandstone, the latter flanked by turrets. These, with the many additions since made under the direction of the proprietor of the castle himself, present altogether an extensive mass of building assuming the castellated form.

This seat of Sir John Lowther stands well in the landscape; but the land around and about it, and particularly that which lies between the castle and the road, does not exhibit the same well-cultivated and rich aspect which I had lately remarked in other parts of Yorkshire.

My peregrination terminated at Middleburgh, whence on the following morning, after crossing the water, I set off by the Clarence railway for Durham and Sunderland, on my way to Hartlepool.

Those who are acquainted with the district will start at the idea of my journeying a distance of nearly fifty miles away from my destination, when Hartlepool laid on the coast conveniently at hand from Middleburgh. But the secret lies in this; that a single coach travels, on alternate days only, the short distance between Stockton or Middleburgh and Hartlepool; and had I adopted that conveyance I must have lost many precious hours in waiting; whereas the Clarence trains travel often in the day and expeditiously; though not quite so much so as in the south; and would wisk me over four times the distance, in infinitely less time than I should have wasted in accomplishing my transference direct from Middleburgh to Hartlepool.

Another consideration swayed me also on the occasion, congenial with the object of my journey. It was the desire of learning something respecting two or three mineral springs in the county, which had been mentioned to me by letters.

To Durham therefore I proceeded by the Clarence railroad; that is to within about six miles of that episcopal see where the railway ends, and from whence a shilling omnibus conveyed me to the city.

Happening to sit in one of the open carriages of the train by the side of a most intelligent gentleman, well acquainted with the country, and apparently connected with some of the mining speculations with which the country is rife, I found the excursion to Durham both pleasant and instructive. As we proceeded, sometimes on a level plain, and again on inclined plains, the country right and left developing itself under our eyes, my travelling companion pointed out to me the various spots of interest, and the little history attached to them.

Wynyard Park appeared conspicuous on our right, beyond Bottle Hill, in the midst of an exceedingly pretty country, with a broad expanse of water before it, sparkling in the sunshine. A little farther lay the extensive grounds and plantations of Hardwicke, in the neighbourhood of which, Mansforth Hall, the small house inhabited by the learned author of the history of Durham, was singled out with a sort of selfcomplacency, by his countryman my informant.

Hardwicke Hall, once the wonder of Durham county for its gardens and temples, and one of the grandest terraces in England, is now used merely as a hunting-box, and its former splendour is for the moment gone.

Turning the eye to the left in the direction of Bishop Auckland, immediately across an extensive and very fertile country, the noble mansion and plantation of Sir Robert Eden exhibited the gratifying contrast of a domain carefully watched and husbanded by its lord, and consequently flourishing.

We were now entering that vast tract of land which covers one of the largest coal-fields in England, from which alone London had, in one year (1837) been supplied with 805,668 tons of coals from nine collieries only, producing to the owners, upon shipping them, 426,332l.—yet costing to the consumers in the metropolis, nearly a million pounds sterling.

As we passed close to Wingate my fellow-traveller did not fail to mention, as one of the examples of the good fortune which will at times attend the purchase of the worst sort of land in this county, the case of the late Lord Howden, one of the best-hearted noblemen in England, and in his time a gallant soldier, who did not long survive the sudden bringing to light of a mine of wealth on his Durham estate. In a tract of many acres of bad land, purchased some years before, his Lordship had found coals, and had sunk a colliery in conjunction with a house of Newcastle. The tract, supposed to cover an almost inexhaustible stratum of coal, extends to about 2600 acres; and a branch rail to the Durham, as well as to the Hartlepool railroad, at once supplies ready means of disposing of the produce. That produce was not likely to fail, said my informant, since the Howden tract was in the immediate vicinity of two other collieries, one of which, the Haswell, had already been worked successfully for two years.

Now that the subjacent strata of this vast estate of Lord Howden, originally purchased at the price of waste or indifferent land, are made to yield gold, its upper surface also will be turned to account, and some of that gold employed to bring the whole tract into a high state of productive cultivation: thus will the owner and the public be benefited in a twofold manner.

We see here another striking illustration of the powerful agency of ready and cheap communications. A quantity of land, amounting to nearly 3000 acres, which before the putting down of any line of railway, had been almost despaired of, or at the utmost had been made to yield but ordinary crops—a land, too, which had changed hands over and over again, without any of the successive owners dreaming of the treasure that lay concealed under his steril acres, or, if suspecting it, unable to convey that treasure where it would be bartered for gold—such a land, I say, by the single agency of a railroad, is about to be converted into a region of inexhaustible riches, from within as well as without.

Further on, and right and left of the railroad on which we

were at the time travelling, another equally striking illustration of this kind was presented to us ; for there lay some of the land on which a noble earl connected by property and his title with the county, had sold to the descendant of a deceased high chancellor, as any common land; although, by borings previously made, the noble proprietor had ascertained that underneath it, rich veins of coal lay concealed. Could his lordship have imagined that at no distant period a line of easy transport for that coal would be made to cross, as it now does, that very land, with a terminus at a seaport, he most assuredly would not have parted with his property, and left the purchaser of it to reap, as indeed he is now doing, the whole benefit of the discovery.*

In like manner, the Lord of Wynyard could not have turned, as he has done, into a large income, the extensive landed property of the Tempest family, but for the branch railway he has established, in communication with the Durham and Sunderland railroads, as well as for the private harbour he has made at Seaham as a shipping terminus, by which an easy and incessant *débouché* is for ever secured to the rich produce of his lordship's collieries.

It is then made manifest that railway communication, by its certainty, rapidity, and consequent economy of time, does more towards creating wealth at home than any other agency which man can command ; since it gives value to that which was valueless before. But it will also give impetus to agricultural enterprise, through the very wealth it creates, which enables us successfully to compel the earth to yield the fruit so much needed by man. Hence as abundance of the earth's produce, and wealth, or capital, the necessary results of it,

---

* Between writing this passage and correcting the press—an interval of time almost too brief for any event—the spirited and high-minded nobleman, here alluded to, has been almost suddenly removed from his territorial possession, and the field of his ambitious views recalled, ere the allotted hour of man, to the home of his forefathers.

if not the only, are at least the principal agents of civilization
—it follows that that government will be the wisest which
shall most encourage and foster the formation of radiating
lines of railway communication between every possible point
of the kingdom.

Apply this principle to a sister kingdom, still a century behind England in every social art and comfort, and that island
will soon be worthy of its present association, and its people
be made happy.   Traverse that island in all directions with
railroads, and the desolate appearance of its surface will soon
change into a rich and productive garden.   Railway communication will do more for the civilization of Ireland than education.   It will give white bread in lieu of potatoes to the
people; and never until that people can eat white bread of
their own growth, will they be in a better position than they
are at present.

CHAPTER XVIII.

BUTTERBY SPAS—DURHAM; HARTLEPOOL.

First view of Durham CATHEDRAL—The Prebend's Bridge—The Durham UNIVERSITY—Modern antique—Students' Rooms—BUTTERBY SPAS—Endless rope Railway—The Collieries—Hetton and its Produce—OFFERTON Spa—Longevity of the people at HOUGHTON-LE-SPRING—Excursion to HARTLEPOOL—The " Home Tour"—Two HEADS better than none—The great Causeway—Hartlepool as it was and as it is about to be—SIR JOHN RENNIE's gigantic works—Sea-bathing Celebrity gone—Chalybeate Spa vanished—Substituted celebrity—The HARBOURS—The Docks—Future Prosperity and present Misery—A CHEMIST and DRUGGIST—The Poor-law Commissioners—The SANDS—Black-hall rocks—A Risk avoided—Awful Situation.

THERE are only two, of the many magnificent cathedral structures in England, that present themselves to the traveller suddenly as it were, upon approaching their respective cities, and in the most imposing manner, towering on high above all surrounding objects, like the cupola of St. Paul's over all the other edifices in London : Lincoln cathedral is one'; the other is this of Durham, towards which I was journeying from the terminus of the railway at Sherburn, mounted on the outside of a lumbering omnibus.

Before any of the dwellings and other parts of the city come in view, as they lie behind lofty and rocky banks, clothed in dark verdure, the body and towers of the cathedral, and the loftier keep of Durham Castle, appeared all at once on the horizon, lit up by the sun of a brilliant day in August.

Oh, for the pencil and pallet of Stanfield to fix this glorious picture! On approaching nearer, and as we cross the Elvit bridge over the Wear, to enter the city, and ascend under the old city-walls to the market-place, the further unrolling of the ground-map of this episcopal See tends to diminish the first impression; yet is every object right and left of the bridge, the new and the old, grouped and arranged in the most picturesque manner imaginable.

Another exceedingly pretty view of the cathedral is obtained from the north end of the Prebend's bridge. The river is here at a bend, sequestered, removed from the bustle of the town, and imbosomed within two lofty and well-wooded banks, dammed up by a wear placed across the stream. The cathedral appears on the opposite bank, towering above its loftiest plantation.

In this secluded spot, the river affords amusement during the summer to the good people of Durham, who assemble once a year on the surrounding banks, dressed in their holiday clothes, to witness a gay regatta that is said to rival those on the grand canal at Venice.

My reason for passing through Durham, and remaining a few hours in that city, after exploring the various objects of interest it offers to a stranger, was a desire to visit the new university, in doing which I received every kind assistance from Professor Johnson, the able teacher of chemistry in that establishment. With him, and with Mr. Shaw, a surgeon in considerable practice in Durham, whom I had casually become acquainted with on the road thither, I went round and examined the various parts of that *young* institution lodged in *ancient* and almost romantic apartments.

It was an excellent idea, that of founding a new university in an old and venerable building; clerical and monastical withal; whereby the *prestige* of such accessaries as those so much boasted of, and deemed so essential to a high, classical, and intellectual education in the two senior sister universities, is at once attained, without waiting for the slow progress of centuries. Hence the university of Durham may be termed " a modern antique."

Professor Johnson escorted us all round, pointing out and explaining the several divisions and arrangements of the college, scattered over a large extent of ground, and through many different old buildings. In our progress along the Gothic corridors, we entered the different rooms of the men (now absent during vacation)—some neat and in good order, others mean-looking, ill kept, and in the same state of confusion in which they had been left.

How easily the mind and disposition of these several absentees might have been gathered from the appearance of their rooms at college. Here, indeed, a species of more sound phrenology than that of the so-called science, might have been exercised, and the disposition of each dweller of these chambers easily and truly read off their walls and flooring, by the mere inspection of their interior condition and arrangement. I tried my hand at this, in two or three instances, and the worthy professor smiled assent and gainsaid me not.

Some of these rooms of the students are in the castle and old archiepiscopal palace, and these have a pretty look out over the castle gardens, with a peep at the river and the surrounding hills. The men can likewise walk round, to a great extent, upon a terrace which was originally a part of the old bastions; or they may descend to the margin of the river, and walk through the shaded groves beneath the lofty walls of the Prebendary's dwellings, under the casements of Mylord Bishop of Chester, or of his Right Reverence of Exeter, or in fine of that of the prelate of St. David's, all three of whom, besides the diocesan, have residence here, as well as in their respective episcopal palaces. In no other cathedral establishment perhaps has it happened before, that four bishops should have an individual right to congregate together.

The great and ancient Refectory, now the Hall, is equal to

some of the best at Oxford or Cambridge, and can accommodate about 400 students; but as yet, not more than 100
have sat down in it.   There is a combination room, which is
very large, and a new room adjoining.

Some of the inner corridors that run round one of the
courts have been much improved of late.   In doing this an
accidental and curious discovery was made, while altering a
window, of some rich Gothic ornaments, with projecting little
columns, and running arches, covering the walls.   These had
been entirely masked with mortar and plaster, which have
since been altogether removed.

Another restoration in which the college authorities were
engaged, is that of the great keep or tower, originally consisting of three stories, but till now appearing to have only
one, in consequence of its being choaked, up to the middle
with rubbish.   In clearing the latter away, the skeleton of a
spermaceti whale was discovered.

As there is a want of rooms for the additional students
expected to attend the university, it is intended to restore the
two stories to the tower, converting them into dwelling and
lecture rooms.   The view from this position is truly beautiful,
extending not only all over the city, encircled by the Wear,
but also far beyond it, over a rich and densely-populated
district.

It was gratifying to hear the learned Professor express himself with satisfaction on the present and future prospects of
this Northern University.

Of the mineral springs in the county of Durham, I have
already described the two most important, and have now
merely to mention a third Spa, which about twenty-five
or thirty years ago enjoyed considerable reputation in the
vicinity of Durham.   I allude to BUTTERBY, a place still
resorted to for its mineral springs, and to which a short but
delightful walk leads the visiter, who on approaching them
enters a most romantic dell, the sides of which are deep, and

shadowed by overhanging wood. There he meets with the "Sweet Well," as the first spring is called from its agreeable taste—or rather from the absence of all taste, in as much as it appears to be a pure water, holding in solution a very small proportion of carbonate of lime.

Further down the dell, on getting nearer to the margin of the river Wear, a second spring is found, the distinguishing character of which is to hold in solution a notable quantity of sulphuretted gas. Its presence, however, does not render the taste of the water particularly disagreeable, owing probably to the combination of moderate quantities of muriate of soda, lime, and magnesia found in it.

Judging by the analysis of this particular water, which I have inserted in my general table, and with which I was favoured by Dr. Clanny, of Sunderland, its author, I should consider it eminently useful as an alterative, and more safe in its internal use as a sulphuretted water than many others of that class.

Its natural temperature is 50°, that of the atmosphere being 63°. It is colourless; gives out a few air-bubbles on agitation; and on being suffered to remain at rest for a few hours, these disappear at last, without troubling the water, or throwing down any sediment, but simply diminishing the intensity of the sulphurous taste and smell.

Dr. Clanny, whom I have just mentioned, while occupying the important post of physician to the Durham Infirmary, published an account of the Butterby or *Beau-trouvé* Spas, to which he had paid great attention. Those of my readers who take an interest in scientific matters of this kind, need hardly be told that the opinion of Dr. Clanny on a subject of this sort may be received with the utmost confidence, as that of an individual perfectly qualified by talent and erudition to express one.

At Butterby, the two springs just described are not the only sources that claim attention; there is a third, even more

interesting in a physical point of view than the others.   This
rises in the very middle of the bed of the river Wear, and is
charged with iron and a large proportion of common salt.
Diluted as this mineral water always is with that of the river
which is for ever flowing over it, hardly any medicinal use can
be made of it, until such time as by enclosure of the spring
all admixture shall be prevented.   In such a case the spring
may be made available, by being administered in combination
with the water from the sulphur well, which seems, as it were,
to lie purposely at hand.

The distance from Durham to Sunderland is only thirteen
miles ; yet the stationary engine railway-carriage, in which I
took my venture, occupied two hours and a quarter in going
over it.   The many stoppages, and the changing of ropes consequent on the system of stationary engines, are the causes
of this delay,—of which I heard people of the county travelling upon it complain bitterly—exclaiming at the same time
against the prevalence of private over public interest.   But as
the ·proprietors of the railroad look for remuneration chiefly
from the conveyance of coals and merchandise, which are neither in haste nor prone to murmur, they laugh at the grumbling passengers, and adhere to their old cumbersome mode of
managing the railroad, which is nearly half a century behind
all other railroads in England.

On our way to Sunderland, we first passed one of Lord
Londonderry's collieries, the produce of which, as I observed
before, is conveyed by a railway proper to Seaham harbour.

We next came to the famed Hetton colliery, where a long
halt took place.   This colliery is one of the most extensive in
England.   It is worked by a company, and not fewer than
1000 men are employed in it.   The excavations have now
attained the extent of three miles, to reach which you must
descend to the depth of nine hundred and sixty feet.   In it
two sets of men, each in its turn, work for eight hours daily,
assisted by   locomotive engine, within those profound and

avernous recesses. In 1837 this colliery threw into the London market 204,668 tons of coals, which fetched the highest coal-market price of that year, namely 24s., besides all the other extra charges.

Hetton colliery is an important colony of itself. The population above ground amounts to nearly six thousand, who have eleven places of worship and seven Sunday-schools. I found the men and their families well lodged in small cottages, provided with fire, and in case of illness with medical attendance. They appeared healthy, and many of the pitmen, still active and at work, were as much as sixty-five and seventy years of age. Wages depend on strength of arms, but speaking generally, the pitmen seldom earned less than twenty, and often as much as twenty-seven shillings a week. They appeared to be orderly, quiet, and perfectly contented, and are always in full work.

It is probable that had I been earlier apprized of the existence of a mineral spring at Offerton, situated on the banks of the Wear, respecting which Mr. Stonow, surgeon at New Bottle, near Houghton-le-Spring, and a company of subscribers, expressed a wish to have my opinion, I should from Hetton have made a deviation to the indicated spot, with a view of examining the water in question. As it is, I can only report, on the authority of Mr. Stonow's letter, that the said water was analyzed at Newcastle, and found to contain three grains and a fraction of carbonate of soda, and one of iron, as the most active ingredients in it.

The situation of the spring is said to be most beautiful, and " wonderfully adapted by nature for a watering-place." Of the purity and salubrity of the air in the neighbourhood of the spring I can entertain no doubt, if it but resembles that of Houghton-le-Spring, where people seem to live " until they forget to die." At the time of my visit at that beautifully sequestered village, the parish boasted of a parson seventy-six years of age, a sexton of seventy-two, a bellows-blower of

eighty, and a sexton's portly rib of ninety ; making a total c
three hundred and sixty-nine years !

Houghton-le-Spring however is famous not only for havin
a very aged rector, but also as being one of the richest recto
ries in the county; and likewise for having been the field c
the apostolic acts of Bernard Gilpin, one of its rectors c
olden times, a man whom his learned contemporaries used t
stile " *Vir sanctissimus.*"

It was as well that the slow and cumbersome train o
which I had embarked was not more expeditious in its move
ment; else all these to me interesting digressions must hav
cost me my place. However, proceeding at length, an
rushing down the inclined plane from Seaton to Ryhope o
the seashore (a species of terrific *montagne russe*, down whic
we rattled at the rate of forty miles an hour with a tre
mulous and unpleasant vibration), we reached Sunderland
from whence I started for Hartlepool on the following day
having in the mean time transacted some business in th
former place.

To Hartlepool, the special object of my summer's excur
sion led me; not only because it was once a sea bathing
place of considerable note, but also because I felt a grea
desire to examine in person the mineral springs long known t
have existed in that place, below high-water mark ; a circum
stance of no inconsiderable interest. How far my expectation
were realized will presently be seen.

Hartlepool is, in too many respects, worthy of particula
consideration to be hastily dismissed. At this moment a
engineering operation of vast magnitude is going on in tha
seaport, which will not only change the aspect of the countr
immediately around it, but also affect property very materiall
in Hartlepool itself, as well as at many of the neighbourin
ports. The author of the " Home Tour in 1835," has ad
mirably and minutely described the great works which ha
been carrying on there up to the time of his visit, when the

ad been suspended, from causes admitted as valid by some
and disputed by others. He saw that line of railroad from
Durham and Sunderland in progress, which has since been
completed, and has given a new turn to the great question
of whether a safe and capacious harbour, as a port of refuge for the shipping on a coast where navigation is dangerous, as well as of export for the mining produce of the northern
counties, is a desirable and a feasible object, and one likely
to prove an advantageous speculation. That question has,
in the mean time, been decided in the affirmative, as far as
regards the eligibility and feasibility of the project,—leaving
but little doubt with regard to its productibility. Not only
have the suspended works been resumed, but they have also
been enlarged, and are now more vigorously pursued than at
any former period.

Sir George Head, then, will rejoice that a plan which his
own sagacity and observations had led him to consider as
" good," and its completion " desirable," is not likely to be set
aside from any caprice or faintheartedness. Look at the returns of the extraordinary progress made by Hartlepool as
a seaport during the last four years only; and the facts alone
which they divulge, will suffice to show the accuracy of my assertion. In a ministerial journal of the 26th of December of
last year, it is officially stated, " that in 1835 there were only
three sloops registered at Hartlepool, and that there were now
1839) ninety vessels, averaging about 245 tons each, and representing a capital of nearly a quarter of a million of money."

An excursion to Hartlepool from Low Haswell, one of the
eleven principal collieries in Durham, which I examined on
my return from a short visit to the mineral springs of But-
erby, is one which I would strongly recommend to every
tourist in the north, who may be desirous of witnessing what
the energy and ingenuity of man can effect, not only in staying the impending ruin and total extinction of a place, once
celebrated " emporium of the see," as Camden calls it, but

also in raising it to an importance far superior to that which it formerly possessed; as most assuredly the operations carried on in that place within the last six years, and now in progress of completion, are calculated to accomplish. It is an excursion I call to memory with the most lively interest.

The first of these operations, and the most influential in producing the results I have glanced at, is the completion of a single line of railway, projected from the end of the Durham junction railroad, through the beautiful district of Castle Eden, and along the summit of that curious causeway or peninsula, which, beginning at Middlethorp, extends about three and a half miles in a straight direction, as far as the north-gate of Hartlepool, with a somewhat rapid downward inclination.

For the space of the two last miles this single railway forms, as it were, the backbone of a ridge, partly natural and partly artificially raised, which becomes narrower as it proceeds onwards to its termination into the ocean, where the town of Hartlepool is seated. Its upper plane is just wide enough to admit that one line of rails and no more. In some parts (that is farthest from the town) the ridge is nearly one hundred feet high, in others only seventy-five, sixty, and fifty feet. On its left the waters of the German Ocean leave a broad sandy shore, along which runs a double and triple parallel line of sandy hillocks, from twenty to thirty feet in height, capable of defending the basis of the ridge from the inroads of the sea. On the right or land side a rich succession of corn-fields appears to a considerable distance, until they merge into a more varied and still further landscape.

Trains of forty and fifty coal-waggons, each of them weighing, with its cargo, fifty hundredweight, are constantly to be seen passing downwards towards Hartlepool, to which the carriages for passengers are linked behind. To one such train of waggons, proceeding from the Thornley colliery, and inscribed with the name of Sir William Chaytor, our carriage was yoked, by means of a single and endless rope, as thick as a man's wrist, travelling over a number of successive iron pulleys, here called sheaves, which are placed immediately under the centre of the waggons and carriages, between the two rails distant from each other about twenty-five feet. Our string of coal-waggons and passenger-carriages, extending over upwards of four hundred feet of ground in length, and weighing a quarter of a million of pounds, made good its descent, of two miles and a quarter, in less than three minutes by my watch!

The endless rope by which the rapid movement is effected is put in motion by a stationary engine, which at the same time pulls up the inclined plane the string of returning empty waggons, to the spot where the two trains, the descending and the ascending, are able to pass each other by means of *sidings*, or short lateral rails. The ascending passengers' train, however, from Hartlepool as far as the level, and again from Hasleton Dean to Castle Eden (a portion of the road on which there is a double line of rails), is dragged up, or sometimes pushed up from behind, by locomotives.

If the tourist, on his way to Hartlepool, departs direct from Sunderland, many are the modes and changes which he will witness in the manner of being forwarded to his destination. The manner altogether is a tedious though an extremely cheap one, and as the levels of the ground vary, so do the means employed to travel over them. Thus, from the sea village of Ryhope, three miles from the first station out of Sunderland, the traveller will be dragged up an elevated plane, by stationary engines working an endless rope, in the way before described, and in that manner will he reach Haswell. Of these stationary engines there is one at every three miles; but even that number would not have been sufficient for the intended purpose, had not the ascending ground been rendered less steep, by excavations made through the soft oolitic rock to a considerable depth.

At Haswell the moving power is again changed, and a single horse, put in front of the whole train, is found to be sufficient to draw the immense loads I have described, along a single rail. This being upon a gentle inclined plane, the animal finds it no difficult task to proceed at the rate of from eight to ten miles an hour, with all that tremendous tail behind him. In this way Castle Eden and its noted iron foundery is quickly passed and left behind.

The train next enters a very extensive and deep excavation, in many places from seventy to eighty feet deep, being alluvium ; it then crosses, over a viaduct, a most picturesque chasm, called Haselden, or Hastleton Dean,—where the sea, to which our back had been turned since leaving Ryhope, again bursts on our view. It is soon after that the long descent to Hartlepool, previously described, begins; before reaching which, however, the drawing horse is removed into a waggon *behind* the train, and the rest of the journey is performed quickly as well as comfortably without him—this being perhaps the only instance in human affairs, where it answers very well to " put the cart before the horse."

The train stops precisely where the excavations for the formation of the new harbour and docks are now proceeding, agreeably to the vast scheme devised by that able engineer Sir John Rennie—a scheme which, including the railway, has already required the sum of three hundred and fifty thousand pounds.

There are two inns at present at Hartlepool, where none existed when Sir Cuthbert Sharp, mayor of that place, published its interesting and antiquarian history twenty-four years ago. The George and the Cleveland Arms stare each other in the face. I selected the latter, and had reason to be perfectly satisfied with my choice. Nowhere in England could a better or a more profuse breakfast be presented to a hungry traveller, as I was, in so expeditious and so neat a manner, and for the moderate charge of one shilling and sixpence

My repast finished, I proceeded to explore the place, and seek for the particular objects I came to examine ; but, alas ! to no purpose.

Hartlepool is in a state of transition. It had once its day as a sea bathing-place. " It is at present a watering-place of considerable celebrity," says Sir Cuthbert, in 1816. That glory is now past.

" Hartlepool," observed Dr. Short, " boasts of by far the best mineral water in the county. It is exceedingly fine, clear, thin, of a pleasant smell, chalybeate taste, smells a little of sulphur, is grateful, and sits light on the stomach, and passes quickly off. It has surprisingly good effects in *scorbutic cases, habitual nervousness, stomach hyppo and hysterics,*" besides a hundred other maladies.

To judge by the number of authors who have written of this mineral water, Hutchinson, Munro, Short, Berkenhout and Eliot, it must have indeed enjoyed a glorious reputation. That reputation is now gone.

Hartlepool is no longer a famous place for either of these two great physical features which before gave it lustre in those respects. We have to record the end of its good days ; but we may also report the termination of its degradation. At no distant period we may have to chronicle its rise and new prosperity. The rail that brought hither the waggons and the black gold from Bradyll and Thornley, has driven the fine company of bathers away; and the excavators who are so much dreaded near the docks and railways in progress, have by their operations given the last blow to the mineral spring, or chalybeate spa, once in existence near the water gate; clearing the coast, at the same time, of the last remnant of sickly dames and invalids.

My occupation, therefore, at Hartlepool was gone. But the contemplation of the eight hundred hardy men whom I beheld at work, engaged in excavating extensive docks, and in remedying the ill effects of that sad catastrophe which Sir

George Head has so vividly described, in 1835, was a sufficient motive for detaining me yet awhile. Sheltered by the
handsome new brick building of the Hartlepool rail-office,
I stood surveying the vast operations of these "dreaded"
labourers, and reflected that by converting a vast tract of
barren land, or a stagnant lake, into one of the finest harbours on this coast, they will be the means of bringing back
to Hartlepool more than its former splendour, and much of
the wealth that now pours into Tynemouth, and the mouths
of the Wear.

This is no dream. The notes of the engineer are before
me, and they tend to explain to the uninitiated, while marvelling at all he sees, the extent as well as intent and purport
of what appears now inexplicable as well as inextricable.

Two great basins, or an inner and outer harbour, the one
containing sixteen, the other thirty acres, with suitable docks,
occupying about sixteen or eighteen acres more, will constitute the port of Hartlepool. Four hundred sail of large colliers will find ample room to float and move about in them.
In case of need, both the harbours may, at any period, be
enlarged.

To cleanse the outer harbour and keep it open, a surface of
two hundred acres of water, collected in a great reservoir
or Slate, lies close at hand, capable of being discharged at
low water by means of sluices. "This is a most powerful
and efficient means for the purpose," observed Sir John
Rennie to me; "the like of which we have not elsewhere in
this country. Ramsgate has only a sluice and power of
eleven acres, and Dovor of twenty acres; and I believe that
there is nothing of similar extent on the continent."

One million and six hundred thousand tons of earth have
already been excavated in the prosecution of this truly
gigantic undertaking, and the total quantity of masonry in
the basins, walls, &c., extends already to 180,000 tons.
Should the remaining part of Sir John's plan be carried into

effect, consisting in raising a great mole or breakwater outside, having five fathoms at low water of Spring tides, Hartlepool would then possess the finest asylum harbour in the
north, for vessels of all classes, so much wanted on this
coast.

With these data and explanations before me, I proceeded
through the huge excavations and embankments, climbing
over some of the heaps of soil, or leaping across many of the
temporary rail-tracks that seemed to intersect the ground
in all directions. A similar scene of bustle and activity,
occupying an extent of flat ground as vast as eye could
encompass, was probably not to be met with, at that time,
elsewhere in England.

Amidst the half finished and the fully completed portion
of the works, one's attention is almost distracted. I halted
on a bridge, struck at the sight of a stupendous dock gateway just finished. It ran nearly due west, with walls cased
in babylonic blocks of stone, and its bed elliptically hollowed,—the sides rose straight and upright,—firm, immovable, and wider apart than in any dock gateway in the
Thames or Mersey. Once within the haven to which this
water gateway leads, hundreds of vessels will lie at peace,
let Æolus or Boreas blow; and either discharge their imported
goods upon the wide quays, now in the course of being
formed with the very materials thrown up from the excavations—or take in the inland produce of the country for ex-
portation.

To expedite both operations the stiff clay, mixed with loose
white sand, brought up from the excavations, is deposited by
the side of the ridge on which the single railroad now runs, to
widen its upper platform, and render a double line of rails
admissible, on which it is to be hoped that locomotives will
supersede altogether the long and tedious process of stationary engines. Such an arrangement will put Hartlepool

in direct communication with the whole of the north and west of England.

What a glorious sight it will indeed be, when the man whose skill has devised and planned the whole, having completed these gigantic works, shall, to crown all, give the word of command that will let in the ocean into the stupendous entrances his genius has created, followed by a long line of decked vessels which will presently be floating proudly and in safety where but a few hours before it would have been destruction for them to have touched ! To see a mighty three-decker launched from a dry dock into the bosom of the deep, is a magnificent and inspiriting sight; yet we have but added another to the myriads of those engines by which man usurps a temporary power over the ocean. But to behold the latter admitted within an artificial estuary prepared for it, that it may be subdued for the safe existence of those very engines the strength and skill of which it laughs to scorn during its moments of ire; to view it imprisoned between lofty walls—its lion-murmurs muzzled, and its surface stilled ;—this is a sight far more inspiriting, and a conquest far superior over the restless element. Such a sight will be worth the journey from London, or any other distant part of the country; and I doubt not but that the opening of Hartlepool New Port will attract thousands of applauding spectators.

After this minute picture of the certain and immediate prospects of Hartlepool, it is hardly necessary to remark, that the present desolate appearance of its semi-abandoned streets and houses will change into a scene of bustling activity, business, and dense population ; and further, that not only will all the already existing modern dwellings, deserted at the epoch of the catastrophe of 1834, be reoccupied—but double and triple their numbers will rise in all directions—for which ample scope is afforded by the state of the land in and about the town. Judging as a cosmopolite, from

all the circumstances of the case, it is not difficult to see that
an investment of money in judicious building speculations at
Hartlepool, would be a safe and lucrative operation.   Accordingly, I found that a building society was about to be formed
in the town, the members of which, by small monthly subscriptions, meant to raise a fund, from which advances could
be made, to be repaid by instalments, with interest, so as to
enable the industrious classes, individually, to build or purchase small freehold or other dwelling-houses.

This is a comforting prospect for the people of Hartlepool,
who have hitherto borne patiently their poverty, or indifferent
fortune—a lot which it is easy to perceive has been more or
less that of every class in the place.   Hence, as I cast my
eyes around me, while walking through the streets, the proofs
of the dismal truth stared me in the face, in a variety of ways,
and I regret to say, even in the case of persons connected
with my own profession.

To what strange occupations has indeed a medical man in
this, as well as in many other distant parts of the country I
have visited resorted, for want of bread, consequent on the
excess of competition from an overstocked market, or from
the casting loose of unqualified and irregular practitioners
among the industrious classes and poorer labourers, by the
Commissioners appointed to carry into effect the New Poor-
laws! Here, within a few paces of the inn, at Hartlepool,
from which I was about to take my leave, a " dispensing
chemist and druggist," who, I understood, gave also advice
with his threepenny powders, showed to what shifts an offshoot of the medical profession is driven to secure bread.
The double windows of his fair-looking shop, besides its
usual characteristic glass flagons, yellow, pink, and blue,
displayed an heterogeneous mass of articles, such as were
never before married together in a similar establishment.
There were scents and toothpowders on the one side, close to
jars of pickled onions and boxes of *genuine* Seidlitz powders.

In the twin window the "true Mexican jet" was strongly recommended to scouring maids; and hard by, there lay French *allumettes* side by side with Congreve lucifers, a case of true Havannahs, and a phrenological head, with its various bumps conspicuous. Against the inside panes of the centre glass-door two printed placards were pendant; on the one, "choice drugs and chemicals," with "bleeding and tooth-drawing," besides "physicians' prescriptions carefully prepared," were inscribed in bold capitals; while the other or fellow placard advertised to the passer by that genuine coffee was imported there.

On leaving Hartlepool, I took to the sands on my return,—it being low water, and the distance along the shore five miles only,—to reach the celebrated clusters, called the Black Hall Rocks, which I was anxious to behold. A walk of so novel a kind to me offered strong temptations. The state of the tide I had ascertained was such, that if I loitered not in picking up the many inviting shells that are found scattered on these sands, or in examining the hundred varieties of fuci, confervæ and ulvæ with which the face of the rocks on the coast is studded, I might reach in time, and so pass through, the perforated rock among the romantic clusters before named, which the force and constant action of the water have separated from the coast, and fashioned so as to appear at a distance like gigantic towers.

Accordingly I began my march, though dissuaded by my landlady of the Cleveland Arms; but I had scarcely proceeded three-quarters of a mile in my lonely excursion, when thoughts and feelings supervened to shake my resolution. It was the 2d of August, the day was intensely hot, and the sun, only an hour removed from its meridian, shone with an intensity of light which the white sand reflected back with a dazzling splendour. I found the sands not so hard as I expected. The way was dreary and solitary; not a human being was in sight. A few distant sails were seen balancing on the waving line of blue, to

my right; and the surf, far ahead of me, was seen to beat against
the fringed coast. Anon this latter seemed to start into the sea
and bar all further progress, until I approached the spot and
discovered a passage. Again it appeared to sink back into
receding inland circles, leaving a broad strand between it and
the incoming tide, which rolled in successive eddies on the
shore, with a rustling noise.

These constant changes in the aspect of the coast portended
the tortuous, long, and dismal course I should have to follow.
The glare of the smooth and dazzling sand, as it reflected the
sun back into my eyes, presently troubled my vision, and made
my brain hot. A few steps farther and the temples beat as if
the hat had been too tight. I doffed this and exposed the
bare head to the western breeze, which blew from between
some chasm in the rocks on my left, or through a break in
that long line of sandhills already mentioned, which, covered
with coarse tall grass, inhabited by rabbits, and here and
there gladdened by the presence of a sauntering sand-bird—
extend, in parts, along the coast.

The sensation in the head, however, was not diminished
by this precaution. Symptoms of fulness in that part kept
increasing apace. *A coup de soleil* is the work of an instant.
It is unexpected, or if preceded by any warning (as I have
often had and profited by, to save myself), it would, in such
a place, come as a warning in vain. To fall unseen and
unknown on the strand, as the rolling tide is within an hour
or two of returning to it, and thus to meet the fate of one
whose cherished image is ever before me, was a possible case
—an event not improbable even—one which might befall me,
and which might remain unknown for many a day after. I
thought of home and those I had left there; and instantly
quitting the solitary strand, along which I dared not retrace
my steps the whole distance I had come, plunged at once
among the sandhills, and past these, with my face to the

west, I gained the narrow tract of cultivated land which lies between them and the foot of that magnificent railway embankment so often mentioned, which now rose nearly a hundred feet above me.

A little rest in one of the fields, and the green aspect of the country around, soon restored my circulation to its former tranquillity. Proper caution and a few efforts enabled me to scramble up the loose acclivity, and gain the summit of that great causeway. But here another danger awaited me, which I had not anticipated, and which, for the moment, presented itself in a much more threatening attitude than the one I had not had the courage to encounter.

It has already been stated that the summit of the ridge, or causeway, is just wide enough to admit of a single set of railway tracks, which occupies the centre. The space left on each side is only of sufficient width for a man to walk upon; but he must be of strong nerves and have a steady head to do so ; for as each margin of the causeway is unprotected by any barrier, and a precipice of sixty, seventy, or even a hundred feet depth yawns below it, it is no ordinary head that can stand the walking upon the very brink of it, along the whole of an uninterrupted line of two miles and a quarter, as straight as the course of an arrow.

To avoid the latter alternative I took to the middle between the tracks, and thus proceeded on my pedestrian tour towards Hasleton, enjoying, from the height whence I surveyed them, the magnificent sight of the ocean on my right, and of the fertile country on my left, which extended to the very verge of the hills on which Durham rose in the distant horizon.

Presently, as I had walked about a mile without meeting a single object in my progress, a small black speck appeared in sight straight before me, and at the farthest visible point, which seemed to occupy the centre of the long and narrow causeway. At first the object, flanked on each side by lofty and dark embankments, seemed stationary, like an insulated rock between them. But as I kept progressing on my way, it appeared to detach itself from the surrounding landscape, and to stand out in front of it, until it left the landscape behind and an empty space besides. The latter kept increasing at every instant as the object got larger and larger, and thus showed that the latter was travelling on the same causeway as myself, and advancing towards me.

Then, and not till then, the frightful thought shot across me, that this was one of the long and heavy trains of loaded waggons, rolling down the inclined railroad on its way to the terminus at Hartlepool—a thought which the total absence of smoke, or of any appearance of fire in a train that was moved without a steam-engine, prevented my entertaining before.

Of the reality of my surmises, and of the awfulness of my position, I soon became convinced, as, with increased velocity and almost noiseless revolution, the rolling train kept nearing me, showing its long line of dark waggons guided by no human hand that could stay its progress on perceiving my danger. Of that danger I became quickly sensible; and in the emergency of the instant, I knew not which way to escape, unless indeed I attempted the perilous experiment of retreating down the precipitous side of the causeway, the bottom of which was, in this part, immersed in an extensive sheet of water. Places there were indeed, here and there, on the summit of the causeway, where the platform swelled out to afford room for the workmen, when employed on the road, or any stray traveller, to retreat to while the trains are passing. But none such were at hand where I stood transfixed almost to the ground, convinced that inevitable destruction awaited me if I continued in the centre of the railway, or serious personal injury if I retreated to the narrow path between the rail and the brink of the causeway. Meantime upon—

" Those single ribs of steel,
  Keen as the edge of keenest scimitar,
  The *lengthened* cars roll'd on.
    *   *   *   *   *   *

Steady and swift the self-moved chariots went,
Poised on their single wheel they moved along,
Instinct with motion ;
Rolling self-balanced on their downward course."

There was not a moment to be lost. I could now distinctly
see and count the loaded waggons ; and as the drumming
noise of their revolving wheels became louder and louder, I
felt sick at heart. What was to be done ? I threw myself
with my face flat on the ground, athwart the narrow path on
the right of the rail, with my arms extended, and quickly
retreating backwards until my legs and body hung pendulous
against the side of the causeway—my head being just above
the edge of it—I kept myself thus suspended by my
arms stretched on the ground, until the whole train had
passed me, its downward velocity fanning the very air on my
cheeks.

" As the cars roll'd on their rapid way,
  I bow'd mine head and closed mine eyes for dread."

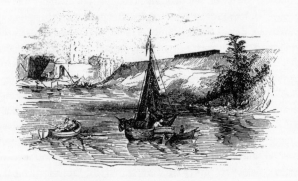

CHAPTER XIX.

SUNDERLAND—TYNEMOUTH—NEWCASTLE.

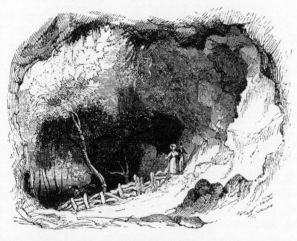

Caves—Castle Eden Dene—Deviation—Strange Characters on the
Road—SUNDERLAND—The Iron Bridge—The Pier—Evening Prome-
nade—Odoriferous Approaches—The Belles of Sunderland—TYNE-
MOUTH—Its Appearance—Sea Bathing-place, or the Brighton of the
Newcastle People—The LIVERPOOL of the North Sea—First and second
Visit to Newcastle—Surprising Aspect of the City—DESPOTISM AND
ARCHITECTURE—The Penny Magazine and a certain fair Authoress—
Accuracy and Blunder—ROBERT GRAINGER—Vast Conceptions—
Extraordinary Results—New Building and new Streets—GREY STREET
and the Column—The Exchange and the Markets—REFORMED CORPO-
RATION—Their love of Jobbing—An American GRAINGER—Parallel
between him and the Northumbrian—GEORGE STEPHENSON—An ami-
able Family—Apology for this Chapter.

" Whoe'er hath loved with venturous step to tread
        The chamber dread
Of some deep cave, and seen his taper beam
Lost in the arch of darkness overhead,
        And mark'd its gleam,
Playing afar upon the sunless stream,
        Where from their secret bed
And course unknown and inaccessible
        The silent waters swell ;—

" Whoe'er has trod such caves of endless night
He knows, when measuring back the gloomy way,
        With what delight refresh'd, his eye
        Perceives the shadow of the light of day ;
How heavenly seems the sky,
And how, with quickened feet he hastens up
        Eager again to greet
The living world and blessed sunshine there,
        And drink as from a glass
Of joy, with thirsty lips the open air."

Of this long but beautiful quotation from the great poet
who supplied me with the few apt lines with which I concluded the preceding chapter, I was forcibly reminded on
emerging from the caverns in Castle Eden Dene.

Having made good at last my walk along the ridge or causeway as far as Heselden or Hasleton, where I was overtaken by a
train of empty waggons on which I got a lift to Castle Eden, I
proceeded to explore its renowned defile, from its upper entrance
within sight of the lofty modern hall in which resides the
daring projector of the Sunderland bridge, down to the gate
which opens on the sea-shore ; being a distance altogether of
about three miles. A little urchin, whom I procured at the
porter's lodge, was my conductor until I found myself fairly
immersed in the midst of romance and wooded gloom ; when,
preferring at all times the luxury of being " alone in solitude," I dismissed him with his expected reward.

A poet, and a poet only, can do justice to the many varied
beauties of this enchanted region. The brilliant tone and
robust pencil of Stanfield might seize and portray some of its

ruly magnificent pictorial features, which appear, as it were,
purposely arranged for the artist, in some of the happiest and
incessantly varying combinations of rocks that seem split
asunder by some geological catastrophe, and hanging woods
which, in many places, actually darken the face of the sun,
and serve to perpetuate night.

A winding and safe road, throughout the whole extent of
this defile, serves admirably the purpose of displaying its
endless beauties to the many hundred visiters who, during
the summer, are admitted by the liberal proprietor to the
enjoyments of this magnificent region, containing some of
the finest scenery in Durham county. Seen from the upper
part of the Dene, not far from where a stream of water
springs from the crevice of a rock, and, forming a natural
cascade, falls into the gunner's pool, the road can be traced
o a considerable distance through the valley below. Snake-
like and in broad coils it rushes down the deep sides towards the bottom of the dell, which is too much steeped in
gloom to reveal its own secrets. Here and there the road is
seen for a moment to right itself upon a level in the shape of
a platform, or to wind round a steep bank covered with trees
and brushwood; but it soon again takes a downward course,
and proceeds to its destination.

Caves, gloomy and unfathomable ; masses of rock, detached and rolled down precipices—among which a stream
of water frets and murmurs—and trees of every species that
please themselves in the soil of Great Britain—such are
some of the features that strike the attention of the visiter,
who in general prefers approaching the Dene, and exploring
it, from the lowest or sea-shore entrance. Gay vehicles
filled with such visiters are seen almost constantly ascending
from below ; and many did I behold on that day, from a
circular terrace that overlooks a hanging wood, and heard
them trying their prolonged halloos, to provoke an echo which
faintly answered to their calls. Gipsy parties are spread
among the steep and grassy slopes, seeking for a spot where

to display their picnic baskets. They gaze upwards at the
azure of the sky, which they can only behold through the
various clumps of trees that hang over them, forming a
refreshing canopy to their repast.

I could have lingered hours in the enjoyment of such a
spectacle as this, and in such a region; but I was warned by the
recollection that the evening was to be spent in Sunderland
and that if I missed the passenger-train, on its return from
Hartlepool, I should have no other conveyance at hand for
that day to carry me thither.

Were it only to behold the span of that stupendous bridge
of iron which, striding over the Wear and its loftiest vessel
under sail, with a length of two hundred and thirty-six feet
and at an elevation of one hundred feet, springs from its
abutments of solid masonry, twenty-four feet thick, one of
which, that to the south, rests on the solid rock, rising twenty
feet above the level of the river—a deviation from my course
to the Northumbrian and Cumberland Spas would have
been at all times excusable. It was to me temptation on the
present occasion—I confess it; and the reader must suffer me
to linger thus awhile on the road from one Spa to another.

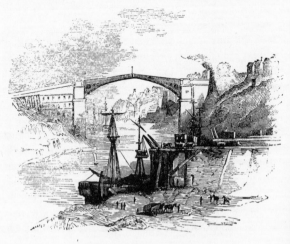

In my present work, I profess not to give a mere catalogue *raisonné* of mineral waters, or to take those who can bear with me from the mere description of one watering-place to that of a second, and a third and a fourth, and so on to the end of the endless list.   Mine is not a treatise on English mineral waters only; neither is it intended to be a strictly scientific account of their chemical composition and medicinal virtues and nothing more.   I should despair of being read were I thus to confine my object; but, taking encouragement from the flattering reception a former analogous publication has met with, in which positive and useful information was blended with light and amusing details of episodical or collateral subjects, I have studied to follow nearly the same plan on the present occasion, and trust I may rely on the same forbearance from my readers.

Curious characters one meets on the road.   I had scarcely taken my place in the Hartlepool train, which had at length worked its way up to the Castle Eden station by means of a locomotive, when two trains, the one of twenty the other of thirty waggons, full of coals, were seen to ascend at the opposite end from Low Haswell, pushed by locomotives.

Turning to a fellow-traveller, who was sitting by my side, and who, with less of the taciturnity than belongs to the Society of Friends, of which he seemed to be a member, had already divulged himself as one of the Directors of the very railroad we were about to travel upon, I inquired how it happened that the passenger-train in the morning was not equally pushed up the steep ascent by a locomotive engine, instead of being dragged by the horribly tedious endless rope.

" Those locomotives belong to the proprietors of collieries," was the reply ; " the company simply permit the use of them in conveying the coals on the railroad at a certain charge each per ton."

" And what might that charge be ?"

" Three farthings per ton and per mile."

I thanked my " friend" for the information which I was in

the act of transferring to my note-book, when, after having
written a few prefatory words, the prices mentioned escaped
my memory. Wishing to be exact, I ventured to ask my in
formant if he had said *three halfpence* a ton and per mile
The silver-headed, square-faced, brown-coated, drab-gaitered
and placid " friend," without moving lips, looked long and
doubtfully for a minute or two at me, and at last exclaimed
" I told thee three *farthings* per ton and per mile ;" and h
turned his back upon me, with marks of something approach
ing to contempt for the dulness of my apprehension.   Th
information, at all events, is worth something, as an elemen
in the consideration of the great Coal question lately agitate
in the metropolis.

The best position from which to contemplate the iron bridg
of Sunderland, is on the brink of one of those numerou
mounds of loose earth which project from the south bank c
the river, immediately over the lower or water road seen fro
thence at a considerable depth below, winding up wide an
steep, from the margin of the river to the level of the princip
side streets of Sunderland, for carts and trucks which go t
and from the shipping.   From that spot the stupendous struc
ture,—one of those projections which show the power of ma
so strikingly, and which well entitle the engineer to exclai
"*Nil desperandum!*"*—looks light and woven like the spider
meshes which that insect has spun in the air, across some va
chasm.

Even though the beholder is here placed at the height c
forty or fifty feet from the river-level, the bridge seems t
him as if suspended in the air, and he must raise his head t
look at it.   Beyond it, and in the immense space defined b
its arch and its lofty abutments, large vessels are seen comin
down the river, and passing under the suspended structur
over which a string of heavily-laden waggons is, at the sam
time, slowly moving along its strong timber-framed pavemen
strewed with marl, limestone, and gravel, yet quivering und

* Such is the inscription on an iron tablet in the centre of the bridge.

the pressure of such a load. Two hundred and sixty tons weight of iron projected and suspended across a wide space, trembling at, yet resisting, the incessant trials to which its strength is subjected every day in the year! Justly will the descendants of Burdon, through whose perseverance, and at whose expense principally, this imposing structure was raised, feel proud of such an ancestor.

Dr. Reid Clanny, who resides in a handsome and wide street leading to the bridge, showed me every civility, and I owe it to him, that in a couple of days I made myself master of every thing worthy of note in a place which, in a commercial point of view, particularly as to the shipping interest, must be regarded as the fourth seaport in the kingdom ; a rank to which it has risen from that of a fishing hamlet, in the course of little more than two centuries. Upwards of 300 new vessels of various burden were launched in Sunderland during the past year.

There is a sort of evening promenade, a marine one, on a noble pier (the south one) at the entrance of the harbour, 650 yards long to its present eastern extremity, and at its widest part 250 feet broad. The top of the pier is eleven feet above high water of ordinary spring tides, and its width between the harbour-wall and the sea-parapet, is divided into two longitudinal parallel portions, one of which, sixteen feet in width, destined for the promenaders, is raised about two feet by means of a continuous range of steps. This platform is paved with large laid blocks of stone, well dressed and fitted together. A handsome parapet, raised a step in height, divides it from the rubble breakwater, formed as a glacis to protect the pier from the south-easterly gales. At my visit this part of the structure was yet in progress. Stones obtained from the limestone quarries of Pollion, situated about three miles up the river on the south bank, are deposited, and when sufficiently consolidated by the action of the sea, the exterior surface of the slope is rough paved with the largest, heaviest, and best-adapted blocks.

There is also a north pier, which has been for the last eigh'
years in the course of rebuilding, on a plan approved of by Si,
John Rennie, and under the superintendence of Mr. Murray
the present engineer of the perpetual commissioners appointec
by act of parliament to watch, enlarge, improve, and protec
the curious and interesting harbour of Sunderland, to which
this town is indebted for its importance.

Mr. Murray, to whom I am indebted for many interesting
details respecting these splendid piers, and of which I regre'
not to be able to avail myself more fully in a work like the
present, is an engineer from whose talents and zeal the good
people of Sunderland, interested in the preservation of their
noble estuary, have reason to expect every thing that is satisfactory. And they truly need it, now that Hartlepool is preparing to dispute, in a few years, the palm of export trade
from Durham county, and other districts in the north.

Like the lastmentioned port, Sunderland has a tidal basir
attached to a dock, lately constructed by a private company ;
but whereas the dock and basins of Hartlepool, as we have seen
will be capable of floating four hundred sail of colliers, this
of Sunderland holds only the fourth part of that number.

A branch railway from the dock joins a railroad called the
Brandling Junction Railway, open during my stay in Newcastle in 1838, which again being connected with the Newcastle and Carlisle railroad, places Sunderland in quick and
direct communication with the Irish sea.

The approach to the pier from the upper part of the town
unfortunately, is through a long dirty street, the prolongation
or tail of High-street, inhabited by the lowest class of people,
principally mechanics and sailors, and from which branch off
to the right and to the left, many very narrow passages or
alleys, those of the latter leading down to the water-side, and
all presenting, at the time of my visit, the very sink of gloom
and filth—an apt nest or rendezvous for typhus and cholera.

Yet in despite of this unfortunate *trajet* to get to the pier
the evening promenade I witnessed upon it was gay and

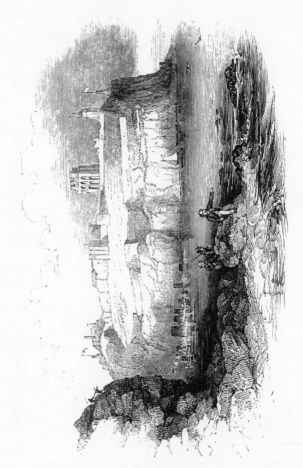

thronged, though of the most motley kind. The physiognomy and appearance of the better sort of women here are calculated to produce a prepossessing effect. There is a peculiar expression in their face, which I had not noticed at Durham, and which approaches almost to what one would call *distingué*. They are moreover frequently tall, but not well made. The men, on the contrary, are short, thickset, light-haired, and not unlike the Hamburgher. There is more than Durham blood in these men and women of the middle and lower classes in Sunderland.

The Northumbrians vaunt their sea bathing-place at Tynemouth. On approaching the mouth of the Tyne from the sea, two projecting headlands, from sixty to seventy feet high, and much less than a quarter of a mile apart, are seen to encompass a receding strand, with firm and fair-looking sands upon it, in front of which, however, many variously-sized, sharp, and swarthy rocks peep out of the water at all times, and render sea-bathing altogether an operation requiring caution. Yet here upon these sands, within this contracted space, on which I espied a few straggling bathing-machines, do the Newcastle people and others from the neighbourhood repair, for the luxury of washing off with muddy salt-water the sooty layers deposited on their skin during the lengthened winter season.

I never saw any thing less inviting, or more discouraging for a bather—any stranger, for instance, who arrives at Tynemouth, either through North Shields, or from South Shields, as was the case with myself—than the appearance of every thing around. The general character of all the three places is that of ugliness—Tynemouth itself perhaps, being the worst, and with the aspect of poverty to boot. Towards the cliffs a few mean-looking houses are let as lodgings during the season ; but there is a great dearth of house accommodation at that period.

The two clever architects, Messrs. Green father, and son, whose celebrated Victoria bridge on the Wear, and the curious

as well as ingenious viaduct on the railway from North
Shields to Newcastle, would alone have stamped them with
the character of men of eminent skill, had they not even
executed the many other great works of which they are the
authors, these gentlemen propose to erect several houses
in the form of two crescents, the one looking north-east, and
the other south-east, on each side of, and on, the lofty cliff
below which the principal sea-bathing takes place as before
stated.   The latter situation has received the name of Prior's
Haven, although placed at some distance from that bold
promontory on which the ruins of an ancient priory, standing with the lighthouse at their north-east angle, like a landmark to sailors, attract the attention of the stranger.   A
parapet, raised breast high, runs round the edge of the cliff,
forming a species of terrace from which a very fine sea-view
is obtained.   Beneath the precipice, the tremendous ledges
of rock, called the *Black Middens*, stretch into the sea to a
considerable distance.

A small and old bath-house, very plain and mean-looking,
is placed at the back of the Prior's Haven, with facilities for
taking warm sea-baths, or getting into a plunging-bath.   It is
to be expected that the opening of the railroad between Newcastle and North Shields will induce a great many more visiters
than heretofore to proceed to Tynemouth, to which an omnibus conveys you, after a rapid journey on railway of sixteen
minutes over a distance of seven miles and a half from Newcastle to North Shields; and it is to be hoped that improvements, equally necessary and important, will be devised, with
a view to render Tynemouth truly worthy of the support of
such of the good people of Newcastle as love sea-bathing
and sea breezes.   By this railroad I made good my way to
Newcastle, taking up my abode, as on a former occasion, at
the Turk's Head in Grey-street.

A second visit to this Liverpool of the North Seas impressed me even more vividly than the first with its importance and striking appearance.   On the former occasion

there was, in aid of my impression, the *prestige* which the presence of nearly two thousand strangers,—philosophers by name,—spouters and men of pleasure by inclination—and gourmands from natural disposition, still all good fellows, assembled to enlighten the good people of Newcastle, was calculated to excite.   Among them, men of an imperishable name in their respective branches of knowledge there were, who shone conspicuous by their works and justified by their example, as really working members, the assumed name of " British Association for the advancement of science"—a name the implied meaning of which did certainly not apply to the majority of the fellows.

Still their united efforts to amuse, or to enlighten, joined to the conspicuous and splendid manner of their reception and treatment by all the easy classes in and about the city, imparted, for the moment, a brilliancy to every object around, which could not fail to impress me, a stranger like the rest, with admiration.

And yet, when on the present, my second visit, I found Newcastle pursuing its ordinary course of busy life, without foreign or meretricious tinselling and excitement to give it a fleeting brilliancy ;—the one day being like the one which preceded it, and like that by which it was followed,—the impression I received of its present and growing importance, and of the prominent station it has nearly taken among the very first cities of the empire, was infinitely more striking than ever.

The reason is obvious.   The one master mind, who, within the short space of four years up to the period of my first visit, had swept away from the very centre of Newcastle, over an area of many acres, scenes of solitude and desolation, and dangerous ravines, and useless orchards smoked into unproductivenes, changing the surface of the earth where such things stood, that he might place on it in their stead a hundred spacious buildings, with façades more elegant, more classical, and more uniform in design than had hitherto been attempted ; opening out, at the same time, more direct and spacious streets, squares, and thorough-fares ;—that master mind, I say, had also in two short years more, so extended his immense operations, and so exquisitely and magically completed those designs and plans which had hardly had any commencement when we first beheld the new city—that the feelings of astonishment and admiration excited at this second visit assumed necessarily a tenfold intensity.

Modern Newcastle would surprise every Englishman pre-viously unacquainted with the place, even though he may have seen and admired the only two other provincial cities that can be compared to it—Edinburgh and Bath—or even after the contemplation of some of the many splendid cities on the continent. Modern Newcastle is a strong illus-tration of the principle which I hold in common with many, that " Despotism is the true creator and encourager of the art of architecture." The will of ONE, capable and deter-mined, is necessary to bring into existence the grandest con-ceptions in that art. Survey all that ancient Greece and Rome, or modern Italy, or the present capitals of the Bava-rian, the Prussian, the Russian, and the French dominions have of truly magnificent buildings, and say whether the single " fiat" of a king, or an emperor, or a pope, or even of the chief magistrate of a republican community, aided by contemporary genius and unbounded means, did not start them into existence. The despotism need not be exclusively that of royalty or political rule—though that be, unquestion-ably, the very best for the object. The despotism of a private individual—his only will, uncontrollable, unsuscepti-ble of any interference, not to be baffled by obstacles and difficulties—backed by all the ready wealth of treasure, or sound credit, that can be needed for carrying vast projects into effect—directed by genius—grand, unique, inspired ;—such a despotism as this is sufficient to produce the wonders in architecture to which applies the principle in question, and such a despotism has enabled the humble apprentice of

a house carpenter to create the marvels which the great majority of Englishmen hardly know to exist in Newcastle.

Know it however they may, if they read ; for within the last
two months that widely-circulated periodical of popular information, the *Penny Magazine,* has in several successive
articles published to the English world a full and able
description of modern Newcastle, and of its numerous edifices
and magnificent streets and monuments, generally superior to
those of other cities in the kingdom—the work of Robert
Grainger, the master-mind to which all my preceding allusions are directed.

Those articles are supposed to have been written by a fair
author whose intellect is as acute as her faculty of hearing is
unfortunately slow. During the stay of the British Association at Newcastle, that lady had sufficient leisure to contemplate all the wonders by which she was surrounded, or those
which were rising before her, and the good fortune of becoming acquainted with the author of them ; none therefore,
either in literary qualification or opportunity, could be better
qualified for the task she has undertaken and ably fulfilled
in the periodical I have named.

But the fair writer has since had, it is supposed, far better
means of performing that task with ability and precision, as
well as of lightening her own labours; for she held in her possession, during several days, a written account of all Mr. Grainger's projects, drawn up by a gentleman intimately connected
with the progress and execution of those projects, and evidently
qualified, as I happen to know from experience, for that duty.
This the open-hearted, candid, straightforward, and successful proprietor had shown her, previously to its being forwarded,
accompanied with a plan, to His Royal Highness the Duke
of Sussex, who, on a recent visit to Newcastle, had requested
to have such an account.

In all that Miss Martineau has there advanced, therefore,
of the former and present state of that city, precision and ful-

ness of information may be expected; and the knowledge of such a fact excuses me from entering, as I was otherwise prepared to do from notes in my portfolio, into a detailed account of Robert Grainger's almost magical achievements. The history of that individual, in every way extraordinary, given by the fair writer in the recent numbers of the *Penny Magazine*, is in substance correct, with the exception of his having designed the works he has so creditably executed. No—that is not the glory of this great man. The writer asks, Whence has he derived his power as an artist? That point she imagines to be still a mystery. But it is no mystery in Newcastle, nor does it detract from Mr. Grainger's great and transcendent merits that he is neither an artist, nor that he has not designed one of the splendid buildings which he has *projected* and *carried into execution*. Whom or how many he may have employed in that department it is hardly necessary to name; since the projects have been wholly from his own creative mind, and were executed entirely under his own inspection and control. Hence his taste, his judgment, and his invention are visible in all the great works which began and were ended at his will. It is he, therefore, who is entitled to the praise of having done all that the wondering inhabitants of Newcastle have seen performing around them for the last six years—of having, in fine, achieved more than any single individual perhaps ever accomplished before.

Mr. Grainger had, after the fashion of other great builders, succeeded in erecting, in the ordinary style, property to the amount of two hundred thousand pounds, in various parts of the town: a square, a royal arcade, and two magnificent terraces; for some of which he had used, contrary to precedents, the excellent material so abundantly found in the neighbourhood, instead of dingy bricks hitherto employed—when the vast conceptions he has since carried into effect for the improvement and embellishment of Newcastle first fixed his attention. Those conceptions embraced almost an entire *bouleversement* of the town, and presented difficulties which none but a daring mind would have ventured to encounter. The natural inequalities of the surface on the line of which our forefathers would have built, no matter how steep the incline, were such as Mr. Grainger could not adopt with his ideas of grandeur, as well as comfort. In effecting the regular levels or gentle inclination which he wished to give to, and which the present streets exhibit, immense valleys required to be filled up, and entire hills to be removed. Some of the former were as much as 35 feet below what was intended to be the finished street as now seen ; and as the foundations which Mr. Grainger was determined to give them were to be placed (as indeed they have been) upon the solid strata considerably below the surface of the valley, there must be several houses with a greater height of masonry below, than appears above the line of the street, many of them being as much as 54 feet in that respect. And such is actually the case with some of the principal houses in Grey-street.

Difficulties of this description, which the perseverance of Mr. Grainger surmounted, may be judged from the fact, that after filling up certain immense valleys with the soil removed from places that rose considerably above the intended level, two hundred and fifty thousand loads were carted off the premises—equal to four and a half millions of cubic feet of soil,—sufficient to cover one hundred and three acres of land one foot thick. The digging and carting alone, exclusive of the sums paid for depositing the soil, cost the sum of 21,500*l.*

But this is not all ; difficulties of another nature, and to a single-handed individual even more formidable, had presented themselves to Mr. Grainger's mind in calculating the execution of his vast projects. Where were the enormous sums requisite to carry them into effect to be found ? Before such an expenditure for buildings and public improvements, even a government has been known to quake and to hesitate.

The old property to be purchased, and to be pulled down, was estimated at 145,937*l.*—to be provided for by the carpenter's apprentice ! Two theatres did this humble individual contemplate to raze to the ground, and a butchers' as well as a vegetable market; and a large mansion, with offices; and one large inn, and eight public-houses ; and about eighty private houses and shops, with a considerable number of workshops, and public and inferior buildings. All these were to disappear at the bidding of the carpenters' apprentice, to make room for more convenient, useful, and splendid structures !

And they *have* disappeared ; while the splendid structures are up and glorious ; and the unknown youngster who called them into existence has provided the means, and expended half a million of pounds sterling in workmen's wages and materials, during the five years that the new streets have been in progress, up to August last.

Behold the result ! in place of the property annihilated, there have been planned and built nine new streets, extending collectively to one mile and the sixth part of another; and these contain three extensive markets, under one general roof, which, with the fourteen entrances from the surrounding streets, comprise an area of upwards of two acres ; they contain also a Central Exchange, since converted into one of the most splendid news-rooms and coffee-rooms in Europe; a new theatre and new dispensary ; a music-hall, a lecture-room, one incorporate company's hall, two chapels, two auction-marts ; ten inns and twelve public-houses; four banks, forty private dwelling-houses of the first class, and three hundred and twenty-five houses with shops : the whole of which already realizes a rental of 18,000*l.* a year, and when completed, will realize, according to valuation, forty thousand, exclusive of many valuable properties sold, such as the markets, the theatre, two banks, and two chapels.

In one word, the new property already created by Mr. Grainger's vast conceptions, first formed in 1833, and still in progress of extension, has been valued at 995,000*l.*, or nearly one million sterling. With an immense stock of honesty, punctuality, and plain open dealing, guided in all his transactions by a fervid imagination and a calm genius, has Mr. Grainger been able to accumulate such a fortune. Towards achieving it, he at first contributed nothing, or very little of pecuniary means, save perhaps a slender sum of five thousand pounds, the marriage portion of an affectionate, intelligent and clever wife, who has been indefatigable in aiding and cheering the partner of her life.

The general appearance of the streets, with their rich and diversified architecture, is particularly striking to the eye of a stranger, and people find it difficult to express the sensation that pervades the mind on a first inspection. Their great extent, their uniformity and expensive decorations, even to the carved work of both houses and shops, all executed in solid stone, of an agreeable and uniform tint, give an idea of magnificence so peculiar and unexpected to those who arrive at Newcastle unprepared for such a scene by any thing they have beholden elsewhere in their journey thither, that the mind cannot help being seized with wonder and admiration.

These feelings are first awakened at the sight of Grey-street, certainly one of the finest double lines of domestic architecture of rich designs and lofty proportions to be found in Europe. Ascending upon a gentle acclivity from south to north, and with a slight curve which detracts nothing from its beauties, this superb street extends to nearly four hundred yards in length, with an average width of eighty feet. In its architectural decorations it is most elaborate, and its different sections formed by the intersecting of the cross streets, comprise separate designs, among which one recognises at once the Corinthian order, after the example of the interior of the Pantheon at Rome, with columns twenty-five feet high; and by its side, the more chaste imitation of the noblest example of the Ionic order, that of the temple of Illysus at Athens; the columns measuring twenty-two feet in height.

Another of the striking features in this street is the new theatre, a building the interior of which is deserving of particular attention, as being in many respects different from similar buildings, and as having a gallery capable of holding fifteen hundred persons.   As it is principally on the attendance of such people as usually frequent that part of a theatre, that the manager depends for remuneration, it was important to have the gallery both spacious and safe.   The bold hexastile portico of this building, which projects across the pavement, with its columns of the Corinthian order placed on pedestals and shafts twenty-nine feet in height, supporting a suitable entablature and pediment, is perhaps the most striking object in Grey-street.

Higher up, and on the same side, however, a portion of an intended splendid square building attracts the attention of the visiter, which is considered the finest piece of architecture among all Mr. Grainger's works.   It is occupied by the new district bank.   Had the whole of the design originally submitted to the corporation by Mr. Grainger on the most advantageous terms been executed, the Newcastle town-court and offices, and the Northumberland assize-courts, now very inconveniently situated in different and remote parts of the town, would have been placed in one grand central building, in the Roman style of architecture, with a portico in front and another at the back, to distinguish the entrance into each of the courts, and projecting over the footpath in each street. But corporations, whether reformed or unreformed, are not of a temperament to keep pace with such a mind as Robert Grainger's, nor capable of appreciating such vast architectural conceptions as he submitted to them ; and so after enduring for some time the indifference of those " liberals," that spirited, though meek individual withdrew his truly liberal offer ; and the people of Newcastle have lost the opportunity of possessing perhaps the most splendid buildings that could have adorned their town.

Mr. John Wardle, who, under the direction of Mr. Grainger, carefully prepared the plans of the proposed pile, is a gentleman who, with Messrs. Green, father and son, both eminent architects and engineers, Mr. Dobson, and one or two other able professional men, has assisted the originator of all these wonders throughout his manifold projects and operations.

I would wish to dwell on some others of those operations ; on the great Central Exchange and News-room for example,* which, within a semicircle of seventy-five feet radius, extended twenty feet beyond the centre point, presents an area of one hundred and fifty feet by ninety-five, the centre of which is a raised platform, encircled by twelve Roman Ionic columns, carpeted, and used as a news-room ; while the broad semicircular space around it, lighted from the roof, curiously wrought, and standing at the height of forty feet, serves as a promenade over a tessellated pavement, that harmonizes with the surrounding wall, its bold entablature, and its columns of imitative Sienna marble.†

* This magnificent building, originally designed as a Corn Exchange, was actually offered as a gift to the *Reformed* Corporation by Mr. Grainger, simply on condition of its being so appropriated. The council declined the offer, and preferred dipping their hands into the people's pocket to the tune of 9600*l.* for a Corn Exchange just built in Nicholas-square.

† A singular oversight occurs in regard to the relative position of the principal or central door, leading by an inner double flight of steps down into the great room. Instead of being exactly placed in the line of the central radius corresponding with the centre point of the encircled platform, this door is considerably on one side of it.

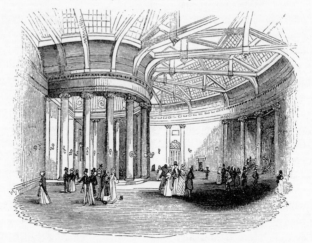

I should also have liked to have pointed out not only the magnitude, but the very happy arrangement of the new markets, which are unquestionably the finest, as well as the most convenient of the kind, in England; and lastly, I might have felt inclined to say a word on that commemorative column, which the reformers directed Messrs. Green to erect and Mr. Baily to surmount with the statue of their patron saint, in Portland stone well oiled, but which column has been left shorn of some of its fair proportions, through the slackening of the primitive fervour of the worshippers, who at last could not muster more than 2350*l.* for the architect, the sculptor, and the builder of the monument altogether!*

* It may be deemed not uninteresting, now that another column is about to rise in the metropolis, to know the exact proportions of the Grey column, especially as they are either not given, or inaccurately given, in other publications. It is of Roman Doric, and measures in height one hundred and thirty-four feet from the ground to the top of the figure, which is thirteen feet high; the shaft is 9 feet eleven inches in diameter and consists of twenty-one courses three feet high. The pedestal is thirty-one feet to the base. The material of which the column is built is a species of millstone grit, hardening on exposure. The statue is of Portland stone, and in three pieces.

All these objects it would have been gratifying to one
fond of architectural pursuits, and a great admirer of Mr.
Grainger's talents, to have described more extensively and
minutely; but I am warned that neither my space nor the
immediate intention of the present work comports with such
learned digressions; and I desist, therefore, from making any
further observations.

I may conclude this imperfect account of the wonders that
have been enacted and are now enacting in architecture at
Newcastle, through the energy of one man, by stating that
the same individual has lately purchased a large estate, consisting of five hundred and seventy acres of land, for fifty-five
thousand pounds, on the banks of the Tyne above bridge;
which he means to convert into a new and extensive fau-
bourg, partly for business—to effect which he is now executing
one of the handsomest and longest quays in England—and
partly for the residence of the wealthier citizens, for whom
handsome detached villas, as well as streets and terraces, have
been already designed.   The scene of bustle I witnessed on
this large tract of ground, occupying a beautiful acclivity on
the left bank of the Tyne, with a corresponding prospect over
the vale, is beyond the power of description.

To facilitate access to this new town (for such it will be),
Mr. Grainger meditates pulling down the present bridge over
the river, and erecting one sufficiently elevated to allow the
largest vessels to mount the stream up to his new and
gigantic wharfs.   When completed, this new creation will
perfectly astonish the people of this country, and with Mr.
Grainger such a creation is the work of a few years only.

This extraordinary person may be compared with the
individual who, according to Captain Marryat, was the
principal moving cause of the springing up of a new and
perfect city in America, near the Erie Lake, named Buffalo,
in the short space of twenty years.   Rathbun (for such was
his name), like Grainger, planned all the streets and squares,

built all the churches, hotels, and public edifices; and, in fact,
every great building worthy of observation in Buffalo was projected and executed by Rathbun. Like Grainger, the American
constructor was quiet and unassuming in his manners; and
and like him too, under an apparent simplicity, he possessed
a mind capable of the vastest conceptions united with the
greatest power of execution. Rathbun entered into contracts
and embarked in building speculations to an amount almost
incredible. In fact, he undertook every thing, and every
thing undertaken by Rathbun was "well done." But here
the parallel must end; for the American Rathbun, as
appears from the sequel of Captain Marryat's statement,
turned out to have used dishonest means to his ends;
whereas the Northumbrian Rathbun has attained his own
equally gigantic ends, justly boasting all along of the honesty
of his means.

Newcastle has always been rich in men of this stamp, who
leaping, as it were, by their own efforts, from an obscure cradle
into a glorious maturity of reputation, end by taking up a
prominent station in society. The examples need not be
quoted,—many of them are of too recent a date not to suggest themselves at once to the minds of my readers. But
one of them occupies too conspicuous a place in the modern
history of human ingenuity not to be especially singled out
in this place; the more so, as in many respects he resembles
his equally-celebrated fellow-townsman Robert Grainger.
My readers will naturally anticipate the name of George
Stephenson, the projector of, beyond comparison, the most
perfect and the most usefully extensive railroad ever constructed—that which connects Manchester with Liverpool;
and of many other equally striking and important public works
besides, since executed. I had the satisfaction of meeting
him in company with the fair members of a most amiable
family residing a short distance out of Newcastle, from whom
I received every mark of kindness.

This great and good man was originally a common pitman, who first showed his skill and ingenuity by cleaning and making clocks for his fellow-pitmen, without having received any instruction; and by inventing a safety-lamp, which gave rise to rivalry and contention of talent between him and Sir Humphry Davy. Mr. Stephenson preserves all the innate simplicity of his manners, and often refers to his early history and humble origin with complacency.

It is possible that some impatient reader may feel disposed to inquire wherefore, into a work on the Spas of England, a long digression on modern Newcastle has been introduced. Though I had twenty reasons for so doing, I will only allege one. Of the many digressions in which I indulged in my work on the Spas of Germany, the public, as well as the critics of the day, accepted with especial favour that which I introduced descriptive of the architectural magnificence of Munich—the work there also of one great directing mind. Should I not then have made myself amenable to the reproach of gross partiality, and of thorough disregard of what I found good in that way in England, if I had passed over in silence that which I knew to be the constant theme of admiration among those who are apt judges in such matters,—foreigners as well as English,—the equally magnificent architectural splendour of the Northumbrian capital?

CHAPTER XX.

SHOTLEY BRIDGE SPA.

In the general map of England, nay, even in some of the local maps, my reader may find it difficult to trace to its proper situation the Spa referred to by the above title; and yet within ten years from this time I predict that no map whatever will be without its name, ay, and in capital letters, too.

An antiquarian, or a geologist, perchance an angler, who recollects the exclamation of the homely poet, Carr—

"Thy minnows, that play when they please,
O Derwent, how happy they look!"

may not be ignorant of such a place as Shotley Bridge,

situated on the river named in the couplet. Sequestered and insignificant as it may hitherto have been considered by others, to them, at all events, Shotley Bridge offered too many objects of attraction ever to be forgotten. But to the lover of mineral hydrology, the place, as connected with any mineral spring, has probably never come under notice, at least out of the county of Durham. And yet in that very county will, ere long, the mineral water of Shotley hold the first rank among its other mineral sources ; and Shotley Bridge will emulate the celebrity of Harrogate, Cheltenham, and Leamington.

The report that such a mineral water had been recently discovered was my principal inducement for proceeding to Newcastle, where I expected to collect that information concerning it which I had in vain tried to obtain at various places during my journey from the south. At Newcastle, however, not only did I learn as much as I could expect respecting it, but chance, and the courtesy, as well as the marked urbanity, of the proprietor of the land in which the spring was discovered, facilitated my object further ; for it put me in direct communication with that gentleman, and enabled me to gain a complete knowledge, from personal inspection, of every particular relating to this new Spa.

For that purpose, I proceeded from Newcastle in a light open carriage, sent by " friend" Richardson, a banker in that city, and the proprietor before alluded to, driven by one of his resident bank-assistants, whose intimate knowledge of the county proved to me a source of much useful information.

And beautiful, truly, are many parts of the county through which we passed. Following the road which runs parallel with the Tyne, on the high ground that forms its northern bank, we soon came in sight of Scotswood Suspension-bridge, thrown across the river near the confluence of the Derwent with the Tyne. This group is, perhaps, one of the prettiest features of the surrounding landscape—itself one of great beauty.*

It is surprising that the citizens of Newcastle have not yet thought of erecting villas on the right of this road—a sort of gentle declivity, having before it a magnificent and most extensive prospect of an undulating, yet highly-cultivated country, far removed from the influence of the dense smoke of Newcastle, and the numerous factories now establishing on Mr. Grainger's gigantic quay. Spreading to the south and south-west, the country displays many lordly mansions, among which that of Ravensworth Castle appears most conspicuous. The sight of that attractive structure, where recent embellishments, yet in progress, are due to the artistic talent of a member of the family, brought to my recollection the affable, courteous, and splendid reception given within its walls, by its lord and his gifted relatives, to the ducal president and many of the members of the British Association in the year preceding.

The suspension-bridge,† just mentioned, is not quite so large as the one at Hammersmith; and near to it is erected another bridge, constructed of wood, and resting upon six short and stout piers, over which the prolongation of the Carlisle and Newcastle railway is to pass in its course to the very verge of the lastmentioned city. The bridge is thrown obliquely across the water.‡

* The design of the bridge, which is a magnificent structure, is another of those happy conceptions of Mr. Green, of Newcastle, which have raised so high his character as an architect, particularly in this class of buildings. The distance between the two points of suspension is 370 feet, with two half aces of 130 feet each, making the total length of the bridge 670 feet. The road is 22 feet wide, and constructed of timber. The two piers on which the four suspending chains rest are in the Norman style.

† The construction of this bridge occupied only two years, and cost 15,000*l.*

‡ While penning this part of the description, I learn, by a letter from

One of the members for Newcastle possesses in this part of the river one of those salmon-fisheries for which the river is so celebrated.

The scenery of the Tyne is expansive and softly undulating, a character which it maintains throughout the course of the river. But when we enter the vale of the Derwent, between Swelwell and Axwell Park, and proceed towards Gibside, the scene changes, and the valley of that narrow and tortuous stream, differing from that of Tyne, becomes contracted, and more romantic in proportion as it gets more contracted.

Crossing at one point of our road the Carlisle and Newcastle railway, my travelling companion alluded to the immense advantages it had produced to both terminal cities in respect to Irish traffic. Connected as he was with the district bank, which has opened an account with most of the Irish banks, he was able to mention one curious illustration of those advantages, in the manner and amount of importation of Irish bacon into England. Formerly, all such commodity, the consumption of which in the north-east counties is very considerable, used to find its way from Ireland to London. But now the facility of a direct and cheaper transport from Ireland to the eastern counties has changed the course of that line of traffic, and the bacon which was formerly offered to the metropolitan market goes now to satisfy the wants of the people of Durham and Northumberland.

Within the last twelve months, bills to the amount of 200,000*l.* had passed through the bank of my informant's employer, to pay for Irish bacon sent to Newcastle. The Irish exporter finding there a price equal to that which he was wont to get in London, and at a much less expense for transport to boot, naturally prefers now the former to the latter

Newcastle, that the archway from the other side, and across the river, and from thence to the turnpike, is now in full operation. By this arrangement, the principal station or terminus of this important railroad is brought within the suburbs of the town.

market. On the other hand, the consumers at Newcastle and
Durham are satisfied that the flavour and substance of Irish
hogflesh are as good as those of the Cumberland bacon,
which they used to purchase before at a somewhat higher
price ; consequently the latter article has been entirely sup-
planted in these parts by the Irish bacon, and is now sent to
London instead, where the consumers have to pay dearer for
their bacon, owing to this change in the line of Irish traffic
consequent on the establishment of the Newcastle and Carlisle railroad.

The farther we advanced towards our destination the more
varied and picturesque became the surrounding landscape.
On our left an Ionic column, surmounted by the figure of
Liberty, rose out of a majestic wood to the height of 140
feet, and seemed, by a strange coincidence, to mark the present
centre of a sad district, where *liberty*-boys, or Chartists, steeped
in gross ignorance—without schools—and with insufficient
religious instruction—were at the time rife with intended mischief. Manufacturers of edge-tools and glass at the several
mills in the neighbourhood, masons, and excavators, formed
the bulk of the troublous and discontented. The pitmen,
once their fellow-conspirators, had just declared themselves
aloof. Those are most vociferous for liberty who have light
pockets and still lighter stomachs ; and the pitmen, who
can earn, with their own and their boys' daily work, as much
as thirty-five and even forty shillings a week, found themselves too snug and well *ballasted* to fly much longer about
the country in search of an uncertain phantom and broken
heads, to the utter neglect of their own certain sources of
livelihood.

By the side of Axwell Park, which I had been skirting ere
I reached Gibside Hall, the residence of one of the members
for Hull, and of a noble Countess—in whose park stands the
column just alluded to,—I was astonished by the appearance

of a well, at which sundry holiday people were quaffing the limpid stream.

I found it slightly impregnated with sulphuretted hydrogen gas, and somewhat ferruginous ; pleasant to the taste, and giving out a few bubbles of free gas. The temperature was 52° F., and the water, perfectly colourless and transparent, is incessantly overrunning its rude stone basin, which, covered on three sides, is accessible on the fourth to all who choose to drink at the fountain-head. Dr. Askew, a celebrated physician, who lived on the other side of the Derwent, published an account of this mineral spring, which, in former times, enjoyed great repute.

Beyond Rowland's-Gill tollgate, the road, which was made by subscription in the course of the last five years, traverses a widely-cultivated country, thickly wooded in parts, following (but at some considerable elevation above it) the narrow Derwent, which is seen to wind its course between two sloping and wooded banks, all the way to Shotley Bridge. It is to commerce again that travellers are indebted for the present excellent road to that important station.

The Shotley Bridge paper-mills, which are perhaps the most extensive in the country, were worked by Messrs. Annandale, who found the old road on the opposite bank very difficult and bad for the conveyance of their materials and manufactured articles. They therefore urged the making of the present new road, began it themselves, and were soon aided by others who have residences in the immediate vicinity

A contributor to the sports of the neighbouring gentry, by his purse and pack of hounds, as well as by his written lucubrations to the Magazine which sportsmen love to patronize, occupies the next important hall we beheld in this species of paradise. Descending by his recently deceased father's side from the historian of Durham, and connected by the parentage of his mother, a high-minded lady, with one of the present members for South Northumberland, the young proprietor of Hamsterley Hall has studied to maintain the high character of his connexions, and has become justly popular.

The celebrated *Chopwell* Woods, once the private property of George the Fourth, when Prince of Wales, and now forming part of the crown lands, range to a great extent in front of Hamsterley Hall, on a steep and picturesque part of the bank of the Derwent through the vale of which, rich and beautiful, the road continues its course, traversing by the way the Roman station at Ebchester, the vestiges of whose *vallum* are still remaining on the Watling-street, or old Roman road, between Edinburgh and London. From this spot, the Watling-street, which descends from the Northumberland moors hither, takes a south-eastern direction to Lanchester, offering here and there many points of interest to the antiquary. In many parts it is still open and intact, but in others covered over. Yet the Scotch drovers, tenacious of their traditional rights, still insist on tracking it, throughout its whole extent, with their cattle, as they find means whereby to feed their beasts, and have lighter tolls *to* pay.

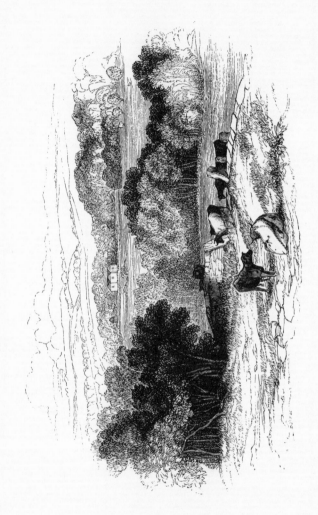

GENERAL VIEW OF SHOTLEY BRIDGE SPA.

We had now reached an eminence, called Westwood, from whence the general view of Shotley Bridge Spa and surrounding scenery, which I have here inserted was taken. A vast dale on the right appears as if hollowed out by some mighty stream of old, whose waters having retired, left two smiling and fertile sloping banks, inclining down to the Derwent.` The undulating surface is mapped in all directions by dense woods of various extent. Here and there a white house, or some superior dwelling, dots the smaller hills, or the champaign country; which affords an occasional view of the river wending its way in curiously fantastic turns, and seeming, by its stream, to cut the vale in twain. Extensive fields highly cultivated and rich in their summer crops complete the locality of the Spa; the rustic dome of which, with its modest pump-room and baths, occupy nearly the centre. In the distance a line of elevated ground bounds the view: it is the Stanhope railway on the left, and the border of the moors, distant about four miles, on the right.

Descending now very gradually, the road traverses a small wood of oak-trees, through which footpaths and sheltered walks have been made, leading to the well; and at length it brings us a little farther into the village of Shotley Bridge.

Having alighted, I proceeded at once to the WELL, passing through the village, which, in its modern parts, the creation of " friend " Richardson, offers the appearance of extreme neatness and comfort. That gentleman' has already built a number of dwelling-houses with shops, all of stone, and roofed over with Cumberland slate. These buildings group well together, and their creamy and rosy tints harmonize charmingly with the rich green foliage of the banks and slopes. He proposes to erect other shops and cottages in the same manner, and so to extend the village. A crescent of handsome houses is to be built on the upland; and planting has been going on in every direction where necessary; the lowlands, by the river-side, being about to be converted into parterres, as flower or kitchen gardens.

There was a new and a handsome hotel in the course of being built at the time of my visit, planned on a large scale, with a suitable set of stables. Since then I learn that it has been completed, and furnished in a manner superior to hotels in general, particularly with good beds. The occupant of the house is well qualified to please his customers, and such was his popularity at the commencement of his career, that the house filled remarkably well during the six weeks it was open before the end of last season.

" Friend" Richardson, equally liberal and endowed with sense, is unsparing in his means and ways to embellish and give importance to this new colony, which promises to be far more fortunate than the colony of Germans, their predecessors of olden times, who settled in this place as eminent sword cutlers, and founded the village. Drinking and evil ways, doubtless the results of gross ignorance and little religion, reduced that once flourishing community to four wretched families only, whose descendants are still to be traced among the larger and happier population of the present village, by the corrupt German structure of their names inscribed over the door of their shops.

Excellent and new lodging-houses, built near the village, afford ample accommodation to the visiters who have hitherto frequented the Spa; but as their numbers are increasing, and will continue to increase, the proprietor of the land offers to sell sites for buildings, above an ornamental belt, lately planted behind the present lodging-houses. The situation of those sites is one of the most favourable, being upon an agreeable slope, commanding a fine view of the opposite hill. I hardly know a more inviting locality for the erection of a private house, particularly with such a landlord, and upon such advantageous terms. In a few years, all these hills will teem with busy dwellings.*

But "friend" Richardson, who is himself a most conscientious, strict, and zealous religionist in his own sect—so much so, indeed, that he has even devoted a part of his own neat and commodious villa for the congregation of his brethren, who flock thither from far and near, to keep the sabbath-day in the strictest and most exemplary observance of their own peculiar religious rites—even he, I am certain, must have felt, ere now, the necessity of providing a suitable place of worship for the larger number of those belonging to the national church, who are either setting themselves down as permanent dwellers in this new and flourishing village, or attend as invalids and visiters during the Spa season. At present an old and small church only can be resorted to by them for the purpose ; but besides being small and inadequate, that place of worship is too far distant from the modern village. A church, therefore, is absolutely called for in Shotley Bridge ; and I know of no impediment in the peculiar position of the excellent individual, who shares with another equally wealthy gentleman, resident in the place, the lordship and property of the village, against his causing to be erected a temple to God for public worship, according to the rites of the church dominant.

Accompanied by my friendly travelling companion, I took the direction to the Spa, along one of the footpaths formed between the village and the entrance to the Spa grounds, the latter of which much resemble a private gentleman's pleasure-grounds. Access to the Spa has been made both easy and pleasant by many subsequent improvements, especially in the opening of new walks to it from the hotel, and

---

* By recent accounts I find that my prediction is in progress of fulfilment, for in the present season (1840) such was the influx of visiters that house-room became scarce—and new buildings have consequently been planned, and are starting into existence.

upper village, along the slope which rises behind it, and
which enjoys a fine view of the country.

The WELL, situated nearly in the centre of an ornamental
garden, about a mile below the village, I found, on my arrival, surrounded by country people from all the neighbouring villages, in their gay holiday-garments, it being Sunday; while the saloon adjoining, as well as the shaded seats
near and about it, were occupied by the permanent visiters to
the Spa.   All of them seemed to be plying the glass freely,
drinking three or four of them full of the water, at short intervals between, without any apparent method or guidance,
but simply from traditional or hearsay directions.

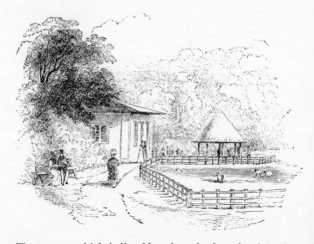

The water, which is limpid and perfectly colourless, issues
in an horizontal stream, through a spout in an upright stone
which covers the well.   It falls into a round, low basin, the
inner surface of which betrays, by its colour, the presence of
iron in the water. This deposition, which is equally observable
on the tile tanks of the bath-rooms, is cleared off by the
attendants from time to time, although they find it extremely
difficult, occasionally, to remove it from the surface, so tena-

ciously does the oxyde adhere. The spring is protected by a simple round thatched roof, supported by slender rustic trunks of trees. Three circular steps lead down to the well.

The temperature of the water I found to be 48° F., after repeated trials; that of the atmosphere in the shade at the time being 76°. The stream yielded a half-pint glassful in twenty seconds exactly, or a pint and a half in one minute. But this supply has since been increased threefold, by the simple operation of lowering the surface around the well one step deeper. Six hundred gallons of the water are now obtained per day, a quantity which, according to a very recent analysis, holds in solution about twenty-one pounds weight of solid contents—making, in all, seven thousand six hundred and sixty-five pounds of solid ingredient in the annual quantity of water yielded by the well.

The analysis I alluded to was undertaken at my suggestion, with Mr. Richardson's immediate consent, by Mr. West, of Leeds, whose analytical chemical skill I have already had occasion to commend. Reasons, not necessary to be specified in this place, had led me to doubt of the accuracy of a printed analysis which appeared on the cards distributed at the Spa, and the result showed the propriety of having a fresh one made. It was impossible to understand the rationale of many of the well-authenticated cases of cure achieved by means of this water, when its former alleged chemical composition was admitted. Thus it will always be found, in mineral hydrology, that the composition of a mineral water may be inferred from the cures it performs; and *vice versâ*, that the nature of diseases benefited by mineral waters being known, the kind of ingredients contained in that water may be readily suspected. With this simple rule to guide me, I have, on many occasions during my recent visits to the mineral springs in this county, found it necessary to insist upon totally new analyses of the several waters being performed by leading chemists; and I have reason to know that the proprietors of those springs, who, in almost every instance, attended to my suggestion, have had occasion to rejoice at the step they had adopted.

As it now appears, the Spa water at Shotley Bridge holds a middle place between the absolute chalybeates and the purgative chalybeate springs of this country. It is an " alterative chalybeate," eminently calculated to relieve and cure diseases of weakness and obstruction in the circulation, glandular affections of the mesentery, dyspepsia, deficiency of tone in the intestines, impurity of blood, or tendency to decomposition, each calculated to produce cutaneous diseases and land scurvy; and, when used as a warm bath, rheumatic complaints have been singularly benefited by it.   The water, in fact, is a most valuable one, containing a large yet manageable proportion of proto-carbonate of iron, with neutral salts sufficient to prevent the inconvenience which mere chalybeates sometimes occasion.   Three distinct muriates, all of them valuable, are present in the water, besides the iron; and in addition to them we find an excess of carbonic acid beyond that which goes to form the proto-carbonate of iron, combined with soda.   The presence of bromine, also, though in minute quantity, and of traces of carburetted hydrogen gas, add to the medicinal efficacy of the water.   In fact, properly studied and properly attended to, the Shotley Bridge Spa water may be made instrumental in the recovery of many disorders which no other water in the country can cure.   The water differs in its composition from all the others I have examined in my recent tour.

Of the many striking examples of recovery from disease, under the mere influence of the Shotley Bridge Spa, I had the means of verifying several by personal inquiry.   An old man, reduced to a state of weakness and emaciation from " constant vomiting, water-brash and heartburn," — such were his words,—and discharged unrelieved from the Newcastle Infirmary, came hither in July, 1838, hardly able to move, and after three weeks of using the water recovered his strength, and returned home " in better health than he had enjoyed for three years."

A woman was confined of twins in 1837, and in consequence of hemorrhage, was much reduced, and had been long under medical treatment. When she reached Shotley Bridge she was under the necessity of remaining in bed for several days. After, however, drinking the water for a few days, she was able to walk, with assistance, to the well, and subsequently regained her colour, flesh, and strength by the continuance of the water, so as to return home quite well.

A very extraordinary case of cutaneous eruption from infancy, which neither medical advice during a course of many years, nor a residence at the sea-side had removed, and in which one of the patient's hands was so sorely afflicted, that it neither could be moved without pain, nor opened or shut without causing it to bleed, was perfectly cured by drinking the Shotley Bridge water for the space of one month.

From the father of the little patient I obtained the following well-authenticated case, which I quote in the narrator's own simple words : " When I brought my child to Shotley Bridge he was so afflicted with the scurvy, that it caused it both to run matter at the eyes and ears, and its face was one whole incrustation, and it also broke out in other parts of the body. We tried medical aid without effect. But we gave it of the Spa water to the amount of one gallon a day before we had done with it, which cured the child in a fortnight ; and so perfect was the cure that in a month's time you would have said the child had not been poorly at all—the skin being quite clear. The child was afflicted from the age of one year and a quarter, and it was three and a half years old when it took the water."

An instance of that disgusting disease, called the chin tetter (*mentagra*), in which both lips were largely involved, and another of a man who was so reduced in strength that he could only speak in whispers, and yet had spent nearly all his fortune in consulting medical men to no purpose, both completely cured at this well, were related to me by Mr. Nicholson, who had ample opportunities of watching the cases.

In fact, the cases illustrative of the good effects of this Spa that came to my knowledge are numerous and important, and I have purposely selected them from among the humbler classes, first, because a medical man can sift these better in all their bearings, and, secondly, because they show the disinterestedness of the proprietor of the spring, who permits all the poorer people to avail themselves of its salutary stream without any charge whatever.

I drank a large quantity of the water at the well. At first it had no prominent taste, but after a short interval the impression of common salt' is awakened ; and on savouring the water, that impression becomes more marked, as well as the *âpreté* of the oxyde of iron. But, besides this, there must be some other ingredient (so I find it noted among my memoranda set down on the spot) present in the water, to impart to it a peculiar softness, which approaches almost to oiliness when being swallowed. The subsequent analysis by West explained the reason of the latter phenomenon. When I drank a large tumbler of the water, previously warmed, I could not help being reminded of the appearance and taste of one of the sources at Ems.

Notwithstanding the presence of carburetted hydrogen, the water has no sensible smell. On standing it becomes turbid, and forms an ochreous deposit ; and when boiled minute crystals form on the surface, and the dry residuum (236 grains in the imperial gallon) effervesces briskly with acids.

Drunk in doses of from three to four half-pint glasses, the water is said to be purgative, and with some to act violently and quickly. Others, however, are obliged to add some Epsom or Glauber salts to render it purgative. Twenty grains of the latter salt to the first glass of the water, which in that case should be drunk quite warm, will suffice to secure a proper effect. *Expertè crede*, &c. Or the same quantity of the dry evaporated salt from the water itself, which I have recommended should be collected from that portion that is now wasted out of the spring, will answer the purpose. This evaporated mass tastes strongly of sea-salt, and when separated from the oxyde of iron, becomes deliquescent. When heated, the water assumes an ochreous appearance. It remains so, and nothing beyond it as long as it is kept in a state of motion; but if suffered to rest it precipitates abundantly the ochreous sediment.

The phenomena presented by the water at its natural temperature contained in a glass tumbler, are even more striking. At first, it is perfectly clear and transparent, as I have said elsewhere, but in an hour or two it turns slightly opalescent. This appearance becomes gradually more intense, and assumes at the same time a brownish or slight claret tinge which, with the opalescence, keeps increasing, while the inner side of the glass and bottom is covered by myriads of air-bubbles, exceedingly minute, and adhering tenaciously to the surface.

To Mr. Richardson belongs the merit of having brought to light this important mineral water. On purchasing his present extensive estate at Shotley, that gentleman was aware of a prevailing tradition in the neighbourhood, that a holy well once had existed on the grounds. By diligent and repeated search, in which he was aided by his clever man of business, Mr. Nicholson, who is an excellent practical geologist, farmer, and miner, the source was at length discovered about three years ago, and forthwith placed in its present flourishing condition, through Mr. Richardson's patriotic spirit and exertions.

In the adjoining saloon or meeting-room a book is kept, wherein all visiters are requested to enter their names. From this register I gathered that about five hundred strangers had come to drink of the water between May and August. That number was increased threefold, nearly, in the last season. Among the names of note contained in the list was that of the author of the "Pickwick Papers."

Not far from this last building is another containing two bath-rooms, with a shower-bath and a dressing-room in the centre. These rooms, as well as the baths themselves, which are lined with white tiles, and have mahogany borders, are as well got up as at the most renowned watering-places. There is nothing superfluous, but every thing useful in the place, and of the best materials. This establishment is but a beginning; and if the liberal-handed proprietor continues, as I doubt not he will, to bestow his care and attention to the further amelioration of the place, in which he has lately taken up his constant abode with his family, going and returning from Newcastle every day; if he will direct the improvements to be carried into effect, many of which I took the liberty of suggesting, both with regard to the grounds around the Spa, and the Spa itself, which ought to be converted into an open well, in order to aerate the water and be surrounded with a handsome iron palisade, to be kept locked, except during the hours of drinking the water; and also, in respect to the bath-rooms, and the position and number of the houses to be erected for visiters,—if, I say, these laudable and politic efforts to deserve popularity are continued, Shotley Bridge will, ere long, be considered as the prettiest village Spa in England—a species of Bruckenau, barring the larger proportion of free carbonic acid present in the latter.

The effect of such a water as that of Shotley Bridge on the system, when used as a hot-bath, is a subject deserving of much consideration; as the continuous application to the skin of a soluble salt of iron, rendered more active by ninety-eight degrees of heat, is never made with impunity. I therefore tested the Shotley Bridge water as a bath on myself. Its appear-

ance in the tank at ninety-eight degrees is exactly like that
of the Kochbrunner at Wisbaden. After twenty minutes of
immersion, my pulse had risen from seventy to seventy-six,
but no other disturbance or excitement in the system took
place ; neither was I sensible of the slightest sensation in
the head. If any thing, I should say that I felt clearer in
that organ, and generally better equipoised in all other parts,
giving me a feeling of great comfort. But as I had experienced much the same sensation in the morning—a circumstance which I attributed to the situation and the exceeding
purity of the air of the place—I cannot say how much the
hot-bath may have assisted in producing my feelings of the
moment.

Now this absence of all species of trouble in the head,
while immersed for half an hour in a steel-water bath at
ninety-eight degrees of Fahrenheit I hold to be with me (as I
observed in another publication) another great proof of the
striking difference between volcanic and *tea-kettle* heat, when
applied to the human body. Had I been in a *thermal* water,
with five times as much steel in it as there is in the water at
Baden (which is the case in this Spa of Shotley), I should
have experienced all the throbbing, fulness, and aching in
the head which that celebrated bath produced on me on
more than one occasion.

Neither was the action of the heart in the least disturbed ;
and I remarked that I did not experience the difficulty of
breathing which an ordinary hot-bath, with a large quantity of
water coming over the chest, usually produces on the first immersion. The immediate effect of the water on the skin is to
render it rough to the touch in two or three minutes. When
the hand is passed slightly over the surface of the body, one
would think that the finest sand was laid between the two. The
skin of the fingers is actually puckered in the water. This
effect is to be attributed to the steel ; but it vanishes as
quickly after wiping the skin dry, and its surface acquires a

soft, satiny feel instead, accompanied by a rosy tint throughout.

The liberality of the proprietor has extended to the charges
usually made at all the Spas; whether for drinking the
water, with the use of the rooms and promenades, or for
the use of the baths. I can only say, in one sentence, that
all these charges are one-third less than in any other
place of the same description. A warm-bath, for instance,
is to be had for two shillings only, and a subscription of *one*
shilling a week entitles the visiter to drink the water, to use
the sitting-room, and read periodical publications in it, and,
lastly, to frequent the carriage-drives and public walks in the
vicinity of the Spa.

The geology of the spring itself, and that of the immediate
neighbourhood, I had an opportunity of studying, accompanied by Mr. Richardson himself, who seems quite an
enthusiast in the cause of mineral hydrology for the benefit
of his fellow-creatures. In the short excursion I made with
him, through and along a most romantic and deep ravine that
crosses the woods immediately above the Spa, and which is
watered by a bourne or *beck,* I could easily notice the stratification of this district, denuded by the wearing action of the
stream. In hot weather, this wild and sequestered walk must
be a luxury to the visiters, such as one does not often meet
so near at hand in other Spas of England.

The strata around the well are covered by moss, with peat
earth underneath, caused, I have reason to believe, by the
water of the spring itself, which, for a century, has been
allowed to overspread the ground around it, without any
direct channel into the Derwent, which runs at a very short
distance from it. Gravel comes next, and beneath it blue
clay of the finest soapy texture. Freestone follows to a
considerable depth, with plates of siliceous stone, and ironstone six inches in thickness. Below these, Mr. Nicholson
informed me, after passing through two or three other minor

strata, limestone is found to the depth of from twenty to thirty fathoms.

Standing upon such rocks as these, it is obvious that Shotley Bridge must enjoy a dry and pure air as compared with the lower parts of the country; nor is this its only peculiarity; for the situation has the further advantage of being sheltered on every side by ranges of hills, supposed to be about 700 feet above the level of the sea, among which Pontop Pike, distant four miles, rises to upwards of one thousand feet in height.

The water is equally as good as the air at Shotley Bridge. Near the village it is found perfectly soft and remarkably pure.

Being situated at equal distances from Durham and Newcastle (fourteen miles), and twelve miles from Hexham, this Spa is within reach of three populous cities and districts, and requires only to be properly known to be appreciated and resorted to. The immediate vicinity of the Carlisle railroad, too, renders its access easy to the people of the west; and the approaching completion of the great Midland railway will afford an equally direct and facile line of communication between the southern and central provinces and this highly interesting Spa.

I would fain have entered into many more interesting details of the neighbouring country; of the mines of lead in the immediate vicinity, particularly that called *Silvertongues*, appropriately belonging to G. Silvertop, Esq., and an object of curiosity to visiters; of the ford in the Derwent, called AL-LANFORD, a name familiar to the readers of the immortal Scott; or of the singular round knoll, called "Arthur's Round Table," thickly wooded, and projecting into the Derwent, which seems actually to writhe around it in many coils, as if angry at the intrusion; and, finally, of the magnificent view which offers itself to the astonished spectator from many of the elevated points on the vertical banks of the

Derwent, whose stream, seen far beneath our feet, takes such strange and so many turns in one confined and particular spot, that its course there measures four miles, though, if taken across between the margins of its outermost turn, the distance would scarcely be half a mile.

All these several attractive features, peculiar to Shotley Bridge Spa, I would fain and ought, in justice to the place, to have dwelt upon. But when I reflect that I have now reached nearly to the conclusion of a thick volume, and have yet before me two-thirds of my long task to accomplish; my heart fails me, and I am compelled to relinquish the gratification of any further lingering in a place from which I derived so much pleasure and information. I therefore close my note-book, lest I should be betrayed into greater prolixity.

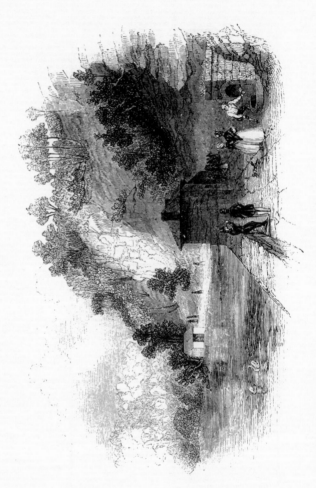

CHAPTER XXI.

GILSLAND SPA.

Attraction of GILSLAND—Coincidences and Recollections—Sir GEORGE
BECKWITH and the Under-Secretary of War and Colonies—Further
suggestions for Shotley Bridge Spa—The Ravine—GEORGE STEVENSON
again—The Stanhope Railway—LIME *versus* COALS—The prettiest
Railroad in England—MUMPS HALL and Meg Merrilies—ORCHARD
House—A Hit at the Incredulous—The Irthing—GILSLAND SULPHUR
SPRING—Indolence—Stratification of Rocks—Physical Character of
the Water—Chemical Composition—Medicinal Virtues—Alentours of
Gilsland—The SPA HOTEL — Subdivision of Company — Men and
Masters but one—The BATHS—Lack instead of excess of Physic—
An Odd Fish—Company at the Spa—Climate—Prevailing state of
health of the Inhabitants.

" RIDING one day with Fergusson they met some miles from
Gilsland a young lady taking the air on horseback, whom
neither of them had previously remarked, and whose appearance instantly struck both so much that they kept her in view
until they had satisfied themselves that she also was of the
party at Gilsland."

Those of my readers who have perused (and who has not ?)
the interesting biography of the great recluse of Abbotsford,
will recognise at once, in the preceding passage, that portion
of it which is meant to prepare them for the short courtship
and speedy marriage of Walter Scott. That courtship began

and ended, in the most gratifying manner for the poet, at Gilsland. There, Scott found a wife, and from that moment a place holding but a local rank among the principal Spas of the north, became suddenly invested with a degree of importance and attraction which secured to it for ever after a renown beyond the pale of its narrow confines.

As warm and enthusiastic an admirer of the "great necromancer of the north" as any of my readers, it was but natural that I should feel anxious to behold a spot so consecrated. I viewed my journey thither as a devout pilgrimage —independently of the less interesting sentiments that induced me to undertake it; and I felt impatient of treading the same ground on which that venturous cavalcade, with Fergusson, described by the biographer, decided the fate of his highly-gifted companion. I therefore prepared to take my departure thither.

The house in which good Mr. Nicholson gave me a most hearty welcome for the night at Shotley Bridge, stands on the summit of a hill at Snowsgreen. From one of its casements I surveyed at early morning an extensive landscape all around me, of the most enchanting description, including those highly interesting spots to which I had driven in the afternoon of the preceding day,—ascending the course of the Derwent, penetrating its upper valley, and looking upon Mugglewitch Wood near us, and towards Sir Charles Monks's Mosswood, farther on in Northumberland. For a Spa, one can hardly desire or even fancy a more romantic neighbourhood.

To what trifling coincidences we are at times apt to attach importance in our estimation? The house I dwelt in for the moment seemed ancient amidst all the scattered new buildings of the Spa, and stood insulated and overlooked the village, like a lordly palace. Its inner apartments, and stiff parterre garden, after the design and fashion, though on a very small scale, of those at Hampton Court, bespoke a foreign taste. I inquired of mine host to whom the house belonged, and in whose state-bedroom I had been lodged for that night: " You have slept," replied Mr. Nicholson, " in the bedchamber of old General Béckwith, whose father, claiming to be descended of the German colonists at Shotley Bridge, erected this house after the taste of his continental ancestors, and reared his son in it till he entered the army, in which, like himself, he rose to the highest rank."

Full twenty-nine years before, that very officer, while commanding-in-chief the king's forces, in the West India Islands, had intrusted to my care, to bring home to England from Barbadoes, the official account of the first outbreak at Caraccas of that great political commotion which was to change entirely the destiny of South America. That account, brought to Barbadoes from Venezuela by the revolted chiefs, who claimed the aid of England (among whom was Bolivar, the very man who was destined to give his name to that emancipated portion of Spanish America) the commander-in-chief had requested me to translate, as the only officer in the English fleet then acquainted with the Spanish language. On committing the despatches into my hands, Sir George Beckwith, the then recent conqueror of Martinique and Guadaloupe, had said, " If ever you come so far northwards, and visit the neighbourhood of Newcastle, you will be welcome under my roof :" and under that very roof was I at the time of inditing this memorandum. That roof still appertains to the Beckwith family, but the gallant host to give the promised welcome is gone !

To render the recollection of this anecdote still dearer and more interesting to me, the despatches and translations to which I have alluded, were delivered by me upon arrival in London, into the hands of one of the then under-secretaries for the colonies; an individual at that time scarcely emerged from his collegiate life, but who, in the course of a few years, since lapsed, unaided by illustrious lineage, has mounted to the highest pinnacle of ministerial power, and acquired an imperishable renown as a statesman, and the head of his party, whether in or out of office.

While I was musing over all these cherished rememberings, my good-hearted landlady had prepared me the morning repast, and good Mr. Nicholson had yoked his trusty nag to a gig which was to convey me to the station of the Carlisle railroad, on my way to Gilsland Spa. I cast a last look from my window over the rich and cultivated lands by which I was surrounded, and which form the joint properties of " friend " Richardson and of Thomas Wilson, Esq., of Shotley Hall, a great lead-mine proprietor, whose father, originally in an humble station, realized a large fortune by discovering, when almost reduced to beggary by mining operations, a solid vein of galena on a property at Alston Moor (Hudgillborn), rented from the Greenwich Hospital.

Respecting this vein, it is asserted that a block of wood was discovered in the centre of it, which is now in the possession of Mr. Wilson, at the Hall. This gentleman, whose elegant mansion, with a park-like ground behind, is on the west bank of the river, close to the bridge, I had not the good fortune of finding at home, he being on a visit to another of his properties. He generally resides here with his aged mother, to whom he is much attached, and enjoys great popularity in the county, as a gentlemanly, intelligent person, conversant with science and many branches of knowledge.

A section of his almost inexhaustible mine, first opened about twenty years ago, and of the strata of the county, was published by the late Mr. Westgatt Foster, agent to Colonel Beaumont. This work is represented as one of great merit, and embraces the whole tract of the mining district in the county from east to west.

After all I am inclined, before parting, to give a hint to these two lords of the manor, or, at all events of the lands around there, respecting the future embellishment and aggrandizement of their favourite village.

From one of the hills at Snowsgreen, called the *Cheiters* or *Chesters*, to the east of the village, Shotley Bridge presents itself at the bottom of a shallow vale, which, from the manner of the expanding declivities around every side of it, that slope down to a gently-undulating and well-cultivated level, mapped with occasional patches of wood, may not unaptly be likened to a gigantic flat and figured basin. The village itself, with its new houses of freestone and shining slates, alternating with groups of trees, pleasingly contrast in their subdued tints with the vivid and variegated colours of the different sorts of culture in the fields adjoining, and afford a far more charming view than can be obtained elsewhere. Houses built on this part of the eminence, or even a little more westwardly, would enjoy one of the most extensive as well as cheerful views in the county, and be sheltered from the cold north and east winds withal. Here it is that I should plant my flag, had I leisure enough to pay a yearly visit to Shotley Bridge Spa.

We arrived, after traversing a vast extent of recently recovered moorland, at the station on the Stanhope and Tyne railway, called *Handgill*, purposely to examine one of the many wonderful engineering features which have stamped George Stevenson as a man of endless resources, and which, in the present case, is worth the long, difficult, and circuitous route we took to see it.

Two sides, N.E. and S.W., nearly, of an immense chasm or ravine have been made available in the direct line of the railway to and from Stanhope, without bridge or embankment or viaduct, by means of a very ingenious arrangement in virtue of which the travelling trains are made to slide down one side, and mount the opposite one, through the operation of a stationary engine, of twenty-five horse power, placed on a platform quite at the bottom of the chasm. The latter is one hundred and eighty-eight perpendicular feet in depth, and its two sides stand at right angles with each other, having each an inclination of thirteen inches for every three feet, to an extent of one hundred and fifty yards.

The train of waggons, loaded with lead or lime, proceeding from Stanhope in the western district, or another train coming from Newcastle in the opposite direction with coals, having reached the termination of the level ground on either side of the ravine, is suddenly stopped, and the foremost waggon (for only one at a time can be operated upon) being unyoked, is turned upon a circle with its side towards the precipice, and slided forward and fixed into a moveable platform. The latter is in waiting on the very brink of the precipice, resting upon the rails with its four wheels, the two foremost of which being of larger diameter than the hind ones, cause the said platform to continue in an horizontal position while sliding down one incline, or ascending the other opposite, with its loaded waggon.

To such as dread the sight of a deep abyss, this rapid manœuvre, performed by a single man, aided by a little boy, who launch down its precipitous side a ponderous load, restrained only by an endless strap in its downward descent, is a spectacle highly exciting to the nerves. Though invited, I had not the courage to commit myself to one of these headlong messengers. One time I had placed my foot on the platform ready to descend with one of them, merely in hopes of seeing afterwards the effect or sensation produced by the ascending train. That sensation is said to be exactly like that experienced in a balloon while mounting into the air. But I contented myself with seeing and admiring the beautiful twofold movements of the ponderous cars.

> " Steady and swift the self-moved chariot went
> Winning the long ascent,
> Or downwards rolling 'gainst the furthest shore."

These trains of lime-waggons from Stanhope, coming to exchange that commodity for Newcastle coals, load in the great quarries at the former place. The limestone is a species of brownish or dark bluish-gray marble, with bivalve shells, taken from the great Stanhope limestone bed, consisting of three strata, divided by indurated clay. The quantity quarried there, either for building-cement or ornamental purposes, or for agricultural uses, is exceedingly large.

Retracing, at length, my steps from the lofty embankment of this curious railroad, down the side of which we scrambled to regain our vehicle, we directed our steps towards the station on the Carlisle railway, opposite Corbridge, where, taking leave of my good conductor, I entered one of the second-class carriages upon the line,—a most comfortable sort of vehicle,—from which I could survey every thing around me.

Unquestionably by far the prettiest railroad in England is this one between Carlisle and Newcastle. It not only traverses a pretty country in every direction, but it is also exceedingly neat and well kept, and its station-houses, built of freestone, are perfect specimens of taste and style in architecture.

It has but a single line of rails throughout the greatest part of its way, except at one or two stations, where there is a double line, and in some other places also for the purpose of enabling the returning trains to pass. It runs nearly all the way from Newcastle to Carlisle upon an inclined plane, ascending gradually from the level of the Tyne at the former place to an elevation of 437 feet at the station at Milton, and again rapidly descending nearly the whole of that height towards Carlisle. In its course it follows the undulating line of the Tyne for a considerable part; but, in some places viaducts or embankments have been thrown up to maintain a level across ravines or extensive valleys; while in other parts cuttings of considerable depth have been found necessary for the same purpose. Among the latter, travellers cannot fail to be struck with what is called the Cowran Cut, which has been made through a hill half a mile in length, in the course of more than the half of which distance the depth of the cutting is from 90 to 102 feet.

Of the many bridges and viaducts which an outside traveller can notice on this railroad, one of the latter, calculated to excite admiration for its architectural beauty, is that across the Corby valley, formed of seven arches, each of forty feet span. Its height from the ground measures seventy and the whole length of the viaduct four hundred and eighty feet. There is also a bridge on this railroad which merits attention ;—I allude to the askew bridge, of great architectural beauty, formed of three arches, of thirty feet span each, which is thrown across the river Gelt at an angle of 26½ degrees.

Besides these striking features, this same railroad possesses the further advantage of passing through a highly-cultivated country, and between undulating and well-wooded hills ; occasionally traversing parks and orchards, and being itself ornamented in many places with well-trimmed hedges and flower parterres on each side. The slopes of the cuttings have been planted with grass, which is kept neatly trimmed, and in the best order imaginable. In fact, as I set out by observing, the Newcastle and Carlisle railroad is by far the prettiest in England, and presents, moreover, various objects of great interest in its immediate vicinity.

As to the traffic of passengers upon it, that may be judged from a single fact, that between Newcastle and Hexham only, upwards of seven thousand persons are said to travel daily.

I halted at the Rose-hill station, eighteen miles short of Carlisle, where I found a charabanc in waiting to convey visiters to Gilsland Spa.

The distance to that sequestered spot, though short, presents two points of attraction which will arrest the visiter in his progress for a while. What stranger, indeed, can have the still-standing hall of the Amazonian Meg Merrilies pointed out to him, as he descends the winding road on his way to a small bridge over the Irthing, and not recollect that under the semblance of a house of entertainment for Scottish travellers straying on the edge of the wild and trackless waste of the " borders,"—the wretched insulated building he beholds often witnessed dark and bloody deeds, and has preserved a traditional celebrity to this day, under the appellation of " Mumps Hall." There it was before me, the miserable thatched hut—its wall now plastered up and tinged with coarse yellow ochre—which Scott has rendered so famous. It still bears the outward token of a house of entertainment ; and, upon an eminence a little way from it, within a few spans of the very earth she so often trod over in terror to the dwellers of Upper and Nether Denton, lies interred its former mysterious tenant.

The other point of curiosity is that singular wall erected by the Roman Emperor Septimus Severus, which, beginning at Newcastle and terminating a little to the west of Carlisle, passes here at a short distance to the south of Gilsland Spa, and to an antiquarian is a source of interesting investigation.

Beyond it a new wide gravelled carriage-road leads to a range of two or three showy buildings, standing upon an eminence, called *Orchard* House, once used as a house of entertainment, fronted with flowered parterres, and facing the broad south. To Mr. Shadforth, the principal proprietor of this estate, I was the bearer of a letter from my friend, the eminent surgeon, and one of the leading practitioners of Newcastle, Mr. Baird, to whom I am indebted for procuring me an agreeable acquaintance, and much of the useful information I obtained at Gilsland.

It is some consolation to one who has been taxed by the incredulous among his brethren, with having too much vaunted the curative powers of mineral waters, whether abroad or at home, to find, that even in places where little or nothing has been done by art or nature to make them desirable, pleasant, or agreeable residences, people of almost every class in this country will, if they are able, flock during the summer months, if there be but some Spa or other in them. Indeed, rather than not follow such a practice, because of the absence of well-established mineral-water rendezvous, hundreds have been known to congregate together wherever a puddle of undrinkable water has been detected, or a " holy well" of undefined virtues has been pointed out by tradition.

The lower and the middle classes of society have their " Spas," as the great of the land have theirs, at home as well as abroad. Now Gilsland is just such a place. It is a nook, or a dell by the side of the river Irthing, which is here shallow, and its stream is like that which one sees issuing from some extensive tanyard—brown as the best London stout, and as frothy. Descending from the moorland-waste on the north a short distance from hence, the Irthing has here scooped out a narrow channel in the form of a crescent, along which it is seen to struggle on its onward way through the broken fragments of millstone grit and plate which strew its bed. A lofty, precipitous, and imposing mass of rocks, a cliff, in fact, nearly one hundred feet in height, forms its north-western embankment. The opposite shore, on the contrary, flat and alluvial, presents some green fields, and is dotted with one or two cottages and other buildings, one of which, called Wardrew House, is fitted up during the season for the reception of visiters. This bank is planted with rows of trees. But this level aspect does not extend far—for assuming soon a gradual ascent, the bank reaches at last a summit nearly level with that of the north-western shore. Both banks are thickly wooded, and their elevation and semicircular form give to the place the aspect of a deep dell, or cup, at the bottom of which the Irthing is heard to rustle by on its stony bed, in form and character like a *Gill;*—whence the name of the Spa.

It is at the bottom of the denuded series of rocks or lofty cliff first described, that the sulphur spring which gives importance to Gilsland, issues in a free and plentiful stream, and is resorted to every morning, soon after sunrise, by a large number of common people from the neighbourhood, as well as by those of the better class of summer visiters temporarily resident here, who are not too idle to leave their bed at so early an hour: for here, as at Harrogate, and at one other English Spa, I found that the ladies, in course of drinking the water, preferred the indolent practice of having it brought to their bedside in bottles or cans, to the more natural and beneficial custom of rising early and repairing to the source itself. The latter is but a quarter of a mile from the principal hotel, at the end of a wide and well-kept zigzag road, shaded with lofty trees running along the side of the cliff down to the border of the river, level with which the spring is found.†

Except in cases of absolute inability from malady, this practice of drinking the mineral waters at home, instead of repairing to the spring for it, obtains nowhere but in England, among the visiters of a Spa, and also in Germany among some few of the English. In this country this objectionable practice was probably first introduced, in consequence of the uncertain and generally wretched weather which prevails during the bathing-season, especially very early in the morning. At Harrogate, for example, during the rainy month of July, I could sympathize with those who felt reluctant to quit their chambers at six o'clock in the morning, to encounter the pitiless storm of wind and rain that drove about the open village or common. But here in Gilsland, such a plea for indolence is hardly admissible. At all events, the practice is

* *Gill*, or *Ghyll*, a mountain stream, confined between steep banks and descending rapidly.

† See the view facing the beginning of this chapter.

a bad one, and in a great measure defeats the object one has in view in repairing to a Spa.

The broad face of the superimposed rocks that hang over the clear and limpid stream of mineral water—rising, as I before stated, to the height of nearly a hundred feet—exhibits, as I observed throughout the tract of country I lately visited from east to south-west, the series of formations which lie over the coal measure. The several beds are here perfectly and strongly marked, and of great depth. Indeed, in reference to what is called, in this district, "plate," I hardly remember having seen beds of that rock under and above strata of freestone, thicker than in this locality. These beds abound in ironstone, and iron nodules, to supply the materials for the chalybeate spring that lies at no great distance from the sulphur spring.

Whence the sulphuretted gas comes with which the latter is impregnated to a degree greater than in any of the like class of mineral waters in the north, is a problem which naturalists affect to consider as a puzzling one. It is evident to the commonest observer that the interior of the whole of this stupendous cliff is bursting with that gas, as, from every horizontal fissure in the lowest strata of the plate level nearly with the river, small streamlets of sulphur-water, with free sulphuretted and carburetted hydrogen gas, are seen to trickle down, leaving its indelible mark of a yellow white upon the subincumbent stones.

The water, I have already mentioned, is clear and limpid ; indeed the finest crystal spring could not be more so. It smells strongly of the gas, and the palate quickly perceives it also. There is no other subsequent taste in it, neither would we expect any, considering the chemical constitution of this water, as published by Dr. Reid Clanny, of Sunderland.*

In about half an hour, an eructation of gas,—such a one as we

* See the General Chemico-Pneumatic Table, at the end of the volume.

may perceive after eating hard-boiled eggs, occurs, and the peculiar taste of that very article of diet, so prepared, continues
some time in the mouth ; a slight headach also is occasionally
experienced after drinking the water.   Its temperature is cold
compared to that of the surrounding atmosphere. Many think
it pleasant to drink, and it does not lie heavy on the stomach.   I have seen a few people make wry faces on approaching the glass; but, unquestionably, owing to the absence of
any large proportion of the muriates, the water is not so disagreeable to drink as the Harrogate water.

It is the practice at Gilsland to drink out of a very small
glass, holding about four ounces, to walk awhile, and to repeat
the dose,—which repetition people here have carried to as great
an excess as some of the Germans have been sneered at for
doing.   The effect of the water *per se* is not aperient, but it
acts rather as a diuretic.   It is said to settle the digestion of
weak stomachs, and to allay irritation in that organ.

Few persons, however, follow a regular course. Most
people come only for a few days, rather on account of the
scenery than the water. Many drink the water for a few
weeks or so, and no longer, and the majority, perhaps, remain a few days only. But even the scenery can hardly be
a source of attraction, as, away from the *Ghyll* and its
wooded banks, and the shaded walks made along them, the
scenes presented, by the locality, are rather those of desolation, to him who is looking for the beautiful and the picturesque.

The geologist, the botanist, and even the antiquarian, may
find interesting occupations in districts near at hand ; but for
distant and perspective views, such as greet the eye in the
vale of the Derwent and near Shotley Bridge—the rich—the
luxuriant—the well-cultivated, and, in many parts, the
romantic aspect of the region we described in a preceding
chapter—those are not to be found here. Turn either towards
the moors northwards, or towards the country which extends

southwards beyond the line of the railroad (here, as every
where along its course, a pretty feature in the landscape) the
eye dwells upon nothing but a vast expanse of hilly country,
gray, sombre, and leaden-coloured ; and seeming, by its outward physiognomy, to reveal the nature of the mineral treasures it conceals within its bosom.

It is near to the brink of the high rocky side of the Irthing
that the only hotel (formerly called Shaw's, but now the Spa
Hotel) open for the accommodation of the visiters, stands with
its long side towards the dell, while its south-western front
is towards the scenery I have just described.   It is but a
sorry " house of accommodation," although all the forms and
fashions of the better and superior class of hotels at well-known
Spas in England are followed—such as fixed charges for
board and lodging to master and man—regular meal-times,
divided into four—drawing-room meetings—and dining-room
etiquette.   But there the comparison ends.   And yet the
liberal proprietor, and, indeed the present tenants under
him, lack neither the will nor the inclination to make the
house comfortable.   The fault lies in the smallness of the
apartments—the somewhat inseparable gloom of the locality
—and, above all, the shortness and unproductive nature of
the Spa season.   Here, at all events, the hotel-keeper is
neither the lord of the place, nor likely to be a very rich one,
as at Harrogate and elsewhere.

There is a practice of dividing the company in the house
into what is called the *Drawing-room*, the *Stone-parlour*, and
the *Hall* company.   The charge accords with those sub-
divisions.   In the first class, the expense per week is as high
as at the best hotels of Harrogate, though the equivalent given
in return is not so good.   There is a difference of one shilling
and sixpence per diem in the next, or second class ; and the
third pays something about three shillings and sixpence per
day, or a guinea per week.

This consideration for the inferior ranks of visiters to the Spa extends at Gilsland, with praiseworthy philanthropy, even in the use of the baths for servants, who are charged much less than their masters, although they bathe in the very same rooms, nay in the very identical tanks. Thus, the bathing goes on alternately, from master to man, and from man to master, with most happy sociality, against which no one seems disposed to grumble. A servant may have the itch (and hereabouts in the north and on " the borders" such a supposition is not preposterous) ;—no matter—in he goes into the sulphur-bath the moment his master has vacated it, and the water can be changed ; and his master, next morning, follows him into the same recipient ! This is primitive.

And so are the baths themselves, as well as the bathing-rooms, erected in the guise of low ordinary cottages, on the very margin of the river, immediately opposite the spring. Nothing can be of ruder aspect, both in and out, than this establishment, and the visiter must be little squeamish, indeed, who can long continue to use such rooms and such bathing-tanks.

In general, and throughout my long and laborious tour to the English Spas, I have had occasion to lament the too busy interference of medicine with the fair use of mineral waters. But here, at Gilsland, absence of medical attendance of every description marks the Spa. Not even a dose of salts can be obtained. It was the practice of a former housekeeper at the hotel, as the present landlady informed me, to keep a supply of medicines, though she professed not to dispense any, but kept them for the occasional service of visiters— some neighbouring surgeon being sent for in case of need, or arriving by chance. At present, however, no such accommodation exists ; and one may awake in the night, in this lonely and retired spot, ill—dying—for want of immediate medical aid—without the smallest prospect of being saved through it. The nearest medical men of character, I am informed, are fetched either from Carlisle, or from Newcastle. Those of the latter city, they tell me, are preferred, though farther away. But the railway has annihilated distinctions of distances, and, therefore, from that city, when required, medical men are sent for express. But the way to get at them upon any serious emergency in the night-time—the rail-train *asleep*, and no carriage, and probably no horse, at hand !

For a watering-place at which a hundred strangers assemble perhaps at one time (and I find from the visiters' book that they seldom amount to so many), this state of things cannot be said to be unaccompanied with danger.

There is, I understood the people to say, an opportunity of sometimes procuring a sort of medical man nearer at hand. Such a one in fact had made his appearance from the neighbourhood, a few hours previously to my arrival. One of the gentlemen whom I met at the supper-table in the hotel, and who seemed to be " all in all " in this little community, mentioned the occasion of that person being sent for. But the village doctor had loitered so long by the way, had tasted so frequently of the border-whiskey, and had heated himself so much, immediately after his arrival, with throwing quoits both over and under his cocked-up leg, stripped of his coat and displaying both " fore and aft " his short corduroys and top-boots and long silver spurs strapped to the ankles, that he was found to be of little professional use after all. Accordingly, having waited some hours without being applied to for his services, the man of medicine prepared to quit Gilsland once more. I saw him mount, or try to mount, his charger, on which he was seated at last by means of a helping hand ; and as he was about to depart, tottering and vibrating to the right and to the left, I heard him bluster out a broken farewell and a hiccup to the company,—the hostlers and the grooms,—one of whom tendered him another " drop " to keep the wind off the stomach during his journey homewards.

My experience of the " doings " at the Spa Hotel, was confined to the having the honour of handing a tall high-cheek-boned, elderly Scotch lady from the drawing-room to the supper-room on the day of my arrival, and of occupying the post of vice-president at the bottom of the supper-table, in virtue of my right as " the last arrived." Here I learnt nothing. But on the following morning, breakfasting at Orchard House, surrounded by a family group which gave me a very favourable notion of a Cumberland fireside, and conversing with Colonel ————, a neighbour, who occupied one of the houses in the same row, called Orchard House,—I obtained some information touching the Spa. It had been but ill-frequented during the last year or two ; but it was expected that the railway would cause an increase of visiters, particularly since the expensive repairs of the hotel, the internal arrangements of which, however, were admitted still to require alteration and improvement.

It was stated also, that the resident inhabitants near and about the Spa, who are born and bred there, are sickly and pale-faced, and that the families of the farmers are not of good constitutions, being liable to consumption. The climate is very trying—few days in the year being free from rain. The snow lies on the ground till mid-spring, and Colonel ————, when he quitted in May, 1839, to proceed to town for the season, left the snow on the bank opposite to his house. Being located on a high ground, and midway between the Irish and German Seas, my host imagined that Gilsland must be exposed to the long sweeping gales that prevail from the south-east and the west ; and, if so, no position can be more unfavourable. Indeed, the waste and high moorlands, close at hand on the north, and the general aspect of the country, to the south of the road, confirm that notion.

If there be any redeeming feature in the position of this "Sulphur Spring," it is the beautiful and romantic character of the deep dell near the bottom of the Gill ; but even this is too confined in extent to make amends, by its various pretty pictures, for the many drawbacks and other unfavour-

able circumstances, attending this establishment for the recovery of health.

Hence I am not surprised that Gilsland is indifferently
frequented, and at best only by very so-so classes of people;
except now and then, when a stray visiter or traveller (like
myself for example) comes to Gilsland for local information,
and takes shelter there for a day or a night—a period amply
sufficient for seeing and enjoying all that there is enjoyable
in the place.

CHAPTER XXII.

SHAP WELLS—BLACKPOOL—SOUTHPORT.

Gaieties of Gilsland — Love, Courtship, and Marriage of Walter Scott—Quick Work—Hint to Mammas—Minor Mineral Springs of Cumberland—Carlisle—Brougham Hall—Voltaire and Mirabeau —Lowther Castle—Scott's Opinion of English Architects—Shap Well—The Spa Hotel—Its Accommodations and Comforts within— Desolate Prospect without—The Well—Its Primitive State—New Bath-house—Shap Well Water—Its Physical Characters—Chemical Analysis—Defects—Medicinal Virtues of the Water—Exaggeration —Reality—Cases in which it is of Use — Medical Attendance— The Penrith Physician—Dennison, the Bone-setter — Climate of Shap Wells — Improvements desirable—Attractions in the Vicinity —Shap Abbey—The Lakes—Waste Land in Westmorland—Earl Lonsdale's Estates — Contrast between Planting and Tilling—The Netherby Estate—Civilization promoted by Tilling—Preston—Its Past, Present, and Future State—Southport—Litham Hall—Black-pool—Sands—Sea-bathers—Hotel and Table d'Hôte.

The gaieties of Gilsland during the summer season must have been far more attractive in 1797, than they are now, or have ever been since ; when we find it recorded, of the former date, that fair damsels, sent thither to improve their com-plexion, rode on their palfreys, and quickly set the hearts of young cavaliers on fire, who ought to have been proof to " first impressions." A ball at that time, unlike a ball at the same Spa nowadays, was a mighty fine field for improving those early impressions ; and if, to boot, something in the shape of a red coat and epaulettes could be sported on those occasions by the swain, why then the result was inevitable.

In the month of July, of the year just mentioned, Walter Scott, who after an excursion to 'the English Lakes, had settled himself quietly in the sequestered Spa at Gilsland for a few days, exhibited in his own case the truth of the preceding remarks. Of all the domestic romances which he subsequently portrayed in his enchanting volumes, none is more romantic than the one he himself enacted at Gilsland, and of which he was the hero. The oldest inhabitants in the place well recollect the Scot lawyer producing himself in regimentals at their balls, and winning the *belle* of the day.

Scarcely had he secured his footing in one of the lodging-houses of the Spa, than the presence of a fair dweller under the same roof fired his poetic soul into admiration, and the composition of those well-known lines—

> "Take these flowers which purple flowing
> On the ruined rampart grew," &c.

A flame so easily lighted, however, blew out as readily, to admit of a still greater conflagration, originating in another quarter. The poet's heart must have been of the most combustible materials, yet not more so than that of the object of his second adoration, "Than whom," observes his biographer, " a lovelier vision could hardly have been imagined." For soon after a first casual introduction at one of those Spa balls to which allusion has just been made, followed by a supper, with its attendant opportunity of whispering pretty nothings, and of offering unnumbered civilities, during which it is to be presumed Scott " popped the question " to his lady-love; we find the Leviathan novelist that was to be, writing to his mother in strains implying that, if his father had no objection to the match, he was pretty certain there were none on the part of that fair lady to a matrimonial alliance " at the earliest convenience !"

Sharp work this for a poet who was quaffing, not of the fountain of Hippocrene, but of the fetid stream of Gilsland—by no means an inspiring beverage ! It is true, there is no date to Scott's epistle to his mother, and his biographer, who found it without any, gives no clue either as to the day of Scott's first meeting with " the lovely vision," or as to that of the fated ball and supper. But, as he has stated that the poet remained in Cumberland until the Jedburg assizes recalled him to his legal duties at the close of September, it is fair to conclude that the beginning, middle, and ending of his amorous negotiation—in other words, that Scott's falling desperately in love, his subsequent courtship, and his settling the question with his intended bride—could only have been the affair of days, or, at most, of a week or so. In that expeditious proceeding the lady-love evidently participated most eagerly, since we find her writing early in October a most confidential, affectionate, and earnest letter to her intended, with the view of putting him in the right course for obtaining from her noble guardian his consent to their matrimonial union.

Now this is as it should be ; else my remarks on the peculiar fitness of Spas, to promote and forward matrimonial schemes, in a far better and quicker mode than is said to be done at a certain great ball in London (now getting out of fashion), would have been without point, and unfounded. But when I say *Spas*, I do not mean your Cheltenhams and Leamingtons and Baths ; but such only as resemble this one of Gilsland, primitive and village-like, where visiters are every thing, and every body else nothing, and where people, assembled from all parts of the world, tacitly agree to live, as it were, *en famille* during their stay.

In this respect, the example set to us by Scott is most triumphant. The happiness that resulted from it to both parties, so casually met, and so soon bound together, is most encouraging ; and I conclude, as I began, by declaring that prudent mammas, who are anxious to see their daughters speedily and well settled in the world, had better look to " the Spas of England."

The Spas of England are many, and there is no lack of such *rendezvous*, in my humble opinion, perfectly legitimate for the praiseworthy object aforesaid. Cumberland alone, the county we are now in, reckons not fewer than thirteen, besides the one at Gilsland ; and, although most of those are but little known beyond the precincts of their own locality, they, nevertheless, attract a certain number of visiters every year.

The majority of these mineral springs of Cumberland are strong impregnations of marine salt, and would be found to contain those two powerful agents, *Bromine* and *Iodine*, if properly analyzed ; for the virtue of some of them in curing scrofulous disorders, as I ascertained on inquiry, can only be well explained by presuming the existence of those two ingredients. A few are of sulphuretted water, like that at Gilsland, and the rest chalybeates.

Of the two former classes, the most remarkable are *Stanger Spa*, a very strong aperient salt-spring, two miles south by east of Cockermouth, near the old road to Keswick ; and another salt-spring like Cheltenham, situated near *Seathwaite*, in the southern part of Borrowdale ; also a sulphur spring at *Slainton*, another at *Shalk-Trot*, and a third at *Biglands*, all three within a very few miles of Carlisle. Of the chalybeates, the most celebrated is the one discovered in 1796 at Kirkbarapton, not far from Carlisle, which is strongly impregnated with iron ; and a second spring at Rockliff, on the way and near to that goal of runaway matches, which is within a stonethrow of that very Spa, at the head of the Solway Firth and rejoices in a farrier-parson for the ceremony.

Carlisle, where I arrived at that bustling inn of mails and coaches, the Bush, in eighteen minutes (a distance of twenty miles, on an inclined plane) by the railway from the Rose-

hill or Gilsland station, detained me at this, my second visit,
but a few hours.   An interview with one or two of my medical brethren, for the sake of obtaining information respecting Gilsland's medicinal efficacy, and other mineral springs
in the county, and a visit to a leading and very intelligent
bookseller, occupied but a small portion of my time.   Engaging afterwards a suitable conveyance, I at once directed
my steps towards the next object of my tour, the principal
Spa of Westmorland—SHAP WELLS.

I was now about to enter one of the most romantic regions
in the north-west of England, with which, however, a previous and more special excursion on my return from Scotland, two years before, had made me well acquainted.

The weather was, at first, unpropitious, lowering and
rainy ; as, indeed, it unfortunately is during most of the
season when one ought to enjoy the Lake scenery of this
enchanting part of the country.   After advancing, however,
a few miles, the rain ceased, and on the mist ascending, the
high peak of Coldbeck fells appeared almost suddenly, close
on the right hand towering to the sky ; with *Saddleback* further south, and between them, and rather behind, the giant
of Keswick—the Alpine *Skiddaw*—rising three thousand feet
above the neighbouring sea.

Penrith was next perceived, seated down in a richly cultivated plain, with Brougham Hall a little way beyond that
small and neat town, and the larger mass of modern Gothic
embattled structures, called Lowther Castle, standing in the
midst of an extensive park, watered by the river Lowther.

My desire to pay a visit to the Hall, which bears the
name of the first orator of our days, was anticipated by
the usual practice of the Penrith postboys who conduct travellers southwards, and who naturally, it seems, inquire of
them whether they will not make a short deviation to the
left of the road, to see the venerable fabric, the work of

various ages, in which occasionally resides the "great Chan
cellor!"

Arthur's round table (one of those natural features, by
the-by, which, like Robin Hood's cave, one meets ever
where in the north) stands not far removed from the Hall, t
add to the temptation.

The Hall, however, will not need such or any othe
adventitious allurement, in future ages, to become an objec
of pilgrimage.   Like the Château de Vernet, BROUGHA
HALL, when the grave shall have swept away prejudice
and political animosities, will be visited by thousands eage
to behold the château of the English Voltaire; he who, t
the encyclopedic knowledge and pungent wit of the Frenc
philosopher, joined the impassioned and flowing eloquenc
of Mirabeau.

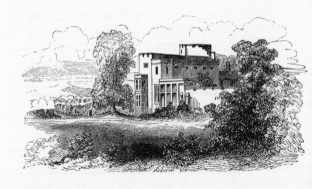

On this occasion I felt satisfied with approaching th
building, and enjoying the prospect from its terrace.   Th
venerable mother of the noble statesman, whose loss h
has since had to deplore, was then lying indisposed at th
Hall; and to have pushed mere curiosity further at suc
a moment would have been an impertinence.   The nob

host, besides, was not in the county at the time, or to his lordship, as no stranger, I should have paid my respects; nor did he reach the Hall until some days after, when that unfortunate accident occurred which had nigh deprived the senate of one of its most splendid ornaments.

At an arrow's-shot length from the modern hall, stands Brougham Castle. Placed near the confluence of two slender river-streams, one of which gives a title to the wealthy lord of Lowther Castle,—and occupying a prominent station on a gentle eminence above those waters,—these vestiges of the feudal possession of *John de Veteripont*, form a group of some interest.

Of Lowther Castle, through the apartments of which, many of them small in size and low roofed (particularly those of the bedroom floor), I wandered with a large party of visiters from the lakes, I would rather eschew offering any remarks, or report the notes I made on the spot. These repeated intrusions on the part of strangers, kindly permitted by the venerable earl and his family, who were, at the time, occupying the castle, must be a source of annoyance to the noble inmates, though they are evidently one of profit to the domestics. But such is the case at all the great mansions in the country.

On the interior of this immense structure, the production of an eminent architect who, when not engaged in Gothic designs, as in this instance, so chastises his imagination and inventive faculty by the severer laws of Grecian simplicity, that hardly any design remains in his works,—one observation seems called for. It refers to the gigantic, square, Gothic hall, around which the various and multiformed small rooms mentioned before have been clustered. That hall, ninety feet in elevation, and not less than sixty feet square, more resembles the central tower of a transept in a cathedral than the *atrium* to a great domestic mansion. That it is handsome of its class, taken in an insulated form, and that it is striking, none can deny; but, is it congruous? is it in character with the apartments around it? or is the immense and principal staircase, which divides at its upper end into two lateral insignificant flights of steps leading to low corridors, proportionate to the parts of the building to which it leads?

Exteriorly this building is not less capricious. In its principal front—extending to four hundred and twenty feet in length towards the north,—numerous towers, round or sexagonal, some high, some low, and all surmounted by embattlements, and pierced with slit-windows, would seem to be erected for the purpose of representiug a baronial castle. But in the south elevation a totally different character, a species of collegiate style, is displayed, in large fretted Gothic windows, in buttresses, and cloisters of the Gothic form.

It would be well for certain English architects of the day, were they occasionally to bear in mind the opinion of the great man whose felicitous matrimony at Gilsland is recorded in the beginning of this chapter; and who, upon the subject of modern Gothic, in reference to some ancient remains of true Gothic grandeur, wrote as follows :—" Several parts of these ruinous buildings might be selected (under suitable modification) as the model of a Gothic mansion, provided architects would be content rather to imitate what is really beautiful in that species of building, than to make a medley of the caprices of the order, confounding the military, ecclesiastical, and domestic styles of all ages at random, with additional fantasies and combinations of their own device." (*Pirate.*) " This is a hit—a very palpable hit."

Returning to the high road, I soon reached the little town of SHAP, whence a smaller vehicle conveyed me three miles further, to the WELLS, leaving on the right the main road for that purpose, and travelling along a cross and tedious carriageway, over bleak downs, to a lonely building standing i a hollow. This is the Spa Hotel, and all that constitutes the Spa besides the Wells.

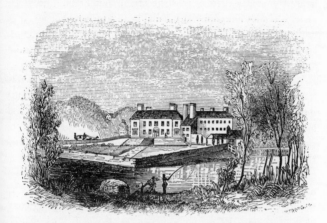

The hotel is a very convenient, commodious, and well-arranged house. It is a recent erection of the venerable earl, who is lord of every thing hereabout. I occupied a double-bedded room facing the south, which would not disgrace a first-rate hotel in London; nay, for cleanliness, abundance of furniture and contrivances, as well as for the excellency of the beds, far superior to most of them. No expense seems to have been spared to make the inmates comfortable. The drawing-room, though not very large, is excellent; and so are the dining and other sitting rooms. In fact every mode of disposing and arranging space for domestic purposes has been evidently studied and thought of with attention. There are as many as sixteen of the best bedrooms, with several more of the second class, and seventy beds altogether,—for which the usual charge is most moderate, as are indeed the charges for every thing else, including those for the warm-baths. Two guineas a week will cover every expense.

A very respectable family (Gibson) occupied at the time the premises as tenants. The landlady, or mistress of the house (for really there is so little of the hotel about it, that an invalid may imagine himself living in a private house), is a mild, pleasing, and lady-like person, with lovely children, and servants of the best description, both as to looks and appearance, and as being well-behaved and attentive.

Something indeed is required within, to make amends for the scene of desolate grandeur that surrounds the place without. Out of my large windows, three successive ranges of heathy downs are seen to swell right and left, and to slope downwards in smooth undulations, until they meet on the margin of a narrow torrent, or *beck*, which travels at a rapid rate, like a mountain stream, over a rocky bed, hissing and chafing amidst the small broken masses of stone that are strewed along its course, and leaving the white foam against each of them. Its tortuous sweeps, as it comes down nearer to the house, concealing here and there portions of the stream behind projecting rocks, serve to give to the whole the appearance of a succession of waterfalls.

In the opening, between two ranges of grassy hills nearest to the house, on which two or three stunted and blanched ash-trees grow, a glimpse is caught of another mountain stream called the Berbeck, the whiteness of whose foam is relieved by the darker swells around it. To these succeed other hills still more barren and rocky than the first ; and the ground rises more steeply as the eye stretches its power of vision over it—ascending higher the further it proceeds, until the prospect is closed by a lofty Fell, running in a south-western direction, the extreme vanishing point of which is a still mightier Peak—the *Shap Fells*—from whose rugged sides have rolled those granite blocks or boulder-stones, which are seen scattered over a great part of Westmorland.

Such is the prospect in the front of the house looking

south. A flat piece of ground between the torrents and the dwelling has been planted in the form of a neat parterre of flowers, and is a cheering ornament to the place.

It is by the side of one of the three *becks* or streams just mentioned, which forms here a succession of leaps as it descends in a nearly direct line from the moors, that the mineral water for which Shap is celebrated, proceeding equally from the upland, tries to mingle itself with the torrent stream; but while in its downward course, along a sloping bank, which has in vain been planted with firs and other trees, the water has been prevented from accomplishing its junction with the Bourne, but on the contrary, has been imprisoned in a square well, fashioned in the rudest style, and covered over on every side but one, where it is protected only by a low door.

The area of this well is about three feet square, and the surface of the water appears always covered with a thin scum, through which bubbles of gas from the bottom are seen to burst from time to time. The colour is that of a very weak solution of soap and water; when held in a glass it precisely resembles that sort of mixture ; or, in other words, it looks as if to a tumblerful of spring-water a few drops of solution of soap had been added. The water is transparent, but not limpid ; several little floating bodies, whitish and milk-like, being suspended in it. The smell of sulphuretted hydrogen is very marked, and its immediate taste slightly saltish ; it feels cold to the stomach, and instantly after drinking a glass and a half, or ten ounces of it, I experienced the same sensations which Harrowgate and other sulphur-waters never failed to produce on me, namely, headach and eructation of the sulphuretted gas. After repeated trials I found the temperature of the water in the well to be 48° F.

No attempt whatever has, as yet, been made to invite invalids to this spring of health—either by facilitating the ac-

cess to it, or by rendering it, and the immediate objects around,
such as to induce people to resort to the source itself to drink
the water or bathe in it. As the well formerly was, when the
waters first became an object of attention, so it is now;
and the vestiges left of a former rude stone bath, show
how little our forefathers have cared for the many luxuries
which visiters to modern Spas expect to enjoy. How people
in such a bleak situation as this, encircled by boulder-stones
and nought else, could deliberately proceed to the miserable
hovel called the Well-house—for it is now exactly as it ever was
—in which the old bath existed, and there bathe in the cold
sulphur-water from the well,—it makes one shudder to think.

The dreariness of the common between Shap and the well,
thoroughly barren even at the most propitious time of the
year in which I visited it, is somewhat appalling—particularly
when traversed during some of those terrific storms which one
seldom witnesses except in highly mountainous countries.

On approaching the termination of the road, the Spa
Hotel is seen to lie in a hollow of a series of moors, and
looks like an island in the midst of an agitated lake of
desolation. Yet the materials of which the handsome house
is built, and the care with which the grounds are kept, give
to the spot a cheering and welcoming aspect.

Midway between the old Well-house and the Spa Hotel, a
bath-house, with convenience for warm and cold bathing,
has been of late years erected. There are two rooms in it,
with two bath-tanks in each—the latter, of wood painted
brown, and exhibiting, by their whitish and opalescent
surface, the action of the mineral water. The building
is good enough for the company which generally frequents
this Spa; not so for the better class to which unquestionably
belonged those few whom I met the preceding evening in the
dining-room, and most of whom were mere *transiters* from
the south, on their way to Appleby, or to the lakes.

In order to facilitate the use of the baths, the mineral water is collected first into a large reservoir, holding about 12,000 gallons, whence a large pipe conveys some of the water to a large iron boiler, while four smaller pipes transmit it cold to the four bath-rooms. I need hardly remark that the use of an iron boiler with sulphuretted water is highly improper.

When heated, the Shap water loses the whitish blue appearance it has at the well, or continues only slightly so. It then tastes at once saltish, has a slight *après goût*, and lies more comfortably on the stomach. Some of the water, which, on its arrival from the Well into the room in which the boiler is kept, and whose temperature was at the time 65°F., had the peculiar bluish opalescent appearance just mentioned, became quite pure and limpid, like the Gilsland water, soon after, and lost nearly altogether the taste, as well as the peculiar smell, of the sulphuretted gas.

The analysis of the Shap water was undertaken by Mr. Alderson, of Westhouse, assisted by Dr. Fife, lecturer on chemistry in Edinburgh. It is somewhat remarkable that the accounts which those gentlemen have published of their analysis make no mention of the presence of sulphuretted hydrogen gas. I am inclined, therefore, to suspect that their examination of the water did not take place at the Well, as ought to have been the case; for the presence of the gas in question in the water is made manifest by its taste and smell—its deposition, its action upon lead and iron—and, lastly, on the oil-paint in the bath-rooms. In fact, it is admitted by all who have tasted or smelt the water, which they compare to the washing out of a gunbarrel.

In other respects the analysis may be correct, and, if so, the combination of the ingredients found in it is a happy one for many medical purposes. Yet I would take Mr. Alderson's pompous eulogium of this water *cum grano salis*.

I can readily believe that a water said to hold twenty-six grains of muriate of lime in a pint measure, may be diuretic, and exercise a powerful influence in the resolution of glandular tumours. But to add that " in cutaneous and impetiginous affections, of the scaly order, the water is *miraculously efficacious*," and that in acute or chronic rheumatism it is " speedily curative," is too near an approach to the region of poetical fancy.

Mr. Alderson says—" In my experience, I have met with no medicated spring more efficacious than the Shap Spa." It is to be presumed that the experience of any medical man who practises in a limited district in Cumberland or Yorkshire, as regards notable mineral springs, can only be small ; how then can he institute such a superlative comparison ? But Mr. Alderson, not satisfied with that, proceeds most emphatically and sublimely in his commendations, ascending, at last, to the highest pitch of eulogium.

I am more inclined to rely on the plain, unvarnished tales I heard in the great meeting-room of the Spa Hotel, where, in particular, a lady and her husband, accompanied by their son, all natives of Westmorland, and well acquainted with the Spa, informed me of the several cures that had come to their knowledge, effected by the Shap Well water. Those cases, principally in the classes of disorders for which sulphuretted waters are beneficially employed, warrant much of the praise given to the Shap Spa, and justify my having detained my readers so long respecting it.

Sequestered as the Spa is, yet, when occasion requires, medical attendance can be procured readily, either from Penrith, or from Shap and Orton, at both which latter places a young physician has lately established himself. Dr. Taylor is the gentleman most commonly sent for from the former place, and I marvelled much at the information I received, that in cases of surgical aid being required, that physician does not scruple to employ the services of Dennison, the notorious bonesetter, of whom most extraordinary stories are related, both in Cumberland and Westmorland.

The occasional consultations with so respectable a practitioner as Dr. Taylor bespeak the presence of company at the Spa of the better class ; and of those, I found registered in the book of visiters between June and August, about two hundred, among whom there were some whose names are conspicuous.

The account of a Spa situated like that of Shap, unaccompanied by a few remarks on its climate, would be incomplete. The air in this region is seldom still; storms of wind are of very frequent occurrence, and the quantity of rain that falls in the course of the year is greater than in any other county in England. According to the observations made with rain gages at Kendal, seventeen miles only to the south of Shap, fifty inches, or four feet two inches of rain appears to be the average quantity that falls in this mountainous region. It is, therefore, somewhat about twenty inches more than the mean quantity of rain that falls in Europe.

A lady sitting before a roasting fire (of which by the by I was glad to partake also) on the sixth of August at Shap, stated in my hearing, that not a single day wholly free from rain, had she passed in the place during the previous month.

The coldness of the air must be excessive during the autumn and spring, which latter season rarely commences before June.

In the winter season, the snow, which lies thick and heavy and late, adds much to the discomfort of the place ; and so prodigious is the quantity that falls and remains on the ground in this immediate neighbourhood, that a considerable sum of money has been paid at times to have a horse track cut through it between Shap and Kendal.

And yet even this desolate region—even the heathy, uncultivated and rudely mountainous vicinity of Shap Wells—might be made the resort of all classes of society, by further improvement and accommodation.   One, and the most urgent of these, is the erecting of a lodge or house of shelter near the cross road that leads to the Spa Hotel from the high-road, and the establishment of a proper conveyance for visiters who arrive by the public coaches, and are set down on that spot, now a barren heath.   At present such visiters, on quitting the public carriage, have to walk three miles and a half to the hotel, and carry their own luggage (perhaps in the midst of torrents of rain), or they must submit to pay pretty heavily for a chaise to convey them from Shap or Kendal.   As for attractions in the neighbourhood, they are neither few nor contemptible; and during a month's residence at the Spa, the visiters need not pass a single day without enjoying some new sight, or the contemplation of some interesting object; besides having the indulgence of capital grouse-sporting on the adjoining moor, by simply applying to Lord Lonsdale for permission.   Horse exercise, so much to be recommended, and too little attended to at Spas, would in this region prove also the best means of making excursions.

One of these would naturally be to the ruins of Shap Abbey —another reminiscence of the many snug settlements by monastic recluses to be met with (and invariably on the most advantageous as well as beautiful spots) throughout the north of England.   Seen from the eastern bank of the Loder, and from a jutting headland thereabout, the first view of the dismantled square tower of the abbey is very striking.   It stands on a green knoll on the opposite side of that river; while the rest of the ruins, by no means extensive, descend towards the noisy and darksome stream, not far from a rude stone bridge, by which it is encompassed, precisely where it sweeps in a semicircle below a rising bank, thickly wooded with old tufty and twisted thorns—the very trees planted by the monks.

Another attractive feature near at hand, is the sweetly

secluded vale of Crosby Ravensworth, particularly if viewed immediately upon our return from witnessing that striking object, Highcup Gill, a valley which, from its singular appearance, has been likened to the tumultuous heaving of a troubled sea, suddenly arrested by a petrifying power, at a moment when the waves, tossed right and left, formed a mighty chasm or hollow trough between.

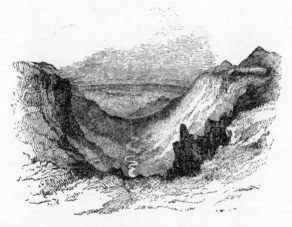

The lakes, however, are, after all, the most inviting of the attractions of this neighbourhood. Many of these, Hawes and Ulleswater, for instance, may be seen, at one view, from an eminence which I reached after an hour's quiet ride, doubling for that purpose the cluster of lofty hills, called Shapfells, the foot of which I skirted, leaving them on my left.

Taking my station, with my back to Rossgill, and my face looking down into the charming vale of Bampton, I enjoyed a spectacle which I marvel much that a Dewint or a Robertson have not made the subject of their pencil. In my case,

z 2

however, the attraction of such a neighbourhood was not
sufficiently strong to induce me to penetrate further into the
enchanting region of the lakes; for I had visited them only
the year before in company with the modest and amiable
author of " Hampden in the 19th Century," and other works,
and I could not now spare the time to revisit scenes to which
even the pen of a Gilpin or a Radcliffe cannot do justice.

But whether we direct our steps to the right or to the left,
although many parts of the country are beautiful and imposing
to look upon, one cannot help being struck, and painfully so,
at the enormous extent of waste and barren moorland which,
in Westmorland as in Cumberland (but much more so in
the former county), meets the eye of the traveller at every
step.   To think that in those two counties nearly half a
million of acres exist still in a wild primitive state, and that
the hand of man has never yet been applied to recover the
smallest portion of it for beneficial purposes, is a distressing
subject of consideration.

The noble earl who is justly acknowledged to be the *primus
inter omnes* in this part of England, has, indeed, in some of the
districts of his extensive demesnes, endeavoured to bring into
use many barren tracts, by planting them with trees.   So did
several of his noble ancestors before him, as we may judge
from the numerous woods, artificially arranged or distributed
in groups, which we meet on the Lonsdale property.   But in
endeavouring to put waste land in cultivation, planting is but
a tithe part of what ought to be done for that purpose; it is,
as compared to tilling, to leave the land in a still half-barren
and unproductive state.

By the latter operation, therefore, principally, ought the
many hundred thousands of acres of waste land in the two
counties which now occupy our attention to be redeemed.   In
that respect, the difference between planting and tilling
is by far, very far indeed, in favour of the lastmentioned

process. It is in its favour, not only on account of what it leads to of beneficial, but also of what it avoids of disastrous results.

The reader will permit me a few short practical remarks on this subject, which is one that forces itself upon our attention every day, as the population is growing apace around us, seeming to defy all calculation, and calling out for bread.

The Lonsdale estates in Westmorland suffered in their timber, during the well-remembered terrific storm of January, 1839, to an extent hardly to be credited. Thousands of lofty trees were felled to the ground, or snapped in twain like a dry splintery deal-board, or were uprooted and laid across the standing trunks of other trees near them. I passed, in the month of August of the same year, through a part of one of the earl's forests, some miles south of Penrith, and was much struck with the appearance of desolation which the still visible effects of that terrible gale had produced. To such disastrous results no tract of land, however extensive, brought into tillage or pasturage from a primitive and wild state, can ever be liable. But the planter of forests, on the contrary, who has carefully reared his trees for twenty or thirty years, deriving no profit from them for the best part of that period, just as he expects to reap the benefit of his operations, or to transmit it to his children, not unfrequently sees the produce of his patient labours, his expectations, and his property, at once demolished by some violent tempest.

This, however, is a purely selfish, and, some may think, an overstrained view of the subject. But there is another and a more philosophical consideration of it which suggests itself; namely this,—that in bringing large tracts of waste land into tillage, we not only benefit mankind pecuniarily, as with the growth of trees, but morally also. Such an operation generally gives rise to the formation of new little communities and villages; it puts poor labourers in the present enjoyment of the necessaries, and even some of the comforts of life; it enables the master to watch over and form the happiness of the many fellow-creatures whom he engages, in one of the most wholesome and beneficial of occupations—an occupation which is to give those creatures bread and sustenance, as the direct produce of the land they have been the means of recovering from waste.

This state of things, in its turn, leads to the formation of schools, the establishment of places of worship, and, consequently, to the extension of civilization. What results better than all these can a good man desire, whom Providence has invested with large territorial seignory? How can the planter of thousands of trees on any waste tract ever expect similar results?

Let us take two examples in illustration of each process. They occur to my mind as mere random recollections of what I have seen or heard in the course of my present tour through England.

A tract of sandy or semi-siliceous soil, extending to nearly six thousand acres, in one of the south-western counties of England (not Cornwall), which had never yielded a blade of grass, or a twig, was planted, in 1818, with Scotch firs, the young plants being about two feet in height at the time. The plantation had thriven to the whole extent of the proprietor's expectations. In thrice seven years it has produced to him by clearings, taking out long sticks, and yearly cuttings, an additional income of some hundred pounds. In the neighbourhood of this large plantation some new houses have been reared, and settlers have been induced to make their dwellings where no human being had been seen to dwell before; attracted, no doubt, by the shelter which the vast forest affords them, as well as by the facility of obtaining timber for their humble buildings, and fuel for their hearths. The population of the district has consequently increased to a certain extent, and land is become more valuable, or, rather, it is valuable now where it was worthless before. But this is all the result; —an increased pecuniary value has been added to a man's patrimony, and at the end of twenty years a hundred human beings, perhaps, have felt the benefit of that addition.

Let us now look upon the other picture. In this very county in which I endite these reflections, and whilst visiting the neighbourhood of Carlisle in search of a sulphuretted mineral spring, called Slainton, south of Longtown, I had before me a plain and extensive proof of the great advantages of tilling waste land, in the actual condition of the Netherby estate, the patrimony of the present distinguished statesman and commoner, member for Pembroke. To him most assuredly it would not have descended in its actual highly-flourishing state, nor with its present magnificent villa, resting on a Roman station, had his ancestor, the Rev. Dr. Graham, been content with simply planting forests for the sake of their timber, on the extensive tracts of waste and bare lands which formed part of his territorial property, instead of raising the latter, by tillage, into a rich, fertile, and, in many parts, beautiful demesne. That demesne at present exhibits every where the marks of prosperity, civilization, and religion, in its extensive corn-mills and corn-fields, its free grammar-schools, and neat places of worship. By such means, and with such results, the worthy divine is known to have quintupled the value of his estates.

Leaving now all these reflections, and the counties that gave rise to them, I hastened on to Preston, with all the speed of one of the numerous mails from the north, which picked me up at Shap, disregarding both Kendal and Lancaster, places I had seen at leisure before.

On a former occasion I had adopted the Bull as my head-quarters at Preston; but having since tried the Victoria New Hotel, which has the double advantage of being out of the smoke of the town, and near to the railway station, I cannot omit recommending it in every way to my readers, in preference to the former house, which has all the inconvenience of a huge country inn.

Of all the rising manufacturing towns in the north, Preston is probably the only one which has contrived to add to its population, its wealth, and its factories, to a very considerable extent, without at the same time having made any corresponding advances in civilization, cleanliness, and ameliorations in the material part of the city. Its streets are as narrow, and as crooked, and as dirty as ever. Very few of its shops, even in Fishergate, the Regent-street of the place, exhibit any appearance of improvement from what they must have been thirty years ago. It possesses no public building, not even a market; and on every Saturday evening the butchers' shambles and other sheds, for the display of every marketable commodity, are set up in a line on one side of the very street just named, nearly to its whole extent, causing filth, confusion, and inconvenience.

It will hardly be believed that there exists no such thing as a public or any other bath, hot or cold, in Preston. There are two ordinary news-rooms in the place—the one a little more aristocratic than the other; yet even the latter is very unworthy of the wealthy people who subscribe to it.

Preston, I repeat it, is fifty years in arrear of the progress of all modern manufacturing towns in England, in the conveniences, the comforts, and the embellishments of life—nay, it is a hundred years in arrear of the steady and somewhat surprising progress of its own manufactures. It is a place slow in improving, and seems to consist wholly of people intent on amassing wealth by commerce, manufacture, and speculation. It would take half a century of steady goodwill, and a considerable expenditure of money, to make Preston what Manchester, Halifax, Bradford, Wakefield, or even Huddersfield, are and have been for a long time.

There is no public spirit in this place; but, *en revanche,* if we are to credit one of their own journals, the *Preston Observer,* there is much of licentiousness, as we are told that one-tenth of the children born during the last quarter of 1839, in the Preston Union, were illegitimate. And yet, to judge from a little episode in the daily routine of the place, to which I was a witness in the green-market, one would feel disposed to consider the Prestonians an intellectual people. A licensed hawker having advertised the importation and intended sale of three thousand volumes of cheap books, had been so successful in his operation, which was carried on in the open market-place, that he felt it necessary to apologize to " the reading public " because his large stock had been exhausted a day sooner than he had anticipated. He promised, at the same time, the literati of Preston, to return soon with a still more splendid supply for their accommodation.

My sole object, however, in halting this time for a few hours at Preston, while on my way to one or two principal watering-places on the coast, was neither to buy cheap books nor to criticise its present condition. I was anxious only to see that splendid collection of fossils, principally of the mountain limestone formation, which has been duly commended by Philipps, and which is the result of a most persevering devotion to geology on the part of Mr. Gilberton, living at the corner of Church-street, in an humble shop, in which he retails drugs. There are upwards of two thousand specimens in the collection, most of them *Geneva,* being specimens of of mollusca, not to be met with in the recent state. Among many other objects, I was particularly struck with the perfect state of a tooth of a bear from Bolland, found at a farm in which Mr. Gilberton had been nursed, and where, as he himself told me, he probably sucked with the nurse's milk the geological mania that has disturbed his mind ever since, to the occasional detriment of his own business.

Although a perfect stranger to this enthusiastic naturalist,

I received from him every mark of attention and civility. Few persons know the treasures of every kind which are to be found in this country, in the hands of private, industrious people, among the humbler classes, devoted to science, antiquities, and sometimes even the fine arts.

As the Manchester people have their favourite sea-bath at SOUTHPORT, so have those of Preston at BLACKPOOL. The former stands on the coast a little south, and the latter a little north, of the entrance into the river Ribble. Southport is buried in sand-hills, and so far protected, that its climate is mild, and suitable even for invalids in the summer. But the sands, which at Blackpool, as at Scarborough, are hard at low water, at Southport are soft and deep when the tide recedes from them, as it does to an immense distance.

Though the two bathing-stations are so near each other, there is only a precarious communication between them. In fine, settled weather, a boat leaves, in the course of the day, Litham for Southport. But if the meditated improvements suggested by Stevenson, should ever be carried into effect, and the Ribble from its entrance up to Preston be widened and deepened in its channel, its banks will be busy with population, and the intercourse between the two become more frequent and regular.

At BLACKPOOL the principal places for residence are the hotels, of which there are some suited to every class of persons, and in which the highest charge for board and excellent living is only five shillings a day, and in some cases, as low as three shillings. But all these establishments are shut up in the winter; whereas at Southport, cottages and private houses are more the fashion than hotels, and are permanently occupied by the families who resort thither, whether for health or the pleasure of bathing.

To the latter watering-place, such as it is, the Manchester factor and artisan—the rich and the " middling comfortable " —repair during two months of the year, either for a week or two's residence, or for a mere frolic.   At that period, one may see the walls of that smoky city placarded with " Cheap travelling to Southport "—" Only five hours to Southport"—" Excursion to Southport;" and vociferations from a hundred throats to the same effect, are to be heard from the top of every species of vehicle in the principal streets.

And no wonder that those who can luckily escape from the soot-inizing atmosphere of Manchester, to plunge into the " wide, wide sea," there to wash off the black deposits on their skin, should eagerly seize the opportunity of repairing even to such a sea bathing-place as Southport.

Precisely the same eagerness actuates the Prestonians, who find Blackpool much more readily accessible than Southport, by a paved road, which for the first ten miles lies through a flat and indifferently-cultivated land, the property of a gentleman occupying Litham Hall, near the neat little village of that name, at the mouth of the Ribble.   But the facility of getting to Blackpool from Preston will be much greater when the Wyre and Preston railway, now in progress, shall be completed.

The first view of the sea on approaching Blackpool is striking, as the first view of that element always is to a traveller just returning from wandering through alpine districts and inland countries.   The busy occupation of the masons, in the prospect before me as I approached the town, bespoke at once the thriving condition of the place.   An increase of building was taking place to the south, and a new colony of visiters and bathers is establishing itself there, under the appellation of South Blackpool.

I slept at Nixon's hotel, one of the oldest establishments, through many generations, in the place.   I had been recommended there by a gentleman, a fellow-traveller on the top of the two-horse coach that had conveyed us hither, from whom I obtained all the information I am able to give on my present subject, which is not from my own observation, and who turned out, on further acquaintance, to be a leading man of law at Preston. The house, to which other dwellings have been added from time to time, has a great extent of frontage W. S. W., and a side of rather a showy appearance to the north, where the principal entrance is. Behind, a very extensive range of coach-houses and stables has been erected.

There are two great rival houses, hotels yclept, in Blackpool, Nixon's and Dickson's—the Capulets and the Montagues—the white and the red rose. The former boasts of a larger and more extended line of buildings, as I before mentioned, conspicuously white from recent painting ; the latter of a more projecting cliff over the strand, and a private terrace with green sward and neat rustic seats, quite still and retired, though fronting the sea. This last hotel is frequented chiefly by the higher class of visiters. At Nixon's the company is less select—or rather it is of a lower grade altogether.

Arrived at Nixon's in the very nick of time for dinner, and the necessary permission having been obtained in my behalf and that of my travelling companion, the aforesaid shrewd limb of the law, we were admitted into a long and lofty apartment having some pretension to the rank of a banqueting-room, in which a long narrow table, groaning under a double line of tin-capped dishes, was awaiting the arrival of the company. A loud-sounding scavenger-like bell soon brought the latter, mob-fashion, into the room ; when I took my place at the bottom of the table, near to my coach companion, who having always been a guest at the Dickson's, or " the upper house," sat himself down here to oblige me, not without symptoms of a curling lip and a turned-up nose.

Such a motley of honest-looking people—men, women, and children, (for there were some whose chins did not reach the edge of the table)—it has never been my fortune to meet under the like circumstance in such numbers before—fifty or sixty in all—except at the anniversary dinner of some dispensary, or at some of your queer banquets at mine host's of the Great Queen-street Tavern, honest and corpulent Mr. Cuff.

Methinks the highest in rank here might have been an iron-founder, from near Bradford or Halifax, or a retired wine-merchant, from Liverpool, who, in the palmy days of *Port*, found the Oporto trade a thriving concern. About a dozen chambermaids acted as waiters, and there was not a vestige of man-servant, at which I heartily rejoiced. It fell to my lot to dissect the chickens for the ladies. Abundance of meat and sauce seemed to be the desirable thing. One whom I had plentifully supplied with leg and pinion, and no small proportion of the parsley-and-butter, sent soon after to crave for the breast, and a little more of the green sauce! The thing was appalling; and the serious and busy manner in which every hand and mouth seemed to be at work during the first ten minutes, *sans mot dire*, plainly showed how palatable was the fare, and how keenly the sea-air and the sea-bathing of Blackpool, had prepared the company for it.

At Dickson's the scene is said to be somewhat more decorous and stately; for there the consuming classes, like the articles to be consumed, are of a different and a better order, although the charge at each place differs only by sixpence; five shillings being the highest price for not fewer than five meals daily.

The bedrooms at Nixon's face the sea, and most of them are desirable. In Dickson's house, which, by the by, is situated farther north, and will consequently be soon deserted, as the colony is travelling southward, there are bedrooms and accommodations of a very superior description, equal to any at Brighton.

Besides these two great hotels, sundry lodging-houses allure the passing strangers, who find in them every desirable comfort.

The town is scattered on a moderately high sandy bank,

terminating abruptly above the sandy beach. In no sea bathing-place have I beheld such an *extent* of superb sands. The cliff, as it is here styled, though it is nothing more than a sand-hill that separates earth from water, stretches nearly due north and south. Upon the very brink of this, good-looking houses have been erected, in a line of a mile and a half in length. Walls of stone have been built in a slanting direction, to keep up this said cliff, and prevent the else inevitable excavation which high water would make—and a little farther north *has* made—giving there a picturesque aspect to the shore.

About the centre of this line, between the extreme north end of the village and the recently-erected south pier, a terrace, nearly opposite Nixon's, has been established, which serves as a marine promenade to the pedestrians as well as equestrians, returning from the sands. Upon the latter I beheld numerous groups and single individuals, scattered in all directions, some walking and others riding, either on steeds or on asses, dotting the extended strand, which looks like the desert of Suez with the parted waters of the Red Sea, murmuring at the distance of half a mile.

Here the visiters bask in the sun ; they trot, or they saunter ; and some vainly try to pick up shells, but shells there are none on this shore. The scene altogether, viewed from the front of the cliff, with the sun brilliantly pouring upon its wide expanse in its fullest glory, is one of far superior beauty to that which Brighton or Hastings, with their terraced palaces, exhibit. The character of the shore alone, its succession of fine sweeping bays, the form of its cliffs, the ruinous castle, and the lofty hills around it, form at Scarborough a more picturesque landscape than we find on the Blackpool coast. But if extent of sea-shore, exquisite beauty of the sands, absence of all rocks, breadth and length, constitute the most striking features of a maritime place destined to collect hundreds of sea-bathers ;—then Blackpool, I say, has not its equal. Blackpool, in fact, as to sea-bathing and sea-sands, is to the west coast of England, what Scarborough is to the east, and Weymouth to the south.

I take it that the manufacturing inhabitants of Lancashire supply most of the company at Blackpool. It is rarely that the superior classes of Preston come hither. They prefer going to roast themselves on the less primitive shores of Brighthelmstone, or under St. Leonard's cliff. None but such as cannot proceed farther south, or farther east, across Yorkshire, take up their abode here.

The bathing, both at high and low water, is excellent, and the charges for the bathing-machines most moderate. From the appearance of the guests on the day of my visit, and still more so of many that I saw wandering along the sea-shore, I imagine that not a few persons repair to Blackpool with the hope of deriving real benefit or relief in severe disorders of outer limbs and internal organs ; since many of them appeared lame, and others had a jaundiced face, or one that bore upon it marks of requiring the cleansing of the Pool of Bethesda.

That they are not all disappointed in their expectations from sea-bathing, if they persevere in it, and live *rightly*, I have no doubt. But the " five solid repasts," and " a *little* of the breast with some more of the green sauce," at the Nixon's and Dickson's, would counteract any good that might be derived from sea-bathing and sea-breezes.

CHAPTER XXIII.

CLITHERO, AND THE CRAVEN SPAS.

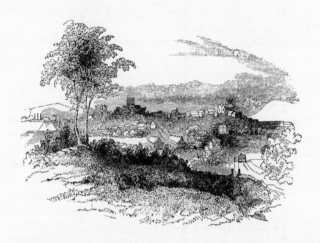

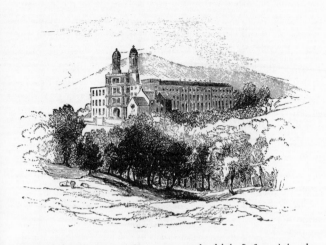

At the termination of a cross-road which I found in the most wretched state of repair, STONYHURST COLLEGE, the place I wished particularly to visit, appeared in view, distant from Preston about fourteen miles in a north-eastern direction. The approach to that showy edifice, destined for the education of Roman Catholic youths, under the direction of the Jesuits,—which to a traveller coming from the east, along the bank of the Ribble, presents itself upon an eminence commanding an extensive view of the Lancashire and Yorkshire hills, is far less romantic, though more stately, when the College viewed from the side of Preston. A long and formal gravel-walk, like an avenue, flanked on each side by a square basin of water, leads to an outer gate in front of the open court before the college.

The remarkable feature in the façade of this building, one half of which bespeaks the Elizabethan style, is the square centre tower rising above the principal gate, and exhibiting in the pillars of its three stories three different orders of architecture. Up the outside of this very tower, did Waterton, the naturalist, climb when a boy and a student in the college ; betraying thus early in life that venturous spirit which he meant to display in subsequent years. The museum of the college, which is, by the by, displayed in this identical tower, contains many proofs of the practical effect of that venturous spirit, in the specimens of South American antiquities for which the college stands indebted to that eccentric traveller.

On the right of the tower the character of the building harmonizes with the church, and the covered cloisters which lead to it from the college. The design of the left wing is more simple, consisting only of three rows of plain, unadorned windows ; but a project is under consideration for altering its front, so as to make it correspond with that on the right.

The structure has been successively enlarged since it became the property of the Jesuits, especially behind the more ancient part, or Elizabethan front, where a large series of buildings — lofty, showy, and with some pretension to Italian architecture—has been erected within the last fifteen years.

In this series of buildings, which extends to 250 feet from east to west, are the principal divisions of the college, devoted to the instruction of the minor pupils, as well as of those more advanced in their studies—called the *Philosophers,*—who are kept distinct from the rest. The *Theologians,* or novice clergymen, who are preparing to take orders, or become members of the congregation of Jesuits. if so inclined, are likewise lodged here.

The provisions made within this part of the college, for a complete education in literature and science are ample, and as far as they were explained to me, likely to promote the ends in view. No expense has been spared to bring together every requisite appliance—whether in chemistry, natural philosophy, astronomy, or mechanics—for the successful tuition of the young people in practical science; and I could not help admiring, not only the beauty and expensive nature of the apparatus provided, but the neatness and method with which they were arranged.

Indeed neatness, order, and cleanliness, seemed to be the great prevailing character of the institution,—whose extensive apartments, school-rooms, the great exhibition-room, the refectory, and the dormitories, I had sufficient leisure afforded me to notice, as well as the silent and quiet regularity with which every operation was conducted.

When I walked through the dormitories, I thought the arrangements made for the comfort, as well as good behaviour, of the scholars, the best imaginable; but I have since had occasion to see something better of the kind, at the new Roman Catholic establishment of Ascott, respecting which I shall have to make some remarks hereafter. The discipline observed is the same in both, although the one is under monastic rule as it were,—the teachers and directors being of the order of Jesus at Stonyhurst—whereas there are only secular priests at Ascott.

The number of pupils was not very considerable at the time of my visit, and I had to regret the indisposition of the principal, the Rev. Mr. Brownhill, who, however, deputed a member of the college to show and explain to me, in the most unreserved manner, the entire establishment.

The physical education of a large number of young boys belonging to the easy classes of society, thus brought together for the purpose principally of cultivating their minds, is an object which was more likely to interest a physician who has, during a long professional life, paid great attention to the subject. I have often had to lament, indeed, that such a subject did not form a sufficiently prominent point of consideration in the collegiate or private education of boys in this country; and I was glad, therefore, of the opportunity of investigating in this establishment how far physical education was attended to.

The division of time, in reference to meals, and the nature of the food allowed, are the first points to be considered. At Stonyhurst that takes place in the following order: Breakfast at a quarter past eight o'clock—milk-and-water with bread ; dinner at half-past eleven—meat, except on meagre days, and some days in the week pastry in addition ; a *goûter* of bread and beer at four o'clock ; supper at six, consisting of bread and cheese, or potatoes,* with, occasionally, meat again. One hour and a half's recreation is allowed after dinner, one hour again after supper, and half an hour for night prayer, and then to bed. To it the boys proceed in regular order and in silence. At the several landing-places on the great staircase, as well as in the dormitories, they are received by one of the sub-prefects, who sits up in turn during the night, to watch over the safety and conduct of the pupils.

During recreation hours, gymnastic exercises are encouraged, for which purpose a large piece of ground is set apart, with all the usual apparatus. The presence of one or more of the assistant-teachers on the playground prevents all possible mischief.

It is this system of *prevention* which seems to distinguish the mode of collegial education adopted in this establishment, and those analogous to it, from that which obtains elsewhere in England, and which is based on the notion that boys should " rough it;" and that it is quite time enough to check mischief or vice when it is actually in operation. In this preventive system, the Moravians resemble the Roman Catholics. Their collegial or school rules also are of that character. " If you take care," say they, " that boys, in the progress of their moral education, shall find it impossible to put in practice any improper thought or vicious inclination, in consequence of the incessant watchfulness exercised over them by the never-failing presence of a superior; and if such a restraint against natural evil propensities be continued throughout the period of their education, the propensities themselves will at last be extinguished ; and it is just as im-

* This is the only objectionable part of the dietary. What can be worse than cheese or potatoes just as we are retiring to rest ?

probable that such boys shall in afterlife evince a tendency to evil-doing, as it would be that they should manifest any cleverness if their mental faculties had been in a similar manner unpractised or restrained."

How far the result of such a system—which, with regard to producing *good* people, has certainly worked well, both with the Romanists and the Moravians, and I may add also with many of the public colleges (not universities) I visited in Germany —has been also successful in, or may be deemed capable of, producing men of genius and of striking or commanding talents, is another question, and one which my experience does not enable me to answer, offhand, in the affirmative. But, as the great bulk of society among the easy classes can only consist of men of mediocre abilities, any system of education that tends to make them *good*, whilst it sufficiently brings forward and makes available their mediocrity of talent, must be the one most desirable for mankind.

Have either Stonyhurst College, or the larger establishment near Birmingham, or, thirdly, the one under the immediate superintendence of the Roman Catholic bishop at Bath, produced any number of men who stand aloof from the common herd, for their immense talents and extraordinary abilities,—as some other colleges or establishments in this country have produced—Winchester, or Eton, or Westminster to wit,—where, certainly, the preventive system flourisheth not, but, on the contrary, the *laissez faire* practice is the prevailing one ? What says the biography of our present great men upon this question ?

The expense of educating a boy at Stonyhurst is fifty pounds per annum, and about twenty pounds extras.

The two divisions of the college mostly deserving of attention at Stonyhurst are the old as well as the new library and the picture-gallery. There are objects in them that would detain a literary man, or one fond of the arts, for many an hour. The latter apartment serves also as a meeting and recreation room for the masters. Many of the pictures, which are principally of the cabinet form, and by very old masters, both German and Italian, have either been sent from Rome or are presents. Chance enabled the member of the confraternity, who was kindly conducting me through the establishment, to pick up, very recently, at a broker's in Wardour-street, for forty pounds, a large well-painted and well-preserved picture, of great interest to himself and brethren, as it represents the chronological tree of the order of St. Ignatius, the founder of the Jesuits, comprising the portraits, three inches in diameter, of all the leading members of that society.

From the picture-gallery a door opens into the private chapel, the altarpiece of which is by Murillo.

The late Lord Arundel left his extensive and choice library, the books of which are mostly bound in white vellum, to this college. These were being neatly arranged in a handsome room in the old building, newly appropriated for that purpose, and, in connexion with the principal library, an oblong oval apartment, having a gallery all round, supported by columns. In the former I was struck with a beautiful copy of *Malvasia's* FELSINA PITTRICE, *vite dei pittori Bolognesi,* 1678. Each life is illustrated by the portrait of the individual painter, engraved in wood; but in the case of about half a dozen of these portraits, the head of the painter, placed within the encircling border, is drawn *à la plume,* in ink. Those of Ercole Procaccini and Pellegrino Tibaldi are in the most spirited style of pen-drawing.

The great gems, however, possessed by the Jesuits in this department of their establishment, are found in a glazed *escrutoire,* in the principal library, which contains some most exquisite objects of art. I shall only specify a crucifix painted on wood by Michael Angelo, in which the *chiaroscuro* and the flesh are quite deceptive, and the blood that streams from the feet seems quick.

I looked with much less interest on the many relics of the great Chancellor More, his seal, and his St. George, presented to the college by the last descendant of that great man, who died at Rome : all these are contained in the same *escrutoire*, with the Gospel of St. John found in St. Cuthbert's tomb, and supposed to be in his own handwriting.

Stonyhurst, after all, is not so much indebted to the comparatively modern establishment of the Jesuits' College, for its celebrity in modern English history, as to the circumstance of its having been the place into which wool-spinning was first introduced in this country.

CLITHERO has a Spa, and to it I directed my steps on quitting Stonyhurst, through a very rural-looking district, principally pasture-land, to the right and left of the Ribble.

The Spa, or Wells, for there are two of them, are situated at about a quarter of a mile from the town, and have not long been made available to their whole extent. They are close to a factory-mill of considerable size, lately erected, and they seem to rise from limestone shale.

The water in both wells is evidently sulphuretted ; but that which I drew from the round well was only slightly so ; whereas the one in the square well exhibited stronger marks of the gas when tasted. To the latter well the public have made good their claim after some squabble, and they avail themselves largely of the privilege of quaffing the water for nothing. The temperature of the water is 48°. It is perfectly transparent, and drank like common spring water—so little saline matter does it contain.

Baths have been established near the wells ; but here again they convey the water in leaden pipes ; so that by the time the water gets to the reservoir the slight quantity of sulphur-gas is gone. In warm-baths hardly a vestige of the sulphuretted gas remains.

The water has been found to be an excellent depurative for all eruptive diseases, and is a great favourite with the better classes of people of Clithero.   Mr. Murray, the travelling lecturer on chemistry, made a superficial analysis, but not a quantitative one, of the water, and states that he found the sulphuretted hydrogen gas abundant, the muriate of soda slight in quantity, the sulphate of magnesia and carbonate of lime small, and of iron only an atom.

Perhaps one of the most striking views of Clithero is that which presents itself on returning from the Spa,—when its castle-keep, and the large house adjoining, formerly belonging to Lord Montague, but now inhabited by the widow of a wealthy agent of the house of Clithero—also the churches and other buildings, seated on as many hills or eminences—seem to group admirably together, interspersed as they are with fields and gardens, and occupying a large extent of ground.

The view of the castle as a centre of this panorama, is interesting in other respects. The town is seen to rest on the slope of the hill below it towards the north ; and, as it spreads, signs of religious toleration, very creditable to modern time, are perceivable throughout the mass ;—for the very picturesque old church, forming the most distant point on the horizon, appears on the right, and St. James's on the left, while the Roman Catholic chapel occupies the centre, flanked by the Wesleyan on one side, and the " Independents" on the other. In the midst of these rises the national school, to which the sum of 300*l.* had been lately awarded—one of the first effects of the recently-promulgated order in council respecting national education.

But if the *proverb* commonly repeated in the place be true to its meaning—namely, that Clithero is celebrated for

" Lime, Law, and Latin,"

this first application of the education money was scarcely needed. That there is something in the proverb as far as lawyers are concerned in it, I had many opportunities of ascertaining. It is doubtful whether a town of the same size, containing about 7000 inhabitants, exists, where the door of every other house, in two or three of the principal streets, as in Clithero, exhibits the awful word " Attorney" on its broad brassplate.

What people in such a place, fattening upon fat cattle (of which, by the by, I witnessed the finest display imaginable in the market-place), and most of them graziers, can have to quarrel about, it would puzzle the very attorneys themselves to decide.

I asked my kind and hospitable conductor, Mr. Garstang, the leading practitioner in Clithero, by whose well informed conversation I profited much, whether he could explain that part of the proverb; but his skill extended not so far. That there is a spirit of mischief in " the honour of Clithero" which must either lead to cudgels or to the attorneys, I had a proof put into my hands, at the time, in the shape of a printed squib—one of a periodical set supposed to be edited by a mysterious trio, who mercilessly attack the *dandini* and the *dandoni* of the place; for it seems that even in the " honour of Clithero," amidst graziers and cotton-millers, such animals do exist.

" As to ' lime,' " said Mr. Garstang, " a trip to Salt Hill will soon convince you that the proverb is correct. Thither we proceeded, therefore, and I can only say, that to a geologist the examination of such an elevated spot, about a mile east of the town, with its extensive quarry of compact shelly limestone rock, would be quite a treat. To me the view from the top of that hill proved one also. On the south-east, " Diamond Hill," rich in crystals of quartz, rose nearly behind me, and close at hand, in the south, was that singularly-formed mountain called Pendle Hill. Salt Hill itself, on which we stood, sloped down to Whally, thus completing nearly a circle, in the north part of which Waddington appeared conspicuous at the foot of Waddington Fell.

But what to an old friend proved more than any other object interesting, was the spire of Browsholme Hall, seen buried amidst its dark green and extensive plantation at a distance, from the lofty staff of which good Lister Palmer, the true friend to the artists of this country, used, in more fortunate times, to display his flag, as a general card of " At Home," that he might show to every one his splendid hospitality. His fame on that score is still great, and the people style him " a princely fellow."

Below, and a little to the left of this once hospitable mansion, is Waddow, embowered in a wood, the property of the late baronet Sir James Ramsden.

" Thus far then," said I to my friendly cicerone, "the two first parts of the proverb are substantiated. What of the last of its members? what of the ' Latin ?' "

" Oh, as for that," replied Mr. Garstang, " the illustration is both simple and true, and you have only to cast a glance at that house which you see there on our right at the entrance of the town, where you perceive a dozen grown up urchins issuing with their satchels of books. That is the Clithero Free Grammar-school, which, under the Rev. T. Wilson, bachelor of divinity, acquired immense celebrity."

Wilson is the author of a theological dictionary, the first edition of which, published in 1782, he dedicated to the great leviathan of English literature. The name of this divine, oddly enough, stands in close association with that of the devil; for, having introduced into his dictionary a definition of that name, which set the faithful, and all the hierarchy of the church, in arms against him, he was forced to recall the work, and alter the obnoxious article in a second edition.

The article ran thus:

" DEVIL. An evil angel, supposed by his pride to have provoked God to cast him down from heaven; all evil thoughts and vicious propensities are imagined to be inspired by him. The word devil, in short, seems in general acceptation, to signify nothing more than that propensity to ill, which is observable in the human mind, and like many occult qualities, is found of great use in the solution of various difficulties. His existence now, like that of ghosts and fairies, seems to be called in question."

After all, the worthy divine had not even the merit of originality in this heterodox declaration; for the encyclopedists of France, at that very time promulgating their dangerous doctrines respecting the Christian faith, had endited the very sentiment, if not the very words, of the learned schoolmaster of Clithero.

Dr. Wilson was a most amiable person, much esteemed by his fellow men, and a high churchman.

I left the Rose and Crown, a very comfortable inn (commercial of course), notwithstanding the bustle of a great fair then at its noontide of business,—directing my steps, first to that very interesting and curious establishment, called Primrose, a short distance from the town, and next to the direct road which was to lead me to others and very important points of my professional excursion.

PRIMROSE, as almost every body who cares any thing about the manufactures of this county knows, is a celebrated establishment, conducted by Mr. Thomson, and his two sons, for printing calicoes. The entire establishment may be compared to a large village, in which square and lofty mills, some five or six stories high, stand in lieu of cottages and ordinary dwellings. It is *daily inhabited* by twelve hundred people, all engaged in working out the many subordinate parts of what seems a simple process—the stamping with indelible colours and designs millions of yards of cotton, and even woollen or merino, and chally cloths. These twelve hun-hundred people receive, on an average, twelve shillings a week wages ; so that a sum equal to seven hundred pounds is paid every Saturday to the temporary inmates of this colony.

Mr. Thomas Thomson, a very intelligent and scientific person, who with his brother, in the absence of their father, conducted me over every part of the establishment, has so little of the ordinary factor about him, that one felt a species of satisfaction in witnessing and hearing the learned explanation he gave me of every operation successively performed at Primrose—a satisfaction we do not usually experience in other manufactories under ordinary guides.

My fair readers, whose gay equipages are lingering at

Harding's, at Waterloo House, or in Regent-street, while they are pondering by the counters of those emporiums over many showy robes of English manufacture, from which they are to make their selection, hardly think by what series of almost interminable operations, the results they so much admire, and to which some officious and stiff-cravated shopman directs their attention, have been obtained. Yet the final, the one operation, which converts some thousands of yards of cotton cloth, previously bleached and prepared, into a surface covered with curious and tasteful designs, and rivalling for colour the brilliant plumage of a tropical bird, is almost magically instantaneous.

But of the details of this process, with which I can have nothing to do, there is only one that seems to require from a medical man a passing remark. I allude to the use of that peculiar gas called *chlorine*, which forms the basis of all bleaching processes, and which is applied to a great extent in a very long but not lofty apartment, on the ground-floor of Messrs. Thomson's establishment; where I found it diffused through the atmosphere, in spite of the precaution adopted, of having every door and window wide open. It was natural then to ask, since I was myself affected at once upon entering the premises, whether the many able-bodied men whom I saw there employed, and who were constantly hovering over the bleaching-vats, suffered from their perpetual exposure to such an atmosphere.

The reply furnished a curious practical illustration of the efficacy attributed of late years to chlorine inhalation in cases of diseases of the lungs. For not only did Mr. T. Thomson assure us that not one of the men so employed suffered in their health, but he added that catarrh, and other complaints of the respiratory organs, were unknown; and that on the contrary, those of the men who happened to catch cold elsewhere, and brought it with them to this place, were not long in casting it off. Certainly the looks of the hardy and robust fellows about me seemed to confirm this statement, which goes to corroborate the value of one of our modern improvements in the treatment of diseases of the lungs, by the topical applications of certain remedies, chlorine gas in particular, to the aerial vessels themselves.

On the exhibition of such remedies applied in the form of vapour, Dr. Corrigan, of Dublin, has published a lucid, philosophical, and satisfactory statement, in which he has moreover proposed a mechanical contrivance, called by him " the Diffuser," for the administration of chlorine, iodine, and other substances, in the form of vapour. Now here, at Primrose, or at any of the great bleaching-establishments, we have, ready prepared, the best and most effectual diffuser of chlorine; and a hint may be taken from it, by adopting, in a suitable apartment, the selfsame process employed by bleachers, for the gradual and imperceptible recovery of persons afflicted with curable diseases of the lungs. There can be no doubt as to the superiority of such a mode of *diffused* exhalation, over that lately attempted to be introduced by means of *confined* inhalers—the employment of which, ineffectual as it is, has proved Laennec's observation to be strictly true,—that inhalation, as a method of cure in diseases of the lungs, has never yet had a fair trial.

To another curious phenomenon connected with the bleaching process, Mr. T. Thomson called my attention. It is the deposition of the successive thin strata of sulphate of lime which takes place in the souring vat, where the pieces of cotton cloth, after having been well steeped in a cold solution of chloride of lime, consisting of 388½ pounds of that salt to 971 gallons of water (which suffices to bleach 700 pieces of calico), are placed for the purpose of removing the lime from them by the application of an exceedingly weak solution of sulphuric acid—the proportions being, I believe, four parts of the acid for every hundred of the water. These depositions, one above the other, form at length a solid thick plate at the bottom of the vat, of half an inch in thickness, so compact, so dense, and so perfectly white, that it is easily polished on its light smooth surface, and then looks like the finest piece of Wedgwood porcelain.   Upon this, expert artists in flower-painting display their talent to advantage, as I witnessed in the performances of their amiable sister, at the house of Messrs. Thomson, where my friendly conductor and myself were most hospitably entertained after the visit.

I required not many hours to reach Skipton, after quitting Clithero; but the desire to see the ancient baronial hall of Bolton, and several curious mineral springs in that neighbourhood, mentioned to me by Mr. West, of Leeds, detained me three or four hours on the road.

Antiquities, particularly of the feudal period, are not much to my taste: still I could not but feel interested at the sight of an exceedingly curious apartment, skilfully arranged and well kept up by its present spirited proprietor, the lineal descendant of the ancient masters of Bolton Hall, who being at the time at home, most kindly devoted two or three hours to show and explain every object of curiosity contained in it.   Among these, the relics left behind by the unfortunate monarch who fled from the field of Hexham Levels, and was sheltered at Bolton Hall, are probably the most curious.   On the present occasion we took refreshments in the very room which had been assigned for the use of Henry by the loyal, steadfast, and illustrious ancestors of my host,—who, in his turn, seemed to feel a sort of loyal pride in taking out of their carved wooden receptacle—to which they had been consigned ever since they had been given as tokens of remembrance—the gloves and boots and spurs of the defeated chief of the house of Lancaster, and even to the silver spoon with which the ill-starred king was wont to travel—no mean luxury in those times.

Mr. L—— next escorted me through the extensive park of Bolton-by-Bolland, and down to the vale of the Ribble, along a precipitous and narrow footpath on the steep and lofty-wooded banks of that river; crossing afterwards a narrow branch of the same, by stepping on a few insulated stones with the help of two branches of trees—as we found that the wooden bridge had been carried away in the night by the

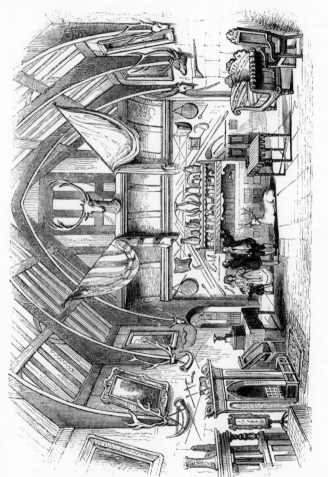

BOLTON HALL, AT BOLTON.

flood. This course we took for the purpose of reaching that part of Ribblesdale—truly romantic—in which the several mineral springs I wished to examine are situated.

Of these I saw three. The first is in a limestone cave, a spring of pure and excellent water issuing from a fissure in the strata, charged slightly with sulphuretted hydrogen gas. It flows abundantly at a temperature of 48 degrees, the external temperature being 60 at this time. The second spring is from limestone beds also, and, at Knaresborough, would be called a petrifying spring, for it incrusts with lime the twigs of trees and blades of grass near it. But the third spring, which I found in a hollow, or conical cup, at the top of a small elevation dependent from a pasture-field, is the one most charged with sulphur, and free from muriate of soda, but remarkable for a soft alkaline taste. None of these waters have been analyzed, or made applicable to useful purposes.

The Ribble, though not so majestic in parts, or so important as the Warfe, is nevertheless a river marked by many interesting features. Here, between the shores of Bolland and those of Gisburne Park, the scenery is perhaps fully as picturesque as that of the Warfe, where the latter runs along a narrow channel, and between high embankments. These two streams, which play a conspicuous part in the topography of Yorkshire, flow in a southerly direction, and for many miles nearly parallel to each other, with a district of country between them of not more than from twelve to fifteen miles. They at length part company as it were—they bid adieu to each other—and assuming very different courses, the one reaches in tortuous windings the Irish Sea, whilst the other hastens to join the shore of the German Ocean, through the Ouse and the Humber. The Great Carn Fell, which rises 2245 feet above those seas, seems to be the parent of both streams.

The little church of Bolton-Bolland, placed nearly opposite to the gates of Bolton Hall Park, is of itself not worth an instant's detention ; but there is a monument in it to a good knight, a Sir Ralph Pudsey, who had three wives and twenty-five children in his lifetime, that deserves to be seen, were it only to view the pretty little darlings carved in stone, " all in a row," by the side of their papa. Such men were particularly valuable at the time of the dreadful slaughters committed by the two rival roses. In our days they would be considered as little short of a scourge to the country. A quarter of a hundred of babes by one man only is rather too prolific a progeny for a starving country.

At a farm further on the road towards Skipton, called *Crickhill*, I halted to examine a very curious, and, perhaps, one of the most abundant sulphuretted springs in Yorkshire. It is found in the middle of a field, removed about six hundred yards from the road, and forming one of the many roundheaded hillocks which, like the waves of a vast atlantic, undulate, with their peculiar features of the oolitic formation, over a vast extent of country.

The soil throughout this district is thin, and bears a short sheep or cattle grass, which clothes these hills in every direction, so as to give them the appearance of a fresh springy hue, even in winter, when the snow is not on the ground. Todd, the master of the farm, is, like every third man in this part of Yorkshire, a grazier. He explained why no part of the land, through which I passed in the morning, bore the smallest vestige of corn. " Why, sir, the landlord, in my case, gets two pounds per acre for the land of my farm, consisting of about one hundred and fifty acres, on which I fatten thirty cattle in the year, and which I sell afterwards at a very considerable profit. Besides, all my farming implements and attendants are my stick and my dog, and these eat none ; and so, long may grazing prosper !"

The mineral water of Crickhill spring is blackened intensely by acetate of lead ; but being wholly unprotected by any canopy or other contrivance, it is not unfrequently diluted or mixed with a large quantity of rain-water. The circular basin in which it surges exhibits at the bottom large depositions of sulphur, and a thin film of the same is constantly floating on the surface, which is frequently broken by the many bubbles of gas that keep rising from the bottom.

As Mr. West analyzed this water, I have admitted it into my general analytical table; but in no other respect does the spring come within the scope of my present work, as Crickhill has not yet been made available as a Spa. Still it may be stated, as an additional corroboration of the efficacy of mineral waters, even when totally divested of every auxiliary resource peculiar to a well-established watering-place, that hundreds of country people flock to this spot, with grazier Todd's permission, to drink of the sulphur-water, in many inveterate complaints—the recovery from which was afterwards testified in person to me.

Before reaching Skipton, where I had another Spa in view, I stopped by the roadside to look at a small, insignificant mineral spring, contained in a stone reservoir, about one foot square and ten inches deep, called Broughton stinking well, which, at one time, was celebrated in the neighbourhood, but is at present entirely neglected. In this basin the water surges in very small quantities from the subjacent shale-rock, at a temperature of 51°, and numerous bubbles of sulphuretted gas are seen to ascend from the bottom of the same.

I am inclined to think, that this must have been the spring of which the historian of Craven recorded that it had a dome over it with a Latin inscription, " *Fontem hunc salutiferum, et perantiquum,*" &c. &c., denoting the sort of reputation it enjoyed eighty years ago. " But now (as the romance-writer would say) the vault which had covered the fountain was broken down and riven—the Gothic fount demolished— and the stream bursts forth from the recesses of the earth in open day."

At Skipton I had the advantage of Mr. Marsden's assistance, a leading surgeon in the place, in my researches after the mineral springs there held in repute, and commonly used in a variety of complaints, by the inhabitants and people from the neigh-

bourhood. Here, again, proofs were exhibited that a new
impetus has recently been given to the treatment of diseases
by mineral waters.

Skipton Spa has been known from time immemorial,
almost, but had, at length, like the mineral springs of every
other place in England, very few excepted, fallen into disuse
—principally owing to the manner in which the common people
had deteriorated its value to others, by using the waters as a
wash to common sores, and for any species of foul disorder
of the skin, in consequence of a right they possessed to the
indiscriminate and gratuitous enjoyment of the spring.

The agents, however, of the Earl of Thanet, who has a land
revenue of about 13,000*l*. per annum hereabout, settled the
question, by declaring the spring to be part of his lordship's
property, it being situated on his estates, and finally demised
it to a worthy medical practitioner in the place, Dr. Dodgson,
who has erected buildings over the spring, and established neat
baths and a pump-room, to the management of which he
has wholly devoted himself—with profit to himself and benefit to others.

The water is in every respect of the same nature as that of
Crickhill, and has been found useful in the same classes of
complaints in which alkaline sulphuretted waters have been
successfully employed. It is, however, but slightly impregnated with the sulphuretted gas, and that little is often still
more diluted and impaired by the infiltration of rain-water
into the spring, and of that which descends from the great
Rumboldmoor, at the foot of which the spring is situated, in
one of those gullies which the many ridges descending from
that upper land, 1300 feet high, form on one side of the great
road from Skipton to Otley.

As every body who remains even a single day at Skipton
proceeds to view its once celebrated castle, I submitted, like
a good traveller, to the custom, and accompanied Mr. Marsden through the semi-antique and semi-modern or renovated
apartments, towers, and dungeons, neither frightened by the

latter, astounded by the second, nor thrown into ecstasy by the appearance of the first. In one of these (indeed the oldest in the castle), which was once the polygonal tower, but now the drawing-room, fitted up in a modern style since the restoration of the castle, in 1650, by Lady De Clifford,—a specimen of the skill of the painters of that age is to be found, in the shape of a large piece of canvass, stretched on a frame, containing family portraits, with others on each of two shutters, originally connected with the principal picture, which admitted of shutting up the family group. A sad state the art of painting must have been in at the time, when one of the proudest and noblest families in the country could not command a higher degree of talent than that of the wretched limner who daubed their faces in this manner.

The historical recollections appertaining to this baronial edifice are the only subjects of real interest of which it can boast. It must be admitted, however, that the several restorations recently made, and the great order in which every thing is kept, places this castellated structure among the most interesting of that class of buildings which have been applied by their modern possessors to domestic uses, or have been converted into country residences.

My good *cicerone* would have fain persuaded me to proceed northwards from Skipton, and after visiting the hospitable mansion of the wealthy heiress and charitable mistress of Eshton Hall, in which I was informed I should have found a magnificent library, advance as far as Malham Tarn and Kilsay,—in order to view its precipitous and perpendicular rock. But such an excursion, however interesting at any other time, I could not at present think of undertaking.

I knew I was in the region of the great limestone district, abounding in caves and fossil remains, which have been examined by Buckland and others. Indeed the extensive region which I allude to is the very field, as I found on inquiry, out of which the druggist of Preston has for years been

2 B 2

making his large collections of fossil remains ; and the method
he has employed for procuring all of them that he can get,
unattended by much trouble and expense or personal inconvenience on his part, bespeaks shrewdness, as well as an
acquaintance with the foibles of womankind. Our collector
buys ready-made women's caps, and tells the good farmers'
wives that if they will let their children and servants rum-
mage about their own neighbourhood, and bring him any sort
of *curious stones* they can find, he will present them with a
cap. Finery and dress are as attractive with the industrious
country housewives as with the most pert lady's-maid in a
nobleman's family ; and accordingly the druggist's scheme
succeeds so well, that he has been enabled to form the extensive geological cabinet of which favourable mention has been
made in a former chapter.

The geology of Craven, through the extensive grazing district of which I was now travelling—the peculiar condition
of the pasturage lands, exhibiting a cold soil unfit for the
growth of corn—the magnificent Hardbank quarry of blue
limestone in the body of a hill called the *How*, close to Skipton
—lastly, the richly-endowed grammar-school in the latter place,
having three masters, very liberally paid, for the instruction
of seventy-five boys—all these various objects engaged
the remainder of the time I had allotted to the examination of Skipton Spa and its auxiliaries. These, however, can
hardly be legitimately presented before my readers in this
place ; and even if introduced, might be deemed by many
too homely to excite interest or curiosity.

But curiosity would at all events be excited, as well as interest, in any traveller attached to architecture, by the
principal hotel in which I would recommend them to dwell
while at Skipton. This was once the residence of the
aristocratic English Palladio, the Earl of Burlington, who so
much honoured his noble caste, [and after whose designs it
was built : in commemoration of which fact the hotel bears
he name of " Devonshire House."

CHAPTER XXIV.

ILKLEY ; OR, THE MOUNTAIN SPA.

An antiquarian Dialogue—Which is the best ?—Should old Abbey Ruins be converted into Parish Churches—BOLTON Park—The WHARFE—The Strid—BOLTON ABBEY—Kirkstall Ruins—A Wish—ILKLEY—Topography—Accommodations—The MOUNTAIN SPRING—Quantity and Quality of the Water—The DOUCHE—Effects of cold Water Pumping on the Author—Disease cured by cold Water—The Peasant of GRÆFENBERG —HYDROSUDOMANIA—Wonders performed.

IN that very hotel, and in its snug little parlour on the left of the entrance-hall, after having parted for the night with my friendly conductor and brother practitioner mentioned in the preceding chapter, and after having committed to the pages of my diary the recollections of a long day, I engaged in conversation with a silver-headed gentleman in black, whose mild demeanour and address, and winning physiognomy, at once stamped him in my mind as a minister of the English church. Each of us, however, kept our own counsels throughout the dialogue, and at the end of a long conference we knew as little of each other's personal history as when we first "broke ice" and began to "exchange thoughts and words."

The prominent topic on which my fellow guest seemed disposed to dwell, was Bolton Abbey, in behalf of which he insisted for a decided superiority over every other monastic house in the north. In this he was only repeating Whittaker's assertion contained in his history of Craven—an assertion from which I ventured humbly to dissent. I had very recently visited ten of the principal among those monastic or abbatial structures,—the glorious vestiges of an age as superior to the present in grandeur of idea and taste for architecture, as it was inferior in general knowledge and liberal sentiments. Among those various ruins, each invested with an almost specific interest, I had in a very special manner distinguished two—Fountains and Kirkstall (of which something anon)—and only the day before our conversation, Bolton priory and abbey had also engaged my attention.   I was therefore in a condition to form an independent and unbiassed notion of their respective merits,—and that notion would not allow me to assent to any unconditional declaration as to the superiority of the favourite abbey of my interlocutor.

I admitted that the situation of that ancient structure was both magnificent and picturesque. The Wharfe, descending at the bottom of a narrow valley overhung by deep and solemn woods, among which huge and perpendicular rocks of gritstone are seen to jut out in various places, bends gently half round a moderately lofty rock, on which stand the ruins of the abbey, modernized and converted into a parish church ! Every thing—every accident—every circumstance in the ground near and about the edifice, which the most imaginative landscape-painter could devise—meets the eye in this sequestered scene. But the eye at the same time rests upon those restorations of our own days in a Gothic structure, the merits of which were its undisturbed ruinous antiquity—its fragmented outline—its ivy-mantled casements half demolished —finally its magnificent and grandiose western window, through which the unintercepted azure of a clear sky was often seen, ere a profane hand stuccoed over its beautiful tracery, and glazed the spaces between the mullions. But the eye falls upon the substituted tower instead of the ancient one of the transept, the want of which is a fatal defect in this edifice. But the eye falls on the humble dwelling of the schoolmaster, and the modernized old school near the magnificent ruins of the priory ; and, worse than all, the eye falls, lastly, upon a slated roof shining with that lilac hue and provoking polish, which bring to mind the every-day buildings erected by an ordinary mason, and destroy those imposing recollections which Bolton's conventual church in its pristine mouldering condition was calculated to excite.

The conversion of the body or principal nave of the abbey into a common parochial house of prayer, has been an error which, it is to be hoped, may not be again committed in regard to other equally important structures of monastic times. As it now appears, Bolton *church* is misplaced in the midst of a scenery the wildest and most romantic that any one can imagine. The sacred edifice should now change places with Kirkstall ruins. How nobly would the dismantled tower and lofty buttresses, and broken cloisters—massive, bold, magnificent—of that striking edifice look, if seated upon the rock on which Bolton Abbey stands ! And how much more suitable to its present character would the latter building find the grassy and unobstructed plain, near a large city, on which all that remains of Kirkstall is now to be seen !

To these arguments, advanced with hesitation, against the alleged superiority of Bolton Abbey, my even-minded, yet tenacious stranger, demurred with much force and learned illustration. He contended, not only that the conversion of the ancient abbey into a modern church was proper, and a great improvement in itself, but also that the landscape had much gained by it. Nay, his zeal in the advocacy of such a measure induced him to wish that Fountains Abbey, and Kirkstall, and Rivaulx, and Glastonbury, and all, in fact, those magnificent ruins which form the only architectural glories of England, might be converted into parish churches by *suitable* restorations !—an idea, by the by, which some tight-laced economist in the Lower House lately reproduced as a great hit, while debating on the question of church extension !

The silver-headed gentleman in black and myself could not quite agree at last ; and having by this time drained to the last drop his very modest glass of something comfortable, and lighted his night-taper, he retired after we had bidden each other farewell, reciprocally unconvinced by each other's argument, as is mostly the case between two litigants.

I learned the following morning that this strenuous advocate for modern Bolton church, was no other than the very author of all its improvements and its historiographer—the Rev. Mr. C—, its most worthy, exemplary, and learned rector.

My approach to the scene I have just alluded to was from Ilkley, on the Leeds road, accompanied by a friend in an open carriage. A delightful drive along an excellent road commanding the Wharfedale, had conducted us down to the sweet village of Addingham in the valley ; from whence we entered on a succession of the most enchanting landscapes that fancy can paint. On our right, beyond the Wharfe, hills and moors, in advance of each other, presented a rich cultivated surface almost to their very summits. Large masses of dense woods dotted the scene, over which the accidents of light and shade, caused by our own everchanging positions, while travelling over a very uneven ground of hills and dales, threw many and varied tints.

At length, on the top of a very steep hill, which descends immediately to Bolton Bridge, we halted where a broad terrace afforded us an opportune situation for that purpose, and surveyed the most striking panorama that had yet offered itself to our view. A vast green parterre lay at our feet, encompassed by a sweep of the Wharfe, which, in this part, describes a semicircle of nearly three-quarters of a mile. It was bounded by hills gradually rising in succession, covered with verdure, and dotted with villages or country residences. Bolton Bridge is seen to stride the Wharfe, and beyond it a woody mass forms a group in a hollow, in the midst of which a small portion of the abbey can be distinguished. No region in Germany—so rich in landscape and views—ever presented to me a more exquisite amphitheatre than this.

We pulled up at the Devonshire Arms, a very neat and modern-looking hotel, standing at the junction of three roads, one of which, the nearest to the inn, leads to the abbey and Bolton Park. This house of entertainment is much frequented, and forms the rendezvous of the Harrogate visiters, as well as of those from Ilkley Spa.

Part of an ancient wall that once encircled the domain of the priory and abbey-lands still exists, in which a breach has been made to admit the visiters to view, as if by a surprise, the ruins of the priory and abbey-church. But we proceeded onward for the present, and having fairly penetrated into the park, drove up and down hills innumerable, through a most enchanting sylvan scene, which reminded us of Hackfall, in Uredale, though here every thing is on a larger and far nobler scale.

We advanced in this manner for the space of three miles along the valley, tracing upwards the course of the Wharfe, the well-wooded embankments of which, richly tinted at the time by the early autumnal colours, seem in some parts to reach an elevation of three or four hundred feet. The valley, now narrow and now expanded, presents a variety of beautiful features. Here it is seen suddenly to enlarge, and then the stream spreads itself over a large area of loose boulder-stones. It then contracts again, and the scene becomes at once as tranquil as that of Fountains Abbey; though the vale has a wider range—its embankments are loftier, and crested with barren rocks—and many of the trees are more magnificent, while the river is larger and more imposing.

At length we reached to where the vale has narrowed its dimensions, so that the greensward between its embankments and the margin of the water has disappeared, and nothing remains but the rocky bed over which the Wharfe is seen coursing. A little higher, the stream is nearly lost, though its presence is vouched by the incessant roaring heard from some deep abyss. It is the gallant stream that has pierced through a large mass of rock, by a fissure or cleft in it, constituting what has been called the *Strid*, of which ever-credulous tradition relates many fabulous stories.

Forming first a fall, and next a whirlpool,—the Wharfe, as it approaches the *Strid*, impetuously rushes through every rocky obstacle, hurrying to its fate impetuous and undaunted. But the struggle is not over after the first successful effort ; for other rocks lower down again deny transit to the waters, and seem to strangle them in their passage. Loud and incessant does the foaming and indignant element murmur over these repeated obstacles and difficulties; but having at length overcome them all, it expands as if to breathe more freely, and is seen to sail along with a smooth surface towards the end of the valley from whence we had been ascending—there to lave the ample amphitheatre in which the abbey is seated.

I have already stated that the latter disappointed us. The prints do not portray the architectural as well as pictorial deformities enacted by the modern hand of man ; and the draftsman, generally selecting his own point of view, exhibits only the few parts which deserve the name of ancient remains. In its best days the edifice never could have been either extensive or striking. The style of architecture is of unquestionable mediocrity, and its general mass and bearing disproportionate, and not congenial to the stupendous scene of which it ought to form the most imposing feature. Here and there, by the help of woody groves, as we quietly sauntered through them on our way back from the Strid, we could catch just as much of the abbey as we could group together with effect, by bringing to bear some of its lighter windows aloft,—or portions of the embattlements and but-

tresses, with the crowning arch of the great eastern window
now towering over the roof of the modern structure.   But a
full or general view of this once renowned abbey, as it now
appears, with closed side-windows glazed by a Skipton glazier,
and roofed by a Cumberland slater, is most fatal to every
sort of pictorial effect.

What would one not give for that miraculous faculty,
which transported from its original to its present site, the
Santa Casa di Loretto, that we might rob my Lord Cardigan
of the highly picturesque remains of Kirkstall, and here plant
them in perfect and harmonious keeping with the magnificent
scenery of the valley, instead of its present unmeaning edifice!   To have converted the abbey of Bolton into a protestant kirk, has been an error of taste as well as judgment.

It was, whilst following the road from Leeds to Ilkley and
Bolton, that we drove by the ruins of Kirkstall, and there
halted, leisurely to contemplate those monastic remains, to
which the historian of Craven has assigned the second place
among those of the north of England,—whether considered
as a feature in a landscape, or as a specimen of architecture.

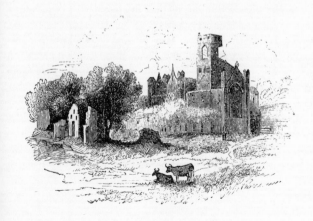

KIRKSTALL is hardly two miles from the extreme north-west point of the town of Leeds, and is a never-failing object of attraction to the passing stranger, who finds every facility afforded him of inspecting both the external ruins and the interior nave and two side-aisles, with their rows of massy clustered columns, having Anglo-Norman capitals to support pointed arches. The latter have been protected since 1806 from depredations and defilement, by gates, kept by a person appointed by the Earl of Cardigan, to whom the remains of the abbey and the ground on which they stand belong.

The lands round the abbey to a considerable extent on the north, east, and west side, are also part of the same manor, which, on the south side, extends to the river Aire. The commonalty of Leeds have not the slightest right whatever round the precincts of the abbey; and even a right of footway through the grounds, which existed up to 1832, was stopped in that year. The whole towering mass, therefore, now stands enclosed and insulated,—an imposing feature in the centre of a somewhat flat and tame landscape—preserved from all those ulterior dilapidations which generally result from the indiscriminate admission of the public to such ruins. To render these still more secure, the late earl, in the course of ten years immediately preceding his decease, caused the erection of buttresses and other repairs, as well as improvements, to be executed under his own direction, by which the several disjointed members of this sacred fabric, admirable for its elegant simplicity, now group and harmonize together in a most beautiful manner.

A further report from an able architect of Leeds, Mr. Chantrell, on the state of the ruins, was made a few years ago, but as yet no step has been adopted to carry his recommendations into effect; and perhaps, as a matter of taste, it will be as well that those ruins be left in their present condition.

It would, indeed, be impossible to desire more picturesque

outlines or more striking masses, than these very vestiges of
Kirkstall present in all directions to the landscape painter.
The ruins are extensive, and more pictorial than those of
Studley, and infinitely more so than those of Bolton, from
being more broken and shaped into more groups, each of a
most fantastic character. Through the wooden railing which
closes the interior, a full view is allowed of its nave, the roof
of which is gone, though the clustered Norman pillars and
arches are intact. The grandeur of desolation is present
within :

> " The long ribb'd aisles are burst and shrunk,
>   The holy shrine to ruin sunk."
>   . . . .
> " The sacred tapers' lights are gone,
>   Gray moss has clad the altar-stone."

Ancient ash-trees, and the magnificent beech, and limes that
reckon some centuries, have grown in the very centre of the
sacred compartments—their massive and columnar trunks
rising above the ruins, and in the summer spreading their
wide branches to canopy them from the sun. In one of
those compartments, whose high-placed windows face the
river Aire, the inner wall is clad entirely with luxuriant ivy.
The walls, like those at Studley, are thick and cased with well
cut and smooth sandstone, but filled with substantial rubble
to give them strength.

The dilapidation is complete; no part of the ancient holy
structure has entirely escaped the ravaging hand of time or
man ; and the scene would be of the most imposing kind,
from the very broken condition of the remains, were it
not for the absence of a congenial landscape around them.
But the want of effect without, from that circumstance,
is amply compensated by that which is excited within, at the
sight of the deserted cloisters, the unroofed chapter, and
silent tombstones.

> " I do love these ancient ruins.
> We never tread upon them but we set
> Our foot upon some reverend history.
> . . . . . . Here in the very court
> Which now lies naked to th' injuries
> Of stormy weather, some men lie interr'd
> Who thought they should have canopied their bones,
> Till domesday."

From Kirkstall we pushed on in the direction of Otley, which appeared as it were suddenly before us, upon reaching the crest of a very long and steep hill, emphatically called here " The Shiven."

There, in the vast green map of the Wharfedale, lay the neat, compact town, refreshing to look upon from its clear stone colour, free from the factory atmosphere we had just left. It unrolled more and more to our view as the carriage kept advancing with a downward course to a hundred feet below the crest of the hill, until the town seemed to divide, into a western and eastern portion, the whole fertile vale.

Northwards, the vale is flanked by the lofty ridges which, under the name of *Jack Hill* and the *Blubber-houses*, mark the southern verge of the famed Knaresborough Forest; whilst on its opposite, or south and parallel embankment, the rugged and almost vertical walls of Rumbold moor rise to an elevation of fourteen hundred feet.

The Wharfe, straight and fleet as an arrow, shot through the town under a light stone bridge; then resuming its fantastic twistings, went on its way to Whetherby and Thorp Arch, decorating, as it coursed forward, many a delightful spot, marked by noblemen's and gentlemen's seats—the Ibbotson's and the Fawkes's and Lord Middleton's, both above and below Otley. In the latter direction its waters proceed to lave the garden-walls of Harewood House, and hasten to mingle, further on, with the stream of the Ouse below Whetherby, leaving on the left the high lands on which are

seated Harrogate and Knaresborough. Westwardly, on the
contrary, or above Otley, the descending current, rioting in
capricious girations, some of which form curious islets, seems
to please itself with lingering and lengthening its course
amidst the wild scenery of Bolton Park and

ILKLEY SPA.

The latter it was my immediate object to visit, and towards
it we directed our steps, passing through the retired and
rural village of Burley. The road, ascending the valley, cuts
in and out the inlets of the descending stream, at the foot of
the great Rumbold moor, and winds through scenery of
exquisite tranquillity, although perfectly romantic.

As we passed Burley the glaring white house of Ilkley
Fountain, stuck, as it were, midway on the steep ascent of
the Rumboldmoor, betokened our immediate approach to
the Spa village ; and the view of Denton park on the opposite
or north ridge, with Middleton, the seat of the Lord of Ilkley,
confirmed that notion.

The effect produced by the sight of that single and insulated building, within which thousands have been known to
quaff the pure stream that gives health, and which to a superficial observer seems almost unapproachable, is one of that
class which can hardly be expressed in words. As the carriage wound up the road, the humble fabric appeared and
disappeared alternately, screened by the tufty and woody
scene which spreads from the margin of the river as far as to
the foot of the hilly range, and even creeps up its precipitous
side to a considerable height. It would be the most attractive object for the moment, were not the attention of the beholder, while scanning the many beauties of this region,
called to a mass of rocks, aping the form of a huge horned
quadruped, which stands as if perched on the summit of a
point or headland of the Rumboldmoor, and before which

a smaller mass, detached like a landslip from its parent rock, rugged and angular, is seen balanced on the edge of a precipice, ready at any moment to roll headlong down the whole declivity of several hundred feet.

How this last colossal boulder-stone was checked in its first and downward career, it is difficult to conjecture : but there it has stood ever since (and Heaven knows since when !) furnishing a subject to the imagination of the good people of the country for likening it to a calf—the parent rock being, of course, the cow. This lofty and almost aerial point—" the cow and the calf"—forms one of the excursions for the boldest of the summer visiters at the Spa of Ilkley.

We halted at the New Inn, a stone building, the last in this primitive and simple village, going towards Skipton. It is superior to two others in the place, both of which, however, had been very full during the season. The New Inn is, for so retired a place as Ilkley, very respectable. There is a large public room in it, and the back looks towards the rich and smiling ascent leading to the moor. In front, the road is a great posting thoroughfare from the West to the East Riding—from Skipton, or even the Lakes, to Leeds and York. As many as thirty dine in this room at a *table d'hôte*, in the summer, when some of the most renowned trout are served up, fresh caught in the Wharfe, such as scarcely any other river in the north is said to rival ; game, also, as may be supposed, is plentiful ; and during grouse-shooting no moor can offer a richer treat than Rumbold side and topping.

There are lodging-houses in Ilkley village sufficiently comfortable, and some that afford the convenience of boarding at a very moderate charge. Water is of the purest sort. Vegetables are in abundance, and milk is excellent, owing to the green pasturage and water-fields near the river. The air is pure and elastic. The north winds are shut out by the lofty range which, from the margin of the north bank of the

Wharfe, ascend for many hundred feet in the direction of Patley Bridge ; while Rumboldmoor guards the village from the south-western gales. The summer is less rainy than in most places in Yorkshire.

The village of Ilkley is purely and intrinsically a rural retreat. It has its church, which, externally as well as interiorly, is not like one of those stone hovels one sees here and there among villages in England,—as far removed from what a house of God should be as possible,—but the contrary. The officiating clergyman exhibits in his person a fair specimen of the salubriousness and exhilarating nature of this favoured region. To such as can make up their minds to be for some time content with going without the luxuries of life, for the sake of the luxuries of health, now or hereafter, Ilkley is just the place for their temporary residence.

But it is not the fashion to dwell more than a fortnight or a month in this region ; although it is perfectly, strictly, and imperatively fashionable for people in [the north to come to Ilkley, or, at all events, to say that they have been at Ilkley. To ignore Ilkley among the higher grades of *factory* society at Halifax or Bradford, Leeds or Huddersfield, Wakefield or Sheffield, and even in the metropolis of the factory world, Manchester, is to bespeak oneself as yet uninitiated into all the mysteries and extent of fashionable life. Ilkley, unknown south of Yorkshire and Lancashire—a *terra incognita* indeed to the southerons of Middlesex—is the Arcadia, or the Malvern of the northern counties ; and I had scarcely put my foot within them, when Ilkley's name was whispered in mine ears, and sundry times repeated every day.

Ilkley fountain, as was before stated, is high upon the side of the Rumboldmoor, consequently distant from the village perhaps three-quarters of a mile ; the ascent is by a rough carriage-road, until about halfway ; then by a winding footpath over the rugged moorside, strewed with large and small boulder-stones.

There is, halfway up the lowermost part of the hill, a range of stone houses, called *Usher's* lodgings, which, with an aspect to the west, are among the best here. They are generally well filled during the season by the superior order of visiters, who, I hear, find the *cuisine* excellent.

The healing waters burst from the rocky mountain-side, in a round and thick stream, at the rate, repeatedly measured by myself, of sixty gallons in a minute; the temperature, 47° F. ; was only eight degrees lower than that of the surrounding atmosphere. It is brilliantly limpid and crystal-like ; but its taste disappointed me, being, like the water at Malvern, which it resembles in other respects, neither sharp nor very sapid. From two to three pints of it are generally drunk by the visiters, who take long and fatiguing walks, round about the mazes of these hills, between the several doses of the water.

But the principal use of these waters is in bathing, or still more for the application of the *douche* to any diseased parts of the body or limb.

There are two baths, the one for male, the other for female patients. They are both open above, occupying a round area, three feet deep, surrounded by a wall. Over a centre room, placed between the two baths, there is a dressing-room ; but all this arrangement is quite in the rough, and the whole building looks very much like one of those stone-built shelters, or houses of recovery one meets on the Alps.

A young girl, about eleven years of age, was being subjected to the *douche*, under the direction of an old primitive dame, who, besides escorting invalids on one of those useful climbing quadrupeds, an ass,—her own property,—serves as a bath-woman also. The application of the *douche* was made directly upon an inveterate sore in one of the young lady's legs, accompanied with an almost total loss of power of moving that limb. The *douche* had been repeated about a week, and the patient admitted to me that she had already derived great benefit from it. I remained until the operation had been finished, and examined the limb. It looked blue, and felt extremely cold ; but she was not sensible of this ; on the contrary, the inward feeling throughout the deadened limb was that of a glow—a feeling which would last, she said, about two hours, and then she was able to move the limb better.

I next submitted my own hand and wrist to the whole weight of the precipitous stream, meaning to retain the limb in that position for five minutes—the time generally considered necessary for efficacious results ; but the pain, principally at the wrist, became, at the expiration of the first minute, so intensely and peculiarly acute, that I withdrew it from the stream. On a second experiment the time was prolonged to four minutes. The first application imparts the sensation of cold for an instant ; it then produces very acute pain for a minute and a half, and at last the sensation approaches that of exposure to ordinary tepid water.

The pulse previously to the *douche,* soon after mounting the steep acclivity, was 108°, and soft ; the heat in the palm of the hand 93° F. After the *douche* it beat 63, and took one minute to ascend to 73 beats. The hand and wrist looked red, they became slowly warm, but upon returning home on foot, they tingled, and felt inwardly hot, although the thermometer marked only 90 degrees of heat of the skin.

This spring has been resorted to for upwards of two centuries. Dr. Mossman, the late Mr. Moorhouse, surgeon of Skipton, and Dr. Hunter, of Leeds, principally on the reports of Mr. Spence, surgeon at Ilkley, have treated of Ilkley fountain ; Dr. Hunter, however, the same able physician of whom I have had occasion to make favourable mention in speaking of Harrogate, is the authority upon whom I principally rely.*   In my

* In his essay on Ilkley, Dr. Hunter states that "The shock, on plunging into Ilkley bath, is excessive, and an irresistible impulse to escape from its influence is the first sensation produced. When this is accomplished, and the bather begins to dress, reaction almost immediately takes place, which is soon followed by a pleasant glow and lightness throughout the whole system. The body feels as relieved from a previous load, and unwonted energy and activity are communicated to the muscles of voluntary motion, while the mental sensations equally participate in the general animation. These feelings continue to a greater or less extent during the day, and are terminated by a night of calm and refreshing sleep. If, however, the body be kept still and quiet, some time after leaving the bath a tendency to drowsiness is perceptible : this seems to arise as well from the previous excitement, as from the ease and freedom from irritation which is almost universally experienced. I prefer assigning it to these causes, rather than to any undue determination of blood to the head or thorax, from observing that headach or similar complaints, are rarely experienced by those bathing in this water.

" Though one of the coldest natural baths to be met with, it is used by the most delicate and infirm individuals, a proper degree of reaction seldom failing to occur. This may justly be attributed to the body being so immediately withdrawn from its action, and to the heat being evolved in the same ratio with the previous cold. Indeed as the benefit derived from every species of cold bathing arises chiefly from the shock sustained, and the subsequent reaction ; by leaving the bath as soon as possible, the necessary excitement must always be more speedily and certainly established. Consequently, where the water is very cold, there is no temptation for remaining in the bath ; persons with great apparent debility are thus enabled to use it with safety ; while, if the temperature of the water were several degrees higher, it might induce them to continue in the bath till the powers of excitement were exhausted.

" In its general effects, this water, used as a bath, is highly invigorating; it promotes the different secretions and excretions, and gives a keen edge to the appetite. In this respect, it excels any water with which I am acquainted. But a share of this quickening power must, in justice, be attributed to the bracing qualities of the mountain breeze, which sweeps along the strath in such ethereal purity.

" Few directions are necessary for the use of this bath. It ought not to be used above once in the twenty-four hours, and for very infirm per-

conversations with that gentleman, at Leeds, I found him strongly impressed with the great efficacy of the water as a remedial agent. Its chemical composition is extremely simple, according to the analysis he has given; being a binary compound only of muriate of lime, and muriate of magnesia, as two to one; with something more than twelve cubic inches of carbonic acid gas in a wine-gallon of the water.

The range of diseases which have been found to derive benefit from this water, includes scrofula in the first place, particularly in that form of it which shows itself in a tendency to suppuration of the glands of the neck and under the jaw; chronic inflammation of the eye; atrophy, and mesenteric diseases, either of children or adults. In deficiency of the vital power, in many cutaneous eruptions, in all stiff joints and muscular contractions, either from sprains, or rheumatic and paralytic affections; in chronic weakness of the general system; in irritability of the stomach, and in some female complaints, accompanied by weakness, the cold water at Ilkley has been found beneficial. I learned that the eminent surgeon of Leeds, Mr. Hay, sends patients to this Spa.

Here, then, is a proper field and an opportune appliance for establishing in this county a branch of that system of cold

sons once in two days will be sufficient. As a topical application, twice or thrice daily will answer every good purpose. For those in good health, or who are tolerably strong, the morning, before breakfast, is the most suitable period for immersion. Weak and debilitated habits generally feel languid till they receive breakfast; for such the forenoon is most proper; the natural heat of the day tending to produce reaction, besides rendering their feelings more comfortable on leaving the bath.—Nothing requires to be stated respecting the period of continuance in the water, as no one, whose external feeling is not completely torpid, will remain in it a moment longer than till he can get out. It should, in all cases, be particularly inculcated upon those using the cold bath, not to desist till, by dry-rubbing, exercise, or the use of warm liquids, they have produced a sensation of heat upon the surface; which will seldom or never fail to be induced by a steady perseverence in these measures."

water cure, or Hydrosudomania, which has of late years become a universal topic of conversation, and a subject of the
most marvellous stories in Germany : I allude to the practice
of the Silesian peasant, Vincent Priesnitz, who has founded,
on the rugged side of the hill of Graefenberg, in Bohemia—a
spot nearly resembling this of Ilkley—a new Hygeian temple,
wherein all diseases are said to be cured by the internal and
external use of cold water, issuing from the recesses of his
native mountain.

That spot has now become the rendezvous of hundreds of
invalids, who resort thither from all parts of Germany (and
the mania is now by means of branches extending further),
to be plunged into water at 46°—urged to run up and down
the mountain-side till ready to drop—wrapt up immediately
after in a coarse woollen envelope or blanket, and made to
sweat by the combined effect of heat without, and the ingestion of gallons of the same cold water within. True it is
that hundreds of people attest the efficacy of this system,
while learned and grave professors have been despatched to
the all-health-giving peasant of Silesia, from Vienna, and
other universities in order to examine and report on the
reality of the proclaimed miracles.

CHAPTER XXV.

BY one of those *tours de force* which theatrical scene-
shifters, romance-writers, and *tourists* are alone permitted
to perform, quitting the rugged side of Rumboldmoor, I am
now travelling upon the exceedingly well-regulated railroad
which from Manchester is to extend to Leeds, principally
under the management of " the friends," who certainly seem to

understand matters of business better than any other class of people; owing, probably, to their deliberate and even-tempered manner of conducting them. As yet the said road goes not beyond Littleborough, a distance of little more than thirteen miles, and it runs unfortunately through an ugly country, the land being of a very inferior description, clayish, and hillocky. The remaining portion of the line, difficult, full of obstacle, and expensive, but penetrating through a country of the most beautiful and picturesque character, through stupendous tunnels and cuttings and along the lovely vale of the Calder,—will, it is expected, be opened for the public service in 1842.

It is remarkable, that since the opening of this first portion of the road, hardly a single accident has occurred on it. Some one of the directors of the company, or a responsible officer, is present at the departure of the train at each station, to keep the several guards in order, who are smart, active-looking fellows, clad in red, and wearing a glazed, round hat, with the name of the railroad in gold letters upon it.

This is the railroad which has proved by experience, that conveying of passengers at a cheap rate yields a higher profit than travellers do by the first-class carriages. Hence the directors have established third-class carriages, precisely for the manufacturing population in the immediate vicinity of the road, which requires cheap conveyance; and they have found that the third pays better than the first class.

Hear this, ye short-sighted mortals of Euston Grove! So dense is the population within three miles on each side of the railway, that there are nearly 1900 inhabitants to the square mile, where as the average population of England is only 250 per square mile. Upwards of 2500 people travel daily over the short distance of thirteen miles by this railroad, in the pursuit of business.

As for my *own* pursuit, in the present instance, it led to a renowned steel-water Spa at Horley Green, near Halifax, once in high vogue, and much extolled by Dr. Garnett, who in his time published a work on the subject. Never doubting but that I should find the mineral spring in question, which all the personal information I could obtain respecting it, and the most recent of the topographical descriptions of the country, induced me to believe was still in existence, I directed my steps first to the thriving city of Halifax, in hopes of there ascertaining the fact, with the friendly aid of Doctor Alexander, junior (author of a treatise on the various modes of bathing), formerly of Scarborough, and now a distinguished practitioner in Halifax, to the infirmary of which place he is one of the physicians.

At Littleborough, a coach received the passengers whom the railway had brought thither, and who intended to proceed farther to the north. Crossing that elevated and bleak region called Blackstone Edge, which reminded me of the desolate heaths of Lammermoor; we soon perceived a most favourable change in the aspect of the country upon entering Yorkshire, and were not long in discovering, a little way beyond Sowerby Bridge, the " Clothier's City," lying in a smiling valley, between two elevated ridges, the North and South Owram. On the extended line of the former, the " Beacon Hill" stands boldly out, and by its direction screens Halifax with its lofty parapets from the easterly winds.

I waited not a moment after my arrival at Halifax, before I set out for

HORLEY GREEN SPA,

accompanied by Doctor Alexander, in whose house I had been most hospitably received ; but alas ! no Spa of any sort was there. The worthy doctor well recollected the spot on which the spring had been, and knew also, that of late years, owing to certain changes in the land property, the spring had been much neglected ; but he was not prepared for its total obliteration from the visible surface—as we ascertained to be the case, upon close inquiries from a guide whom we engaged near the spot, as well as upon our own inspection of the site.

There lay before us, in a corner of a field, the vestiges of what seemed to have been a Spa-house, and a sort of dispersed streamlet appeared to meander along the surface; but the mingling of other streams from the upper fields, made it impossible to distinguish the mineral from the ordinary water. Of this entire dilapidation, even Doctor Alexander, living within two or three miles of the spot, seemed not to be aware.

The loss of a spring, known of old to possess powerful properties, was much to be deprecated in a place like Halifax, and its surrounding populous district; inasmuch as no class of people require more, or derive greater benefit from, mineral and strengthening waters, than the labourers closely and daily confined for hours together, in the heavy atmosphere of a manufactory, a coalpit, or a foundry. It was therefore agreed between us, that every step should be taken for the recovery of the lost spring—that water when so recovered, should be submitted to Mr. West for chemical analysis, and that certain measures which I pointed out to ensure the success of the operation, should be adopted.

I could answer for the zeal and activity of my excellent brother practitioner,—and he, in his turn, was quite certain that the proprietor of the spring, Mr. Drake, of Nidd Rock, near Ripley, upon a proper representation being made to him on the subject, would co-operate in recovering the mineral water, and placing it by suitable measures, in the same flourishing condition in which it formerly stood, according to Dr. Garnett's published " Account of Horley Green Spa."

In these expectations I was not disappointed. The Spa is restored—the water is now again collected for use—and the analysis by Mr. West confirms, in the fullest manner, the

notion of its great power and peculiarities as a chalybeate—
first vaunted by Dr. Garnett. For all this the inhabitants of
Halifax, and all those who will not fail to reap benefit from
the restored Spa, are indebted to Dr. Alexander, and to the
liberality of Mr. Drake, the latter of whom, from the first
moment of my visit down to the period of the rediscovery of
the mineral water, and its analysis by West, has gone hand-
in-hand with that physician in endeavouring to obtain the
results which have since rewarded their united efforts.

The Horley Green mineral water springs from the east side
of a hill at the distance of a quarter of a mile from Horley
Green, and is about a mile and a quarter north-east of Halifax.
The soil around consists chiefly of clay-plates, shale and
pyrites, the latter of which are so plentiful, that some works
for obtaining green vitriol were erected in the neighbourhood
some years since. Coal-mines exist also in abundance; and a
rivulet which runs below the locality of the spring, derives its
name of Redbeck from the ochry deposit in its bed and sides.

The temperature of the water at present is about 49 degrees,
and its specific gravity, according to Dr. Garnett, was 1.0031,
at the temperature of 60 degrees Far. On the 27th of May,
1840, a bottle of the fresh water was submitted for my
examination. It had been perfectly colourless and transparent when first drawn from the well; and it continued so after
its arrival in London for some days, at the expiration of
which it began to throw down a light yellowish deposit, which,
in the course of a little more time, assumed a greenish tinge.
The taste of the water was then less intensely styptic than when
drunk immediately at the spring. That taste is astringent
and gently sub-acid; but the latter character quickly disappears, whereas that of astringency lingers a longer time on
the palate.

The water in Dr. Garnett's time was not long in acquiring
a prodigious celebrity, and to the many cases in his own
practice successfully cured by it, were soon added several

others from Dr. Percival, the eminent physician, of Manchester, and the late Dr. W. Alexander, a relative of my friend. Its reputation continued until the absurdities of the Brunonian system on the one hand, and the purely chemico-yatraleptic theories on the other, so absorbed and engaged the attention of the medical world, that mineral waters fell almost at once into general disuse. We are now endowed with a little more of good sense in our professional endeavours to cure disease; nor can we any longer scorn the apparently simple, yet efficacious means offered to us by nature for that purpose.

A suitable building, the design of which I have seen, is now erecting for the protection of the spring, the south wing of which will embrace the well, and the rest of the house be appropriated to the purposes of the Spa. As the supply of water is abundant, and its impregnation with green vitriol, or sulphate of iron, far exceeds that of all other chalybeates now resorted to as such (being of not less than seventy-four and a half grains of the crystallized salt in the gallon), I trust that bath-rooms will be erected for private and public bathing. There should be two bath-rooms for the former purpose, for either sex; and a plunging cold-bath of proper dimensions for the latter object. Three or four dips during the summer-months, in a water of this description, at its natural temperature of 49 degrees, will be found to constitute one of the most powerful means (guided by discretion and skill) which a medical man can resort to for restoring impaired vitality—for bracing relaxed muscles and weak joints—and for strengthening the frame generally of people who are enfeebled by hard labour, or over-exertion of any kind. The recent analysis by Mr. West, I have inserted in the general table.

During my visit I had an opportunity of learning from the mouth of some of those who had derived benefit from the Spa in former days, its effects in verminous disorders, in complaints of the stomach and weak state of the intestines, as well as in irregularities of the female constitution.

With regard to its internal use, the great strength of the

Horley Green water as a chalybeate, at once indicates the classes of disorders for which it will be found useful in practice. Dr. Alexander himself is already engaged in making judicious and well-directed observations on its effects on the constitution of certain patients, and if his experience (for which his opportunities as a medical officer to a public infirmary are considerable) should confirm but the half of the virtues ascribed to the Horley Green Spa water, since its original discovery about sixty years ago, a little time before Dr. Garnett published his account in 1789 (as I little doubt will be the case), Dr. Alexander and I will have reason to rejoice that my mission of the summer of 1839 led to the investigation, and ultimately to the successful restoration of the Spa.

By a recent letter from that physician I learn that he has already employed the Horley Green water in a case of green sickness (*chlorosis*) with marked benefit, and in another of amenorrhœa with equal advantage.   Dr. Alexander very justly thinks that this water will prove to be the best form of ferruginous medicines we possess—infinitely superior to the carbonated chalybeates ; and I may add that it contains that form of the salt of iron which a justly-celebrated practitioner at a very fashionable Spa, to be hereafter described, is very fond of administering, where he does not prescribe instead his own magnetic oxide of iron.

We may now, therefore, confidently add to the list of the most important Spas in the northern group, this *unique* one near Halifax, whose inhabitants I feel convinced will reap great benefit from re-establishment.

Were I not warned by the increasing bulk of the present volume, and the prospect of what is yet remaining of materials for a second, I should have rejoiced in the opportunity of entering into some interesting details respecting the improving city of Halifax, and its delightful position in one of the most romantic districts, as well as neighbourhoods, in Yorkshire. I should have wished, in particular. to have dwelt on its old church in the spirit of an antiquarian ; or upon that striking and imposing quadrangle called the *Piece* Hall, or clothiers' exchange, the inner court of which surpasses in area and effect, from its surrounding porticoes and colonnades, any thing of the sort I have seen in Yorkshire. I should also have liked to have said a word on the museum of the Philosophical Society, and the musical hall, a spacious apartment, ninety feet long, divided into three compartments capable of being thrown into one, which serves for public meetings cr assemblies ; and probably I might have alluded, by way of contrast to that terrible gibbet-law which led, in this town, to the invention of a more expeditious instrument of death, improperly ascribed by the Scots to the Earl of Morton, under the name of *Maiden,* and which was afterwards adopted by Guillotin in France. Nor should I have forgotten to commend in due terms the order and neatness which I noticed in the interior of the Public Infirmary.

All these things it would have been more satisfactory for me to have described—my materials for that purpose being ample, and the novelty of many of the objects warranting their introduction in this place. But the reason I have already assigned precludes the possibility of such digressions, however interesting.

Of the beauty of the country around Halifax—which is principally bold and imposing in its character—I ought also in justice to descant. For position, Halifax is by far the most favoured of the manufacturing towns in Yorkshire. Its neighbourhood is enchanting, with a dash of the romantic in it. I myself beheld, with the same interest which one feels on hearing some exquisite old ballad sung by a minstrel, the Robinhood pillars, or palace, carved out of the solid rock on the face of an almost perpendicular hill, in the vicinity of Horley Green Spa.

The Elizabethan Hall, not a great way from it, called Scout Hall, and the curious embowered dell in which is the

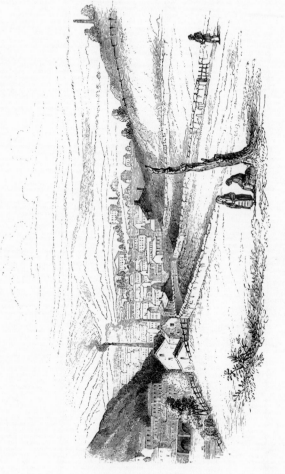

GENERAL VIEW OF HALIFAX.

entrance into a coalpit drained by means of one of the most primitive and simplest forms of trail pumps imaginable ; also Robinhood Well, with its waters charged with carbonate of lime, and some traces of magnesia, well adapted to cure acidity of the stomach ; and, lastly, High Sunderland and Shibden Hall—each of these engaged my especial attention ; but I should despair of conveying to my readers the feelings which those places excited, or the varied and interesting views to be enjoyed from them.

The appearance of Halifax, seen from the top of a hill called " the New Bank," in North Owram, is probably one of the most striking, and is the one selected as an illustration to the present chapter, because it embraces part of the road leading to the newly-recovered Spa—a road which in future years, will become much frequented during the Spa season. I am indebted for the original sketch to my kind hostess, the lady of my medical friend and correspondent.

The aspect of the houses, owing to the uniform drab tint peculiar to the freestone of the country, with which they are built, and even roofed, is pleasing and refreshing to the eye ; and in this respect, as well as in many others, Halifax is far preferable to Leeds or Manchester, with their heavy and fiery brick buildings. Being, moreover, interspersed with groups of trees and small gardens, which display 'much taste ; and also surrounded by the villas and private residences of many of the most wealthy citizens, the general tone of the place is calculated to create at once a most favourable impression on the beholder.

Altogether, I was much pleased with Halifax and its environs, its situation, its scenery, and, above all, its pure air (notwithstanding the presence of so many manufactories), and the visible effects of that most necessary element of life on the health and appearance of the inhabitants.

I speak this in my professional character ; for, as it is more than probable that a mineral water so peculiar in its composition, and so powerful as that of Horley Green, and one the like of which is not to be found certainly in two-thirds of the extent of this kingdom, will be resorted to for the cure of diseases that can only be benefited by such an agent,—it is important that I should state my opinion of a town in which invalids will have to reside during their course of mineral water, before suitable houses are erected nearer to the spring, on some of the beautiful and picturesque sides of the hills by which the Spa is surrounded : a consummation much to be desired, and which may yet be accomplished.

To render a sojourn at Halifax very agreeable, there are other and various means besides those already alluded to, exclusively belonging to nature ; and among the latter, by the by, I ought not to forget to mention the many interesting geological excursions for which the immediate neighbourhood of the town furnishes sufficient motives.

During a short visit that I had the honour of paying to the Archdeacon of Craven, vicar of Halifax, I learned from that reverend person, who is himself versed in science, and is the bosom friend of two of the great scientific luminaries of Cambridge, that the country around was rich in geological accidents and facts.

The career of this eminent and exemplary divine, like that of his still more fortunate brother—one of the present prelates of the English church—is full of interest and encouragement to such as, being lowly placed by fortune upon entering the world, know how to raise themselves to the highest dignities, by talent and the exercise of every virtue. The archdeacon, besides being himself a distinguished dignitary of the church, enjoys the patronage of eight chapelries in Halifax parish, one of the largest in England, containing not fewer than 150,000 inhabitants.

Society affords, perhaps, fewer resources in Halifax, than one would be led to expect ; considering the large number of opulent families resident in or about the place. There is not much intercourse among the various sections of the community; and although six great public balls are given in the very handsome Musical Hall already alluded to, few families of distinction are known to attend them, as there is found among them a spirit of etiquette, and a disinclination to mix, which are not at all favourable to that species of assemblies.

Society at Halifax would seem to be divided into two classes—those who give dinners, and those who only receive company in the evening. Among the latter, there is often a very objectionable *mélange*, while to the former belong the select and the exclusive few. To the houses of one or two of these I was introduced by my friendly conductor; and when one has beheld the situation, internal aspect, and pleasure-grounds of such a residence as the *Shay*, inhabited by one of the wealthier merchants of Halifax,—or seen the house of another of the primates of the place, Mr. Waterhouse, situated on a green knoll, of the same highly-cultivated ridge that overlooks the ravine, the Calder, and the canal,—it is impossible not to conclude that Halifax contains within itself the elements of comfort, luxury, and all the conveniences of an easy life.

This is no mean consideration for an invalid of consequence, who may be advised by his physicians to come hither in order to try the Horley Green Spa water;—nor is it less important that invalids in general should know, that in the beautiful and highly-cultivated valley, watered by the Calder and called the Elland basin, they will find a milder climate for the winter than in any other part of Yorkshire—with many very neat and nice houses, felicitously placed on the same acclivity, down which slopes Ellbank park and wood.

It is through this delightful region that the projected railway line of communication between Manchester and Leeds will pass, in the direction of the axis of the valley —marking its progress through many of the sweetest villages in these parts.

I have yet to describe other Spas in Yorkshire, which I visited after leaving Horley Green. The number of mineral springs in that county is very considerable ; and to attempt to give an account of the whole of them would be a bootless task. In my own case, besides those already described, I also visited and examined three or four others, on which I shall make only a few passing remarks.

I allude first to LOCKWOOD SPA, situated at about a mile west of the flourishing town of Huddersfield, to which I proceeded in company with Dr. Alexander; next to SLAITHWAITE, some miles further in a south-western direction ; and thirdly to ASKERNE, not many miles north of the cleanest of all the towns in Yorkshire, Doncaster.

But these Spas I cannot undertake to bring before my readers in any other than a superficial manner. Far more interesting ones claim our attention in other and distant parts of England ; and after all, the three mineral springs just enumerated so nearly resemble each other in their most prominent chemical characters, that when one of them has been described, little could be said of the other two which would not be considered a repetition.

From this observation, I ought perhaps to except the last of the three mentioned Spas, namely,

ASKERNE;

where the water, strongly impregnated with sulphur,* surges

---

* So strongly does this water emit its sulphuretted effluvia, that Dr. Edward Chorley, of old a physician at Doncaster, perpetrated upon it the following epigram :

> " The devil when passing by Askeron
> Was asked what he thought thereon :
> Quoth Satan—' Judging from the stink,
> I can't be far from home, I think.' "

from an extensive bog or quagmire, covered over with a short sward, near the margin of a small lake or pond. This water has the very objectionable taste of a *vegetable* sulphuretted water, instead of that of the sulphuretted water which, as in the case of Gilsland Spa for example, springs from a shaly rock, limpid and colourless, and is, unlike the Askerne water, free from all decomposed vegetable fibres.

A species of Tuffa is found near the surface, which sufficiently denotes the sort of soil from whence the sulphur water oozes. It consists of a congeries of the reedy stems of gramineous grasses, incrusted with depositions of carbonate of lime, and nothing else.

Askerne, moreover, lies in a flat and unpromising locality, and so little success does it seem to meet with, that the Park Hotel, the principal inn of the place, at the time of my visit, which was at the termination of the season of 1839, was compelled to close its doors for want of a superior class of customers.

I tasted of all the waters in the place (for there are several), down to the one most recently discovered, two hundred yards to the south of Coes' South Parade Bath, in a green field,—which seems to be a water not only the most strongly impregnated with sulphuretted hydrogen of any in England, but one which is disgusting to look at, as well as to drink, from its greenish tint.

I cannot say that I was favourably impressed with what I either tasted or saw at this Spa; and the blunder again here committed, of transmitting a strong sulphuretted water through leaden pipes, convinced me that no scientific person presides over the establishment. I found that all the water-bibbers here are compelled to have recourse to the addition of Epsom salts to the water, if they wish it to act as an aperient.

When, on my return from it to Doncaster, I conversed with the very intelligent physician of that place, Dr. Scholfield,

2 D 2

on the subject of the employment of the Askerne water in disease, he candidly admitted that he knew little from personal experience of its virtues—that both the water and the place were objected to by invalids, yet that in some cases of obstinate cutaneous disorders it had proved decidedly beneficial.

There is a neat Spa-house at Askerne, which is much frequented by the poor, and a bath-house for the better classes of visiters, called the Old Manor-house Baths, placed upon the border of the lake, which plays a conspicuous part in the landscape. The writer of a fanciful and poetical account of Askerne, which I have seen, takes the trouble of discussing the point, whether this place had been known to the Romans as a bathing-station, and is candid enough to admit, though with great sorrow, that the evidence is not strong in favour of such a supposition. He need not have been at such pains to argue the question, for the Romans have invariably shown too much discrimination, and the most accurate tact, in selecting and fixing upon natural spots and springs for medicinal purposes. The nation who colonized Aix-la-Chapelle, established baths at Baden, and who settled near the *Aquæ Solis* of Bath, would never have planted their tents on the margin of a quagmire, covered though it be with green herbage, and inundated by sulphurous water, the result of vegetable decomposition. The Romans would not have established baths on the Pontine marshes.

Dr. Edwin Lankester, of Campsall, near Askerne, however, is about to publish a little work on that Spa, which will be an improvement upon the only work now extant on that water, by Brewerton, a member of the Society of Friends residing at Bawtry, where he died about nine years ago ; and as he has also employed the chemical aid of Mr. West, of Leeds, to analyze afresh the water, I regret the less my want of space for the notes I had taken on the spot, on the same subject.

With respect to

LOCKWOOD,

it is a Spa, situated on the left bank of the Holm, which winds its way under a precipitous rock forming the opposite bank, and is an old sulphur-well, utilized recently by a company of subscribers, who have erected a neat cursaal and suitable bath-rooms, with a tepid plunging-bath besides. The water is derived from a well, a couple of yards below the surface, which is kept constantly covered—a vent-pipe alone being plunged into it through the ground for its ventilation. The water is plentifully supplied to the public, at the rate of four gallons for one penny, and used by the inhabitants in the neighbouring town of Huddersfield for making tea, to which it is said to impart an excellent flavour. In my general table I have inserted the most recent analysis of this mineral water, which belongs to the class of slightly sulphuretted alkaline springs.

It is gratifying to me to find that local experience of the efficacy of such a water as this, though mild in its composisition, has induced people to confide in its use for the cure of many disorders, particularly those of the skin, which ordinary medicines fail to remove. This is an additional demonstration of the goodness of my cause, who contend that nature has not spread mineral waters so profusely throughout the globe without a salutary intention, did we but interrogate her properly on the subject, and avail ourselves, with skill and discrimination, of the boon she tenders.

Even a blunder, committed in pure ignorance, in one of the bath-rooms at Lockwood, serves to exhibit the power of this water on disease. A sorely-afflicted plumber and glazier of Huddersfield, having exhausted his purse and his patience under the care of successive medical men, for the removal of a cutaneous disorder of the most troublesome as well as disgusting description, had recourse to the Lockwood Spa water, and was cured. In thankful gratitude, the honest tradesman, finding the bath-room, which had so often received him, in a very indifferent state of repair, offered to put it in good order free of any charge to the company, and, accordingly, not only repaired it, but also embellished it. But, alas! in so doing, he painted his own bath with lead-colour—which must alter the nature of the gas peculiar to the water and change the character of the latter—thereby depriving himself of any benefit he might require from it hereafter.

SLAITHWAITE

is a somewhat analogous water, which is distributed and used in an establishment like that at Lockwood, except that the baths are rather too small. The water rises in the bed of the river Colne, and is now confined within a well or reservoir of solid masonry, from which an *iron* pipe (a blunder again) conveys it to the baths, comprised within an elegant building above which is a large news-room. As in the case of Lockwood, the mineral water is derived from the shaly limestone beneath the lofty moorland which crests the Blackstone Edge with reference to Slaithwaite, as it does the Farnley Tyas heath with regard to Lockwood.

It will be seen, by inspecting my analytical table, that the Slaithwaite water is richer in alkaline salts than any of the waters in the north, hitherto described. The proportion, also, of the carburetted hydrogen is very considerable, and this gas is emitted in so pure a state from the water, that it may be readily collected and burnt. Here, as at Lockwood, the dense population of manufacturers, and other mechanics, furnish the larger part of the visiters who frequent the Spa—the efficacy of which has been attested to me by more than one invalid who had recovered his health through its means.

The truth of this fact, and the need of so powerful an aid in freeing the poorer classes of their community from trouble-

some and disabling disorders, have so convinced the wealthier
inhabitants of the advantage to be derived from the gratuitous
distribution of the mineral water to the afflicted poor, that a
subscription charity for that purpose has been established at
the Spa. This is as it ought to be, and the propagation of this
information ought to stimulate others to follow the benevolent
example at other watering-places.

An advertisement in one of the Leeds newspapers, one
day, excited my curiosity to visit a mineral spring, said to have
been discovered two years previous, at a place otherwise famous,
called CALVERLEY, and supposed to resemble the powerful
steel water at Sandrock, in the Isle of Wight. To Calverley,
therefore, I felt it my duty to proceed on leaving Bradford,
where I bade a friendly farewell to Dr. Alexander, after having
changed vehicles. Nor was I sorry to fleè from that terrific
atmosphere which, at the very moment of traversing the
infernal region of Wibsey Lowmoor iron-works in order to
reach Bradford, so began to tickle my trachea and constrict the
air-passages in my lungs, that I felt as much suffocated as if
a bundle of lighted matches had been held under my nose.

Alas! for those who must dwell in such a pelagus of sul-
phureous effluvia. And yet, on looking around me, among
the dense population that paraded up and down the narrow, black, fuliginous, and gloomy streets, many of them
ascending with almost perpendicular acclivity, I could detect
no evil result on " the human face divine," from such an
atmosphere. On the contrary, the fair sex appeared well-grown
and very showy—the children good-looking and healthy.

The condition of Bradford is dreadful. Lowmoor iron-
forges most extensively spread their suffocating exhalations on
the one side, and at a very short distance from the town on
the road to Halifax or Huddersfield. On the other side,
Bowling Iron *Hell* (for it is one truly) casts a still denser atmosphere and sulphurous stench, much nearer,—indeed, close

at home,—for it is but a short way out of the town on the right of the road to Leeds. At eve the view of these volcanic regions is awful: and Vesuvius in a dark night, up-pouring its first preliminary fitful flames which illumine the area around it, not unaptly may be said to resemble those which rise unceasingly in this place, showing more distinctly the thick covering of black and dense smoke that overspreads the hills on which the forges are erected.

Add to these two awful neighbours—these fields of never-failing combustion—three or four collieries at work within a span of the town, and its own hundred pyramidal or obelisk-like chimneys, which bespeak as many factories—and then for a moment imagine what atmosphere must that be, within which devoted Bradford is enveloped!

Bradford is in every way inferior to Halifax in the disposition of its houses, in buildings, in locality, and in comforts as a permanent residence. It is wanting, too, in water-courses for the conveyance of merchandise or the assistance of the manufactures. At night the town presents a mass almost theatrical to behold. Whichever way the eye turns, whether on the lofty hills that surround the town, or on the crest of ascending streets; large square buildings, whose black and massive outlines stamp themselves on the gray arch of heaven behind, appear like the palaces of Saladin, glittering with the magic and blazing light of gas through their hundreds of square casements.

I was glad to learn from good authority, that the depravity said to reign paramount among the miserable beings who work at their hard and unwholesome task in this part of Yorkshire, and of which so dismal a picture has been drawn by Dr. Wade, existed only in his heated and demagogic imagination. Of the generally favourable state of their health also, Dr. Outhwaite, of Bradford, assured me. I regretted not to have seen more of this highly-respectable physician.

CALVERLEY

can only be reached by a deviation from the high-road leading to Leeds. The cross-road follows the crest of a hill immediately above the Aire, into the beautiful and fruitful vale
of which it peers from a considerable height, commanding the
view of many interesting objects—Kirkstall ruins amongst
them. This digression of about a mile and a half amply
repays the trouble. How few travellers think of these by-
road excursions; or ever dream that, whilst following the
beaten track, they may miss the most charming scenery or the
loveliest prospect!

Calverley spring is in an open field, a little below the village.
It was discovered in boring for a mine in a coalpit, through
the aluminous shale strata. The water is a supersulphate
of alumine and iron, and resembles that of the Sandrock, as
was before stated. By dint of paragraphs in the public
journals, thousands of people were made to flock to the spot,
there to drink the water, on paying a small charge for each
person.

It is in the colliery of Mr. Suttlefe that the spring surges,
but the stream is contested by many; at present it is fast
losing its fashion. At the vicarage of Calverley, where I was
hospitably received, I had the water brought to me, and
with it a statement of an analysis of its contents made in
London, bearing the approving signatures of Drs. Prout and
A. T. Thomson. That analysis differs materially from the
one given in " White's History of the West Riding ;"* but
deeming it accurate only from the circumstance of the two
respected physicians just mentioned having affixed their

---

* The difference is so great, that whereas the one represents carbonate
of iron to be one of the ingredients in the water, the other states that it is
sulphate of iron instead. The total sum of the ingredients also varies in
each. In the one, a gallon of water is said to contain thirty-seven and
a half grains ; in the other, forty-five of solid contents. Neither analyze-
takes notice of the gaseous principles.

names to it, and not from any belief I have in the skill of the analyzer, I have inserted it in my analytical table.

Farmer Thornton, who brought me the water, collected in one of his fields, into which it finds its way out of the colliery, where the spring was originally tapped at a depth of thirty yards from the surface, assured me that the supply would be plentiful if properly attended to. It now trickles down from his field into a small rivulet or *beck*, and thence goes into the Aire, where it is lost. No use is at present made of it. Its taste is subacid—*âpre*, like a very unripe crabapple—it puckers up the inside membrane of the mouth —it is quite transparent, and has a slight golden tint.

On finding myself in Calverley, " All's one, or One of the Foure Plaies in one, called a Yorkshire tragedy,"—generally placed among the minor dramatic poems of Shakspeare,—came strongly to my mind. The tradition of that dreadful deed is yet vivid in the village, and the rooms, still stained with the blood of the victims, in which the unnatural and foul act was perpetrated, are frequently pointed out to travellers, and supposed to be still haunted by the reckless spirit of the criminal.

On the site of the largest part of Calverley Hall, however, a number of cottages have been erected; and of the tragical scene of action, nought now remains but the ill-fated chamber in which a furibond and jealous husband, and a gamester, plunged into the heart of his lady and babe the murderous knife, still reeking with the blood of his eldest son! That murderer was the last seignorial master of the ancient hall of Calverley; and the castle of York never enclosed, in the course of its long existence, a greater culprit than the principal actor in the dreadful scene called the Yorkshire tragedy, who forfeited his life within that fortress on the 5th of August, 1604, to the violated laws of nature and man.

Leaving a spot so desecrated, and which, in spite of the

strong chalybeate spring lately discovered, will never rise to the rank of a fashionable watering-place,—I hastened to the capital of the manufacturing districts of the county, where it was my intention to terminate the first part of my tour and visits to the Northern Spas of England.

LEEDS,

on a rainy day, as it was my fate to encounter, presents an aspect of filth through its streets perfectly appalling to a pedestrian, even though he may have had the benefit of experience in the purlieus of the great city. In this respect Leeds is infinitely worse than Manchester.

On such days we must not venture down the numberless narrow and intricate passages and lanes that, right and left of Briggate, the main artery of the town, spread in zigzag direction, forming perfect labyrinths; for there the maze is beyond conception. In this respect, however, Leeds offers only a repetition of what may be observed elsewhere in England. The *water lanes* of Sunderland, the *chairs* at Newcastle, the *cellars* at Manchester, the *yards* at Preston, the *courts* and *alleys* of St. Giles's and Seven Dials, or the *alentours* of Whitechapel, are only facsimiles of each other, for unspeakable filth and foul air; and they are not worse than Leeds in those respects; " Swine-gate" and the " Isle of Cinders" to wit.

The great difference that strikes one on a first view, between the two vast emporiums of wool and cotton, in both of which red brick buildings constitute the most conspicuous masses, seems to be this: that whereas at Leeds, factories and tall chimneys are interspersed with private houses; at Manchester, private houses are interspersed with tall chimneys and factories. In Leeds, hardly a single acre is to be found, a thousand yards square, which looks like an ordinary paved

city, with streets flanked by good houses, uninterrupted
by bits of rough ground, by deserted mills, and dilapidated
dwellings. Except in the heart of the town, empty spaces
and waste portions of ground seem to be the order of the day.
On some of these, a sort of short coarse grass seems to grow,
amidst every species of rubbish ; and the sheep which are
allowed to wander about and feed upon it, look very much
like so many ambulatory *popes-heads*, that have just been
used to cleanse the foul flues of the factories.

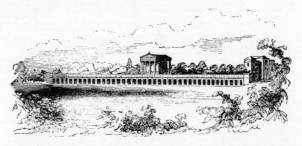

Of the modern buildings that mostly attract attention, besides the lofty Ionic colonnade of the commercial rooms,
erected by Clarke, the cemetery is perhaps the most showy,
though, as usual, it looks finer in print than in reality. Such
as it is, however, the general aspect of that region of death,
which, with marked toleration is opened to the departed of
every denomination of religious worship without distinction,
is solemn and imposing, as far as it has been completed. Its
small Ionic temple, with a portico of four columns, is of good
proportions. It seems to rest upon, and occupies the centre
of, a semicircular and elongated terrace, the lofty wall of
which presents a number of divisional gates, leading to a
corresponding number of catacombs.

Externally, the entrance into the cemetery is grand, and
borrowed from the Egyptian architecture ; while within, and on
each side of it, a handsome house, after the Italian style, has

been erected for the residence of the officiating minister and his assistant; but so contrived that, in approaching the dominion of death from the town, those dwellings of the living do not obtrude on the sight to break the solemn impression of the place—being concealed behind the ponderous piers of the Egyptian gateway.

As a medical man, setting aside the feelings of philanthropy to which, in common with my fellow men, I may lay claim, I rejoiced during my recent extended tour through England, to behold at last the pernicious custom of burying the dead amidst the living, giving way to the enlightened practice of almost every civilized nation, of collecting the mortal spoils of departed citizens without the walls of the city, in an appropriate Necropolis. The impetus once given to the latter practice, it has steadily been gaining ground with the inhabitants of the principal cities in this country.

Of the very many benefits that must accrue to society from such a change, it is not the least gratifying or valuable that the establishment of cemeteries has given fresh impetus to architectural imagination and skill, as well as to sculptural talent; both of which have thus a new field open for their operations, as in the case, for instance, of this cemetery of Leeds, of those at Liverpool and Newcastle, and the many others recently established, including those of the metropolis.

Unquestionably the merit of first having started the idea of erecting a grand Necropolis for the capital belongs to the late Francis Goodwin, architect, whose splendid project for an establishment of this description, which should contain fac-similes of nearly all the most renowned temples of Athens and Rome, eclipsed every thing that had before or has since been projected or executed.

Poor Goodwin ! I knew him well. With a sanguine temperament, a highly sensitive complexion of mind, coupled to great imagination and unrivalled skill in the art of design, he came with his project some years too soon, and overshot the intellect and comprehension of the public. All his efforts proved unavailing; his labour was cast away; and his time, unremittingly devoted to the making and maturing of his plans, greatly to the injury of his other professional interests, was wholly lost. The public responded not to his appeals; and after many unsuccessful efforts to bring his vast conceptions into operation, he died at last, disappointed, mortified, and broken-hearted!

Alas! it is too often so with genius. Its fate is to point out to others the path of glorious originality and undreamt-of improvements, to be itself disregarded, scouted even, nay, persecuted; while, on the other hand, mere sciolists and aping imitators coming after, reap the whole benefit of the magnificent projects and inventions. Thus it has been with regard to the public cemeteries that have of late years started into existence in many parts of this country. They are but puny imitations of the magnificent project of poor Goodwin; and, like every thing else in the fine arts in England, they tend to show that if the country does produce men of transcendent genius, the nation is neither capable nor willing to embrace to the fullest extent, and in all the magnitude that appertains to them, their brilliant and splendid conceptions.

Woodhouse Moor, a clayish and swampy plain, by the side of the cemetery, is not unaptly the parade of the belles of Leeds, who come hither to witness cricket-matches, and be present at reviews. It is right that the bustle and riot of gay life should be rifest in the vicinity of the region of the tombs, within which all worldly concerns and pleasures must at last be buried.

This moor is the highest part of Leeds. Having a north-west horizon, of a pleasing character, and the lovely village of Headingly in sight, people are tempted hither in fine weather; and some even plant their residence on the spot, erecting new ranges of dwelling-houses, as in the case of the so-called Hanover and Lyddon squares.

A new and wide road of approach leading thence into the town is now in progress. It passes by many a waste piece of ground, on which the wealthy clothiers are hastening to build their villas, away from the dreadful atmosphere of their mills. In their eagerness to testify how gladly they make the change, they bestow the inspiriting and refreshing denominations of *Springfield*-place and *Mount Pleasant* on their new abodes.

But even favourable situations like these are but a half-and-half region, in the estimation of people *à plus grande prétention* in Leeds, who push further their own extension from the smoke of the town, and get upon Headingly's smiling banks, on which insulated suburban villas, graced with the names of the opulent Marshals, the Stanfields, the Gotts, and other families, are made to start into existence, facing the merry dale of the Aire, and constructed of freestone —that spurns the vulgar stare and blushing ornaments of brickwork.

In the vicinity of this favoured part of the town, a huge wall caught my attention, which I found on inquiry to surround the Zoological Gardens. The locality, and the internal arrangement of these pleasure-grounds, so far as it could be carried into effect, are praiseworthy. But at the present moment things are at a standstill, and the subscribers have withheld their further countenance from the establishment, in consequence of a resolution which has closed the gardens entirely on Sundays.

It is not easy to imagine a more injudicious or impolitic resolution on the part of those who wish well to such institutions, than that of closing them on the only day on which the industrious classes of citizens can and ought to have some proper and useful recreation, after the hours consecrated to divine worship. If it be admitted that exercise in the open air is necessary to maintain people in health, and that the contemplation of nature's varied and infinite beauties contributes to that object also, as well as to instruct and ennoble the human mind ; if it be not denied that general and useful knowledge is best obtained through the eyes, and that to render any point of information easy of acquisition, it is better to familiarize people with its peculiar objects, by repeated inspection ;—then the excluding of those whom we wish so to benefit, inform, and instruct, from an establishment best calculated to produce all these effects, on the only day on which their weekly occupations will permit them to attend it, is, to say the least, to act in direct violation of principles admitted to be sound and philosophical.

The exclusion, therefore, is injudicious; but it is also impolitic. It is so, on the score of economy ; it is so, on the score of morality. Unquestionably, if the only day on which the friends of the actual supporters of an institution like a Zoological Garden, or the supporters themselves, can attend it, be declared a *dies non*, and the establishment be shut against them, the latter will withdraw themselves from it, and cease to subscribe—as they have done at Leeds. A large portion of the funds will thus " cease and determine," and the operations, perhaps the very existence of the institution, will be placed in jeopardy.

Certain it is, that were such a measure to be adopted by the Zoological Society of London—judging from the names upon their present prodigious list of members—nearly four-fifths of them would cease to be such, by withholding their subscription. Why should they not, indeed ? In subscribing, their object was to enjoy the appliances of the institution. To those they can only have access on the day of rest from labour or occupation, and on that day the doors are closed against them ! Is it wonderful—nay,· is it not natural—that they should then withdraw altogether from the concern ?

And if they do not withdraw, yet are denied on a particular day an attendance upon the grounds, which is un-accompanied by tumult, profanation, or uproariousness, but which, on the contrary, tends to keep the people congregated together, orderly, well-behaved, and observant of all the proprieties of life—is not then a most capital chance thrown away, of promoting and encouraging the exercise of certain moral virtues on the part of that portion of the community which most of all requires them?

If it be pretended that the admission of a large number of people within the enclosure of a garden on a Sunday, is a desecration of the Lord's day, then the same rule should be applied to every other public garden, and to the parks also, all of which ought in such strictness to be closed on the sabbath. It can be no more an infraction of that holy day to walk in one garden than in another; and if in the one there are many objects of interest to excite curiosity, collected from the most important kingdoms of nature, while in the other nothing but a vain and indecorous staring at each other takes place,—the reason for closing the latter is infinitely more valid than any which can be urged for closing the other; for in that, at all events, the wonderful works of the Deity, and the endless varieties of animal creation, can be duly contemplated.

In fact, if a preacher were every now and then to take up his argument for redeeming evil-minded persons, and such as are idle in the worshipping of God, out of their ignorance of his miraculous works—he might, with surpassing effect, select his examples from among the wonders of the animal creation, and send his congregation, after the discourse, to a Zoological Garden, where such a one exists, for the best illustrations of his subject.

The plea that certain persons, in their capacity of servants to the establishment, must, if that establishment be kept open on a Sunday, be prevented from attending a place of worship on that day, ought to have little weight, inasmuch as it must ever depend on their own spontaneous good will whether, even if the gardens be closed during the hours of divine worship, they will attend those holy places. But besides, such a plea would apply to so many analogous cases, that it would be obviously impossible to act in accordance to it. Why—in the very house of God, on the sabbath-day, a certain number of male and female attendants are constantly occupied, during divine service, with their individual duties, which are perfectly inconsistent with the true exercise of devotion.

In Leeds, in particular, a prohibition to the middle and industrious classes from attending the Zoological Garden would have the worst effect, as the people are fond of viewing and examining any number of objects capable of conveying information to them; a fact which I had a very satisfactory opportunity of ascertaining when I attended the gallery and saloon of the Leeds public exhibition, where many a thousand objects of art, skilfully displayed, seemed to be a never-ceasing source of interest to all the visiters present.

Leeds is not without its mineral spring. An alkaline and very slightly sulphuretted water peculiar to the town, and indeed hawked about the streets every day, or supplied to families regularly, is one which has enjoyed considerable reputation for many centuries, I may say. The supply is abundant, and drawn from a suburb of Leeds, on the south side of the Aire, at a village bearing the name of Holbeck; hence called *Holbeck water*. It is not only drunk medicinally, but used also for domestic purposes, especially for making tea, the flavour of which it is supposed to enhance considerably.

In the supply of ordinary water Leeds has always been deficient, and is so still. It used to be drawn from the river high up in the stream; but the multiplication of dyers and manufacturers on the banks so soiled the water that the Leeds people, like men of sense, are just about completing an arrangement for drawing water from springs and other sources in the country, and ten thousand pounds had been subscribed towards it.

Two other important objects engaged my attention at Leeds; the state of the church, and the woolcloth factory.

The parish church of St. Peter, now in course of being rebuilt on its ancient site, but on a more splendid scale, after the designs of Mr. Chantrell, the very able architect of Leeds, which will be, in appearance, grandeur, and internal service, almost a cathedral, first attracted my notice as I returned from the York railway station, and drove past it.

The eminent divine who for some years has been vicar of this densely-populated town, has exerted the great influence of his name, his pulpit eloquence, and his character with all those of his own communion among the inhabitants, in hopes of giving to Leeds a parish church worthy of its rank as the principal emporium of, perhaps, the most important species of manufacture in England. In this object the pious zeal of Dr. Hook is likely to be amply satisfied, and in a short time hence it will not again be observed of Leeds parish, that while the dissenters possess not fewer than thirty-two places of worship in the town, among which some are of an imposing size; and the Roman Catholics have two chapels, besides the lately erected and very splendid structure, called " St. Ann's Catholic Church," which comes nigh to the cathedral form and character,—the members of the church of England could not boast of a sacred edifice equal in magnitude and design to the catholic temple, and were satisfied with the old cruciform structure of St. Peter's, and its square embattled tower of Norman origin, as their first and principal place of worship. Henceforth, modern St. Peter's will command admiration for its imposing mass and richness of design, even though there be among the seven or eight other subordinate protestant churches or perpetual curacies in Leeds, one or two that are very favourable specimens of architecture.

A visit to a woolcloth factory, or mill, is one of the most interesting occupations for a stranger in Leeds. I devoted some hours to it under the friendly guidance of one of the partners in an eminent and extensive firm; and though every operation I witnessed, from the sorting of the raw material to the folding of and preparing for market a superfine piece of cloth, was shown and explained, according to the clear, methodical and successive order in which it takes place,—I confess I was bewildered at the sight of so much complicated machinery, extensive contrivances, ingenious devices, and improvements in mechanics, which appeared necessary to produce an apparently simple result.

Three long months does the completion of a single piece of the finest woollen cloth require—as much time nearly as it takes to wear it out, if converted by some modern Stultz into coats. An idea may thus be formed of the extent and variety of labour which such a manufacture involves, and of the number of hands it demands; and yet one of these pieces of the finest sort, with a beautiful gloss upon it, although died in the wool, will be sent out from the factory at fifteen shillings per yard, to the general merchant or wholesale dealer, who is himself satisfied with the profit of one shilling a yard upon his purchase-money when he re-sells it to the retailer.

It would seem to be the latter trafficker, therefore, who benefits most, and for whose advantages all this immense machinery, population, capital, and ingenuity, are principally put in motion; it is for him who retails to the public at twenty-two or twenty-four shillings a yard, a handsome cloth which cost him but sixteen, thus making a profit of from forty to fifty per cent. And this without risking any capital himself; often taking long credit from the wholesale merchant; and not unfrequently paying nothing, by becoming a bankrupt. Such an arrangement, though inherently unjust, is one which must be submitted to by the manufacturer if he means to get a market for the goods he produces.

After all, however, the Leeds clothiers are men of wealth, as the Marshalls and the Gotts may testify; one of whom, among the latter, hesitated not in sinking a capital of 40,000*l.* within the last few years, for the erection of a triple parallel range of gigantic cloth-mills! I recollect sitting at dinner one day by the side of one of these opulent men of the broad cloth, and inquiring of him how his brother was, whom I had not seen for a year or two—" Oh," was his answer, " he has retired from business, and been occupied in looking out for an estate of 200,000*l.* to purchase." The said brother had, to my knowledge, been engaged in his factory very little more than thirty years before, principally during the late war!

The time had at length arrived for leaving the Northern Spas, and the magnificent country which has supplied me with the principal subjects of the present volume.

I quitted Yorkshire with regret. In the whole range of my travels in England, I have not seen a county which, take it all in all, can be compared to this. Yorkshire is a kingdom of itself, with all the resources of one, and with capabilities inexhaustible. For extent of area, it surpasses every other county, and is nearly equal to the aggregate area of the two largest counties in England, Lincolnshire and Devon. In population, it is not only superior to Lancashire and the metropolitan county, which are the next most densely inhabited provinces, but it nearly equals that of some of the kingdoms of Europe, such as Würtemberg, Saxony, or the Hanseatic towns; while it surpasses that of the sovereign duchies of Baden and Tuscany. As an agricultural county, its importance may be deduced from the number of its inhabitants engaged in the cultivation of the land, which, according to the census of 1831, amounted to 85,660, or to one person in every sixteen of the whole population. A number of people in Yorkshire, very little short of this, namely, 76,060, busy themselves in manufactures of every description; while not fewer than 13,211 persons are engaged in professional pursuits, or in banking, or in the cultivation of science and the *belles lettres*,—showing that in Yorkshire, at all events, knowledge and talent are consistent with opulence.

Nature has showered its choicest gifts on this fortunate portion of the British dominions. Yorkshire possesses every thing desirable, except an Italian sky or a Lisbon climate. Level lands that yield food for men, and pasture for animals in abundance, with very little trouble, cover a large extent of the whole area, and in some places exhibit the richest cultivation, equal at times to that of the choicest garden. Scattered in the middle plains, one sees dense forests dotting the great map of the country; whilst on the mountain-tops, or within the caverns of Alpine ranges, or beneath the gentle and rounded undulations that rise from the plain, most plentiful supplies are found of building and ornamental stone, of metalliferous substances, and of that most important of all combustibles, coal.

In rivers, what other county is superior? In canal navigation, what other part of England is better provided? Of highways and byways, where do we find any better? Its valleys are rich, smiling, and extensive; they teem either with modern towns and villages, or with the remains of ancient cities and stations. In scenery of the most romantic character, few other counties can vie with it. Of interesting ruins of bygone monastic splendour, no single county besides can reckon so many; neither can any competitor be found for equality in the number and grandeur of its seignorial residences. As to its race of men, whether for personal appearance, stature, or hardiness, are they not looked upon as some of the finest in the kingdom?

Nor let us forget to add to all these blessings vouchsafed by Providence to the county of York, the not contemptible one of being provided with many mineral springs as sources of health, which it has been the main object of the present volume to make known to the public, in a more detailed and ample form than has hitherto been done. In the pursuit of that object, the author has not only become well acquainted with the fair region he has just summarily described, but with many most excellent, exemplary, and learned men also—the recollection of which, and of whom will ever prove to him a source of happiness and gratification.

END OF VOL. I.

WHITING, BEAUFORT HOUSE STRAND.

From the Holy Mountain

From the Holy Mountain

A JOURNEY
IN THE SHADOW OF
BYZANTIUM

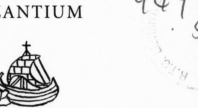

WILLIAM DALRYMPLE

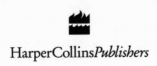

HarperCollins*Publishers*

HarperCollins*Publishers*
77–85 Fulham Palace Road,
Hammersmith, London W6 8JB

Published by HarperCollins*Publishers* 1997
Copyright © William Hamilton-Dalrymple 1997
Map and illustrations © Olivia Fraser 1997

The author asserts the moral right to
be identified as the author of this work

A catalogue record for this book
is available from the British Library

ISBN 0 00 255509 3

Set in Postscript Minion with Photina display by
Rowland Phototypesetting Ltd,
Bury St Edmunds, Suffolk
Printed and bound in Great Britain by
Caledonian International
Book Manufacturing Ltd, Glasgow

For my parents,
with love and gratitude

ILLUSTRATIONS

vii

The Monastery of Mar Saba.
Fr. Theophanes, Guest Master of Mar Saba, at the monastery gate.
St Paul and St Antony breaking bread. Detail of icon at the Monastery of St Antony, Egypt.
The same scene carved on a Pictish symbol-stone, St Vigeans, Dundee.
Fr. Dioscorus discusses the latest sighting of St Antony, Monastery of St Antony, Egypt.
The desert between Asyut and the Great Kharga Oasis.

COLOUR

Between pages 406 and 407

The Monastery of Simopetra, Mount Athos.
Fr. Christophoros and his cats, Monastery of Iviron, Mount Athos.
Haghia Sophia and Haghia Eirene, Istanbul.
The Fishponds of Abraham, Urfa (Edessa).
Qala'at Semaan, the Basilica of St Symeon Stylites, Syria.
A flock of sheep in the wilderness of Judaea.
The ancient fortress, Monastery of St Antony, Egypt.
The necropolis of Bagawat, the Great Kharga Oasis.

ACKNOWLEDGEMENTS

The journey recorded in this book took place over a single summer and autumn, but incorporates a few episodes from two visits, to Israel and Egypt, made earlier in the year. The identity of a great many people has been disguised, particularly in those sections dealing with Turkey, the Israeli-occupied West Bank and Egypt. I sincerely hope that no one comes to any harm through what I have written.

A great many people have helped me during the four years this book took to write. I would particularly like to thank the following, without whom it could not have come into being: Abbas, Mohammed Sid Ahmed, Canon Naim Ateek, Abdullah and Noah Awad, Leila Badr, David Barchard, Andrew Berton, Robert Betts, Gaby Bostros, Dr Sebastian Brock, Derek and Eileen Brown, Yvonne Lady Cochrane, Con Coughlin, Alkis Courcolas, Hew Dalrymple, Fr. Jock Dalrymple, His Beatitude Diodoros I Patriarch of Jerusalem, Abouna Dioscuros of the Monastery of St Antony, Alistair Duncan, Eustathios Matta Rouhm Metropolitan of the Jazira and Euphrates, Mike Fishwick, Robert Fisk, Kadreya Foda, Robert Franjieh, Archie Fraser, Jenny Fraser, John Freely, Patrick French, Dr Nicholas Gendle, Sami Geraisi, David Gilmour, Charlie Glass, Philip Glazebrook, Giles Gordon, Juan Carlos Gumucio, Malfono Isa Gulten, Harry Hagopian, Roy Hange, Milad Hanna, Richard Harper, Bernard Haykel, Sarah Helm, Dr Isabel Henderson, George Hintlian, Jill Hughes, Mar Gregorios Yohanna Ibrahim Metropolitan of Aleppo, His Holiness Mar Ignatius Zaki Iwas Patriarch of Antioch, Fr. Jeremias of the Monastery of Iviron, Walid Jumblatt, Mansour Khaddosh, Nora Kort, Robert Lacey, Fr. Emmanuel Lanne, Dominic Lawson, Tony Mango, Dr Philip Mansel, Peter Mansfield, Philip Marsden, Sally Mazloumian, Dr Otto Meinardus, Sam Miller, Bishop Mesrob Mutafian,

Mark Nicholson, Maggie Noach, John Julius Norwich, Anthony O'Mahony, Dr Andrew Palmer, Dr Philip Pattendon, Fr. Michele Piccirillo, Hugh Pope, Rebecca Porteous, Tom Porteous, Annie Robertson, Max Rodenbek, Sir Steven Runciman, Dr Bernard Sabella, Assem Salam, Dalia Salam, Archbishop Georges Saliba, Professor Kamal Salibi, Victor Samaika, Anthony Sattin, Neville Shack, His Holiness Pope Shenoudah III, Antoun Sidhom, Fania Stoney, Jane Taylor, Fr. Theophanes of the Monastery of Mar Saba, Timotheos Metropolitan of Lydda, Tony Touma, Christopher J. Walker, Bishop Kallistos Ware, John Warrack, Zhogbi Zhogbi.

I would particularly like to thank Alan and Brigid Waddams, who not only looked after me in Damascus but also lent their house in Somerset, where much of this book was written and edited.

I am also very grateful to Cistercian Publications (Kalamazoo, Michigan and Spencer, Massachusetts) for kind permission to quote from *John Moschos: The Spiritual Meadow*, translated by John Wortley, © Cistercian Publications, 1992.

My greatest thanks are, however, reserved for Olivia, friend, lover, adviser, illustrator, editor-in-chief, occasional travelling companion and beloved wife.

Finally, I would like to acknowledge the unique contribution of my daughter Ibby, born soon after the return from this journey, who provided a many-splendoured distraction throughout its writing, but for which this book would certainly have seen the light of day at least six months earlier.

WILLIAM DALRYMPLE
Provis, Somerset, November 1996

I

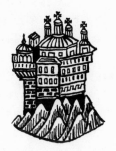

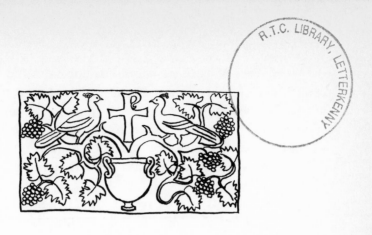

The Monastery of Iviron, Mount Athos, Greece
29 June 1994. The Feast of SS. Peter and Paul

My cell is bare and austere. It has white walls and a flagstone floor.
Only two pieces of furniture break the severity of its emptiness: in
one corner stands an olive-wood writing desk, in the other an
iron bedstead. The latter is covered with a single white sheet,
starched as stiff as a nun's wimple.

Through the open window I can see a line of black habits: the
monks at work in the vegetable garden, a monastic chain-gang
hoeing the cabbage patch before the sun sets and the wooden
simandron calls them in for compline. Beyond the garden is a
vineyard, silhouetted against the bleak black pyramid of the Holy
Mountain.

All is quiet now but for the distant breaking of surf on the jetty
and the faint echo and clatter of metal plates in the monastery
kitchens. The silence and solemnity of the place is hardly designed
to raise the spirits, but you could hardly find a better place to
order your mind. There are no distractions, and the monastic
silence imposes its own brittle clarity.

It's now nine o'clock. The time has finally come to concentrate
my thoughts: to write down, as simply as I can, what has brought
me here, what I have seen, and what I hope to achieve in the next
few months.

My reference books are laid out in a line on the floor; the pads containing my library notes are open. Files full of photocopied articles lie piled up below the window; my pencils are sharpened and upended in a glass. A matchbox lies ready beside the paraffin storm lantern: the monastery generator is turned off after compline, and if am to write tonight I will have to do so by the light of its yellow flame.

Open on the desk is my paperback translation of *The Spiritual Meadow of John Moschos*, the unlikely little book which first brought me to this monastery, and the original manuscript of which I saw for the first time less than one hour ago. God willing, John Moschos will lead me on, eastwards to Constantinople and Anatolia, then southwards to the Nile and thence, if it is still possible, to the Great Kharga Oasis, once the southern frontier of Byzantium.

This morning, six days after leaving the damp of a dreich Scottish June, I caught ship from Ouranopolis, the Gate of Heaven, down the peninsula to the Holy Mountain.

We passed a monastic fishing boat surrounded by a halo of seagulls. Opposite me, three large monks in ballooning cassocks sat sipping cappuccinos under an icon of the Virgin; over their grey moustaches there rested a light foam of frothed milk. Behind them, through the porthole, you could see the first of the great Athonite monasteries rising up from sandy bays to crown the foothills of the mountain. They are huge complexes of buildings, great ash-coloured fortresses the size of small Italian hill-towns, with timber-laced balconies hanging below domed cupolas and massive, unwieldy medieval buttresses.

The first monastic foundation on Athos was established in the ninth century by St Euthymius of Salonica who, having renounced the world at the age of eighteen, took to moving around on all fours and eating grass; he later became a stylite, and took to berating his brethren from atop a pillar. Some two hundred years

4

later – by which time St Euthymius's fame had led to many other monasteries and *sketes* springing up around the saint's original foundation – it came to the ears of the Byzantine Emperor that the monks were in the habit of debauching the daughters of the shepherds who came to the mountain to sell milk and wool. Thereafter it was decreed that nothing female – no woman, no cow, no mare, no bitch – could step within its limits.

Today this rule is relaxed only for cats, and in the Middle Ages even a pair of Byzantine Empresses were said to have been turned away from the Holy Mountain by the Mother of God herself. But 140 years ago, in 1857, the Virgin was sufficiently flexible to allow one of my Victorian great-aunts, Virginia Somers, to spend two months in a tent on Mount Athos, along with her husband and the louche Pre-Raphaelite artist Coutts Lindsay. A letter Virginia wrote on her visit still survives, in which she describes how the monks had taken her over the monastery gardens and insisted on giving her fruit from every tree as they passed; she said she tasted pomegranate, citron and peach. It is the only recorded instance of a women being allowed onto the mountain in the millennium-long history of Athos, and is certainly the only record of what appears to have been a most unholy Athonite *ménage-à-trois*.

This unique lapse apart, the Holy Mountain is still a self-governing monastic republic dedicated to prayer, chastity and pure, untarnished Orthodoxy. At the Council of Florence in 1439 it was Athonite monks who refused to let the Catholic and Orthodox Churches unite in return for Western military help against the Turk; as a result Constantinople fell to the Ottomans within two decades, but Orthodoxy survived doctrinally intact. That deep pride in Orthodoxy combined with a profound suspicion of all other creeds remains the defining ideology of Athos today.

I disembarked at Daphne, caught the old bus to the monastic capital at Karyes, then walked slowly down the ancient foot-polished cobbles, through knee-high sage and clouds of yellow butterflies, to the *lavra** of Iviron.

The monks had just finished vespers. As it was a lovely balmy

---

* Explanations of all ecclesiastical and technical terms can be found in the glossary.

evening, many were standing around the courtyard enjoying the shade of the cypresses next to the *katholikon*. Fr. Yacovos, the guestmaster, was sitting on the steps of the domed Ottoman fountain, listening to the water dripping from the spout into the bowl. He stood up when he saw me enter the courtyard.

'Welcome,' he said. 'We've been expecting you.'

Yacovos was a garrulous, thick-set, low-slung monk, bearded like a brigand. On his head, tilted at a jaunty angle, sat a knitted black bonnet. He took my bags and led me to the guest room, where he poured a glass of ouzo and offered me a bowl full of rose-scented *loukoumi*. As he did so, he chattered happily about his life in the merchant navy. He had visited Aberdeen on a Cypriot ship in the winter of 1959, he said, and had never forgotten the fog and the bitter cold. I asked where I could find the librarian, Fr. Christophoros. It had been Fr. Christophoros's letter – surmounted by the great Imperial crest, the double-headed eagle of Byzantium – that had originally lured me to Athos. The manuscript I was looking for was in Iviron's monastic library, he had said. Yes, it had survived, and he would try to get the Abbot's permission for me to see it.

'Christophoros will be down at the Arsenal at this time,' said Fr. Yacovos, looking at his fob watch, 'feeding his cats.'

I found the old man standing on the jetty, holding a bucket full of fishtails. A pair of enormous black spectacles perched precariously on his nose. Around him swirled two dozen cats.

'Come, Justinian,' called Fr. Christophoros. 'Come now, Chrysostom, *wisswisswisswiss* . . . Come on, my darlings, *ela*, come . . .'

I walked up and introduced myself.

'We thought you were coming last week,' replied the monk, a little gruffly.

'I'm sorry,' I said. 'I had trouble getting a permit in Thessaloniki.'

The cats continued to swirl flirtatiously around Christophoros's ankles, hissing at each other and snatching at the scattered fins.

'Have you managed to have a word with the Abbot about my seeing the manuscript?'

'I'm sorry,' said Christophoros. 'The Abbot's away in Constantinople. He's in council with the Ecumenical Patriarch. But you're welcome to stay here until he returns.'

'When will that be?'

'He should be back by the Feast of the Transfiguration.'

'But that's – what? – over a fortnight away.'

'Patience is a great monastic virtue,' said Christophoros, nodding philosophically at Kallistos, a rather scraggy, bow-legged old tom-cat who had so far failed to catch a single fishtail.

'My permit runs out the day after tomorrow,' I said. 'They only gave me a three-day *diamonitirion*. I have to leave by the morning boat.' I looked at the old monk. 'Please – I've come all the way just to see this book.'

'I'm afraid the Abbot insists that he must first question anyone who . . .'

'Is there nothing you could do?'

The old man pulled tentatively at his beard. 'I shouldn't do this,' he said. 'And anyway, the lights aren't working in the library.'

'There are some lamps in the guest room,' I suggested.

He paused for a second, indecisive. Then he relented: 'Go quickly,' he said. 'Ask Fr. Yacovos: see if he'll lend you the lanterns.'

I thanked Christophoros and started walking briskly back towards the monastery before he could change his mind.

'And don't let Yacovos start telling you his life story,' he called after me, 'or you'll never get to see this manuscript.'

At eight o'clock, I met Fr. Christophoros outside the *katholikon*. It was dusk now; the sun had already set over the Holy Mountain. In my hands I held the storm lantern from my room. We walked across the courtyard to the monastic library, and from his habit Fr. Christophoros produced a ring of keys as huge as those of a medieval jailer. He began to turn the largest of the keys in the topmost of the four locks.

'We have to keep everything well locked these days,' said Christophoros in explanation. 'Three years ago, in the middle of winter, some raiders turned up in motorboats at the Great Lavra. They had Sten guns and were assisted by an ex-novice who had been thrown out by the Abbot. They got into the library and stole

7

many of the most ancient manuscripts; they also took some gold reliquaries that were locked in the sanctuary.'

'Were they caught?'

'The monks managed to raise the alarm and they were arrested the following morning as they tried to get across the Bulgarian frontier. But by then they had done much damage: cut up the reliquaries into small pieces and removed the best illuminations from the manuscripts. Some of the pages have never been recovered.'

Three locks had now opened without problem; and eventually, with a loud creak, the fourth gave way too. The old library doors swung open, and with the lamps held aloft, we stepped inside.

Within, it was pitch dark; a strong odour of old buckram and rotting vellum filled the air. Manuscripts lay open in low cabinets, the gold leaf of illuminated letters and gilt haloes from illustrations of saints' *Lives* shining out in the light of the lantern. In the gloom on the far wall I could just see a framed Ottoman *firman*, the curving gilt of the Sultan's monogram clearly visible above the lines of calligraphy. Next to it, like a discarded suit jacket, hung a magnificent but rather crumpled silk coat. Confronted dragons and phoenixes were emblazoned down the side of either lapel.

'What is that?' I whispered.

'It's John Tzimiskes's coat.'

'The Emperor John Tzimiskes? But he lived in the tenth century.'

Christophoros shrugged his shoulders.

'You can't just leave something like that hanging up there,' I said.

'Well,' said Christophoros irritably, 'where else would you put it?'

In the gloom, we found our way past rank after rank of shelves groaning with leather-bound Byzantine manuscripts, before drawing to a halt in front of a cabinet in the far corner of the room. Christophoros unlocked and opened the glass covering. Codex G.9 was on the bottom shelf, wrapped up in a white canvas satchel.

It was a huge volume, as heavy as a crate of wine, and I staggered

8

over to a reading desk with it, while Christophoros followed with the lamp.

'Forgive me,' he said, as I lowered the volume gently onto the desk, 'but are you Orthodox or heretic?'

I considered for a second before answering. A Catholic friend who had visited Athos a few years previously had warned me above all never to admit to being a Catholic; he had made this mistake, and said that had he admitted to suffering from leprosy or tertiary syphilis he could not have been more resolutely shunned than he had been after that. He told me that in my case it was particularly important not to raise the monks' suspicions, as they have learned to distrust, above all their visitors, those who ask to see their manuscripts. They have long memories on Athos, and if the monks have never forgiven the Papacy for authorising the ransacking of Constantinople during the Fourth Crusade over eight hundred years ago, they have certainly not forgotten the nineteenth-century bibliophiles who decimated the libraries of Athos only a century ago.

The English traveller the Hon. Robert Curzon is still considered one of the worst offenders: after a quick circuit around the monastic libraries of Athos in the late 1840s (in the company, I am ashamed to say, of my great-great-uncle), Curzon left the Holy Mountain with his trunks bulging with illuminated manuscripts and Byzantine *chrysobuls*; in his travel book *Visits to Monasteries in the Levant* he writes of buying the priceless manuscripts from the Abbot by weight, as if they were figs or pomegranates in an Ottoman market. Worse still is the memory of the German bibliophile Herman Tischendorff. Some twenty years after Curzon's trip to Athos, Tischendorff left the Greek Orthodox Monastery of St Catherine's in Sinai with the *Codex Sinaiaticus* – still the earliest existing copy of the New Testament – tucked into his camel bags. Tischendorff later claimed that he found the various leaves of the manuscript in a basket of firewood, and that he had saved it from the monks, who were intent on burning it to keep them warm in winter. The monks, however, maintain to this day that Tischendorff got the librarian drunk and discreetly swapped the priceless manuscript – which, like Curzon's plunder,

9

duly found its way into the British Library – for a bottle of good German schnapps.

Noticing my silence, Christophoros asked again: What was I, Orthodox or heretic?

'I'm a Catholic,' I replied.

'My God,' said the monk. 'I'm so sorry.' He shook his head in solicitude. 'To be honest with you,' he said, 'the Abbot never gives permission for non-Orthodox to look at our holy books. Particularly Catholics. The Abbot thinks the present Pope is the Antichrist and that his mother is the Whore of Babylon. He says that they are now bringing about the Last Days spoken of by St John in the Book of Revelation.'

Christophoros murmured a prayer. 'Please,' he said, 'don't ever tell anyone in the monastery that you're a heretic. If the Abbot ever found out, I'd be made to perform a thousand prostrations.'

'I won't tell a soul.'

Christophoros relaxed slightly, and took off his glasses to polish them on the front of his habit. 'You know, we actually had another Catholic in the monastery earlier this year?' he said.

'Who was that?' I asked.

'He was a choirmaster from Bavaria,' said Christophorus. 'He had a beautiful voice.'

I eased the book up onto a reading stand, and began to unbutton its canvas cover.

'He said our church had wonderful acoustics,' continued Christophoros, arranging the lamps on the desk. 'So he asked Fr. Yacovos if he could sing a *Gloria* inside the *katholikon*, under the dome.'

'What did Fr. Yacovos say?'

'He said that he didn't think he could let a heretic pray *inside* the church. But just this once he said he would let him sing a little *alleluia* in the porch.'

I had now got the protective canvas off, and the beautifully worked leather binding gleamed golden in the light of the lantern.

I opened the cover. Inside, the text was written in purple ink on the finest vellum – strong, supple and waxy, but so thin as to be virtually translucent. The calligraphy was a beautifully clear and cursive form of early medieval Georgian. According to the library's detailed catalogue, the volume had bound together a number of different early Byzantine devotional texts. The first folio I opened was apparently a shrill sermon by St Jerome, denouncing what he considered the thoroughly pagan practice of taking baths: 'He who has bathed in Christ,' fumed the saint, 'does not need a second bath.'

Only towards the end, on folio 287 verso, did I come to the opening lines of the text I had come so far to see. Its author was the great Byzantine traveller-monk John Moschos, and the book had been compiled at the end of his life as he prepared for death in a monastery in Constantinople, 1,300 years ago.

'In my opinion, the meadows in Spring present a particularly delightful prospect,' he wrote. *'One part of this meadow blushes with roses; in other places lilies predominate; in another violets blaze out, resembling the Imperial purple. Think of this present work in the same way, Sophronius, my sacred and faithful child. For from among the holy men, monks and hermits of the Empire, I have plucked the finest flowers of the unmown meadow and worked them into a crown which I now offer to you, most faithful child; and through you to the world at large . . .'*

Turning up the lamp, I opened a fresh page.

In the spring of the year 578 A.D., had you been sitting on a bluff of rock overlooking Bethlehem, you might have been able to see two figures setting off, staves in hand, from the gates of the great desert monastery of St Theodosius. The two – an old grey-bearded monk accompanied by an upright, perhaps slightly stern, and certainly much younger companion – would have headed off south-east through the wastes of Judaea, towards the fabulously rich port-metropolis of Alexandria.

It was the start of an extraordinary journey that would take John Moschos and his pupil, Sophronius the Sophist, in an arc across the entire Eastern Byzantine world. Their aim was to collect the wisdom of the desert fathers, the sages and mystics of the Byzantine East, before their fragile world – already clearly in advanced decay – finally shattered and disappeared. The result was the volume in front of me now. If today in the West it is a fairly obscure text, a thousand years ago it was renowned as one of the most popular books in all the great literature of Byzantium.

Byzantine caravanserais were rough places, and the provincial Greek aristocracy did not enjoy entertaining: as the Byzantine writer Cecaumenus put it, 'Houseparties are a mistake, for guests merely criticise your housekeeping and attempt to seduce your wife.' So everywhere they went, the two travellers stayed in monasteries, caves and remote hermitages, dining frugally with the monks and ascetics. In each place, Moschos seems to have jotted down accounts that he had heard of the sayings of the fathers, and other anecdotes and miracle stories.

Moschos was taking to an extreme the old Orthodox tradition of the wandering monk. In the West, at least since St Benedict introduced the vow of stability in the early sixth century, monks have tended to be static, immured in their cells: as the saying went, 'A monk out of his cell is like a fish out of water.' But in the Eastern Churches, as in Hinduism and Buddhism, there has always been a tradition of monks being able to wander from guru to guru, from spiritual father to spiritual father, garnering the wisdom and advice of each, just as the Indian *sadhus* still do. Even today, modern Greek Orthodox monks take no vow of stability. If after a period of time in a monastery they decide they want to sit at the feet of another teacher in a different monastery, possibly in a completely different part of Greece (or indeed in Sinai or the Holy Land), then they are free to do so.

The Spiritual Meadow was a collection of the most memorable sayings, anecdotes and holy stories that Moschos gathered on his travels, and was written as part of a long tradition of such *apophthegmata*, or Sayings of the Fathers. However, Moschos's writings are infinitely more evocative, graphic and humorous than those of any of his rivals or contemporaries, and almost alone of the surviving examples of the genre, they can still be read with genuine pleasure.

For as well carrying a still potent spiritual message, on another level the book can be enjoyed today simply as a fascinating travel book. Moschos did what the modern travel writer still does: he wandered the world in search of strange stories and remarkable travellers' tales. Indeed his book can legitimately be read as the great masterpiece of Byzantine travel writing. For not only was Moschos a vivid and amusing writer, he also had an extraordinary tale to tell.

Reading between the lines of John Moschos's memoirs, it is clear that he and his friend were travelling in dangerous times. Following the collapse of Justinian's great attempt at reviving the Empire, Byzantium was under assault: from the west by Avars, Slavs, Goths and Lombards; from the east by a crescendo of raids by desert nomads and the legions of Sassanian Persia. The great cities of the East Mediterranean were in fast decay: in Antioch, huts full of refugees were springing up in the middle of the wide Roman avenues which had once buzzed with trade and industry. The great Mediterranean ports – Tyre, Sidon, Beirut, Seleucia – were becoming idle; many were reverting to little more than fishing villages.

As the physical world fell into decay, thousands left their families, intent, like Moschos and Sophronius, on becoming monks and hermits in the desert. Yet even in the great monasteries there was no safety: frequently the two travellers arrived at a destination to find that the abbey where they intended to spend the night had been torched by raiders, and the monks massacred or led off in great stumbling caravans to the slave markets of Arabia. It was not a picture of total holocaust: in those isolated areas of the Empire unaffected by the Persian wars, the monastic scriptoria and workshops were hard at work producing some of the most beautiful Byzantine manuscripts, ivories and icons ever designed. But these oases of monastic calm were exceptions. John Moschos's writings make clear the horrifying, almost apocalyptic, nature of the destruction he witnessed around him.

In 614 A.D. the travellers' own home monastery of St Theodosius was burned to the ground by the marauding Persian army, and all their brethren – hundreds of unarmed monks –

13

were put to the sword. Shortly afterwards Jerusalem fell and those who survived the massacre – including the city's Patriarch – were led off as slaves to the Sassanian capital of Ctesiphon. From then on John and Sophronius continued on the road as much refugees as travellers. They took shelter in Alexandria, and when the Persians massed outside the city walls, the pair managed to get onto the last galley out of the beleaguered city.

The following year, the two pilgrims finally reached the shelter of the great walls of Constantinople. There, just before exhaustion brought about his death, Moschos completed his travel memoirs. *The Spiritual Meadow* received an ecstatic reception across the Empire. Within a generation or two it had been translated into Latin, Georgian, Armenian, Arabic, and a variety of Slavonic languages; to this day many of its anecdotes are common currency among monks and peasants across the Orthodox world.

Most surviving Byzantine texts from the period have a curiously opaque quality: we read either of the flitting shadows of a hundred upstart emperors, rising suddenly through palace coups and disappearing equally rapidly via the assassin's dagger; or else of saints so saintly as to be virtually beyond comprehension. Nor, for all its often hypnotic beauty, does the surviving corpus of Byzantine art much help in visualising the world that gave it birth. There are the great mosaics at Ravenna with their celebrated portraits of Justinian and Theodora accompanied by their retinues of eunuchs and admirals, generals and bishops, courtiers and sycophants; the same intrigue-ridden court familiar from the written sources. But away from these two isolated Ravenna panels, Byzantine art is strictly non-secular, strictly transcendent. Across the broken apses and shattered naves of a hundred ruined Byzantine churches, the same smooth, cold, neo-classical faces of the saints and apostles stare down like a gallery of deaf mutes; and through this thundering silence the everyday reality of life in the Byzantine provinces remains persistently difficult to visualise. The sacred and aristocratic nature of Byzantine art means that we have very little idea of what the early Byzantine peasant or shopkeeper looked like; we have even less idea of what he thought, what he longed for, what he loved or what he hated.

Yet through the pages of *The Spiritual Meadow* one can come closer to the ordinary Byzantine than is possible through virtually any other single source. Although it often seems a fairly bizarre book – an unlikely fricassee of anecdote, piety and strange miracles – as a historical text it adds up to the most rich and detailed portrait that survives of the Byzantine Levant immediately before the advent of Islam. Through its pages forgotten monasteries rise suddenly from the sand; even a great metropolis such as Byzantine Alexandria – from which not one building, indeed barely one wall, has survived – is brought back to life, peopled by credible characters, villains and eccentrics.

Most intriguing of all are the tales which tell of the more humble folk, the sort who normally slip through the net cast by the historian. One typical story tells of a muleteer from Rome whose donkeys trample and kill a small child at an inn. He takes ship to the Holy Land and flees to the desert, where he is overcome by remorse and tries to kill himself. Only when a lion refuses to savage him does he reconcile himself to the possibility of divine forgiveness. We meet a repentant Alexandrian grave-robber who claims he was seized by a corpse whose shroud he had tried to steal (he was not released until he promised to take up a more respectable profession); a novice who, overcome with desire, pays a visit to the brothel in Jericho (he is quickly struck down by leprosy); a merchant's wife from Ascalon who is forced to prostitute herself after her husband's ship goes down.

Some of the figures are oddly familiar. One story revolves around a Byzantine version of Fr. Christophoros, an animal-loving monk from a suburban monastery outside Alexandria who not only feeds the monastery's dogs, but also gives flour to the ants and puts damp biscuits on the roof for the birds. Other characters are rather more exotic than anything you are likely to find today, such as the monk Adolas who 'confined himself inside a hollow plane tree' in Thessaloniki, cutting 'a little window in the bark through which he could talk with people who came to see him'.

Moschos is an unpredictable narrator. He was a champion of Orthodoxy at a time when it was challenged by a dazzling variety of heterodox currents circulating through the caravan cities of the East, and Monophysites, Jews, Manicheans, Zoroastrians and Gnostics all receive short shrift from a man whose tolerance of the beliefs of others was clearly every bit as limited as that of his modern successors on Mount Athos. Yet there is also a carefree scholar-gypsy feel to *The Spiritual Meadow*, and an endearing lightness of touch and gentle sense of humour evident in its stories. One of my favourite tales concerns a novice from Antinoe in Upper Egypt 'who was very careless with his own soul'. When the novice dies, his teacher is worried that he might have been sent to Hell for his sins, so he prays that it be revealed what has happened to his pupil's soul. Eventually the teacher goes into a trance, and sees a river of fire with the novice submerged in it up to his neck. The teacher is horrified, but the novice turns to him, saying: 'I thank God, oh my teacher, that there is relief for my head. Thanks to your prayers, I am standing on the head of a bishop.'

Of course to the modern eye much of the world described in *The Spiritual Meadow* is not just curious: its beliefs and values are so strange as to be virtually incomprehensible. It was a world where eunuchs led the imperial armies into battle; where groups of monks were known to lynch and murder pagan ladies as they passed in their litters through the fashionable bazaars of Alexandria; where ragged, half-naked stylites raved atop their pillars; and where dendrites took literally Christ's instruction to imitate the birds of the air, living in trees and building little nests for themselves in the upper branches.

But what is perhaps most surprising about the Eastern Mediterranean as it emerges from the pages of Moschos is the fact that it is Christian at all. In the popular imagination, the Levant passes from a classical past to an Islamic present with hardly a break. It is easy to forget that for over three hundred years – from the age of Constantine in the early fourth century to the rise of Islam in the early seventh century – the Eastern Mediterranean world was almost entirely Christian. Indeed, at a time when Christianity had barely taken root in Britain, when Angles and Saxons were still sacrificing to Thor and Woden on the banks of the Thames and in the west the last Christian Britons were fighting a rearguard action under a leader who may have been called Arthur, the Levant was the heartland of Christianity and the centre of Christian civilisation. The monasteries of Byzantium were fortresses whose libraries and scriptoria preserved classical learning, philosophy and medicine against the encroaching hordes of raiders and nomads. Moreover, for all the decay, the Levant was still the richest, most populous and most highly educated part of the Mediterranean world: three quarters of the revenue of the Byzantine exchequer came from the eastern provinces. They contained the main centres of industry and within living memory their ships and caravans had conducted a hugely profitable trade with the Orient; even in the chaos of the late sixth century that trade had still not entirely disappeared. There was nothing in the West to compare with this high Eastern Byzantine culture. In the late sixth century, Byzantium was still the focus of the entire Eurasian land mass.

It was not to remain so for long. John Moschos was an almost exact contemporary of Mohammed. When Moschos died in 619, the Empire was still ruled, however shakily, from the Veneto to Southern Egypt. But a few years later, Moschos's young companion Sophronius saw the eastern half of the Byzantine dominion shatter and fragment. In his old age Sophronius was appointed Patriarch of Jerusalem, and it was left to him to defend the Holy City against the first army of Islam as it swept up from Arabia, conquering all before it.

Fresh from the desert, the Arabs were not very adept at siegecraft: when stalled outside Damascus, the great army of the Prophet had to borrow a ladder from a nearby monastery to get over the walls. But with the Imperial legions already ambushed while crossing the River Yarmuck, there was no prospect of relief for Jerusalem. After a siege lasting twelve months Sophronius prepared to surrender, with only one condition: he would hand Jerusalem over to no general. The Holy City would surrender only to the Caliph himself.

On a February day in the year 638 A.D., the Caliph Omar entered Jerusalem, riding upon a white camel. The Caliph wore the filthy robes in which he had conducted his campaign; but the

Patriarch was magnificently dressed in his robes of Imperial silk. Sophronius handed over the keys of the city and through his tears was heard to murmur: 'Behold the abomination of desolation, spoken of by Daniel the Prophet.'

He died, heartbroken, a few months later. He was buried in the ruins of the Monastery of St Theodosius; in the next niche lay the body of his friend, teacher and travelling companion John Moschos. Sophronius had faithfully honoured his friend's last wish: that his embalmed corpse be carried from Constantinople to be buried in what was left of his own home monastery, at the edge of the deserts of the Holy Land.

I first read about John Moschos in Sir Steven Runciman's great three-volume *History of the Crusades*. Intrigued by a passing reference to *The Spiritual Meadow*, I wrote to Runciman and received – by return of post – a reply in Edwardian copperplate asking me over to the historian's medieval tower house in the Scottish Borders. One cold April day I drove under grey cloudbanks, through the barren sheep tracts of Annandale and Eskdale, to take up the invitation.

Runciman has always been a most undonnish don: he has been besieged by Manchu warlords in the city of Tianjin, but escaped to play a piano duet with the Emperor of China; he has lectured Ataturk on Byzantium and been made a Grand Orator of the Great Church of Constantinople; he has smoked a *hookah* with the *Celebi Effendi* of the Whirling Dervishes and, by reading their tarot cards, correctly predicted the death of King George II of the Hellenes and Fuad, King of Egypt.

He is well into his nineties: a tall, thin, frail old man, still very poised and intellectually alert, but now physically weak. He has heavy-lidded eyes and a slow, gravelly voice, with a hint of an old fashioned Cambridge drawl. During lunch, Runciman talked of the Levant as he knew it in his youth: of Istanbul only a month after the last Ottoman was expelled from the Topkapi, when there

were camels in the streets, when there were still hundreds of
thousands of Greeks in Anatolia, and the Turks still wore the red
tarboosh; of the Lebanon, 'the only place I've seen books bound
in human skin'; of the monasteries of Palestine before the Zionists
expelled half the Palestinians and began to turn the country into
an American suburb; of Egypt when Alexandria was still the most
cosmopolitan city east of Milan.

Later, over coffee, I broached the subject of John Moschos and
his travels. What had attracted me to *The Spiritual Meadow* in
the first place was the idea that Moschos and Sophronius were
witnessing the first act in a process whose dénouement was taking
place only now: that that first onslaught on the Christian East
observed by the two monks was now being completed by Christianity's devastating decline in the land of its birth. The ever-
accelerating exodus of the last Christians from the Middle East
today meant that the *Spiritual Meadow* could be read less as a
dead history book than as the prologue to an unfolding tragedy
whose final chapter is still being written.

Islam has traditionally been tolerant of religious minorities: to
see this, one has only to contrast the relatively privileged treatment
of Christians under Muslim rule with the terrible fate of Christendom's one totally distinct religious minority, the unfortunate
European Jews. Nevertheless that Islamic tradition of tolerance is
today wearing distinctly thin. After centuries of generally peaceful
co-existence with their Muslim neighbours, things are suddenly
becoming difficult for the last Christians of the Middle East.
Almost everywhere in the Levant, for a variety of reasons – partly
because of economic pressure, but more often due to discrimination and in some cases outright persecution – the Christians
are leaving. Today they are a small minority of fourteen million
struggling to keep afloat amid 180 million non-Christians, with
their numbers shrinking annually through emigration. In the last
twenty years at least two million have left the Middle East to make
new lives for themselves in Europe, Australia and America.

In Istanbul the last descendants of the Byzantines are now leaving what was once the capital city of Christendom. In the east of
Turkey, the Syrian Orthodox Church is virtually extinct, its ancient

19

monasteries either empty or in the process of being evacuated. Those who have made it out to the West complain of protection rackets, land seizures and frequent murders. In Lebanon, the Maronites have now effectively lost the long civil war, and their stranglehold on political power has finally been broken. Most Maronites today live abroad, in exile. The same is true of the Palestinian Christians a little to the south: nearly half a century after the creation of the State of Israel, fewer Palestinian Christians now remain in Palestine than live outside it. According to a Palestinian Christian writer I talked to in London, things have got so bad that the remaining Christians in Jerusalem could be flown out in just nine jumbo jets; indeed there are now said to be more Jerusalem-born Christians living in Sydney than in Jerusalem itself. In Egypt, the Copts are also profoundly troubled and apprehensive: already facing a certain amount of discrimination under the current regime, they are well aware that things are likely to get much worse if President Mubarak falls and an Islamic revolution brings the fundamentalists to power.

Everywhere, in short, the living successors of those Christian merchants, monks and bishops visited by John Moschos now find themselves under intense pressure. Yet when I began to research into Moschos's travels, I discovered that despite this great Christian exodus, a surprising number of the monasteries visited by Moschos and Sophronius still – just – survived.

The monasteries on Mount Athos and in Coptic Egypt are apparently relatively healthy. Elsewhere, in south-east Turkey, Lebanon and Palestine, these timeless islands of Byzantium, with their bells and black robes and candle-lit processions, are said to be occupied by an ever-diminishing population of elderly monks whose heavily-whiskered faces mirror those of the frescoed saints on the monastery walls. The monks' vestments remain unchanged since Byzantine times; the same icons are still painted according to the same medieval iconographic rules. Even the superstitions have endured unaltered: relics of the True Cross and the Virgin's Tears are still venerated; demons and devils are still said to lie in wait outside every monastery wall. In the early fifth century Bishop Parthenius of Lampsacus reported that he had been attacked by

Satan in the form of a black dog; on my last visit I was told an almost identical story by an old Greek monk in the Holy Sepulchre. A couple of years ago there was great excitement in a Coptic quarter of Cairo, when the Virgin was clearly seen floating over the towers of the Church of St Damiana.

Driving back home from Runciman, I knew what I wanted to do: to spend six months circling the Levant, following roughly in John Moschos's footsteps. Starting in Athos and working my way through to the Coptic monasteries of Upper Egypt, I wanted to do what no future generation of travellers would be able to do: to see wherever possible what Moschos and Sophronius had seen, to sleep in the same monasteries, to pray under the same frescoes and mosaics, to discover what was left, and to witness what was in effect the last ebbing twilight of Byzantium.

The wooden *simandron* has just begun to call from the church; matins will begin in ten minutes.

Soon it will be dawn. The first glimmer of light has begun to light up the silhouette of the Holy Mountain. The paraffin in my lamp is exhausted, and so am I. The day after tomorrow I must leave Athos; ahead lies four or five days' travel across Thrace to Constantinople, the great Byzantine capital where John Moschos completed his *Spiritual Meadow*.

The *simandron* is being rung for the second time. I must shut this book and go down to the church to join the monks at prayer.

II

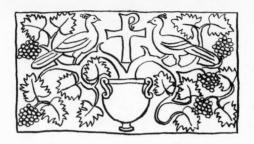

PERA PALAS HOTEL, ISTANBUL, TURKEY, 10 JULY 1994

After the penitential piety of Mount Athos, arriving here is like stepping into a sensuous Orientalist fantasy by Delacroix, all mock-Iznik tiles and pseudo-Ottoman marble inlay. A hotel masquerading as a Turkish bath; you almost expect some voluptuous Turkish odalisque to appear and disrobe behind the reception desk.

I ate breakfast in a vast Viennese ballroom with a sprung wooden floor and dadoes dripping with recently reapplied gilt. The lift is a giant baroque birdcage, entered through a rainforest of potted palms. On the wall nearby, newly dusted, is a framed diploma from the 1932 Ideal Homes Exhibition, signed by the Mayor of East Ham.

The Pera Palas was bought by the Turkish government last year, and attempts to renovate the old structure seem to have started manically, then been abruptly given up. In the dining room the gilt is so bright you have to wear sunglasses to look at it; but upstairs the carpets are as bald as the head of an Ottoman eunuch.

The hotel has a policy of naming its bedrooms after distinguished guests, which has unconsciously acted as a graph of its dramatic post-war decline: from before the war you can choose to sleep in Ataturk, Mata Hari or King Zog of Albania; after it there is nothing more exciting on offer than Julio Iglesias.

At dawn the Sea of Marmara appears like a sheet of silver, with the stationary ships sitting as if welded to its surface. Now, at night, it becomes invisible but for the lights of passing ships and the distant lamps of Uskudar and Kadi Koy – Byzantine Chalcedon – shining across the Bosphorus.

From the old Byzantine Acropolis to the waters of the Golden Horn, the yellow glow of the sulphurous streetlights silhouettes the city's skyline, with its minarets and rippling domes and cupolas. The perfect reflections of the great Ottoman mosques and palaces that form in the water below are intermittently shattered by skiffs and caiques crossing and recrossing the Hellespont. No other city on earth has so magnificent a position. With its remarkable configuration of hills and water, sitting astride the land and sea routes connecting Europe with Asia, the Black Sea with the Mediterranean, and commanding one of the greatest anchorages in the world, there could be no more perfect position for a great imperial city.

For over a thousand years Constantinople was the capital of Christendom, the richest metropolis in Europe and the most populous city west of the great Chinese Silk Route terminus of Ch'ang-an. To the Barbarian West Byzantium was an almost mythical beacon of higher civilisation, the repository of all that had been salvaged from the wreck of classical antiquity. In their sagas, the Vikings called it merely Micklegarth, the Great City. It had no rival.

From the Great Palace on the shores of the Sea of Marmara Justinian, probably the greatest of the Byzantine emperors, controlled an empire that ran from the walls of Genoa clockwise around the Mediterranean to the Pillars of Hercules at Ceuta, embracing Italy, the Balkans, Turkey, the Middle East and the North African littoral. From Constantinople armies were dispatched to build a line of border fortresses on the Tigris, to repair the walls of Rome and to reconquer North Africa from the Vandals. Architects were ordered to construct basilicas in the marshes of Ravenna, on Mount Zion and in the sands of the Sinai. When the Emperor ordered Anthemius of Tralles and Isidore of Miletus to build the greatest church in the world and dedicate it to Haghia Sophia, the Divine Wisdom of Christ, stone was specially brought from as far afield as Libya, the Lebanon, the Atlantic coast of France, Mons Porphyrites in the distant deserts of Southern Egypt and the green marble quarries of Hellenic Sparta.

Half a century later, when John Moschos arrived in Constantinople, the city probably had a population of around three quarters of a million; it was said that seventy-two different tongues could be heard in its streets. Coptic monks rubbed shoulders with Jewish glassblowers, Persian silk traders and Gepid mercenaries who had walked to the city after padding across the ice of the frozen Danube. In the city's great markets and bazaars, Aramaic-speaking Syrians would haggle with Latin-speaking North Africans, Armenian architects and Herule slave traders who knew only some debased dialect of Old German. Goldsmiths, silversmiths, jewellers, ivory carvers, workers in inlay and enamel, weavers of brocade, sculptors and mosaicists all found ready markets for their wares. Already, by the second quarter of the fifth century, the city boasted five imperial and nine princely palaces, eight public and 153 private bath houses; by the time of Justinian there were over three hundred monasteries within its walls.

Few who were brought up in this most cosmopolitan and sophisticated of cities could bear to leave it for long. 'Oh, land of Byzantium, oh thrice-happy city, eye of the universe, ornament of the world, star shining afar, beacon of this lower world,' wrote a twelfth-century Byzantine author forced to absent himself on a diplomatic mission, 'would that I were within you, enjoying you to the full! Do not part me from your maternal bosom.'

After its fall to the Turks in 1453 the importance of the city was, if anything, increased. For the next two hundred years the Ottoman Empire was the most powerful force in all Eurasia, and Constantinople again became the Mediterranean's greatest port. The sixteenth-century Grand Vizier Mehmed Sokollu Pasha simultaneously planned canals between the Don and the Volga, and the Red Sea and the Mediterranean; one day he might send armaments to Sumatra to thwart the Portuguese, the next choose a new King of Poland to thwart the Russians. He ordered pictures and clocks from Venice, decorated his capital with one of the most beautiful mosques ever built, and commissioned an eleven-arched bridge over the River Drina which was only recently destroyed by Croatian bombs.

The achievements of early Ottoman Constantinople were built on the foundation of religious and ethnic tolerance. The great majority of senior Ottoman officials were not ethnic Turks, but Christian or Jewish converts. At a time when every capital in Europe was ablaze with burning heretics, according to the exiled seventeenth-century Huguenot M. de la Motraye there was 'no country on earth where the exercise of all Religions is more free and less subject to being troubled, than in Turkey'. It was the gradual erosion of that tradition of tolerance under the tidal wave of nineteenth-century nationalism that as much as anything finally brought down the Ottomans.

The end result of that sterile hardening of attitudes is that Istanbul, once home to an inspirational ferment of different ethnicities, is today a culturally barren and financially impoverished mono-ethnic megalopolis, 99 per cent Turkish. The Jews have gone to Israel, the Greeks to Athens, the Armenians to Armenia and the United States. The great European merchant houses have returned home, the embassies and the politicians moved to Ankara. For all its magnificent monuments, for the first time in two millennia, Istanbul now feels almost provincial.

It is ten years since my last visit to this city. Since then much has changed: many of the old wooden houses with their intricately latticed balconies have been swept away and replaced by grey apartment blocks. A smart new tram rattles around Sultanahmet, past new flotillas of Russians squatting on the pavements trying to sell their sad piles of Soviet junk: shapeless jeans, hideous shirts and sub-standard leather jackets. There is a blight of seedy news-stands filled with a surprising profusion of Turkish hard porn (there is even a glossy called *Harem*; one notices these things after a week in the celibate purity of Athos). The most striking change of all, however, is the rise of the Islamic right, which this sort of thing has helped to bring about. On every wall are election posters for the hardline *Refah* party, which recently won the municipal elections both here and in Ankara; there is now serious talk of them sweeping into power nationally at the next election. In the meantime many of the young men have taken to wearing thick, moustacheless Islamic beards, while their womenfolk are increasingly shrouded in veils.

In many ways, Turkey's development since the Second World War seems to have followed exactly the opposite course to that of India. There Gandhi tried to wean the whole country onto *dhotis*, non-violence and spinning wheels; the result was crass materialism and the almost daily burning of brides in 'kitchen accidents' if they fail to deliver the new moped or colour television promised as dowry. In Turkey Ataturk tried the reverse approach: he banned the fez, outlawed the Arabic script and tried to drag the Turks kicking and screaming into Europe. The result: a resurgent Islamic movement, mullahs being cheered in the mosques whenever they announce that the earth is flat, and the sophisticated career women of Istanbul competing with each other to wear the most all-enveloping veil or medieval-looking *burkha*.

ISTANBUL, 17 JULY

This afternoon I walked along the Golden Horn to the Phanar, the oldest surviving institution in the city and the nearest thing the Greek Orthodox have to a Vatican. For in a series of humble buildings surrounded by a modest walled enclosure in Istanbul's backstreets lives the successor of St John Chrysostom, the senior Patriarch to millions of Orthodox Christians around the world.

The Patriarch's secretary, to whom Fr. Christophoros had given me an introduction, was out. So while I waited for him to return

I drank tea in a small, dark *chahane* nearby: sawdust on the floor, the acid stink of cheap Turkish cigarettes stinging the nostrils, the incessant thump of heavy hands on wooden card-tables; unshaven, unemployed men playing game after game of poker. Outside a man in a waistcoat, flat cap and dirty apron pushed a handcart of fruit along the cobbles. It could have been a Bill Brandt photograph of the London East End in the thirties.

I walked back to the Phanar an hour later. The Patriarch's secretary had still not returned, but this time I did manage to speak to a member of his staff. Fr. Dimitrios was initially suspicious and evasive, but after reading Fr. Christophoros's letter he took me up to his office overlooking the Patriarchal church. There we talked about the city's dwindling Greek minority, the last descendants of the Byzantines left in what was once their capital city.

According to Fr. Dimitrios the population of Istanbul was still almost 50 per cent Christian at the end of the nineteenth century. The tumultuous events of the first quarter of the twentieth century – the fall of the Ottoman Empire, the Turkish victory in the 1922 Greco–Turkish War and the expulsion of all the Greeks in Anatolia in exchange for the Turkish population evicted from Northern Greece – did not alter this. By the terms of the 1923 Treaty of Lausanne, the 400,000 Greeks in the city and its suburbs were specifically allowed to remain in their homes with their rights and property intact.

All this changed in 1955 when Istanbul played host to the worst race riot in Europe since *Kristallnacht*. In a single night, with the police looking on, thousands of hired thugs descended on the city's Hellenic ghettos. Almost every Greek shop in the city had its windows broken; cemeteries were desecrated; the Tombs of the Patriarchs were destroyed; seventy-three Orthodox churches were gutted.

'I was still a baby,' said Fr. Dimitrios. 'The rioters came into our house, but my mother had wrapped me up in the Turkish flag so the rioters did not harm me; instead they just broke the windows and the furniture then moved on. Afterwards the government said it was just a few ignorant people, but that's not true: the riots were very well organised, all over Istanbul.'

'I don't understand what the Turks would gain by organising such a pogrom,' I said.

'The Greeks still controlled the commerce of the city,' replied Dimitrios. 'They wanted to drive us out and take over our business. They succeeded. By 1965, when I was ten, the Greek population had sunk to around seventy-five thousand. Today there are only – what? – five thousand Greeks left. All my childhood friends, everyone I grew up with, they've all moved away.'

Dimitrios shrugged his shoulders.

'I love this city, of course: it is my home. But frankly life is impossible here if you are not a Turk. The boys get abused on their military service; they are always sent to the most dangerous postings on the Kurdish front line. Then afterwards, when they come out, they can't get government jobs. If you live here you have to spend your life pretending you are Turkish. Those Greeks who have stayed have started calling themselves Turkish names: if you're called Dimitrios, you change your name to Demir; if your name is Fedon, you ask your friends to call you Feridun.'

Dimitrios said that the war in Bosnia – with Orthodox Serbs committing atrocities against Muslims – and the recent resurgence of Islamic fundamentalism in Turkey, had made everything much worse. The Phanar windows were broken by stones on an almost daily basis, while its perimeter walls were regularly covered with spray-painted threats such as 'Patriarch you will die!' Moreover, there had been a renewed bout of grave desecration at the disused Greek cemetery at Yenikoy; blazing rags soaked in petrol had been thrown over the Phanar walls, starting a small fire; and three small firebombs had gone off a month previously in two nearby Greek girls' schools and the Church of the Panaghia.

But the most serious problem, said Dimitrios, revolved around the Phanar gateway. In 1821 the Greeks sealed the main door of the Phanar after the Sultan had hanged the then Patriarch, Gregorios, from its lintel. The Turks always considered the sealing a snub, and recently the *Refah* party had revived the issue by threatening to break open the gate by force. Then last month, on the eve of the anniversary of the fall of Byzantium to the Ottoman Turks, a huge bomb was found planted next to the gate inside

31

the main courtyard. It was defused in time, but had it gone off not only the gate but the entire Phanar would have been reduced to a large crater.

'They left a note near the bombs,' said Dimitrios. 'I've got a translation somewhere.'

He rummaged around in his drawers and drew out a file. From it he took a single sheet of foolscap. 'Read this,' he said.

FROM THE GENERAL HEADQUARTERS OF THE FIGHTERS OF LIGHT

Our administration has targeted the Patriarchate and its occupying leader, who behind what he considers insurmountable walls takes pleasure in the shedding of the blood of the Muslim people of the East, and to this end he is working on suspect and fiendish plans. We will fight until the Chief Devil and all the occupiers are chased off; until this place, which for years has contrived Byzantine intrigues against the Muslim peoples of the East, is exterminated. Occupiers disappear! These Lands are ours and will remain ours. We warn you one more time: there is no right to life for those who are occupiers.

Until the Greek Patriarchate and the Devil, the ridiculous Bartholomaios who wears the robes of the Patriarch, disappears from behind the thick walls where he plans his fiendish intrigues, our fight will continue. Patriarch you will perish!

Long live our Islamic Fight! Long live our Islamic Liberation War!

THE CENTRAL HEADQUARTERS OF LIGHT

'After this,' said Dimitrios, 'our young have finally become convinced that there is no future for them here.'

'I can see their point.'

'Now it's just the old who remain. Our priests here are sick and tired of funerals. A single baptism – or rarer still, a marriage – is the event of the year.'

I asked whether the Phanar was getting enough young priests coming up to keep the place going.

'The Turks closed our only seminary in 1971,' replied Dimitrios. 'It's cut the bloodline of our existence. A decade from now, when the older bishops have all died, there will be no clergy left. After 1,500 years, the Ecumenical Patriarch will have to leave Constantinople.' Dimitrios sighed. 'A century ago this was the centre of Greek Istanbul. Today there are no Greeks at all left around here. On a very good Sunday the Patriarch may still get a hundred people in this church. On a bad one he can't even fill the first two rows of pews. Come down and see what it's like at vespers.'

'Who will be there?'

'I fear just you, me and the angels.'

Fr. Dimitrios's apprehensions were justified. The service had already begun. One old bishop was standing at a lectern chanting hymns for the saint of the day. The other officiating priest, a bent-backed octogenarian, clanked a thurible from behind the iconostasis. There was no congregation in this, the senior church of Eastern Christendom, the Orthodox St Peter's; not one person occupied the empty pews. After a few minutes the bishop gave the dismissal and both old men quickly left the church.

'Look at your watch,' said Fr. Dimitrios. 'Exactly 4.15. It never takes a minute longer when it's an empty church. Our priests don't feel inspired. In fact they feel almost embarrassed.'

From the Phanar I walked through the old city to the Armenian Patriarchate in Kum Kapi, overlooking the Sea of Marmara. In London, Armenian friends had told me horror stories about the fate of the sixty thousand Armenians left in Istanbul: that *Refah* party activists had taken to slopping buckets of human urine into Armenian church services, as well as regularly vandalising the graveyards and churches. My friends had told me that the parish councils hushed these things up for fear that they would be accused of 'making anti-Turkish propaganda', but I hoped that the staff of the Patriarchate might at least be able to confirm or deny what I had heard.

The Patriarchate was a lovely wooden Ottoman building with a pediment and slatted louvres. After a short wait I was shown in to a plump Armenian priest, who called for tea and chatted happily about his trip to England twenty years previously. But when I turned the conversation to politics he just raised his palms and shrugged, indicating clearly – if wordlessly – that it would be undiplomatic for him to comment.

As I was leaving, I mentioned that I had just been to the Phanar: 'Watch out, then,' he whispered. 'The Phanar is full of informers. Your phone will be tapped and they've probably followed you here. Don't leave your notebooks – or anything valuable or incriminating – in your hotel room.'

The old Middle Eastern paranoia, one of the strongest legacies of the Ottomans, a shadow which falls uniformly from the Danube to the Nile. I smiled, but – as always happens after such a warning – did find myself looking behind me on my way back, to see if I was being followed.

Of course, there was nobody there.

ISTANBUL, 20 JULY

John Moschos did not like Constantinople, and he makes this dislike quite apparent in *The Spiritual Meadow*. One of his Constantinople stories concerns the astonishing sexual appetites of the Emperor Zeno; another is about a priest in the capital who 'was indulging in murder and dabbling in witchcraft'; a third is an anti-Semitic rant against a Jewish glassblower who tries to burn his eldest son to death after the boy announces that he plans to convert to Christianity. There are several other such tales, all designed to show the Byzantine capital – 'the city where the wicked rulers lived' – in a very dim light.

In some ways, Moschos's reaction is a little surprising. After all the monk admired the other two great Byzantine metropolises – Antioch and Alexandria – for their learning, and this was something in which the Imperial capital also excelled. Certainly Constantinople's university could not compare with that of Alexandria, but ever since the Emperor Theodosius II endowed a number of chairs in subjects such as medicine, grammar, rhetoric, law and philosophy, it had grown in size and stature, its reputation augmented by the presence nearby of the city's great public library.

Shortly before John Moschos arrived in the capital, his friend and mentor Stephen the Sophist had been lured to Constantinople from the School of Alexandria, where for many years he had lectured on medicine, philosophy, astronomy, astrology, horoscopy and ecclesiastical computus. Stephen should have been able to introduce Moschos to Constantinople's leading luminaries, men like the great historian Theophylact Simocatta; yet there is no indication in Moschos's writing that he met any particularly inspiring figures during his stay in the city.

There was another attraction which should have recommended Constantinople to Moschos: its extraordinary number of sacred relics. Moschos comments on the existence of such relics in almost every place he writes about; only in Constantinople does he omit to mention the number of holy objects on show in the churches, even though the capital's collection was the finest in Christendom. In one shrine alone, that under the Porphyry Column in the Forum of Constantine, were secreted the holy nails used in the crucifixion, the axe with which Noah built the Ark, and the *Dodekathronon*, the twelve baskets in which had been collected the left-over loaves and fishes from the feeding of the five thousand, which had been miraculously rediscovered by the dowager Empress Helena near the Sea of Galilee. Elsewhere in the city could be found the Crown of Thorns, the head of John the Baptist ('complete with hair and beard', according to one source,) the bodies of most of the innocents murdered by King Herod, and great chunks of the True Cross.

However dubious their pedigrees may seem to our eyes, to the

Byzantines relics were objects of priceless value. To see or to touch them was to come into direct contact with a God who was otherwise almost unimaginably distant and inaccessible. Relics were holes in the curtain wall separating the human from the divine. By contemplating them, and by reaching out and touching them, the Byzantines felt they were reaching through the great barrier which separated the visible from the invisible, the mundane from the transcendent. Gregory of Nyssa, a century before Moschos, described the emotion felt by ordinary Byzantines when they touched a sacred relic: 'Those who behold them embrace them as the living body [of the saint] itself; they bring all their senses into play and shedding tears of passion address to the martyr their prayers of intercession as if he were alive and present.'

Moschos must have had good reason to dislike a city full of such precious and holy objects, and a quick reading of the sources gives a good idea of what it was. For it seems that even by metropolitan Byzantine standards, Constantinople was a deeply degenerate place. When Justinian legislated on the Empire's brothels, the law he published contained a preamble which gives some details about the state of the capital's morality. Agents, it seemed, toured the provinces luring girls – some of them younger than ten years old – into their clutches by offering them fine clothes and shoes; once in the capital they were made to sign contracts and provide guarantees for their attendance at their bordello. Otherwise the unfortunate girls were kept imprisoned inside the whorehouses, shackled to their beds.

Nor was Constantinople's aristocratic elite renowned for its marital fidelity. Asterius of Amasia scolded his congregation: 'You change your wives like your clothes, and build new bride-chambers as casually as stalls at a fair.' St John Chrysostom blamed the city's famously lascivious theatre: 'When you seat yourself in a theatre and feast your eyes on the naked limbs of women, you are pleased for a time, but then, what a violent fever you have generated! Once your head is filled with such sights and the songs that go with them, you think about them even in your dreams. You would not choose to see a naked woman in the marketplace, yet you eagerly attend the theatre. What difference does it make if the stripper is a whore? It would be better to smear our faces with mud than to behold such spectacles.'

St John Damascene was even more shocked by what he heard of the 'city filled with impiety'. Constantinople was the setting of dances and jests, he wrote disapprovingly, as well as of taverns, baths and brothels. Women went about with uncovered heads and moved their limbs in a provocative and deliberately sensuous way. Young men grew effeminate and let their hair grow long. Indeed, complained the monk, some went so far as to decorate their boots. In such a climate even the bishops grew foppish. The *Ecclesiastical History* of Socrates talks of Bishop Sisinnios, who 'was accustomed to indulge himself by wearing smart new garments, and by bathing twice a day in the public baths. When someone asked him why he, a bishop, bathed himself twice a day, he replied: "Because you do not give me time for a third." '

The chief witness for the prosecution must, however, be Procopius, Justinian's official court historian. For most of his adult life, Procopius faithfully produced volume after volume of oily sycophancy, praising Justinian for his skill as a general, his taste as a builder and his wisdom as a ruler. Then quite suddenly, towards the end of his life, it seems he could stand it no more. He cracked, and the result was *The Secret History*, a short volume of the purest vitriol, in which the old historian sought to correct the honeyed lies he had been writing for thirty years. Justinian's reign, he wrote, had been an unmitigated disaster, leading to fiascos on many fronts, but above all to a situation of unparalleled moral anarchy. And he knew who to blame: Justinian's wife, the scheming Empress Theodora. Brought up in a circus family,

> as soon as she was old enough she joined the women on the stage and promptly became a courtesan. For she was not a flautist or a harpist; she was not even qualified to join the corps of dancers; but she merely sold her attractions to anyone who came along, putting her whole body at his disposal . . .
>
> There was not a particle of modesty in the little hussy: she complied with the most outrageous demands with-

37

out the slightest hesitation. She would throw off her clothes and exhibit naked to all and sundry those regions, both in front and behind, which the rules of decency require to be kept veiled and hidden from masculine eyes ... In the theatre, in full view of all the people, she would spread herself out and lie face upwards on the floor. Servants on whom this task had been imposed would sprinkle barley grains over her private parts, and geese trained for the purpose used to pick them off one by one with their bills and swallow them.

She used to tease her lovers by keeping them waiting, and by constantly playing about with novel methods of intercourse, she could always bring the lascivious to her feet; so far from waiting to be invited by anyone she encountered, by cracking dirty jokes and wiggling her hips suggestively she would invite all who came her way, especially if they were still in their teens. Never was anyone so completely given over to unlimited self-indulgence. Often she would go to a dinner party with ten young men or more, all at the peak of their physical prowess and with fornication as their chief object in life, and would lie with all her fellow diners in turn the whole night long: when she had reduced them all to a state of physical exhaustion she would go to their menials, as many as thirty on occasion, and copulate with every one of them; but not even so could she satisfy her lust.

And so it goes on, for (in the Penguin edition) 194 pages. It seems likely that Procopius had some personal grudge against the Empress, who may have been responsible for blocking his promotion or somehow harming his career. Even so, it is a remarkable testimony. At the end of the book, Procopius tells of Theodora's attempts in her old age to control prostitution. Overcome with guilt for her former sins, she closed the brothels, bought up all the prostitutes, and put them in a former Imperial palace which she converted into a Convent of Repentance.

38

But, notes Procopius, this was one of Theodora's less popular enterprises. According to him, the girls found this new way of life so dull that most 'flung themselves down from the parapet during the night' rather than be turned into nuns.

In the cool of the evening I walked over to the Hippodrome. In what was once the stalls, where the violent Byzantine circus factions once knifed it out, large Turkish ladies in headscarves now sit quietly gossiping on park benches. Their husbands squat nearby, under the chestnuts, cracking pistachio nuts. The occasional salesman with a glass cupboard on wheels wanders past, hawking paper cones full of chickpeas. Gulls hover silently overhead. It is strange to think that the hippodrome once held 120,000 people – double the present-day capacity of Wembley Stadium.

The obelisk of the Emperor Theodosius still stands in the centre of the old racetrack, rising from the plinth where it was placed in the 430s. A carving on the side shows the cat's-cradle of ropes and pulleys which was used to raise it. On another face is carved a picture of the Emperor in the imperial baldachin overlooking the races; these are illustrated at the base with a series of small relief carvings of what look like horse-drawn bathtubs.

Between the Emperor and the charioteers stand his bodyguard, a remarkably effeminate gaggle of fops with long floppy 1970s fringes, every bit as willowy as St John Damascene's blood-and-fire sermons might have led one to expect. Certainly these gentle cosmopolitans not only look remarkably unthreatening, they appear to be much more interested in the races than in guarding the Emperor. Here could lie part of the explanation for the large number of successful assassination attempts in Byzantine history.

At the end of the Hippodrome, then as now, rises the great dome of Justinian's Haghia Sophia, the supreme masterpiece of Byzantine architecture, and still, in the eyes of many, the most beautiful church ever built. No other Christian building is so successful in transporting one to the threshold of another world, or so dazzlingly intimates the imminence of the transcendent. In the golden haze of its interior, with its extraordinary play of light and space, precious stone and mosaic, under a dome that blazes like the vault of Heaven, even the solid walls seem to cease being barriers and become like passages into a higher reality. When it was first built in the 530s, Procopius, in one of his finest passages, described the overwhelming effect it has on the visitor. 'So bright is the glow of the interior that you might say that it is not illuminated by the sun from the outside but that the radiance is generated within,' he wrote in *The Buildings*. 'Rising above is an enormous spherical dome which seems not to be founded on solid masonry, but to be suspended from heaven by a Golden Chain. Whenever one goes into this church to pray, one understands immediately that this work has been fashioned not by human power and skill, but by the influence of God. And so the visitor's mind is lifted up to God and floats aloft, thinking that He cannot be far away, but must love to dwell in this place which He himself has chosen.'

The power of the building has not been diminished by fourteen hundred years of earthquakes and rebuildings, the destruction of much of its mosaic, the stripping of its altars, nor even a city fire which caused molten lead from the dome to run down the gutters in a flood of boiling metal. As you stand in the narthex you can see even the gossiping tour groups falling silent as they enter the dome chamber; if anyone talks they do so in a hushed whisper. The sacred breaks in on the mundane; and one immediately understands what a Byzantine monk must have felt when he touched a relic or gazed at a sacred icon: for a moment the gates of perception open and one catches a momentary glimpse of the Divine. Here, as nowhere else, one is transported back to the mental world of the Byzantium of John Moschos.

Yet the miraculous preservation of this one building – judged by the Byzantines themselves as their most perfect creation – can easily blind one to the amount that has been lost. Geography apart, John Moschos would not recognise much in this city if he came back today. Of the five hundred churches and monasteries which once decorated the land rising up from the Golden Horn, the remains of less than thirty survive, most of them rebuilt and converted into mosques.

This morning I visited the site of St Polyeuctes, once the greatest church in the whole Christian Empire; Justinian was said to have built Haghia Sophia in an attempt to match it. It would have been a familiar monument to John Moschos; indeed it was probably in a monastery attached to some great church like this that he lodged when he came to the city to finish *The Spiritual Meadow*.

The church fell into disrepair, and after the Turkish conquest of 1453 it collapsed and was forgotten. In 1960 it was accidentally rediscovered. Briefly it became famous again, and art historians and archaeologists triumphantly announced that many of the innovations of Justinian's reign were pre-empted by the work at St Polyeuctes.

Thirty years later the various archaeological reports are gathering dust, and St Polyeuctes seems to be returning to the earth. The ruins are an open latrine, and stink too badly to be examined at any length; only the most desperate Turkish tramps linger in its portals. Meanwhile the famous capitals – supposedly the first of the characteristic Byzantine basketwork impost-capitals that were to reach their fullest glory in Ravenna – are scattered around a nearby playground, where they provide seats for courting Turks. This means that anyone who wishes to study this crucial phase of early Byzantine sculpture is forced to spend an afternoon peering like a pervert beneath the legs of entwined couples.

Secular Byzantine architecture has fared even worse. The great Theodosian land walls, in their day the most sophisticated defensive military architecture the world had ever seen, are still there; there is also the great fourth-century aqueduct of Valens and a pair of superb arcaded cisterns dating from the time of Justinian. Yet not one single house from Byzantine Constantinople still stands. Even the two largest Imperial palace complexes, the Great Palace and the Palace of Blanchernae, have disappeared but for a few arches, a line of windows, some buried foundations and a few splendid floor mosaics.

I spent much of the afternoon in the Mosaic Museum, admiring what has survived. All the work there dates from the late sixth century – just after the reign of Justinian – and is from the Great Palace, which once occupied the slope behind the Blue Mosque. These then are the very floors that the Emperor Heraclius must have paced as he heard of the Persian capture of Jerusalem or the fall of Alexandria.

The initial impression is of the unexpectedly persistent Hellenism. The style of most of the mosaics is pastoral and bucolic, and their warm naturalism seems at first to have more in common with the delicate frescoes of Pompeii than with the stiff, hieratic inhabitants of later Byzantine icons or the unsmiling *Pantocrators* which overwhelm the domes of so many medieval Byzantine churches. It is only after you have been in the museum for some time and look a little closer at the pastoral idylls that you begin to worry about the mental state of the mosaic-makers, or perhaps that of their patrons.

At first sight a horse appears to be giving suck to a lion: the perfect symbol of peace, like the Biblical wolf lying down with lamb. Only when you look closely do you see that what is actually happening is that the lion is ripping the stomach out of the horse and biting off its testicles. Another lion rears up and attacks an elephant, but misjudges his leap and impales himself on a tusk. A wolf tears off the neck of a deer. Two gladiators in leather hauberks and plus-fours await the charge of a pink tiger (the tiger is already badly wounded in the neck, and blood is pouring out of its mouth). Elsewhere a winged gryphon swoops down and rips the back of an antelope; another gobbles up a lizard.

One can only speculate what induced the head mosaicist to make his creations so psychopathically violent: after all, with assassinations and palace coups as frequent as they were, it can hardly have been very calming for the Emperor to have to walk over these scenes of gruesome blood-letting day after day. On the other hand they are certainly a blessed antidote to the gloomy piety of most Byzantine literature: those endless saints' *Lives* with their heroic ascetics resisting the lascivious enticements of demonic temptresses. Indeed, after enduring one of the Patriarch's two-hour sermons on chastity, the Emperor may actually have been relieved to return to these lively scenes of carnage and mayhem.

On the way back I passed through the Gulhane Gardens surrounding the Topkapi Palace. As I passed I was surprised to see that the basilica of Haghia Eirene appeared to be open. This was unexpected because, for some reason best known to the Turkish authorities, this magnificent building, one of the very greatest Byzantine churches surviving in the city, is normally kept resolutely locked. This time, however, the door was open and a couple of sophisticated-looking Turkish women were sitting chatting in the porch.

I thought I would take the opportunity to have a look at the church, but as I wandered past the women one of them called out: 'I'm sorry, you can't go in there. It's closed.'

'It looks open.'

'I'm afraid you need a special pass to go in. For security reasons.'

'What do you mean?'

'There are VIPs inside.'

'Politicians?'

'No. Models.'

'Models?'

'Today they are having a beauty contest.'

'In a church?'

'Why not? All Turkey's top models are there. They are currently changing into Rifat Ozbek bikinis.'

Hagia Eirene is the worst possible place to have a beauty contest: it is dark, gloomy and badly lit. But the Greeks desperately want this church back, and the Turks will go to any length, however absurd, to annoy their hereditary enemies. No doubt, however, the Greeks play similar games with the abandoned mosques of Salonica. They would probably do the same to those in Athens, too, had they not bulldozed the lot in the 1920s, in a sadly characteristic outbreak of virulent nationalism.

By ferry to the island known to the Turks as Buyuk Ada, and to the Greeks as Prinkipo. Hazy, all-enveloping heat. Boys bathing by the Bosphorus. The scent of sea-salt, hot wood, rotting fish. We pull away from the Golden Horn, pass around the wooded ridge of the Topkapi Saray, and head out across the narrow stretch of water that separates Europe from Asia.

The other passengers: beside me, a sad-eyed conscript, perhaps eighteen years old, in ill-fitting fatigues. Small moustache. Cropped hair. Gazes vacantly over the sea. Perhaps he is on his way to do his military service on the Kurdish front.

Opposite, a girl in a lilac headscarf and long Islamic raincoat. She is earnestly studying an English-language pharmacology textbook: 'Chapter Two – Drug Permeation'.

On the bench at the back, an old labourer with toothbrush moustache and no teeth. Unbuttoned flies. Cigarette hangs from the side of his mouth.

Shady-looking character in tight T-shirt. Stubble chin. He clacks worry beads from the palm to the back of his hand, and darts furtive looks around him. Fare dodger?

Shaven-headed sailor in war-movie sailor's suit. Thickset and swarthy. His cap is on his knee. Drags deeply on a cigarette, then loses interest and throws it overboard.

Moving from bench to bench: a blind violinist, led by his son who bangs a small wooden hand-drum. Both wear flat caps.

Various salesmen selling Coke, biros, potato peelers, Rolex watches (fake), Lacoste socks (fake), Ray-Ban sunglasses (also fake) and Bic cigarette lighters (apparently genuine, but of the poorest quality). I buy a Coke and it turns out to be a fake too: tastes of warm deodorant.

Halfway through the voyage another fearsome-looking head-scarf-and-raincoat lady appears at the top of the stairwell and begins to harangue us all. I assume she is telling us to vote *Refah*, or ticking off those few middle-aged women who are not wearing a veil. But I'm quite wrong. Her daughter is in hospital and she needs money for medicine. The passengers give generously, especially the old labourer with the open flies, who extinguishes his cigarette to dig deep in his pockets.

The Byzantines used Prinkipo as a prison, and exiled a succession of crooked chancellors and plotting princes to its monasteries. The Ottomans turned it into summer resort, and so it remains: a thin line of lovely slatted wooden houses, with carved balustrades and lattices, prettily painted in cream and light blue. But the site of one of the old monasteries is still an active shrine, and it was there that I was heading. Fr. Dimitrios had told me about it. The Shrine of St George was an example, he said, of something which was once common, but is now rare: a holy place sacred to both faiths, where Greeks and Turks still pray side by side.

Because of a local by-law cars are banned from the island, so at the jetty I hailed an old horse-drawn phaeton. We trotted along the cobbles, up the hill, with gardens and orchards on either side. Apples and apricots hung heavily on the trees; bougainvillaea and jasmine blossomed over orchard walls.

A century ago Prinkipo was exclusively Greek, and today one or two old Hellenes still cling on to their houses: large, ostentatious wooden buildings with pediments and pillars. Occasionally, as we passed the manicured lawns, we caught glimpses of old Greek women sitting in the shade of magnolia trees with shiny green leaves and thick creamy flowers; some were sewing, others sipping glasses of sherbet.

We drove out of the town and up the mountain; pine forests replaced orchards and thick carpets of pine needles rotted in the wheel-ruts. Other than the clip-clop of the horse and the rattle of other phaetons taking farmers and pilgrims back into town, it was completely silent.

After twenty minutes, the driver dropped me beside a graveyard at the bottom of the dusty path leading up to the shrine. Before climbing the hill, I looked inside. It was the last Greek graveyard in Turkey still in use. I wandered through the unkempt memorials, overgrown and unswept, carpeted now, like the road outside, by a thick muffling of pine needles. Many of the headstones were decorated with photographs. Paradoxically, I found that it was these photographs of dead people from a deserted graveyard which, more than anything else, brought to life the world of the Greek Istanbul which had been ended by the 1955 riots.

Fr. Dimitrios had described those who had left – the Greeks who formed such an influential minority in the Istanbul of the nineteenth century – as cosmopolitan, artistic and well educated; but the photographs, less nostalgic, revealed a prosperous petit-bourgeois society of shopkeepers and spinsters: moustaches and double chins, waistcoats and fob watches, bald spots and pinces-nez; line upon line of plump, suspicious men, grown prematurely old in their confectionery shops, moustaches bristling in late Otto-man indignation; pairs of old ladies shrouded in funereal black, plain and bitter, all widows' weeds and pious scowls.

Walking up the hill, among the ebb and flow of pilgrims, I marvelled at what I took to be thick white hibiscus blossom on the bushes near the summit. Only when I reached the top did I see what it really was: on every bush the pilgrims had tied strips of cloth, primitive fertility charms, to the branches. Some were quite elaborate: small cloth hammocks supporting stones or pebbles or small pinches of pine needles. Others were tangled cat's-cradles of threads wrapped right around the bushes, as if packaged for the post.

Inside the shrine it was just as bizarre. At some stage a fire had half-gutted the building, leaving charred rafters and singed window frames standing in the open air. But the rooms, though half exposed and quite unrestored, were filled by a continuous trickle of supplicants. The two nationalities were praying side by side; but they were not praying together. The Greeks stood in front of the icon of the mounted saint, hands cupped in prayer. The Turks put prayer carpets on the floor and bent forward in the direction of Mecca. One veiled Muslim lady scraped with long nails at a tattered nineteenth-century fresco of the saint, then with her fingertip touched a fragment of the paintwork to her tongue.

'The Muslims also believe in St George,' explained a young Greek student I met waiting by the jetty half an hour later. 'They hear St George is working miracles so they come here and ask him for babies. Maybe they don't know he is Greek.'

'They probably think he is Turkish,' said her friend.

'Probably,' said the first girl. 'They think everything is Turkish. I've heard boys say Haghia Sophia and the Hippodrome were built by the Seljuk Turks.'

'They don't know history,' agreed the second girl. 'One day some boy asked my sister, "Why did you Greeks come here? All you do is make trouble." She said, "We didn't come: you did."'

'They even think Homer was one of them,' sighed the first girl. 'They say he was a Turk and that his real name was Omar.'

ISTANBUL, 1 AUGUST

11 p.m.: I have just returned from supper with Hugh Pope, Turkey correspondent of the *Independent*. We ate in a fish restaurant at Bebek, five miles up the Bosphorus, overlooking Asia. Talk soon turned to the Kurdish war currently raging in the southeast.

'At least fifty people are being killed every day,' he said. 'Unless at least two hundred are gunned down, I don't even bother calling the Foreign Desk.'

Hugh told me that the previous December, when the *Independent* sent him to Diyarbakir, he managed to get through to the largest of the surviving Syrian Orthodox monasteries in the southeast, Mar Gabriel. The day before he arrived, a lorry had hit an anti-tank mine two hundred metres from the monastery's front gate. As he drove up, the charred corpse of the driver was still sitting in the burned-out skeleton of the truck, hands welded to the wheel. The mine had apparently been placed by the PKK, the Revolutionary Kurdistan Workers' Party, and was thought to have been aimed at village guards – in the eyes of the PKK, collaborators with the Turkish government – passing on their way to the neighbouring village of Güngören. Although the mine's target did not seem to have been the monastery, it dramatically brought home to the monks how vulnerable they were to being caught in the crossfire between the PKK and the government.

According to Hugh, the Kurdish guerrillas dislike the Suriani Christians as much as the local government does, accusing them of being informers, just as the authorities accuse them of being PKK sympathisers. Moreover, the Kurds have much to gain by driving the Suriani out: they can then occupy their land and farm it themselves.

Yet the problems faced by the Christians and the Kurds have similar roots. The Ottoman Empire was administered by a system which allowed, and indeed thrived on, diversity. Each *millet* or religious community was internally self-governing, with its own laws and courts. The new Turkey of Ataturk went to the opposite extreme: uniformity was all. The vast majority of Greeks were expelled, and those who remained had to become Turks, at least in name. The same went for the Kurds. Officially they do not exist. Their language and their songs were banned until very recently; in official documents and news broadcasts they are still described as 'Mountain Turks'.

It is this ludicrous – and deeply repressive – fiction that has led to the current guerrilla war. Because of it the rebels of the PKK are now involved in a hopeless struggle to try and gain autonomy for the Turkish Kurds, something Ankara will never allow. More than ten thousand people have been killed in the south-east of Turkey in the last five years, and great tracts of land and around eight hundred villages have been laid waste in an effort to isolate and starve out the guerrillas. At least 150,000 Turkish troops are tied down in the mountains of the south-east, fighting perhaps ten thousand PKK guerrillas. At the moment the government seems to have the upper hand, and it is said the average life expectancy of a guerrilla is now less than six months.

Hugh says that the fighting, though currently intermittent, is expected to reach a new climax in the coming weeks: summer is the fighting season.

I plan to set off to the south-east next week. Antioch – modern Antakya – is on the edge of the trouble. Once there it should be easier to judge how bad things really are: it is virtually impossible to gauge the difficulty of getting to the Syrian Orthodox monasteries from here, and the situation changes from day to day. *Inshallah* it should be possible to get through without taking any unreasonable risks. Hugh has given me the name of a driver in Diyarbakir who last year was willing – for a price – to drive him into the war zone.

He also raised the question of whether I should get a press card. On the one hand, he says, the authorities in the south-east hate all journalists: last year his wife was beaten up by the police in Nusaybin when she produced her card. On the other hand, he says that no one will believe me if I say I'm a tourist – no tourist has gone anywhere near the south-east for three or four years now – and if I have no Turkish ID he tells me that there is a real possibility that I could get arrested for spying.

On my return from supper I asked the advice of Mettin, the hotel receptionist, whose home is in the south-east. He seems to think my plans are hysterically funny. 'Don't worry, you'll only get shot if you run into a PKK roadblock, and only get blown up if you drive over a landmine. Otherwise the south-east is fine. Completely safe. In fact highly recommended.'

Becoming serious, Mettin said that if the police did not arrest me, and if I did not drive over any landmines, there was always the delightful possibility of being kidnapped by the PKK. This happened last year to three British round-the-world cyclists. They were not in the least harmed, but as the guerrillas cannot light fires – that would reveal their whereabouts to the army – the hostages were forced to live for three months on snake tartare and raw hedgehog.

'The tourists should consider themselves lucky,' said Mettin. 'If it had been Turkish soldiers that had fallen into the PKK's hands, they would have had their dicks cut off. *Then* the PKK would kill them. Roasted them over a fire or something. Very slowly. Chargrilled them.'

'And this sort of thing still goes on?'

'These guys are committing mass murder *right now*,' answered Mettin.

'But they only do that to Turkish soldiers, right?'

'You can't be too careful in the east,' said Mettin, twirling his moustache. 'As they say in Ankara: Kurdistan is like a cucumber. Today in your hand; tomorrow up your arse.'

ISTANBUL, 3 AUGUST

My last day in Istanbul; tonight the train.

This morning I went to the Phanar to say goodbye to Fr. Dimitrios, and to collect the letters of introduction he has written to the *hegumenoi* (abbots) of the Greek monasteries in the Holy Land and Sinai.

Running down the stairs from Fr. Dimitrios's office, I knocked into a visiting Greek monk who was crouching in the doorway leading into the courtyard, feeding the sparrows. I apologised and we fell into conversation. He said he had been to England once but did not like it much. 'It was so sad,' he remarked. 'All the churches were closed. In Ipswich I went. Not one church was open. Not one!' He added darkly: 'I read in a magazine that the head of the Satan Cult lives in England.'

He disliked London and was unimpressed by Buckingham Palace. In fact only two places really appealed to him. One was Kew: 'Your Kew Gardens! So beautiful! So lovely! I would feed the squirrels and bring them nuts.' The other was a shop in Lambeth which sold religious trinkets. From his suitcase the monk produced a small plastic hologram of Christ. 'It is so beautiful, no? It is by a Swiss artist and is based on the exact likeness of Jesus. Some of the other monks think it is not pleasing to look

50

at, but I do not understand why. Walk around: look! Now our Lord is smiling! Now he is showing his sobriety! Now he is dead. Now he is risen! Alleluia! It is so beautiful, no? I carry it with me always.'

A night ferry across the black Bosphorus to Hyderpasha, the Anatolian railhead of the old Berlin to Baghdad railway that T. E. Lawrence spent so long trying to blow up. Tomorrow to Ankara to pick up my press card.

On the train the conductor had no record of my reservation. But he asked me my nationality, and when I told him, I thought I saw a brief flicker of terror cross his face; certainly, I was immediately upgraded to first class. Only when I sat eating supper in the station restaurant did I discover the reason for this uncharacteristically flexible behaviour: there was a European Cup soccer match that evening between Manchester United and Galatasaray, and the television news was full of the English visitors' traditional pre-match activities: trashing restaurants, picking fights, beating up innocent Turks and so on. For the first time I felt grateful for English football's international reputation for hooliganism: it seemed that my compatriots from Manchester had unknowingly guaranteed me a first-class berth for the night.

NIGHT BUS BETWEEN ANKARA AND ANTIOCH, 6/7 AUGUST

4.15 a.m.: This is a horrible way to travel. It is nearly dawn, and the first glimmer of light has illuminated an expanse of flat plains covered by a wraith of thin mist. The rutted roads, the bracing crash of the long-defunct suspension, the snoring Anatolian peasants: these one expects and can bear. What is intolerable is the deliberate regime of sleep deprivation imposed on all passengers by this driver and his henchman, the moustachioed Neanderthal of a conductor.

Every other hour we pull in to some seedy kebab restaurant. The lights are put on, we are shaken awake and a Turkish chanteuse is put on the Tannoy so loud that we have no option but to vacate the bus. The driver and his friend disappear behind the scenes to pick up their commission from the restaurant owner, while we are all expected to make merry with plateloads of malignant kebabs or, even more horrible in the middle of the night, bags full of sickly-sweet Turkish delight.

Worse is to follow. On returning to our seats, the Neanderthal marches down the aisles, gaily shaking *eau de cologne* over the outstretched hands of the passengers. This can be quite refreshing at three o'clock on a hot afternoon; but it is irritating beyond belief at three o'clock in the dull chill of the early morning. And so on we trundle, rattling and shaking like a spin dryer, smelling like a tart's boudoir, tempers rising steadily with each stop.

6 a.m.: We pull in to a particularly run-down *kebabji* which, with horrible inevitability, has suddenly materialised from nowhere amid the grey wastes of Anatolia. We stumble out of the bus and obediently line up for our breakfast, smelling like a collection of extras from some spectacular epic of an after-shave advertisement. Too weak to argue, too tired to care, I join the queue and load my plate with some slurry that must once have been an aubergine.

8 a.m.: Issus, site of Alexander's great victory over the Persians. It may be one of the turning points in world history, but it's a miserable-looking place now: a scrappy village with a petrol pump, a derelict electricity station and the statutory seedy restaurant over which hangs a terrible smell of grease and dead animal.

My neighbour in the bus, a garrulous traffic policeman from Istanbul, made the mistake of eating a kebab at the last stop and is now being noisily ill in the street; he has attracted a small circle of onlookers who appear to take the view that this is the most interesting thing to have happened in Issus for several months. Despite the early hour, it is already hot and muggy. We're through the Cilician Gates and heading into the plains. On the far side of the road parties of bedraggled peasants are standing in lines, hoeing the dead ground beside the cotton and tobacco fields – or at least some are: most have put down their implements to watch my friend's streetside evacuations.

The men here are a rough-looking bunch, scowling, ill-kempt and unshaven. But – looking around the motley crew filling the tables around me, and glimpsing my own reflection in the mirror – who are we to talk?

9 a.m.: Antioch: a gridiron of dirty alleyways surrounded on three sides by the crescent cliffs of Mount Silpius. As we leave the bus for the last time and stumble into the glare of the bus station the smirking Neanderthal offers us a last splash of *eau de cologne*. I shake my head, but get the horrible stuff poured all over me anyhow.

BUYUK ANTAKYA OTELI, ANTIOCH, 11 AUGUST

Cleansed, vowing never again to go on a night bus, nor ever again to touch *eau de cologne*, I went to bed for the rest of the morning, lulled to sleep by some of John Moschos's more soporific miracle stories: tales of doughty Byzantine hermits fending off the advances of demonic temptresses and saucy 'Ethiopic boys'.

With the exception of the mosaics in the museum and a few fragments of the much-rebuilt town walls, it seems that barely one stone remains from what was once the third greatest metropolis in the Byzantine Empire and briefly, under Julian the Apostate, its capital. Of the city's famous buildings – Constantine's Golden Octagon, the Council Chamber where Libanius declaimed, the great hippodrome that could seat eighty thousand people – nothing now remains. Like Alexandria, its traditional rival, Byzantine Antioch is now just a city of memory, forgotten but for the conjectures of scholars.

There is a reason for this. The city is built in the centre of an earthquake zone and has been levelled again and again, at least once every two hundred years. Today it is a sleepy, provincial place, architecturally undistinguished but for a few fine late-Ottoman villas decorated with carved wooden balustrades and with vines tumbling over the shuttered windows. Other than the occasional archaeologist, no one really bothers to come to Antioch any more: not the Turkish politicians, not the journalists, not the tourists, not even the PKK.

It is odd to think that all Europe, much of the Middle East and the entire length of the North African coast was once ruled from this little market town, today a forgotten backwater even by Turkish standards. Perhaps one day Los Angeles or San Francisco will be like this.

When John Moschos visited Antioch in the 590s, there were already many signs that the city was in serious decline. The School of Antioch, once one of the most sophisticated of all theological schools, was no longer in its prime. The days of John Chrysostom and Theodore of Mopsuestia were long past, even though it was probably at this time that Theodore of Tarsus came to the city to receive his training in the Antioch tradition of Biblical exegesis, a training he later brought with him to Anglo-Saxon England when he was appointed the seventh Archbishop of Canterbury. Antioch's port, Seleucia ad Pieria, was beginning to silt up, and the great trade of the Mediterranean had begun passing the city by. The bazaars were empty but for local agricultural produce, and refugees were setting up shacks where once great caravans of merchants traded in silks and spices from Persia, India and the East.

Moreover, corruption had set in, and the city had the most dubious reputation. When the Emperor framed a troublesome Bishop of Antioch for consorting with a prostitute, no one for a minute doubted the bishop's guilt. The Antioch theatre was famed

54

for its great aquatic spectacles featuring (as one source puts it) 'large numbers of naked girls from the lower classes', and the city's eighteen public baths were as disreputable as any in the Empire. St John Chrysostom, later the scourge of Constantinople, began his career as moral watchdog in Antioch, where he attacked the institution of 'spiritual partnerships' between monks and nuns and for good measure went on to accuse the city's upper-class women of habitually exposing themselves before the eyes of their servants, 'their softly nurtured flesh draped only in heavy jewellery'.

But it was sorcery that was the declining city's greatest vice. In an age when demons were considered to fill the air as thickly as flies in a Turkish market (Gregory the Great always used to recommend making the sign of the cross over a lettuce in case you swallowed a demon that happened to be perched on its leaves), in Antioch things had come to such a pass that demonic activities were rife even among the clergy – or so it was whispered. The Antioch hippodrome was a famous centre of such witchery: not only were all kinds of magic practised there against horses and charioteers, but the galleries were packed with nude classical statues believed to be the haunt of those demons who specialised in exciting the carnal passions. Indeed the Byzantine version of the Faust tale involved a Jewish necromancer leading a presbyter to the hippodrome in the middle of the night. The Presbyter has been sacked from his position as *oikonomos* (treasurer) by the new bishop. The necromancer succeeds in conjuring up Satan himself, who promises to help the presbyter regain his former position if he first agrees to become the Servant of Darkness, and kisses his cloven foot in submission. The presbyter does as he is bidden, and sells his soul to the Devil.

Surrounded by similar stories, the worried Antiochians looked for guidance not to their clergy, nor to the Byzantine governor or the *magister militum*. Instead they turned to St Symeon Stylites the Younger, a renowned hermit who had set up his pillar a few miles outside the city. From there he issued a series of dreadful threats and warnings to the faithful, calling on them to repent and mend their ways.

His powers were remarkable. According to his anonymous hagiographer the dust from his clothes was more powerful than roasted crocodile, camel dung or Bithynian cheese mixed with wax – apparently the usual contents of a Byzantine doctor's medicine chest. This dust could cure constipation, cast leprosy on an unbeliever, bring a donkey back to life and restore sour wine to sweetness. It was clearly a particularly handy thing to have on board ship in the event of a storm. A certain Dorotheus, a cleric at Symeon's monastery, sailed during the forbidden period of the year in the midst of winter, trusting to the protection of his stylite master. Far out to sea, however, the vessel ran into a tremendous storm which lashed it with waves so high they rolled over the deck. The Captain was in despair, but Dorotheus took some dust which had been blessed by St Symeon and sprinkled the ship with it; 'a sweet fragrance filled the air, the churning sea was pacified, a fair wind filled the sails and safely brought the ship to its destination.'

Symeon was clearly not a man to be trifled with. An Antiochian brickmaker who privately voiced his view that Symeon's miracles might not be the work of God but instead of the Devil found that his hand promptly turned putrid, and 'it was only after he shed many tears of repentance that he was forgiven and restored to health'. Symeon could have an equally dramatic effect on other parts of the body. Moschos tells a story of a renegade monk who gave up the habit, left his monastery in Egypt and settled in Antioch. One day, on his way back to town from a trip to the coast, the ex-monk decided to visit Symeon's pillar. He had no sooner entered the enclosure than the stylite pointed him out amid the crowd of assembled pilgrims: 'Bring the shears!' cried Symeon, miraculously divining his visitor's monastic past. 'Tonsure that man!'

Packing him off back to his Egyptian monastery, Symeon promised the man a sign that he had been granted divine forgiveness. It duly arrived: one Sunday, back in his cloister, when the monk was celebrating the Eucharist 'one of his eyes suddenly came out'. This, oddly enough, was considered a good thing, at least by Symeon's more ardent admirers. 'By this sign,' comments a breathless Moschos, 'the brethren knew that God had forgiven him his sin, just as the righteous Symeon had foretold.'

After lunch, refreshed, I set about trying to find a driver willing to take me to what remains of the stylite's pillar on the Wonderful Mountain, a few miles south of modern Antakya.

In the main bazaar – a vaulted Ottoman street that still follows the line of the old Byzantine *corso* – I met a pious and thickly bearded driver named Ismail. He owned an ancient and much repainted Dodge truck, currently coloured lemon-yellow. We haggled for long enough for both of us to feel we were being swindled, and after Ismail had attended midday prayers we drove off in the truck, jolting out of Antioch, heading due south.

Olives were everywhere: long regimented lines of trees forming neat chequerboard patterns against the ash-coloured soil of the hills. But for the occasional minaret poking up beyond the groves and the groups of baggy-trousered peasants loading firewood onto carts, it could have been Umbria. In the valley to our left shepherds and their barking dogs were leading herds of long-eared goats and sheep, bells tinkling, through the mulberries and aloes. Within a few minutes the perfect pyramid of Mons Mirabilis rose up through the morning haze.

Bouncing off the main road onto a track, we climbed a dry *wadi* in a cloud of dust. We passed an old couple with mattocks in their hands, hoeing a barren terrace. The track continued to spiral steeply upwards; slowly a great vista opened up around us. Ahead lay the distant metallic glint of the Mediterranean; to the south, Mount Cassius and the olive groves of Syria; to the north, the hot, flat, plains of Cilicia. Immediately below us, through the heat haze, we could see the meandering course of the sluggish Orontes, and on either side lines of dark green cypresses.

When John Moschos came here, all the peaks within view were crowned by stylites, and competition between them was rife: if one was struck by lightning – something that clearly happened with a fair degree of frequency – the electrocuted hermit's rivals would take this as a definitive sign of divine displeasure, probably indicating that the dead stylite was a secret heretic. Judging by what Moschos has to say in *The Spiritual Meadow*, visiting these pillar saints was a popular afternoon's outing for the pious ladies of Antioch's more fashionable suburbs. The most chic stylite of all was undoubtedly Symeon, whose pillar lay a convenient palanquin's ride from the waterfalls of Daphne, the resort where Antony took Cleopatra for their honeymoon.

Today it seems that no one comes to Symeon's shrine. There are only a handful of Christians left in Antioch, and they have better things to worry about than the ruins of a forgotten hermit. The broken pillar is surrounded now by the ruins of the churches, monasteries, pilgrims' hostels and oratories that sprang up around it, a crumbling panorama of collapsed walls and fallen vaults. The only intruders are shepherds looking for somewhere to shelter their flocks during storms. Even the dirt track no longer reaches the pillar. I left Ismail bobbing up and down on his prayer carpet at the end of the path, and climbed up to the summit on my own.

Rising to the crest of a hogsback ridge, I could see above me the lines of honey-coloured masonry that marked the exterior wall of the stylite's complex. But it was only as I got much nearer to the ruin that I began to take in the true scale and splendour of the building: high on that empty hilltop with the wind howling over the summit lay a vast cathedral, constructed with great skill out of prisms of finely dressed stone. It was built with deliberate extravagance and ostentation: the basket capitals of solid Proconessian marble were lace-like and deeply cut; the pilasters and architraves were sculpted with an imperial extravagance. It was strange: a ragged, illiterate hermit being fawned over by the rich and highly educated Greco-Roman aristocracy; yet odder still was the idea of a hermit famed for his ascetic simplicity punishing himself in the finest setting money could buy. It was like holding a hunger strike in the Ritz.

I clambered into the basilica over a pile of fallen pillars and upended capitals; as I did so a thin black snake slithered from a marble impost, through a patch of poppies, down into the unseen dark of an underground cistern. I sat down where it had been lying, and opened up *The Spiritual Meadow* to read Moschos's description of the teeming crowds that once thronged the site to look at Symeon, to hear his pronouncements and, possibly, even to be healed. Once the road between Antioch and the coast was jammed solid with devotees and pilgrims coming from all over the Mediterranean world. Now it was just the snake and me.

The complex was based on that of the original St Symeon Stylites, St Symeon Stylites the Elder, who first ascended his pillar near Aleppo a century earlier in an effort to escape the press of pilgrims around him. His pillar was originally just a refuge from the faithful; only by accident did it become a method of voluntary self-punishment and a symbol in itself. The building around the original St Symeon's pillar was erected by the Emperor after the stylite died, so that his pillar became a relic and the church which enclosed it a huge reliquary. But here on Mons Mirabilis there was a crucial difference: the church was built around a living saint. In one of the most unlikely manifestations of Christian piety ever witnessed, it was a living man – a layman, not even a priest – who was the principal object of reverence in the church.

The stump of the pillar rises still from a plinth in the middle of an octagon, around which are stacked tiers of stone benches. In a normal Byzantine episcopal church such stone benches, reserved for the senior clergy of the church and called the *synthronon*, would be placed around the apse and would look onto the altar. But in this church conventional worship was relegated to the flanking side chapels; here the main nave looked not towards the altar (and thus to God) but towards the saint himself. The stylite had become like the Christian version of the Delphic oracle: raised up on his pillar at the top of the highest mountain, a literal expression of his closeness to the heavens, he spoke what all assumed to be the words of God. The Byzantines were constantly haunted by the spectre of heresy, but no one in Antioch ever seems to have suggested that in behaving in this way the stylites or their followers were doing anything in the least bit uncanonical. Even when the Egyptian monks tried to excommunicate Symeon, the rest of the Byzantine Church assumed – perhaps not inaccurately – that they were just motivated by jealousy: after all, the stylites had rather stolen the desert fathers' thunder.

The sun was lowering in the sky, sinking towards the Mediterranean. In the distance, to the east, lightning played on the horizon. But even though it would soon be dark I lingered in the ruins, pacing through the complex in the dusk and wondering at the oddness of the world John Moschos inhabited: sophisticated enough to build this astonishing classical basilica, yet innocent enough to believe that these strange, ragged men shrieking from their pillars were able to pull aside the heavy curtain of the flesh and gaze directly on God. Standing on their pillars, they were believed to be bright beacons of transcendence, visible from afar; indeed in some cases we hear of disciples claiming to be unable to bear the effulgence of the holy man's face, so bright had it become with the uncreated light of the divine.

The Byzantines looked on these stylites as intermediaries, go-betweens who could transmit their deepest fears and aspirations to the distant court of Heaven, ordinary men from ordinary backgrounds who had, by dint of their heroic asceticism, gained the ear of Christ. For this reason Byzantine holy men and stylites became the focus for the most profound yearnings of half of Christendom. They were men who were thought to have crossed the boundary of reality and gained direct access to the divine. It is easy to dismiss the eccentricities of Byzantine hermits as little more than bizarre circus acts, but to do so is to miss the point that man's deepest hopes and convictions are often quite inexplicable in narrow terms of logic or reason. At the base of a stylite's pillar one is confronted with the awkward truth that what has most moved past generations can today sometimes be only tentatively glimpsed with the eye of faith, while remaining quite inexplicable and absurd when seen under the harsh distorting microscope of sceptical Western rationality.

Back in Antioch, the incipient storm had not yet broken and a stuffy afternoon had turned into a heavy and swelteringly hot night. In the backstreets, many families had settled themselves outside, laying straw mats and old kilims out on the pavements. Grandmothers sat on stools at the back, knitting; women in head-scarves brought out steaming pilaffs to their cross-legged hus-bands. The richer families sat in a semi-circle in front of televisions, often placed on the bonnet of a conveniently parked car. The noise of televised gunshots and the murmur of Turkish soap operas mingled with the whirr of cicadas.

I got Ismail to drop me off, and wandered in the dark through the narrow streets, under the projecting wooden balconies of the old houses and the vine trellising of the bazaars. Down alleys, through arched doorways, you could catch glimpses of the hidden life of the courtyard houses: brief impressions of bent old ladies flitting from kitchen to zenana; old men in flat caps gossiping under palms, sticks in their hands.

After nearly an hour I found a café with a marble Ottoman fountain, and there I washed off the dust of the afternoon and settled down to drink a glass of *raki*. From inside came the acrid smell of Turkish tobacco and the sharp clack of dominoes. Gnarled old men with moustachless Islamic beards pushed barrows of figs and pomegranates along the cobbles. Flights of dark-skinned teenagers kicked balls amid the uncollected rubbish of unlit alley-ways; smaller children pulled toys made of old crates, with wheels cannibalised from long-rusted prams or bikes. Through the dark, from another part of town, came the thump of drums from an unseen circumcision ceremony.

Later, walking back to the hotel, I took a wrong turning and stumbled by accident across the Greek Orthodox church. It was a substantial eighteenth-century building, Italianate and flat-fronted, with a small belfry facing onto the courtyard. The whole complex lay hidden by a discreetly narrow arch, and was guarded by an old Turk in a pair of baggy *charwal* trousers.

The priest was away in Istanbul, but from the doorkeeper I learned that the Christian community now numbered only two hundred families. In his lifetime, he said, as many as fifteen thousand Christians had left the town for new lives in Syria, Brazil, Germany and Australia. As with the Istanbul Greeks, it was just the poor and the old who were left. If I wanted to know more, he suggested, I should try to find the Italian Catholic priest who had recently come to live in the town; he didn't know the address, but had heard it was somewhere nearby in the old Jewish quarter.

It was not difficult to find him. Everyone seemed to know about the Italian. Fr. Domenico turned out to be a missionary friar from Modena. He was a tall, thin man with a lined, ascetic face and a distant, rather disconcerting gaze. He lived on his own and was finishing his supper when I interrupted him.

He had been in Turkey for twenty-five years, he said, and now thought of it as home, although each year he still crossed the Mediterranean to spend a fortnight with his elderly parents.

Like the gatekeeper at the Orthodox church, Fr. Domenico was gloomy about the future of Christianity in the city. 'Antioch was one of the first centres of the Early Church,' he said. 'St Peter and Paul both preached here. According to the Acts of the Apostles it was in Antioch that the disciples were first called Christian. But now there are barely two hundred Christian families left.'

'What will happen to them?' I asked.

'They are better off than the Greeks in Istanbul,' said Fr. Domenico. 'They are too few to be a threat. The Turks do not mistreat them. But the community will die out. The young are still emigrating, mainly to Brazil. Christians may have been here since the time of the Apostles, but I doubt whether there will be any here at all in twenty years' time.'

I asked what the Antioch imams thought of his activities in their town.

'When I first arrived they came to see me and asked, "What do you believe in?" So I showed them some books in Turkish. One was a hymn book which contained the words "Jesus Son of God". They were scandalised, and half of them left then and there muttering about blasphemy. But two or three imams stayed on for tea and we discussed theology. They accused me of using the wrong gospels and said that only the Gospel of Barnabas was true.'

'The Gospel of Barnabas?'

'It's an apocryphal late-medieval gospel written by a Christian who converted to Islam. The Muslims like it because it says Jesus is a good man and a prophet but not the son of God. I told them that the Gospel of Barnabas was medieval and that its author obviously knew nothing, because he describes Jesus going up to Jerusalem by boat. We argued all day. Since then I've had no real trouble.'

I asked whether he had converted anyone in all the time he had been in the country. He shook his head. 'Not one,' he said, smiling. 'There are only ten Catholic families here, all Maronites who came from Lebanon in the last century. But in the mountains there are many Armenians who have pretended to be Muslims ever since the massacres of 1915. Sometimes they come and get baptised by me, even though I am a Catholic. On their papers they say they are Muslim, but they know – and I know – the real situation.'

As I was leaving I asked Fr. Domenico whether he was lonely living on his own in a foreign country, a representative of what was now thought of as a foreign faith. He shrugged: 'What is loneliness?' he said.

The Buyuk Antakya Oteli is a remarkable example of the provincial Turkish talent for spending large sums of money building a very good hotel, then, in a matter of months, letting it decay into a morass of broken gadgets, leaking geysers and fraying electrics. There are no bulbs in the light sockets, no ballcocks in the lavatories, no water in the taps, no handles on many of the doors.

On returning from Fr. Domenico's, I found a trail of red ants leading into my room, and a small rivulet of water from the flooded cistern snaking out of it in the opposite direction. The red plastic telephone was dead but the cockroach in the defunct shower unit was not. Worst of all, the air conditioner was bellowing hot muggy air into the room with a noise like a marching band. I went back down to Reception to try to get it fixed, and while standing around waiting for help I noticed an envelope in my pigeonhole.

It was from the manager, and contained two bits of bad news. The first was a brief note answering my query about the different ways of getting to the next stop on the way to the Tur Abdin: Urfa, the ancient Edessa. It appeared there was no train and only one bus service: inevitably it left late in the evening and arrived in the early hours of the morning – another night-bus journey. The second item was more ominous. It was a cutting from the English-language *Turkish Daily News* and concerned a PKK raid on a village near Midyat, the principal town of the Tur Abdin. There had been a firefight; two village guards had been killed and five others taken hostage by the Kurdish guerrillas and spirited away to the mountains.

I got out my map and searched for the village. It lay only a couple of miles from the monastery of Mar Gabriel, where I hope to spend much of next week.

HOTEL TURBAN, URFA, 12 AUGUST

The night bus dropped me off at a roundabout on the outskirts of Urfa at 3.00 a.m., and drove off into the night. Disorientated with sleep, it took a few minutes for it to sink in that I was alone, standing in the dark, at a considerable distance from the centre of town. Cursing the weight of the books in my baggage, I wandered through the deserted and dimly lit streets searching for a hotel.

Forty minutes later I arrived outside the Hotel Turban, and rattled like a madman on the door. After a while the owner appeared in his pyjamas. He seemed understandably surprised to see me standing there at four in the morning, hammering on his front door and howling to be admitted. For several minutes he peered warily through the glass, before his curiosity finally got the better of him and he let me in. I filled in a flutter of registration forms, and was admitted to a dingy room lit by a single, naked lightbulb. The room was filthy and contained only a plastic chair and a metal bedstead. But I was long past caring and immediately fell asleep on the bed, fully clothed.

I was woken by the light from the open window six hours later. It was not yet mid-morning, but already it was very hot. Outside, I could hear the tap-tapping of copper engravers at work in the bazaar outside. I shaved in a grimy basin at the top of the stairs, then went out into the glare.

Urfa was a proper Silk Route bazaar-town, straight out of the *Arabian Nights*: a warren of covered alleys loud with a Babel of different tongues – Arabic, Persian, Kurdish, Turoyo, Turkish. Everywhere the air was heavy with thick clouds of kebab-smoke and the smell of grilling meat. Through the shadows, lit intermittently by shafts of sunlight breaking through the skylights, passed a surging crowd of wild, tribal-looking men: lean, hawk-eyed, hard-mouthed Kurdish refugees from Iraq in their baggy pantaloons and cummerbunds; sallow Persian pilgrims from Isfahan in flapping black robes; weatherbeaten *Yuruk* nomads from the mountains above Urfa; stocky Syrian Arabs in full *jellaba* and *keffiyeh*. Herds of fat-tailed sheep wobbled through the medieval arcades. Outside a tea house a party of nomad women, all dressed in different shades of purple calico, were sitting around a silver tray covered with white saucers full of oily vegetable delicacies. Their heads were shrouded under swathes of elaborate turban wraps, but their faces were uncovered and their cheeks were tattooed with crosses and swastika designs. Behind them a cauldron of pilaff steamed on a fire.

Urfa has always been a frontier town, filled with an explosive mix of different nationalities. At the time of John Moschos it lay on the most sensitive frontier in the world, separating the two great powers of late antiquity: Persia and Byzantium. As one of only two legal crossing points from East to West, Edessa – and especially the members of its large merchant class – grew plump on the trade which passed between the pair of hostile empires. From Byzantium the Persians bought gold and manuscript vellum; from Persia the Byzantines purchased Indian spices, Chinese silk and, above all, dark-skinned Asian slave girls. The Imperial treasury became rich from the customs duties – 12.5 per cent – levied on this merchandise, and checks at the border were rigorous. When Apollonius of Tyana, a pagan sage and wonder-worker, returned from a missionary journey to India and the East, he was asked by the Imperial customs officer what he had to declare, and replied: 'Temperance, virtue, justice, chastity, fortitude and industry.' The customs officer had heard all this before. 'Where have you hidden the girls?' he demanded.

Merchants were not the only people to cross the divide. Edessa was one of the great Byzantine university towns, and the scholars it attracted from Persia and beyond led to a rich cross-fertilisation of ideas in its lecture halls. There was a marked influence of Persian and Indian ideas on Edessa's theology, and its theological school became notorious for the dangerous heterodoxy of its teachings. In this cosmopolitan environment the city's most notorious heretic, Bardaisan of Edessa, was able to write an accurate account of the dietary regimes of Hindu priests and Buddhist monks, while Indian stories and legends came to be written down in unexpected new Christian incarnations: it may have been through Edessa that the *Life of the Buddha* passed into Byzantine (and ultimately Western) monastic libraries.

It was not a one-way traffic. There was a School of the Persians in Edessa, and in the sixth century no fewer than three Patriarchs of the Persian-based Nestorian Church were recorded as having spent much of their youth in Edessa studying Greek medicine and philosophy. Built as it was on the philosophical faultline that ran between the Eastern and Western worlds, Edessa became a great crucible fizzing with strange heresies and exotic Gnostic doctrines. One sect, the Elchasiates, believed that two gigantic angels had appeared to their founder, Elchasaios, and told him that Christ was reincarnated century after century, and that each time he was born of a virgin. The angels also instructed Elchasaios that his followers should venerate water as the source of life, and passed on a mystic formula to be used whenever members of the cult were bitten by a mad dog or a snake. To add to the richness of the mix, the Elchasiates observed the ancient Jewish Mosaic laws, circumcising their male children and scrupulously keeping the Sabbath, as well as holding out against new-fangled innovations to the New Testament such as the Letters of St Paul.

More unorthodox still were the Marcionites, who took a rather different attitude to Judaism: they believed that the stern Jehovah of the Old Testament was different from – and indeed was the enemy of – the true, kind, creator-God of the New Testament. If this was so, then, logically, the heroes of the Old Testament were actually villains: all over Edessa Marcionite churches rang with praise of Cain, the Sodomites, Nebuchadnezzar and, above all, the Serpent of the Garden of Eden.

In contrast, the Messalians, bitter enemies of the Marcionites, looked on the Cross as the object of their loathing, and refused to revere Mary as the mother of God. They strongly believed that it was possible to exorcise demons through prayer: if you prayed hard enough, they maintained, the demon would exit from the nose as mucus, or from the mouth as saliva. Once this had happened and the believer had achieved union with the Holy Spirit, he could henceforth do whatever he liked: no amount of sin and debauchery could harm his soul, as it was already part of God. A breakaway group from the Marcionites, the Carpocratians, took this view to an extreme: they maintained that to achieve true freedom the believer must scrupulously ignore the distinction between what is good and what is evil.

Straitlaced clerical visitors to Edessa were horrified to discover that Orthodoxy – true Christianity as understood elsewhere in the Christian world – was regarded by many in Edessa as only one among a considerable number of options available to the inquiring believer, and that the teachings of all these different sects tended to be regarded as equally valid. As in the very early Church of the first century, doctrine was still in a state of continual flux, and no one interpretation of the Christian message and no single set of gospels had yet achieved dominance over any others. Indeed in Edessa in the sixth century the Orthodox were known merely as Palutians, after a beleaguered former bishop of the town. Visitors were appalled: if it were possible to understand Christianity in so many radically different ways in one town, what would happen if these heretical tendencies were to spread across the Empire?

Strange things certainly went on in Edessa. In 578, the year in which John Moschos set off on his travels, a group of prominent Edessans – including the provincial governor – were caught red-handed performing a sacrifice to Zeus. Even worse, many Edessans openly professed themselves Manicheans, members of a cult so weird and inventive – even by local standards – that it was unclear whether Manicheans were heretical Christians, heretical Zoroastrians, Pagan survivals or a completely new religion altogether.

In Edessa it seems that any belief or combination of beliefs was possible – as long as it was inventive, unorthodox, deeply weird and extremely complicated. But what such a flourishing proliferation of different faiths highlights is the fact that it was only by a series of historical accidents – or, if you like, the action of the Holy Spirit – that the broad outlines of our own understanding of Christianity came to be seen as accepted and established, and that Manichean, Marcionite and Gnostic ideas came to be deemed heretical. After all, a theologian as intelligent as St Augustine of Hippo could spend several years as a champion of Manicheism before being won over to what we now regard as more acceptable beliefs. In the uncertain world of early Christianity it does not seem impossible that the Manichees or the Gnostics could have won the day, so that on Sundays we would now read the Gospel of Philip (which emphasises Jesus's lustily red-blooded attachment to Mary Magdalene) and applaud the Serpent of the Garden of Eden. Churches would be dedicated not to 'heretics' like St John Chrysostom but rather to Manichean godlings such as the Great Nous and the Primal Man; reincarnation would be accepted without a second thought, and Messalian mucus-exorcisms would take place every Sunday after evensong.

For months before I set off on this journey, while waiting for my wife to recover from a burst appendix and the succession of operations which followed it, I sat by her hospital bed reading about the bizarre percolation of heresies that once flourished in the Edessan bazaars. But it was only this afternoon, coming out of the bazaar and stumbling by accident across the old Edessa museum, that I was actually able to picture the *milieu* in which this whirligig of strange theologies could flourish. For there in the garden of the museum lay the finely-carved stone images of late antique Edessans who may once have subscribed to some of the heresies that circulated so promiscuously in the city between the first and seventh centuries A.D.

On the left as you entered the sculpture garden stood a figure dressed like a Roman senator, complete but for his missing head. It was an Imperial Roman sculpture the double of which you might expect to see in any archaeological museum from Newcastle to Tunis, from Pergamum to Cologne. Classical superciliousness was expressed in every inch of the man's bearing: one arm hung loose, the other was hitched up to his breast by the fold of his toga; one leg was pushed slightly forward, the shoulders were pulled slightly back. The robes fell easily over a slight but firm physique. The head may have been missing, but the figure's bearing still managed to give the impression of effortless Imperial superiority, the same pose that was adopted by the late Victorians to portray their empire-builders (and whose statues, sometimes similarly headless, now lie tucked into similar corners of museums across India). Who was this toga-wearing plutocrat? A governor posted to the East from his home in Alexandria, Antioch or Byzantium? Some Imperial functionary's ambitious nephew or promising younger son, sent briefly to the Persian frontier before being promoted to a senior position at the Imperial court?

Three feet to the right of the Roman, but representing a world many thousands of miles to the East, stood another male figure, this time in the dress of a Parthian noble: the long flowing shirt and baggy pantaloons, drawn in tight at the ankle, that are still worn with little alteration as the *salvar kemise* of modern Pakistan. Unlike the Roman, this Edessan nobleman was thickly bearded and his hair piled high over his head in a topknot. A sword lay buckled at his waist and he wore a pair of Central Asian ankle boots. The same figure could be seen in a hundred Kushan sculptures across northern India, Afghanistan and Iran; he stood here between the Tigris and the Euphrates, but he would have been equally at home beside the Oxus, or even further to the east, the Yamuna.

Near this Parthian warrior stood a third figure, who represents the typically Edessan synthesis of both the other sculptures. He was also wearing Parthian dress, but his face and hairstyle was Roman: cropped short, with a tightly clipped beard; moreover he did not wear Parthian boots but a pair of Roman sandals. He appeared lost in thought, and held not a sword but a book. He looked bourgeois, educated and highly literate, cross-cultural and probably multilingual. Here then was exactly the sort of character who could have fitted happily into one of those hybrid Edessan cults, their Christian skeleton fleshed out with Indian- or Persian-inspired mystical speculation.

Throughout the rest of the sculpture garden there was a vivid impression of the different cultures that converged at this Imperial crossroads: busts of grand Palmyrene ladies, perhaps courtiers of Zenobia, mysterious and semi-veiled, their identities hidden behind defaced Aramaic inscriptions; Hittite stelae – long lines of bearded men in peaked witches' caps; semi-pagan Seljuk friezes of the Lord of the Beasts; Arabic tombstones; Byzantine hunting mosaics; Roman *putti*; early Christian fonts covered in tangles of lapid vine scrolls.

But perhaps most intriguing of all were those pieces which could have come from any of the great cultures that converged at this point. One sculpture in dark black Hauran basalt showed a magnificently winged female figure, her robes swirling like a Romanesque Christ, as if caught in some divine slipstream. Her navel was visible through her diaphanous robes; one breast was loose, the other covered; there was a terrific impression of forward movement. But her head was missing, and now no one will ever know whether she was a Roman Victory, a Parthian goddess, a Manichean messenger of Darkness or simply a Gnostic archangel.

I slammed the logbook shut.

Night had fallen. I was still sitting in a tea house near the museum; it was hot and muggy, and mosquitoes were whining around the sulphurous yellow lights of the streetlamps. In the background there was the incessant burr of cicadas. Tucking my notes under my arm, I set off back towards the hotel.

On the way I stopped in at the Ulu Jami, which at the time of John Moschos, before its conversion into a mosque, was the cathedral of the Orthodox. Now all that remains of the Byzantine period is an arch, a few fragments of the east wall and the base of the octagonal minaret, once the cathedral tower.

As I was trying to see where the Byzantine masonry ended and the Turkish masonry began, the old blind muezzin came tap-tapping along the path from the prayer hall. Unaware that I was in his way, he brushed past me and, arriving at the door at the base of the minaret, fumbled as he tried to get the right key into the keyhole. Eventually there was a click, and soon I heard the tap-tapping as he wound his way up the stairs.

When he got to the top, the muezzin switched on the microphone a little before he was ready to sing the call to prayer. The sound of his breathless wheezes echoed out over the rooftops of Urfa. Down in the courtyard, under the fir trees, the faithful gathered, several of the old men seating themselves on the upended Byzantine capitals to exchange gossip before going in to pray.

Then the *azan* began: a deep, nasal, forceful sound, echoing out into the blackness of the night: *Allaaaaaaaaaah-hu-Akbar!* The words came faster and faster, deeper, louder, more and more resonant, and from all over Urfa people began to stream into the mosque. The call went on for ten minutes, until the prayer hall

71

was full and the courtyard deserted again. The blind *muezzin* stopped. There was a moment of silence, filled only by the whirring cicadas.

Then the muezzin let out a great heartfelt wheeze of a sigh.

Back at the hotel, I put a call through to the Monastery of Mar Gabriel. By good fortune it was Afrem Budak who answered. Afrem was a layman who had lived in the monastery for many years and assisted the monks. We had corresponded, had friends in common, and most important of all, Afrem spoke fluent English.

I told him I hoped to be with him in three days' time, on Thursday night, the eighteenth. He said the road was open, but warned me to be careful. Apparently since the PKK raid I had read about in the *Turkish Daily News*, the army had been out in force. There should be no problem, he said, as long as I was off the roads by 4 p.m., when the Peshmerga guerrilla units begin coming down from the mountains for the night. Afrem also advised that I take the longer route to the monastery, via Midyat: apparently the short cut via Nisibis is unsafe, being often and easily ambushed.

Unsettled by all this, I went and had a Turkish bath in a subterranean vault next to the hotel. For forty minutes I sat in the steam being pummelled black and blue by a half-naked Turk in a loincloth: my legs were twisted in their sockets, my knuckles cracked and my neck half-dislocated from my torso. It was extremely uncomfortable, but I suppose it did at least succeed in taking my mind off the coming day's journey.

A perfect morning. A storm during the night cleared the air, and it has dawned fresh and cool and clear: a blue sky, a gentle breeze and the whole town looking renewed and refreshed; a faint scent of almond blossom after the rain.

In the early-morning cool I walked through the slowly waking town. At the end of the bazaar, above the eggbox semi-domes of the baths, rose the walls of the ancient citadel, and nestling below these crags, surrounded by a rich thicket of willows, mulberries and cypresses, lay the Fishponds of Abraham, Urfa's most extraordinary survival.

Few of the heresies which flourished in late antique Edessa outlasted the early centuries of the Christian era. Suppressed by the fiercely Orthodox Byzantine Emperors of the late sixth century, then extinguished by the arrival of Islam, a few last embers of Gnostic thought crossed the Mediterranean to reach the southern shores of France in the eleventh century, where they inspired the Cathars – until the Cathars were in turn massacred by the 'crusade' of Simon de Montfort.

Yet some vague memories of these strange cults do linger on in some of the more inaccessible corners of Mesopotamia. In the mountains around the upper Orontes, it is said that the heretical Nusairi Muslims still profess doctrines that derive from the neo-Platonic paganism of late antiquity. Similarly, on the lower Tigris near Baghdad, a secretive sect called the Mandeans claim to be the last followers of John the Baptist, and still practise a religion that represents a dim survival of some early Gnostic sect. There is nothing like that left in Edessa, which is now solidly Sunni Muslim; nevertheless the fishponds do represent a last living link with the city's heterodox past.

The principal pond is a long, brown, rectangular pool fed by its own superabundant spring. Up and down its edge walk tribesmen taking the air with their womenfolk – great walking tents who stagger along in the midday heat, a few steps to the rear of their husbands, smothered under huge flaps of muslin.

On one side of the pool lies an elegant honey-coloured Ottoman mosque from which springs an arcade of delicate arches; on the other is a shady tea garden, surrounded by a screen of tamarisks and lulled by the coo of rock doves and the rhythmic clatter of backgammon pieces. I took a seat and ordered a cup of Turkish coffee; it arrived on a round steel tray accompanied by a saucer of melon seeds and a plate of sweet green grapes. I nibbled the seeds and waited to see what would happen at the ponds.

Every so often one of the tea drinkers would walk up to a boy sitting outside the mosque, buy a packet of herbs from him, and throw a pellet into the pool. Immediately there would be an almost primeval churning of the waters – a horrible convulsion of fin and tail and hungry yellow eyes – as the carp jumped for their food, jaws open, tails flailing.

Close-up, the fish looked like miniature sharks, with slippery brown-gilt scales, great thick bodies and cavernous mouths. They streaked greedily through the water, tails slashing as they leapt to grab the pellet – terrifying the smaller fish, who did their best to swim as far away as they could for fear they might themselves become targets of their larger cousins' appetites. Some of the slower movers were blotchy with bites and the white fungus infections that had taken root in the gashes. Cannibalism is apparently the only danger these fish face, for they are held to be sacred, and believed to be the descendants of fish once loved by Abraham; it is said that anyone who eats them will immediately go blind.

An old imam from the mosque was drinking a glass of tea at a table beside mine. One of his eyes was clouded with a trachoma, and when he smiled he revealed a wide horizon of gum. He invited me to sit, and I asked him about the legend of the creation of the pool.

Father Abraham, said the imam, was born in a cave on the citadel mount, where he lay hidden from its castellan, Nimrod the Hunter. Nimrod nevertheless tracked down Abraham's cradle, and using the two pagan pillars on the acropolis as a catapult, he propelled the baby into a furnace at the bottom of the hill. Luckily the Almighty, realising that his divine plan for mankind was in danger, intervened at this point and promptly turned the furnace into a pool full of carp. The carp, obedient to divine promptings, came together to form a sort of lifeboat. They caught the baby and carried him to the poolside. In his gratitude, Abraham promised that anyone who ate the carp would go blind.

I heard several other versions of the story while in Urfa, most of which tended to contradict each other in the details, but which all agreed on the broad outlines of the tale, one way or another linking Abraham, the citadel, the pond and the carp, with a walk-on part for Nimrod the Hunter. While the Book of Genesis does quite specifically mention Abraham's visit to Haran, only twenty miles from here, quite why Nimrod should turn up in Urfa is a mystery. His brief appearance in the Bible after the Flood in no way links him either to Abraham or to Urfa, yet the imam firmly insisted that it was Nimrod who founded the town, and raised its walls and palace: a bizarre dogleg from both Biblical and Koranic tradition.

But the true history of the fishponds as disentangled by historians is no less bizarre than the versions I heard by the pool. Apparently the ponds may well go back to the era of Abraham, and even the taboo on the consumption of the fish seems to be a remarkable survival from ancient Mesopotamia. For historians are unanimous that the origins of the fishponds are not linked to Islam, nor even to early Christian or Jewish legend. Instead it seems almost certain that they are a relic of one of the most ancient cults in the Middle East, that of the Syrian fertility goddess Attargatis.

The second-century writer Lucian of Samosata, the only reliable ancient source for the goddess's cult, describes the worship of Attargatis as being centred on the adoration of water – naturally enough for a fertility cult that grew up in a desert. In the goddess's temples, statues of mermaids stood on the edge of ponds in which – then as now – swam fish of immense size. The fish were never eaten and were so tame, claimed Lucian, that they came when summoned by name. Attargatis's altar lay in the middle of the lake, in which devotees used to swim and perform erotic ceremonies in honour of the Goddess of Love and Fertility.

When Edessa was converted to Christianity, the new religion

took on much of the colouring of pre-existing pagan cults in the town. The priests of Attargatis used to emasculate themselves; as late as the fifth century A.D. the Christian Bishop of Edessa was still frantically trying to stop his priests from taking knives to their own genitalia. In the same way, astonishingly, the fishponds seem to have succeeded in making the transition from being sacred to an orgiastic pagan fertility cult to being holy to Christianity instead.

In 384 Egeria, the abbess of a Spanish nunnery, arrived in Edessa on her epic pilgrimage to Jerusalem and was invited for a poolside picnic by the bishop. Had she read Lucian's description of the fertility ceremonies performed by the fishponds she might have suspected the bishop's intentions. As it was, clearly ignorant of the ponds' pagan origins, she recounts that they were miraculously created by God and were 'full of fish such as I had never seen before, that is fish of such great size, of such great lustre'.

After the Arab conquest the fishponds continued to attract reverence, but under a new Islamic guise; Islam thus became the third faith to which these fish have been sacred. The name of the religion and the sex of the deity has altered with the centuries, but the fish have remained sacred age after age, culture after culture. It is a quite extraordinary example of continuity despite surface change: as remarkable as finding Egyptians still building pyramids, or a sect of modern Greeks still worshipping at the shrine of Zeus.

In my reading I have found only one reference to these sacred fish ever being eaten. This occurs in the imperious dispatches of the Rev. George Percy Badger, an Anglican missionary who passed through Edessa in 1824 while attempting to persuade the local Christians that what they really wanted to do was to abandon two thousand years of tradition and join the Anglican communion. He was not impressed by Edessa. The Ottoman troops there were 'a cowardly set of poltroons on horseback'; the women 'were excessively ignorant, untidy and not over clean in their persons or habits'; and as elsewhere in the Levant there was a 'severe lack of English clergy ... I had ample opportunity to explain the doctrines and discipline of our church, of which they were profoundly ignorant ... and they seemed pleased when I promised to send them a stock of books on our ritual.' There was not even any rhubarb to be had in the Edessa bazaars, the one thing which recommended Diyarbakir to Badger, for there at least 'Mrs Badger could not resist her home associations' and had made a 'good rhubarb pudding'.

In Edessa Badger visited the fishponds. Dismissing Muslim superstition he commented that: 'the Christians often partake of the forbidden dainty, the fish being easily secured in the streams which flow from the pond through the gardens. They generally cook them with a wine sauce,' notes Badger approvingly, 'and declare them excellent.'

I climbed to the citadel and looked down over Urfa. On every side the hills were brown and parched. It was nearly noon, and beyond the town's limits nothing moved except the shimmering heatwaves and, in the distance, a single spiral of wheeling vultures. But the town itself was a riot of greens, reds and oranges: trees and gardens backing onto flat-topped Turkish houses, with the whole vista broken by the vertical punctuation of a hundred minarets. Some of these were the conventional Turkish pencil-shape, others were more unusual: the Ulu Jami retained its Byzantine octagon, while a square campanile rising above the fishponds with four double-arched horseshoe openings may once also have been the bell-tower of an early medieval church.

But there are no functioning churches in Edessa any more. Although legend has it that Edessa was the first town outside Palestine to accept Christianity – according to Eusebius, its King Abgar heard about Jesus from the Edessan Jews and corresponded with Him, accepting the new religion a year before Christ's Passion – there has been no Christian community here since the First World War. For in 1915 the governor began 'deporting' the Armenians: rounding them up in groups, marching them out of town with a 'bodyguard' of Ottoman irregulars, then murdering them in the discreet emptiness of the desert. Fearing this treatment would be extended to the rest of the Christian community, the two thousand remaining Christian families in the town barricaded themselves into their quarter and successfully defended themselves for several weeks. But eventually the Ottoman troops broke through the makeshift defences. Some Christians escaped; a few were spared. More were massacred.

On my way back to the hotel I passed the old Armenian cathedral. Between 1915 and last year it was a fire station; now, as I discovered, it is being converted into a mosque. The altar has been dismantled, leaving the apse empty. A *mihrab* has been punched into the south wall. A new carpet covers the floor; outside lies a pile of old pews destined for firewood. Two labourers in baggy pantaloons were at work on the façade, balanced on a rickety lattice of scaffolding, plastering the decorative stonework over the principal arch. I wondered if they knew the history of the building, so I asked them if it was an old mosque.

'No,' one of the workmen shouted down. 'It's a church.'

'Greek?'

'No,' he said. 'Armenian.'

'Are there any Armenians left in Urfa?'

'No,' he said, smiling broadly and laughing. His friend made a throat-cutting gesture with his trowel.

'They've all gone,' said the first man, smiling.

'Where to?'

The two looked at each other: 'Israel,' said the first man, after a pause. He was grinning from ear to ear.

'I thought Israel was for Jews,' I said.

'Jews, Armenians,' he replied, shrugging his shoulders. 'Same thing.'

The two men went back to work, cackling with laughter as they did so.

A bleak journey: mile after mile of blinding white heat and arid, barren grasslands, blasted flat and colourless by the incessant sun. Occasionally a small stone village clustered on top of a tell. Otherwise the plains were completely uninhabited.

Diyarbakir, a once-famous Silk Route city on the banks of the River Tigris, was announced by nothing more exotic than a ring of belching smokestacks. The old town lies to one side, on a steep hill above the Tigris. It is still ringed by the original Byzantine fortifications built by Julian the Apostate in the austere local black basalt, and their sombre, somehow unnatural darkness gives them a grim and almost diabolic air.

The Byzantines knew Diyarbakir as 'the Black', and it has a history worthy of its sinister fortifications. Between the fourth and seventh centuries it passed back and forth between Byzantine, Persian and Arab armies. Each time it changed hands its inhabitants were massacred or deported. In 502 A.D. it fell to the Persians after the Zoroastrian troops found a group of monks drunk at their posts on the walls; after the subsequent massacre, no fewer than eight thousand dead bodies had to be carried out of the gates.

Today the city retains its bloody reputation. It is now the centre of the Turkish government's ruthless attempt to crush the current Kurdish insurgency, and indeed anyone who speaks out, however moderately, for Kurdish rights. In Istanbul journalists had told me that Diyarbakir crawled with Turkish secret police; apparently in the last four years there have been more than five hundred unsolved murders and 'disappearances' in the town. One correspondent said that shortly after his last visit, the editor of a Diyarbakir newspaper who had given him a slightly outspoken interview had an 'accident', tumbling to his death from the top floor of his newspaper offices; after this the political atmosphere became so tense that local newspapers could only be bought from police stations. No one, said the journalist, dared to speak to him, other than one shopkeeper who whispered the old Turkish proverb: 'May the snake that does not bite me live for a thousand years.'

As we drove, I wondered if my taxi driver would prove equally tongue-tied, so I asked him if things were still as bad as they had been. 'There is no problem,' he replied automatically. 'In Turkey everything is very peaceful.'

As we passed along the black city walls, I noticed a crowd gathering on the other side of the crash-barrier. Armed policemen in flak jackets and sunglasses were jumping out of jeeps and patrol cars and running towards the crowd. I asked the driver what was happening. He pulled in and asked a passer-by, an old Kurd in a dusty pinstripe jacket. The two exchanged anxious words in Kurdish, then he drove on.

'What did he say?'

'Don't worry,' said the driver. 'It's nothing.'

'Something must have happened.'

We pulled up in front of a huge green armoured car that was parked immediately in front of my hotel; from the top of its glossy metallic carapace protruded the proboscis of a heavy machine gun.

'It's nothing,' repeated the driver. 'The police have just shot somebody. Everyone is calm. There is no problem.'

That evening I found my way through back alleys to Diyarbakir's last remaining Armenian church.

In the mid-nineteenth century the town had had one of the largest Armenian communities in Anatolia. Like the Jews of Eastern Europe, the Armenians ran the businesses, stocked the shops and lent the money. Like the East European Jews, their prominence led to resentment and, eventually, to a horrific backlash.

In 1895, during the first round of massacres, 2,500 Armenians were clubbed to death, shut up in their quarter like rabbits in a sealed burrow. When the English clergyman the Rev. W. A. Wigram visited the town in 1913 he reported seeing 'the doors still splintered and patched in the houses which were stormed by the rioters ... and the ghastly bald patch in the midst of the city where the Armenian quarter was razed to the ground and has never been re-erected to this day'. He warned that further massacres were an ever-present danger; and his prophecy was proved horribly accurate only two years later. During the First World War the sadistic Ottoman Governor of Diyarbakir, Dr Reşid Bey, was responsible for some of the very worst atrocities against Christians – both Armenian and Syrian Orthodox – to take place anywhere in the entire Ottoman Empire: men had horse-shoes nailed to their feet; women were gang-raped. One Arab source close to those who carried out the 1915 massacres in Diyarbakir Province estimated the number of murdered Christians across the governorate as 570,000: a high, but not entirely unbelievable, estimate.

Yet despite all this, a handful of Armenians were said still to cling on in the city, and my architectural gazetteer, written in 1987, said that one Armenian church was still functioning. I found the compound easily enough, and was astonished by the size and magnificence of the church: it was inlaid with fine sculptural panels and looked large enough to contain maybe a thousand people. It was only when I looked through the grilles on the window that I realised the church was now a ruin. Holy pictures still decorated the walls; a gilt iconostasis still separated nave from sanctuary; a book stand still rested on the high altar. All that was missing was the roof.

I found a family of Kurdish refugees huddled in the lee of the west porch, cooking a cauldron of soup on an open fire. I asked if they knew what had happened, but they shook their heads and explained that they had only been sheltering there for a few days. They directed me to the door of a house at the back of the compound.

Inside lived two Kurdish brothers, Fesih and Rehman, and in a little annexe to one side, a very old lady called Lucine. Lucine was an Armenian. One of the brothers went to get tea, and I tried to ask the old lady what had happened to the church. She didn't reply. I asked again. It was Fesih who answered.

'It fell in last winter,' he said. 'There was no one left to look after it. A heavy fall of snow brought the roof down.'

'Does she not like to talk about this?' I asked.

'She can't speak,' said Fesih. 'She hasn't said a word for years. Since her husband was killed.'

Lucine smiled absent-mindedly and fingered a cross around her neck. She rearranged her headscarf. Then she walked off.

'Her mind is dead,' said Fesih.

'We look after her now,' said his brother, returning with three glasses of tea. 'We give her food and whatever else she needs.'

'What about her family?'

'They are all dead.'

'And other Armenians?'

'There are none,' said Fesih. 'There used to be thousands of them. Even when I was small there were very many. I remember them streaming out of here every Sunday, led by their priest. But not now. She is the last.'

We talked for twenty minutes, but Fesih would not let me stay to finish my tea.

'You must go now,' he said firmly. 'It is not good to be on the streets of Diyarbakir after nightfall. It's getting dark. You must hurry. Go now.'

Seeing what had happened in the last few months to the Armenian churches of Edessa and Diyarbakir – one in the process of being converted into a mosque, the other collapsing into a state of roofless ruination – reminded me of my first encounter with the increasingly rapid disappearance of Turkey's Armenian heritage.

In the summer of 1987, a year after following Marco Polo's route from Jerusalem to Xanadu, I returned to eastern Turkey to fill out my notes on the region, before setting about writing a book on the journey. The previous year I had spent a happy afternoon in Sivas, admiring the old Seljuk colleges there, and had noticed that in front of the Shifaye Medresse there lay a most unusual graveyard where tombstones inscribed in Ottoman Turkish, Armenian and Greek were all jostled together side by side.

On reflection I decided it must actually have been a lapidarium, or sculpture garden, rather than an ecumenical graveyard, for at no period have Muslims and Christians ever been buried side by side. But whatever it was, when I returned the following year the Armenian stones had all disappeared. The removal of perhaps fifteen heavy slabs and memorials would have been a considerable operation, and it had clearly taken place very recently, for the grass was still depressed and discoloured where they had rested; but when I asked the custodian where they had gone, he resolutely denied that any such stones had ever existed. I could probably have persuaded myself that I was mistaken and that the stones were my own invention, had I not actually written quite full descriptions of them in my notebooks the previous year. It was all very strange.

A week later I left Sivas and went to see a cousin who was working as an agricultural engineer in Erzerum, attempting to reintroduce silk farming to the region. Over dinner one night I happened to mention what I had seen, whereupon my cousin said that he had had a similar experience himself only the previous month. He told me that for four years he had been in the habit of taking an annual fishing holiday in the village of Maydanlar in the hills to the north of Tortum. On previous occasions he had admired a magnificent collection of early medieval Armenian cross-stones (known as *khatchkars*) which lay piled up near the village well; but this year the stones had all vanished. When he asked the villagers what had happened to them they became visibly nervous and would not tell him; it was only when he was alone with one old man that he learned what he believed to be the real story. Government officials from Erzerum had come through the village the previous month; they had asked the villagers for the whereabouts of any Armenian antiquities, and then proceeded to smash the stones up. Afterwards they had carefully removed the rubble.

I had heard other similar stories of the mysterious disappearance of Armenian remains, and the following year, working as a journalist on the *Independent*, I was able to investigate the subject in some detail. The trail led from the Armenian community in Paris, through Anatolia, to the library of the Armenian community in

Jerusalem. By the end I had amassed a body of evidence which showed the alarming speed at which the beautiful, ancient and architecturally important Armenian churches of Anatolia were simply vanishing from the face of the earth.

An incomplete inventory of actively used Armenian churches compiled by the Armenian Patriarchate of Constantinople in 1914, immediately before the genocide, recorded 210 Armenian monasteries, seven hundred monastic churches and 1,639 parish churches, a total of 2,549 ecclesiastical buildings. A 1974 survey of the 913 buildings whose locations were still known found that 464 had completely disappeared, 252 were in ruins and only 197 remained in any sort of sound condition. Since then there had been several new discoveries, but the condition of most of the others had continued to deteriorate dramatically. Many still standing in 1974 had begun to crumble, while some extremely beautiful buildings had collapsed and completely disappeared.

There was nothing very sinister in the cause of the condition of many of the buildings. Some had been damaged by earthquakes; and the explosion of Turkey's population had caused a demand for building materials which the churches readily supplied; others had been fatally undermined by Turkish peasants digging for 'Armenian gold', the legendary El Dorado of riches supposedly buried by the Armenians before they were 'deported' in 1915.

Nevertheless it was clear that the Turkish antiquity authorities had not exactly gone out of their way to stop the Armenian monuments from falling into decay. During the 1980s numerous Seljuk and Ottoman mosques and caravanserais had been restored and consolidated, but this treatment had not been extended to one single Armenian church. The Armenian monastery on the island of Aghtamar in Lake Van, arguably the most famous monument in eastern Anatolia, had belatedly been given a guardian, but this had not stopped the building's decay: five of the main sculptures – including the famous image of Adam and Eve – had been defaced since the guardian's appointment, and there had been no attempt to consolidate the building in any way. One British architectural historian I talked to maintained that there was a 'systematic bias' in what the Turks restored or preserved.

84

Moreover it was clear that academics – both Turkish and foreign – were strongly discouraged from working on Armenian archaeological sites or writing Armenian history. A British archaeologist (who, like almost everyone I talked to on this subject, begged to remain nameless) told me, 'It is simply not possible to work on the Armenians. Officially they do not exist and have never done so. If you try to get permission to dig an Armenian site it will be withheld, and if you go ahead without permission you will be prosecuted.' The truth of this was graphically illustrated in 1975 when the distinguished French art historian J.M. Thierry was arrested while making a plan of an Armenian church near Van. He was taken to police headquarters where he was fiercely interrogated for three days and three nights. He was released on bail and managed to escape the country. In his absence he was sentenced to three months' hard labour.

Fear of this sort of thing severely restricts the investigation of Armenian remains and leads to a kind of selective blindness in those scholars whose professional careers demand that they continue to work in Turkey. In 1965 plans were announced for the building of a huge hydro-electric scheme centred on the Keban dam, near Elazig in the south-east of the country. The artificial lake this created threatened a number of important monuments, and a team of international scholars co-operated in the rescue operation.

Five buildings were of particular importance: a pair of fine Ottoman mosques, a small Syrian Orthodox church, and two Armenian churches, one of which contained exceptional tenth-century frescoes. The rescue operation is recorded in the *Middle East Technical University (Ankara) Keban Project Proceedings*. The report describes how the two mosques were moved stone by stone to a new site. The Syrian Orthodox church was surveyed and excavated. The two Armenian churches were completely ignored. Although the most ancient and perhaps the most interesting of the threatened monuments, they did not even receive a mention in the report. They now lie for ever submerged beneath the waters of the lake.

Those who flout the unspoken rules on Armenian history still find themselves facing almost ludicrously severe penalties. In early December 1986 Hilda Hulya Potuoglu was arrested by the Turkish security police and charged with 'making propaganda with intent to destroy or weaken national feelings'. The prosecutor of the Istanbul State Security deemed that her offence merited severe punishment, and asked for between a seven-and-a-half- and fifteen-year jail sentence. Her crime was to edit the Turkish edition of the *Encyclopaedia Britannica*, in which was included a footnote reading: 'During the Crusades the mountainous regions of Cilicia were under the hegemony of the Armenian Cilician Kingdom.' It would be impossible to find a respectable academic anywhere in the world who could possibly take issue with the historical accuracy of this statement, but in the view of the prosecutor, Potuoglu was guilty of distorting the facts on a politically sensitive issue: the *Britannica* quickly joined the index of forbidden books, along with such other politically dubious publications as *The Times Atlas of World History* and *The National Geographic Atlas of the World*.

During the 1970s and early 1980s it was clear that the censorship of publications dealing with the Armenians had been dramatically stepped up. The reason for this was the rise of ASALA – the Armenian Secret Army for the Liberation of Armenia – which in the early eighties began attracting international attention with a series of terrorist attacks, directed mainly at Turkish diplomats. The resulting publicity succeeded in bringing the issue of the Armenian genocide back onto the political agenda. This culminated in 1987 in the passing of a resolution in the European Parliament which recognised that the refusal of Turkey to acknowledge the Armenian genocide was an 'insurmountable obstacle' to the consideration of its bid to join the European Community.

The Turkish government argued that although some Armenians may have been killed in disturbances or deportations during the First World War, so were many Turks. Moreover, the Turks insisted, there were never very many Armenians in Anatolia in the first place, and the numbers supposedly massacred – around one and a half million – actually exceeded the total Armenian population of the Ottoman Empire. In 1989 the previously classi-

Above The oldest surviving manuscript of *The Spiritual Meadow*, Monastery of Iviron, Mount Athos.

Right Byzantine fops watching chariot racing. Obelisk of Theodosius, the Hippodrome, Istanbul.

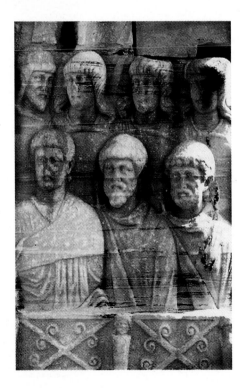

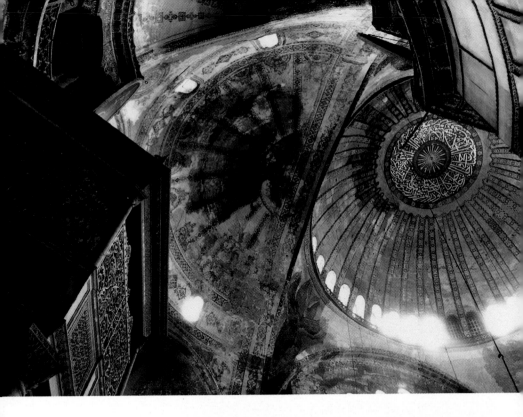

Above The domes and semi-domes of Haghia Sophia, Istanbul.

Right Turkish workmen converting the Armenian cathedral into a mosque, Urfa (Edessa).

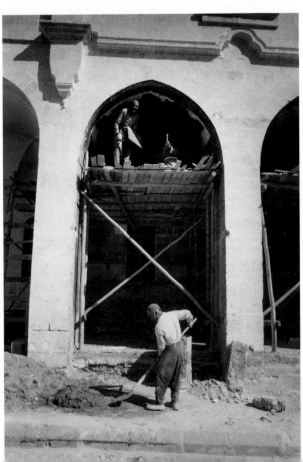

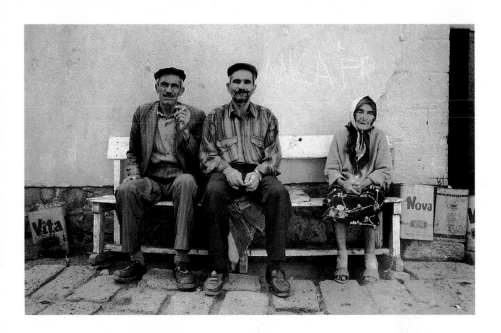

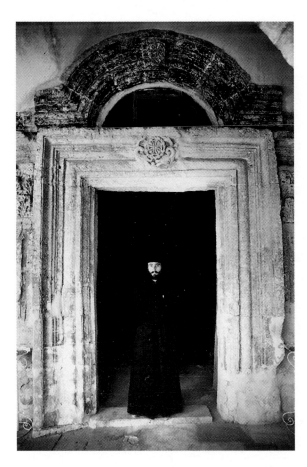

Above Fesih, Rehman and Lucine. The last Armenian in Diyarbakir, with her two Kurdish guardians.

Left A monk of the Monastery of Deir el-Zaferan, Tur Abdin, Turkey.

Below The last two monks at the Monastery of Salah, Tur Abdin.

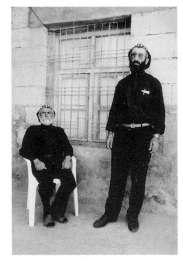

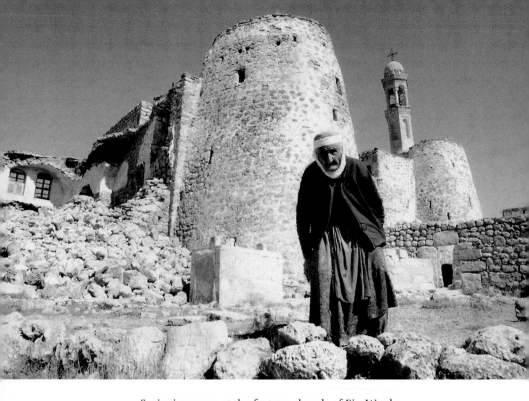

Suriani woman at the fortress church of Ein Wardo.

The Mausoleum, Cyrrhus, Syria, looking out over the olive groves of the Kurd Dagh.

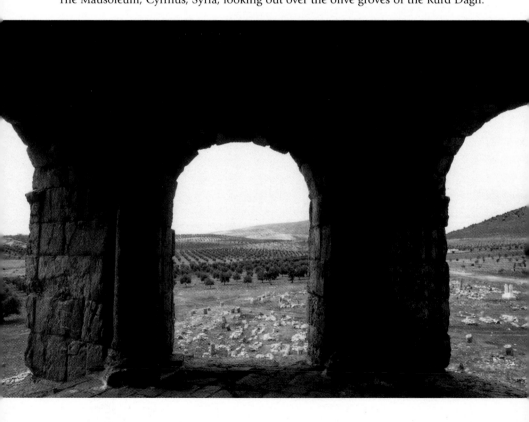

fied Ottoman archives relating to the period were opened up to a select group of Turkish scholars and combed for material to prove the Turkish case. The Turkish Foreign Minister claimed that when the process of declassification is complete, 'allegations of an Armenian massacre will be no more than a matter of political abuse'.

None of this, of course, created a particularly favourable environment for the conservation of the principal legacy left by the Armenians in Turkey, the hundreds of Armenian churches and gravestones which still littered eastern Anatolia. It is probably no coincidence that it was at exactly this time that reports of deliberate Turkish government destruction of Armenian remains began to multiply. The stories were always difficult to corroborate, for what witnesses there were in these remote regions tended to be illiterate Turkish peasants, and after the destruction of a building it is extremely difficult to distinguish what is alleged to be dynamiting from what could well be earthquake damage.

There are however a small number of intriguing incidents which are difficult to explain away. At Osk Vank, for example, the village *kaymakan* (headman) told J. M. Thierry that a government official from Erzerum had come to the village in 1985. The official asked for help in destroying the church, but the *kaymakan* refused, saying it was far too useful: his people used it as a garage, granary, stable and football pitch.

Another case concerns the once magnificent group of churches sitting astride a deep canyon near Khitzkonk, south-east of Kars. In photographs taken at the beginning of the century, five superb churches can be seen. After the massacres the area was closed off to visitors, and was not reopened until the 1960s. When scholars returned, only one church, the eleventh-century rotunda of St Sergius, was still standing; the other four were no more than one or two courses high. Two had been completely levelled and the stones removed. The peasants told of border guards arriving with high explosives. More reliable witness to what had happened was contained in the remaining building: the cupola was untouched, but the side walls had been blown outwards in four places where small charges appeared to have been laid.

Certainly Armenian scholars are convinced that a deliberate campaign is under way to destroy all evidence of the Armenians' long presence in eastern Anatolia. As my friend George Hintlian, curator of the Armenian Museum in Jerusalem, put it: 'You can attribute disappearing churches to earthquakes, robbers, Kurds, Islamic fundamentalists, men from outer space or anything else you care to blame. The end result is exactly the same. Every passing year another Armenian church disappears and for this the Turkish authorities can only be pleased. They have already changed all the Armenian village names in eastern Anatolia; the churches are all we have left. Soon there will be virtually no evidence that the Armenians were ever in Turkey. We will have become a historical myth.'

THE MONASTERY OF MAR GABRIEL, TUR ABDIN,
18 AUGUST

Mas'ud, the driver I had been recommended, turned up at the hotel at seven in the morning.

We left Diyarbakir by the Mardin Gate and drove down into the brilliant green of the river valley. The Tigris, at its lowest in midsummer, was no wider than the Tweed at Berwick. Its banks were marshy with reeds and lined by poplars and cedars; beyond stretched fields of ripe corn. A fisherman on a flat skiff was spearing fish, like the gold figure of Tutankhamen in the Cairo museum; nearby children were wading in the shallows.

A little downstream, a black basalt bridge several hundred yards wide spanned the river. The central piers – built of great blocks of stones each the size of a coffin – were early Byzantine; the outer ones were more delicate, the work of Diyarbakir's Arab conquerors: the fine kufic inscriptions they carved to record their work still decorated the upper registers. I had just got out my camera to take a picture of the bridge, with the grim black bastions of Diyarbakir crowning the hill in the background, when Mas'ud hissed at me to stop: 'The men in the white car are plainclothes security police,' he said.

I looked where he was indicating. A little behind us a white Turkish-made Fiat had pulled in opposite the fishing skiff. The passenger door was open and a burly Turk was standing looking at us. 'They followed us down from the hotel. If you photograph the bridge they may arrest you.'

I was unsure whether Mas'ud was imagining things, but still put the camera away and got back in the car. We drove on; the white car stayed where it was.

The road followed the slowly meandering banks of the Tigris; soon the walls of Diyarbakir slipped out of view behind a curve in the river. We passed a ford where a shepherd was leading a string of long-haired Angora goats over the rushing water; nearby a party of peasants were dressing a vineyard full of young vines. On either bank the land was rich and fertile; above the sky was bright blue, and a light breeze cooled the already intense heat of the sun. It was difficult to imagine that this peaceful, plentiful countryside held any threat to anyone.

Then, turning a corner, we saw a barricade blocking the road in front of us. A group of men in ragged khaki uniforms, some topped with chequered *keffiyehs*, stood behind a line of petrol cans. Some held pistols, others snub-nosed sub-machine guns; a few held assault rifles.

'Police?' I asked.

'*Inshallah*, village guards,' said Mas'ud, slowing down. 'Just hope it's not PKK. You can't tell at this distance. Either way, hide that notebook.'

We slowed down. The men walked towards us, guns levelled. They were village guards. The leader exchanged a few words with Mas'ud and waved us through without checking our documents. But at a second checkpoint a few miles later we were not so lucky. The commando at the barricade indicated that we should pull in. We did as we were instructed and parked beside a large single-storeyed building.

The building had once been a police station but had now been

taken over by the army. Troops were milling around in full camouflage. To one side, in front of a fortified sandbag emplacement,
stood a six-wheeled Russian armoured personnel carrier; on the
other were two light tanks and four or five Land-Rovers with their
canvas back-covers removed and heavy machine guns mounted
over the cabins.

The commando took our documents – Mas'ud's ID and my
passport – and left us waiting in a corridor, saying he had to get
permission from his superior before we could proceed. After half
an hour a telephone rang, and shortly afterwards a group of maybe
twenty soldiers jumped into the Land-Rovers and set off at speed.
We continued to stand in the corridor.

Eventually we were admitted to a room where an officer was
sitting behind a desk. He spoke a little English, told us to sit down,
and offered us tea. Then he asked me what I was doing and where
I was going. I told him my destination, but following the advice
of the journalists in Istanbul, I did not produce my press card,
which I kept in my pocket. The officer scribbled down a few
details, repeated the advice that we should be off the road by four
at the latest, and handed back our documents.

'Be careful,' he said.

We saw what he meant a few miles later. By the side of the
road lay the fire-blackened hulk of a car. It had been burned the
previous week, said Mas'ud, at a PKK night-time roadblock.

Soon after we passed the skeleton of the car, the road left the
Tigris and the landscape began to dry out. The vines disappeared
and were replaced by fields of sunflowers; a few coppices filled
the valley bottoms. Then they too vanished and we entered a plain
of rocky, barren scrub. A convoy of six APCs passed us from the
opposite direction. We drove on, passing a succession of roadblocks and more armoured convoys.

Shortly before lunchtime we drove through Mardin, then turned
off the main road onto a track; over a hillock, surrounded by
silver-grey slopes of olive groves, rose the unmistakable silhouette
of the melon-ribbed cupolas of Deir el-Zaferan, the Saffron Monastery.

Until the First World War, Deir el-Zaferan was the headquarters of the Syrian Orthodox Church, the ancient Church of Antioch. The Syrian Orthodox split off from the Byzantine mainstream because they refused to accept the theological decisions of the Council of Chalcedon in 451 A.D. The divorce took place, however, along an already established linguistic fault-line, separating the Greek-speaking Byzantines of western Anatolia from those to the east who still spoke Aramaic, the language of Christ. Severely persecuted as heretical Monophysites by the Byzantine Emperors, the Syrian Orthodox Church hierarchy retreated into the inaccessible shelter of the barren hills of the Tur Abdin. There, far from the centres of power, three hundred Syrian Orthodox monasteries successfully maintained the ancient Antiochene liturgies in the original Aramaic. But remoteness led to marginalisation, and the Church steadily dwindled both in numbers and in importance. By the end of the nineteenth century only 200,000 Suriani were left in the Middle East, most of them concentrated around the Patriarchal seat at Deir el-Zaferan.

The twentieth century proved as cataclysmic for the Suriani as it had been for the Armenians. During the First World War death throes of the Ottoman Empire, starvation, deportation and massacre decimated the already dwindling Suriani population. Then, in 1924, Ataturk decapitated the remnants of the community by expelling the Syrian Orthodox Patriarch; he took with him the ancient library of Deir el-Zaferan, and eventually settled with it in Damascus. Finally, in 1978, the Turkish authorities sealed the community's fate by summarily closing the monastery's Aramaic school.

From 200,000 in the last century, the size of the community fell to around seventy thousand by 1920. By 1990 there were barely four thousand Suriani left in the whole region; now there are around nine hundred, plus about a dozen monks and nuns, spread over the five extant monasteries. One village with an astonishing seventeen churches now only has one inhabitant, its elderly priest. In Deir el-Zaferan two monks rattle around in the echoing expanse of sixth-century buildings, more caretakers of a religious relic than fragments of a living monastic community.

Nineteenth-century travellers who visited Deir el-Zaferan often thought it looked more like a fortress than a monastery, and they had a point. Standing under the great ochre battlements, I hammered on the thick, heavily reinforced beaten-metal gate while Mas'ud locked the car. After a few minutes a young monk's bearded face peered suspiciously at us through an arrow-slit. Soon afterwards there was a rattling of bolts and chains and the gate swung open. Abouna Symeon stared at us with amazement.

'You had no trouble getting here?' he said in English.

I described our journey.

'Things are very bad at the moment,' he said. 'We have not had any visitors for many months. No one will come. There is no security in these mountains.'

Abouna Symeon led us up a dark gallery which opened into a wide and shady cloister. In the bright light of the cloister-garth a flat-capped (but barefoot) gardener was watering pots full of geraniums and anemones. To his side rose an astonishing arcaded portico, supported on two deeply cut pilasters rising to a pair of elaborate Corinthian capitals. It was late Roman, yet, astonishingly, it was still employed for its original purpose, and was inhabited by the direct spiritual descendants of the original builders. Here bands of classical acanthus decoration, of a quality equal to the finest Byzantine sculpture surviving in Istanbul, covered sanctuaries in which the Aramaic liturgy was still chanted, unchanged from the day they were built. It was odd to think that these barren and remote hills, now terrorised by troops and guerrillas, and home only to poor and illiterate peasant farmers, were once places of considerable sophistication.

'It is beautiful,' said Abouna Symeon, coming up behind me. 'But for how much longer? Maybe the next time you come sheep will be grazing here.'

'Is that likely?'

'All our people are leaving. One by one our monasteries and our Christian villages are emptying. In the last five years – what? – twenty villages around here have been deserted. Perhaps nine are left; maybe ten. None has more than twenty houses. If the door were open – if the rest of our people could get visas for the West – they would all go tomorrow. No one wants to bring up their children in this atmosphere. They want to go to Holland, Sweden, Belgium, France. Not many years are left for us here.'

We walked through the cloister. At one end sat another monk, a much older man, wearing the characteristic Syrian Orthodox black hood embroidered with thirteen white crosses representing Jesus and his apostles. He was bent over a desk, peering short-sightedly at the page in front of him, and in his hand he held a pen. As we drew near I saw that he was writing in Aramaic with a thick, broad-nibbed pen. I was just about to introduce myself when he looked up.

'You are Mr William?'

'Yes . . .'

'And this is Mr Mas'ud?'

'Yes. How . . . ?'

'The police telephoned from Mardin five minutes ago to see if you had arrived. They said we should phone them when you got here.'

'They followed us from the first checkpoint as far as Mardin,' said Mas'ud. 'Another white car.'

'We were being followed again? Why didn't you tell me?'

Mas'ud shrugged: 'Always they do this.'

As we were speaking the telephone rang again. Symeon went to answer it. Mas'ud and I looked at each other.

'That was the police again,' said Symeon on his return. 'They told us to find out where you are going and to tell them when you leave.'

'You must see the monastery and leave quickly,' said the old monk. 'We don't want the police in here.'

'Anyway, you haven't got much time if you are to get to Mar Gabriel by nightfall,' said Symeon. 'For your own sake you must hurry.'

We left the old monk at his writing desk and Symeon took us down some stairs into the darkness of a vaulted undercroft. It was built of huge quoins with a stone roof, and constructed without mortar. Inside it was hot and damp. We stood in silence, waiting for our eyes to adjust to the semi-darkness.

'This was built about 1,000 B.C.,' said Symeon. 'There was a pagan sun temple here before the monastery. Then when Christianity . . .' He broke off suddenly. 'Listen,' he said. 'That banging. Can you hear?'

In the dark of the crypt we listened to a distant clash of metal against metal.

'It's the front gate again,' said Symeon. 'But who can it be?'

We climbed the stairs and Symeon sent the gardener off to see who had come. We were now standing next to a great Roman doorway, above which was sculpted an equal-armed Byzantine cross, set in a classical laurel wreath which in turn rested on a pair of confronted dolphins.

'What's this?' I asked.

'In the sixth century it used to be the medical school. It was famous even in Constantinople. Later it became a mortuary. We call it the House of Saints.'

He took us inside. In the middle of the room, a ribbed dome rose from a rectangle of squinches. The walls were lined with an arcade of blind arches, each niche forming a separate burial chamber.

'All the Patriarchs and all our fathers are buried in here,' said Symeon. 'It is said the monastery contains the bones of seventeen thousand saints.'

He led us through a rectangular Roman doorway into the small, square monastery church. Every architectural element was decorated with an almost baroque richness of late antique sculpture: over the omega-shaped sanctuary arch, friezes of animals tumbled amid bucolic vine scrolls and palmettes; feathery volutes of wind-blown acanthus wound their way from the capitals to the voussoirs of the arches, and thence down exuberant and richly carved pilaster strips. The church was sixth-century, yet the architectural tradition from which it grew was far older: the same decorative vocabulary could be seen on Roman monuments two hundred years earlier at Ba'albek and Leptis Magna. At the time of its construction, this sculpture must have appeared not just astonishingly rich; it must also have seemed deliberately conservative, even nostalgic, a deliberate attempt at recalling the grand old Imperial traditions during a time of corruption and decline.

At this point the barefoot gardener reappeared with the new visitors. They were three men, all Turks, dressed in casual holiday clothes: T-shirts, slacks and trainers. They ignored us and began looking around the cloister, making a great show of examining the pot plants and the architecture. It was only when the back pockets of all three men simultaneously burst into crackles of static from hidden walkie-talkies that what was already obvious to Mas'ud and Abouna Symeon became clear to me: the men were plainclothes security police.

A few minutes later, I was still looking at the extraordinary sculpture in the church when the old monk, Abouna Abraham, appeared at the door. He seemed anxious and began nervously turning off the lights, indicating as politely as he could that my visit should be drawing to a close. Abouna Symeon, however, was determined not to be intimidated by this latest batch of uninvited visitors, and asked me upstairs to see the rooms of the old Patriarchs. I followed him up the steps onto the roof terrace.

'Look!' said Symeon. 'On the top of the ridge. Do you see: the ruins of five more monasteries.'

I looked up to where he was pointing. On the rim of the crags high above Deir el-Zaferan rose the jagged silhouette of several lines of ruins.

'On the left, do you see that cave? That's the Monastery of St Mary of the Waterfall. And those ruins? That's the monastery of St Jacob. Next to it, that's St Azozoyel. Then those cells: that's St Joseph, and the last one – another St Jacob's.'

'So many monasteries . . .'

'Two hundred years ago there were seven hundred monks on this mountain. The community has survived so long – survived the Byzantines, the Persians, the Arabs, Tamurlane, the Ottomans. Now there are just the two of us left.'

'Do you think you'll be the last?'

'God alone knows,' said Symeon, leading me over to the other side of the terrace. 'But I certainly hope I'll outlive Fr. Abraham.'

From the battlements we looked south, over the olive-covered hillsides, past the monastic vineyard and on down to the flat plains of Mesopotamia. We stood in silence.

'It's very lovely, isn't it?' said Symeon. 'When I went abroad to do my studies it was this view I always remembered when I thought of home: these vineyards stretching away into the distance.'

'Does the monastery make its own wine?'

'The fundamentalists don't like us doing it. In Dereici village ten miles from here they shot a Christian winemaker. After that most of the village vintners abandoned their vines. But that's not why we stopped. The old monk who used to superintend the vintage died six years ago. Now the grapes are too small and bitter for wine. They're a lot of work and there are simply not enough Christians left in the villages to help us harvest and dress the vines properly. Even the man who is looking after them now is off to Germany next month. His relatives are all there already, and his visa has finally come through.'

'Is the exodus speeding up?' I asked.

'Certainly,' he said. 'It's partly economic. Life is hard here at the best of times, and the stories of the wages and social welfare payments they get in Sweden and Germany have got around by now. But our people also have political problems. I can't ever remember things being as bad as they are at present. Our people are caught in the crossfire between the government and the PKK. And now there is the Hezbollah too.'

'Here? I thought the Hezbollah were in Lebanon.'

'They've just set up here. The authorities seem to tolerate them as a counterweight to the PKK. They help the government in many ways, but of course they hate the Christians. Three or four months ago they kidnapped a monk in Idil district. He was on his way to officiate at a wedding when two gunmen in a car stopped the minibus he was on and ordered him out. They buried him up to his neck, and later hung him upside down in chains. They kept him for two weeks, until a ransom was paid.

'Sometimes the Hezbollah kidnap Christian girls from remote farms and villages and force them to marry Muslims. They say they are saving their souls; it happened to four girls last year. Another Hezbollah unit has taken over Mar Bobo, a Christian village near here: about ten or fifteen gunmen live there now. They've seized the roof of the church as their strongpoint, and they make the Christian women wear veils. They say we should go back to Europe where Christians come from, as if we were all French or German, as if our ancestors weren't here for centuries before the first Muslim settled here. Now our people live in fear. Anything can happen to them.'

'Can't you tell the police?'

'If anyone did the Hezbollah would kill the family . . . Wait: look!'

Fr. Symeon pointed to a dust cloud now rising on the track from Mardin.

'More visitors.'

'It's the army,' said Symeon. 'Two Land-Rovers.'

Below us, Mas'ud had also spotted them and was rushing over to his car.

'What's he doing?' I asked.

'I think he's turning his tape machine off. It was playing a Kurdish nationalist song. The soldiers might have arrested him if they heard it.'

The Land-Rovers pulled to a halt by the monastery walls, and armed soldiers began to pour out, some carrying heavy machine guns.

'My God,' said Symeon. 'Is it war?'

But the soldiers did not enter the monastery. Instead they fanned out into the olive groves, jumping over the fence. One soldier kicked down a gate as he passed; another began to throw stones at a pomegranate tree, attempting to dislodge the ripe fruit. Symeon shouted down at them to stop: 'Use the gate! Don't break the fence.'

He turned to me: 'Look at them! Breaking the tree to get at the fruit. Smashing our fencing. This is too much.'

'Is this all because of my visit?'

'I fear so,' said Symeon.

'I'm sorry,' I said. 'I'd better go.'

'You must go anyway. The sun is beginning to go down. You won't get to Mar Gabriel unless you leave now.'

We walked down through the cloister to the car.

'I'm very sorry for all this,' I said.

'Just make sure you tell the outside world what is happening here,' said Symeon. 'Go quickly now. God be with you.'

Mas'ud pulled away. When I looked behind me I could see the short black-robed figure of Symeon gesticulating at an officer, as the soldiers closed in around him.

The shadows were lengthening into a deep blue slur, spreading softly over the ridges and gullies of the Izlo Mountains. In the narrow river valleys shepherds were leading their flocks through rich groves of fig, walnut and pistachio trees. Women were fetching cooking water from roadside pumps; donkeys with bulging pack-saddles were ambling along the road. It was so easy to forget the troubles: only the continuous gauntlet of checkpoints and the occasional shell of an incinerated vehicle lying abandoned by the roadside reminded one of the dangers that the imminent twilight would bring.

We were making good time. It had just passed 4.30 and we were nearing Midyat, the nearest town to Mar Gabriel. In the distance on the left we could see the church towers of the Christian half of the town, flanked on the right by the minarets of the new Muslim quarter. On the edge of Midyat a large checkpoint had been erected, with a strip of sharpened nails laid out across the road like a fakir's bed in a cartoon; behind it stood a slalom of oil cans. A line of bored soldiers were sitting in the shade, watching the cars zigzag through the obstacles. We were three quarters of the way through before one of the men – an officious looking conscript with a shaven head – decided to pull us in.

The man asked for our documents. He looked through my passport, pausing suspiciously at one of my Indian visas as if he had just uncovered conclusive evidence of my Kurdish sympathies. He examined Mas'ud's ID, turning it over with a growing sneer on his face. Then he asked Mas'ud for the documents concerning the car. Mas'ud fumbled around in the glove compartment looking for them. It was clear we were in for trouble.

The conscript chose to take exception to something written on Mas'ud's driving licence, and spent the next forty-five minutes cross-questioning him. I began to look nervously at the sinking sun and the minute hand on my watch. Eventually Mas'ud passed over a large banknote, folded up in his ID card. The man looked at it, and for an awful five seconds I thought he was about to expose Mas'ud's attempt to bribe him. But he slipped it into his pocket without his colleagues seeing, and after complaining about the state of Mas'ud's tyres, let us go. Mas'ud drove away muttering violent Kurdish curses under his breath.

It was now after 5.30. The sun was sinking behind the hills as we headed into the desolate country on the far side of Midyat. The road was now little better than a track; it contained no other traffic and was surrounded by no signs of habitation. There was no noise, no birdsong. It was completely silent; unnervingly so.

It was only when I began to look carefully at the shadowy country through which we were passing that I realised what it was that was so unsettling about it. It was not just barren: it had been deliberately laid waste. The olive groves on the upper slopes were not naturally so twisted and gnarled: someone had actually burned them, so that their skeletons formed a charred and jagged silhouette on the skyline. It was like a Paul Nash picture of Arras or Ypres in 1916. We were passing through scorched earth.

'The soldiers have done this,' said Mas'ud.

'Why?'

'If they think the PKK are using trees or buildings for cover, the army burns them. It's partly to hurt the guerrillas, partly to punish the local people for allowing the PKK to use their land. Further east, around Hakkari, whole districts have been laid waste. Many villages have been destroyed.'

Eventually we rose over the crest of a low hill. There was just enough light to distinguish ahead of us the crenellated ghost of Mar Gabriel's monastery. The huddled buildings stood alone and exposed on a bare and stony hillside, surrounded by a high wall; as we drew near the rising moon silhouetted the cupolas and spires of the churches, and illuminated a tall tower to one side.

A moonwashed gateway rose out of the gloom; and from beyond

came the faint but comforting sound of monastic chant. A porter opened the narrow wicket, and as we unloaded our baggage from the car, the monks and nuns began to stream out of vespers. In the lead was the Archbishop; and a little behind him, dressed in a blazer, was a layman. He came up and introduced himself. It was Afrem Budak, to whom I had talked on the telephone. He was welcoming, but clearly also a little angry.

'You should have been here at least an hour ago,' he said quietly, shaking his head. He took my rucksack. 'The risks you take yourself are your business. But you could have got us all into trouble if something had happened to you.'

THE MONASTERY OF MAR GABRIEL, 23 AUGUST

I am sitting outside my cell, under a vine trellis. For the first time I am sleeping in a monastery which John Moschos could have stayed in, hearing the same fifth-century chant sung under the same mosaics. Facing me is the south wall of what is probably the oldest functioning church in Anatolia. It was built by the Emperor Anastasius in 512: before Haghia Sophia, before Ravenna, before Mount Sinai; it was already eighty years old by the time St Augustine landed at Thanet to bring Christianity to Anglo-Saxon England. Yet some parts of the monastery date back even earlier, to the abbey's original foundation in 397 A.D.

There is only a handful of churches anywhere in the world this old. It is incredible that it has survived at all, but that it has survived intact and still practising when Persians, Arabs, Mongol and Timurid hordes have all come and gone, Constantinople has fallen to the Turks and Asia Minor has been completely cleared of Greeks – this is little short of a miracle.

One of the monks, Brother Yacoub, has just dropped by, and handed me a bunch of grapes freshly picked from the trellis. He is now standing behind me, watching me write. After years of visiting ruined churches across the length of Anatolia, finding these monks wearing almost identical robes to those John Moschos may himself have worn, still inhabiting a building of this antiquity, feels almost as odd as stumbling across a long-lost party of Roman legionaries guarding some remote watchtower on Hadrian's Wall.

I had had my first unforgettable glimpse of the interior of the churches and buildings of Mar Gabriel on the night of my arrival. After our baggage was brought in, the monastery gate was locked and bolted behind us. I ate supper with the monks in their ancient refectory and afterwards drank Turkish coffee in the cool of a raised roof terrace near the Archbishop's rooms. By nine o'clock the monks were beginning to return to their cells, and Yacoub, a gentle novice of my own age, offered to show me around before I retired for the night.

Yacoub led the way, holding a storm lantern aloft like a figure in a Pre-Raphaelite painting. The electricity supply had failed some time before, a common occurrence, explained my guide, due sometimes to 'load-shedding' by the electricity company, and sometimes to the PKK's irritating habit of blowing up the region's generating stations. I followed Yacoub down a wide flight of stairs, along a vaulted corridor and into the thick, inky blackness of the crypt. In the flickering light of the lantern, shadows danced along an arcade of arches.

'This is the Cemetery of the Martyrs,' said Yacoub. 'During the Gulf War this was our bomb shelter. On the floor there: see that capping stone? That's where Mar Gabriel's arm is buried.'

'What happened to the rest of him?' I asked.

'I'm not entirely sure,' said Yacoub. 'In the fifth and sixth centuries our monastery used to fight many battles with the local villagers for the remains of our more saintly fathers. Sometimes monks were killed trying to defend our stock of relics.'

'And you think maybe the villagers got the rest of Mar Gabriel?'

'Maybe. Or perhaps one of the monks hid the rest of the body and took the secret of its resting place with him to the grave.'

'Do the villagers still take an interest in your relics?' I asked.

'Certainly,' said Yacoub. 'And not just the Christians: we get Muslims and even Yezidis [Devil-propitiators] coming here to pray to our saints. Many of the Muslims in this region are descended from Suriani Christians who converted to Islam centuries ago. They go to the mosque, and listen to the imams – but if ever they are in real trouble they still come here.'

Yacoub bent down with the lantern and pointed to a small aperture below the capping stone of the grave. 'You see here? This is where the villagers come and take the dust of the saint.'

'What do they do with it?'

'It has many uses,' said Yacoub. 'They keep it in their houses to get rid of demons, they give it to their animals and their children to keep them healthy during epidemics . . .'

'They actually eat the dust?'

'Of course. It is pure and full of blessings.'

'What sort of blessings?'

'If ever they dig a new well, for example, they place some of the dust of the saint in it so that the water will remain pure for ever.'

I told Yacoub that in Istanbul I had seen barren women come to a shrine of St George if they wanted children. Did the same happen here?

'Mar Gabriel is good for sickness and demons only,' replied Yacoub. 'If they want children they go upstairs.'

'Upstairs?'

'To the Shrine of St John the Arab. Come, I'll show you.'

Yacoub led the way out of the crypt. At the top of the stairs, in a niche covered by a close-fitting arch of dark basalt, stood a small plinth, similar to the one downstairs.

'This is his tomb,' said Yacoub. 'Or rather it is the tomb of his torso.'

'The villagers have been at your bones again?'

'No. The nuns this time.'

'The nuns?'

'Yes,' said Yacoub. 'They are in charge of the tomb, and they keep St John's skull in their quarters.'

'What on earth do they do with it?'

'When the local women come, the nuns fill a bowl of water and place it for an hour on the tomb. Then they take St John's skull and, saying the appropriate prayers, they fill the skull with water, then pour it onto the woman's head. This makes the lady have a baby.'

'And people believe all this?'

'Why not?' said Yacoub. 'The nuns think it never fails.'

Yacoub led me out of the shrine into the starlight outside. 'At the moment, because of the troubles, not so many are coming,' he said. 'But before, in the days of peace, there would be long queues every Sunday: people would come from as far as Diyarbakir, especially after they were married. Now of course it is dangerous to travel. Also the Hezbollah are telling the Muslims that they must not come to a Christian shrine.'

We walked over to the main church and Yacoub opened the great door. Amid the herringbone patterns of the brick vaults, the light of the storm lantern picked out the glittering mosaics with an almost magical brilliance. As we drew nearer, the shapes of crosses, vine scrolls and double-handled amphorae glinted in the dancing flame. With Yacoub still holding his lamp aloft, we passed through the sanctuary and into a small side-chapel. In the back wall were two openings, one near the ceiling, the other at shin-height.

'At the end of his life Mar Gabriel walled himself up behind here,' said Yacoub. 'His food was put though that hole at the bottom. If he wanted to take communion he would stick his hand through there at the top.' Yacoub pointed to the upper hole. 'Mar Gabriel was a great ascetic,' he said. 'Behind that wall he punished his flesh in order to liberate his soul. Come and see what I mean.'

Before I had time to demur, Yacoub had pushed the lamp through the small lower aperture and wriggled in after it. Left in total darkness, I had no option but to follow. Lying flat on my back and pulling in my stomach, I found I could just fit through the hole. Yacoub extended a hand and helped me to my feet.

'Look here,' he said, pointing to a narrow slit in the wall.

'Sometimes our Holy Father Mar Gabriel felt he was not being hard enough on himself, that he was sinking into luxury. So he would squeeze into this slit and spend a month standing up.'

'Why?'

'He used to say no slave should sit or lie down in the presence of his master, and that as he was always in the presence of his Lord he should always stand up. At other times, to remind himself of his mortality, he would bury himself in that hole in the corner.'

'That's a bit extreme, isn't it?'

Yacoub was already on the floor, about to wriggle his way back to the church.

'I don't understand what you mean,' he said, before disappearing into the blackness. 'Mar Gabriel was a very great saint. We should all try to follow his example.'

The day at Mar Gabriel starts at 5.15 with the tolling of the monastery bells, announcing the service of matins. After four days enjoying the monks' hospitality but sleeping late, I thought I had better make an appearance. So this morning when the bells began to peal, rather than covering my head with the nearest pillow, I rolled out of bed, dressed by the light of a lantern, then picked my way through the empty courtyard towards the echo of monastic chant.

It was still dark, with only a faint glimmer of dawn on the horizon. In the church the lamps were all lit, casting a dim and flickering light over the early Byzantine mosaics of the choir. I kicked off my shoes by the door and stood at the back of the church. To my right four nuns dressed in black skirts and bodices were prostrating themselves on a reed mat. Ahead of me a file of little boys stood in line, listening to an old monk. He had a long patriarchal beard and stood chanting from a huge hand-written codex laid on a stone lectern to the north of the sanctuary. Each phrase rose to a climax, then sank to a low, almost inaudible conclusion.

Slowly the church began to fill up; soon the line of boys stretched right across the length of the nave. Another monk, Abouna Kyriacos, appeared and walked up to the sanctuary. He started chanting at another lectern, parallel but a little to the south of the other, echoing the old monk's chant: a phrase would be sung by the first monk, then passed over to Kyriacos who would repeat it and send it back again. The chant passed from lectern to lectern, quick-paced syllables of Aramaic slurring into a single elision of sacred song.

By now some of the older boys had also begun to go up to the lecterns and were standing behind the monks, joining in with them. The chant rolled on, as deep and resonant as Gregorian plainsong, but with a more Oriental feel, the strangely elusive monodic modulations reverberating under the rolling Byzantine vaults.

Before long an unseen hand was pulling back the curtains from the sanctuary; a boy holding a smoking thurible rattled its chains. The entire congregation began a long series of prostrations: from their standing position, the worshippers fell to their knees, and lowered their heads to the ground so that all that could be seen from the rear of the church was a line of upturned bottoms. All that distinguished the worship from that which might have taken place in a mosque was that the worshippers crossed and recrossed themselves as they performed their prostrations. This was the way the early Christians prayed, and is exactly the form of worship described by Moschos in *The Spiritual Meadow*. In the sixth century, the Muslims appear to have derived their techniques of worship from existing Christian practice. Islam and the Eastern Christians have retained the original early Christian convention; it is the Western Christians who have broken with sacred tradition.

The white light of dawn was filtering in through the great splayed Byzantine windows in the south wall. Inside the church, the tempo of the chant was now sinking. The curtains closed; silence fell. A last eddy of prostration passed through the congregation. The Archbishop appeared and the boys queued to kiss his cross.

Slowly the church emptied; from outside you could hear the birds stirring in the vine trellising.

However alien and eccentric Eastern asceticism sometimes seems, it had an extraordinary influence on the medieval West; indeed the European monks of the early Middle Ages were merely provincial imitators of the Eastern desert fathers. The monastic ideal came out of Egypt, that of the stylite from Syria. Both forms travelled westwards, stylitism, amazingly enough, getting as far as Trier before being abandoned as impossible in a northern climate, with the aspiring German stylite eventually yielding to pressure from his bishop to come down before he froze to his pillar. It was as clear and unstoppable a one-way traffic, east to west, as the reverse cultural invasion of fast food and satellite television is today.

What has always fascinated me is the extent to which the austere desert fathers were the models and heroes of the Celtic monks on whose exploits I was brought up in Scotland. Like their Byzantine exemplars, the Celtic Culdees deliberately sought out the most wild and deserted places – the isolation of lonely bogs and forests, the bare crags and islands of the Atlantic coast – where they could find the solitude that they believed would lead them to God.

Moreover, despite the difficulties of travel, the links between the monastic world of the Levant and that which grew up in imitation of it in the north of Europe were unexpectedly close. Seventh-century Rome had four resident communities of Oriental monks and many Eastern church fathers travelled 'beyond the Pillars of Hercules' to the extreme west. Theodore, the seventh Archbishop of Canterbury, was a Byzantine from Tarsus who had studied at Antioch and visited Edessa; his surviving Biblical commentaries, written in England, show the extent to which he brought the teaching of the School of Antioch and an awareness of Syriac literature to the far shores of Anglo-Saxon Kent.

Many other more anonymous figures seem to have followed in his footsteps. The 'seven monks of Egypt [who lived] in Disert Uilaig' in the west of Ireland were proudly remembered in manuscripts of the Irish Litany of Saints, along with coracle-fulls of other nameless 'Romani' (i.e Byzantines) and 'the Cerrui from Armenia'. All these diverse figures seem to have found their way to the most extreme ends of the Celtic fringe, where they were revered for centuries to come: indeed so holy was the reputation of these travelling Byzantines that according to the Irish Litany of Saints even to read their names over a sick man was believed to prevent 'boils, and jaundice and the plague and every other pestilence'.

If an intermittent flow of living monks from east to west was possible, then the flow of inanimate books was greater still. Up to the eighth century, *The Life of St Antony of Egypt* by Athanasius of Alexandria was probably the most read and imitated book in Europe after the Bible, and what was true of manuscripts in general was particularly true of manuscript illumination: that early Irish and Northumbrian gospel books took as their principal model work from the Byzantine east Mediterranean is now beyond question.

At Cambridge I spent my final year specialising in the study of Hiberno-Saxon art, and what above all pushed me on to try and get through to the Tur Abdin was the knowledge of the extent to which the early medieval art of Britain was indebted to the artists of the scriptoria of the monasteries there. For though these monasteries now lie forgotten and half-deserted in an obscure corner of a predominantly Muslim country, some scholars believe that work produced in the Tur Abdin may well once have provided the inspiration for the very first figurative Christian art in Britain.

As I lay on my hard monastic bed, unable to sleep, I turned over in my mind an art historical controversy I had once studied in some detail. The debate revolved around a most intriguing tale.

In the mid-sixteenth century Stephanos, the Catholicos of Armenia, prepared to make a journey which he hoped would change the history of the east Mediterranean. Finding his Patriarchal seat of Echmiadzin surrounded on the east by the resurgent Persian Empire, and on the west by the new Ottoman dynasty, he saw his people facing the same fate as had befallen the Byzantines a century earlier: conquest followed by a bitter subjection under the dusty sandal of Islam. Like the Byzantine Emperor Manuel II

Palaeologus, the Patriarch saw only one hope for his people: that he should travel to Europe, somehow forge an alliance with the West, and so surround the Turkish armies in a Christian pincer movement.

Manuel had travelled to the West in vain: though he had acquiesced to many of the doctrinal demands of the Catholic Church at the Council of Florence, and had even been received with honour by King Henry IV of England at a grand banquet at Eltham on Christmas Day 1400, he came back to Constantinople empty-handed, without securing the dispatch of a single Western knight to defend the eastern frontiers of Christendom. Fifty years later, in 1453, his successor Constantine XI Paleologus died fighting on the walls of Byzantium as the Turks finally burst into what had once been the capital of the Christian world.

Catholicos Stephanos thought he could do better; and he hung his hopes on the support of the Pope, Paul III Farnese. Stephanos's spies had told him that Pope Paul had made it his special pontifical objective to liberate the oppressed churches of the Orient. They also told him that the Pope had a special interest in the study of scripture, and that he had called a council of scholars to establish once and for all the authentic text of the Bible. Stephanos knew that if he was to succeed in his mission he would have to establish a personal rapport with the Pope, and for this reason he cast around for a suitable present for the Roman Pontiff. Eventually his advisers hit upon a brilliant idea.

Someone in Echmiadzin had heard that in the libraries of the monasteries of the Tur Abdin there lay an astonishing collection of early Christian gospel manuscripts. One of these was a copy of the *Diatessaron*, a very early and very unusual gospel harmony – the four canonical gospels united into a single life of Christ – originally composed by the priest Tatian in the early second century A.D. For a century or so the *Diatessaron* had been the standard New Testament text in use in the Church of Antioch, but as copies of the original gospels became more widely available, it slipped out of common use and eventually came to be seen as a heretical text. At some stage it seems to have been ordered that manuscripts of Tatian's work were to be destroyed, and only in the obscure recesses of a few remote monastic libraries did copies of the *Diatessaron* survive.

Stephanos sent an envoy hundreds of miles south from the Caucasus to Mesopotamia to locate one of these last *Diatessaron* manuscripts. When eventually one was found, it was agreed that a local scribe, a Syrian Orthodox priest, should copy out the text. It was this copy that was taken to Rome by Stephanos. According to a colophon in the manuscript, the scribe was a native of Hasankeif, a town on the Tigris, a few miles south of Diyarbakir near Deir el-Zaferan. The overwhelming likelihood is that the original manuscript from which the papal copy was made came from the monastic library of Deir el-Zaferan.

In the event the Catholicos's embassy to the West was a fiasco. Stephanos never saw the Pope, and within a century his people, like the Byzantines before them, had been conquered and their land divided between the Persians and the Turks. The copy of Tatian's *Diatessaron* was never presented to the Holy Father, only getting as far as the office of his secretary. Later it found its way from the Vatican to the Bibliotheca Medicea Laurentiana in Florence.

Four hundred years later, in the winter of 1967, the Danish art historian Carl Nordenfalk was at work in the Laurentian Library when he came across the manuscript and began to browse through its pages. Suddenly he found himself staring at a set of illustrations that made him stop dead in his tracks. Nordenfalk was a specialist in Celtic manuscripts, and he saw immediately that these illustrations in the *Diatessaron* were iconographically identical to those in the first of the great illuminated Celtic gospel books, the Book of Durrow. The *Diatessaron* pictures also had a close relationship with a slightly later Celtic manuscript, the Gospels of St Willibrord.

In the Book of Durrow each gospel is preceded by a whole-page illustration showing the sacred symbol of the Evangelist who wrote the book (in this early case, a man to represent St Matthew, an eagle for St Mark, a bull for St Luke and a lion for St John). Most scholars would accept that these paintings in the Book of Durrow, probably executed in the last years of the sixth century A.D., are the first figurative paintings in British art.

Although the style of the *Diatessaron* and the two Celtic Gospel Books are very different – as you would expect from two manuscripts drawn centuries apart – the poses of the symbols, the angles at which they were drawn and the attitudes they strike are identical with each other, and totally different to anything else in Christian iconography. Moreover, both sets of manuscripts open with nearly identical full-page illuminations showing a double-armed cross embedded in a weave of intricate interlace. The same pattern also found its way onto a Pictish cross-slab, the Rosemarkie Stone, which still lies on the Beauly Firth, a few miles north-east of Inverness.

It took several months of intense study before Nordenfalk felt confident that he had worked out how an obscure mid-sixteenth-century copy of a manuscript from eastern Turkey could have such a close relationship with a pair of Celtic gospel books which were probably illustrated on the isle of Iona, off the distant west coast of Scotland, some eight centuries earlier.

Nordenfalk's thesis was that the illustrations of the Book of Durrow were based on an earlier copy of the *Diatessaron* which had somehow reached Iona from the Levant in the early Middle Ages. He even had a suspect for the carrier of the manuscript from east to west.

In his *History*, the Venerable Bede records that one winter night at the very end of the seventh century, a Frankish galley on its way back from the Holy Land was wrecked off the coast of Iona; a storm had blown the ship around the north coast of Scotland until it came to rest, as fate would have it, on the shores below the island's abbey church. Bede records that on board the vessel was a Gaulish nobleman named Arculph, who dictated a description of the holy places of the Levant to Adamnan, Iona's Abbot. (A copy of the manuscript of Arculph's descriptions, entitled *De Locis Sanctis*, later reached Bede's own scriptorium in Jarrow and became a source of much future Anglo-Saxon comment – both factual and legendary – on the eastern coast of the Mediterranean from Constantinople to Alexandria.) 'It is extremely tempting to assume,' wrote Nordenfalk, 'that [a copy of] the illustrated *Diatessaron* was among the books in Arculph's baggage.'

The realistic portraits in such an Eastern manuscript would have come as a revelation to Celtic monks familiar only with the geometric whorls and trumpet spirals of pagan Celtic art. Nordenfalk proposed, not unreasonably, that the arrival of the *Diatessaron* was the spark which ignited the almost miraculous blaze of Celtic book illumination during the seventh and eighth centuries, a process which culminated in such masterpieces as the Lindisfarne Gospels and the Book of Kells.

In his excitement Nordenfalk went on to make several other, much wilder claims for the Florence *Diatessaron* which were later questioned by rival academics. But the core of his thesis has never been successfully challenged. There can be no doubt that the miniatures and interlace patterns of the Florence *Diatessaron*, a manuscript originally illuminated in a monastic scriptorium some-where in the Tur Abdin, comes from the same family of manu-scripts as those contained within the Book of Durrow and the Gospels of St Willibrord.

Somehow, perhaps in the baggage of a shipwrecked Frankish nobleman, a set of pictures probably originally drawn in a monas-tery in eastern Turkey came to form the seed from which sprung the first Christian figurative paintings ever drawn in the British Isles. It is a considerable cultural debt, and one that is little known, and certainly unrepaid.

This evening, an hour before vespers, the monks, the novices and the schoolchildren got out the ladders and began the harvest of Mar Gabriel's pistachio trees.

The orchards stood on a ripple of narrow terraces sloping down from the front gate of the monastery. On the lower terraces the grapes were growing black with sweetness and the sheaths of the almonds were near to bursting; but the pistachio trees were so ripe that they would clearly rot if they were not picked that week. So the boys swarmed around the pistachio trees, trying to clamber up into the boughs without using step-ladders, pulling themselves up and swinging over to the ends of the branches. There hung the clusters of green buds which enclosed the soft white nuts. The boys plucked at the trees and threw down the buds to the novices who stood below, holding tin buckets.

As they scrabbled around, the harvesters were chatting to each other in Turoyo, the modern dialect of Aramaic still spoken as the first language of the Suriani. It had a completely different sound to Turkish or Kurdish or any other Anatolian tongue I had ever heard, sounding instead far closer to the guttural elisions of Hebrew or Arabic. Jesus must have sounded much like this when, as a boy, he spoke Aramaic in the carpenter's shop at home or chatted to his friends beside the Sea of Galilee.

After half an hour plucking at the buds, I took a rest and looked on from the edge of the terrace. Afrem came over to join me. He pointed out the burned earth of the slopes of the Izlo Mountains ahead of us, dramatically lit up now in the last light of the sun. 'You see over there?' he said. 'Those were all olive groves. Now they have been burned. It will be years before any trees that are replanted will be ready to harvest.'

'You think there will be a chance to replant them?'

'We have to hope,' he said. 'Without hope we cannot live.'

Yacoub came up and joined us. He put down his bucketful of pistachio buds and sat with his legs dangling over the edge of the terrace.

'We should be thankful,' he said. 'Here they've only burned the trees. Further east, towards Hakkari, they've been clearing all the villages too: seven or eight this year alone. Since the trouble with the PKK began ten years ago they have cleared many Muslim villages, and nearly twenty-five Christian ones.'

Afrem said that a refugee from one of the destroyed Christian villages, a priest, Fr. Tomas Bektaş, was being sheltered by the monastery until he found somewhere to live. He said I should talk to him, and promised to introduce me after dinner.

Afrem kept his promise. After we had all eaten in the monastic refectory – the normal bracing Suriani dinner, a haunch of boiled goat with salty porridge and sticky rice, followed by *pekmez*, a thick slurry of pressed grapes considered the greatest of delicacies in polite Suriani society – the monks withdrew as usual to take coffee on the roof terrace. Fr. Tomas was sitting a little to the side. He was an unremarkable-looking man with a small toothbrush moustache and a nervous tick which made him wink his right eye every few seconds. Afrem had warned me that the clearance of his village had led to Fr. Tomas having a major nervous breakdown from which he had yet to fully recover, and that the priest might not want to talk about what had happened to his village: 'He will get nightmares again,' said Afrem.

In the event, however, Fr. Tomas poured out his heart without hesitation. I sat back on my stool, and the priest talked. 'It was the middle of winter,' he said. 'One day an army officer in a Land-Rover dug his way through the snowdrifts. We gave him tea and then he simply told us that we had twenty days to leave. At first we did not understand what he meant. He said we had all been helping the PKK, that we had been supporting them with food and giving them guns. It was all nonsense, of course: what business do we have with the Kurds?

'The next day I went to the sub-governor in Silopi and pleaded for Hassana, but he would not receive me. His assistant said, "He does not want to speak." So I had to return to my village and tell my people that we had to leave, that there was no choice.

'We all left on the last day, all two hundred of us: thirty-two families in all. My family was the last. I was the priest: I had to make sure they all left safely.

'They came in the evening: five Land-Rovers packed with troops. They did not apologise or give compensation: they simply burned the empty houses and destroyed the gardens. There were no better gardens in Turkey. We had springs and water and earth and flowers and vegetables. The gardens were the livelihood of the village. Now they are barren and destroyed.

'Afterwards some Muslim village guards detained seven Suriani shepherds. They accused them of being Armenian sympathisers of the PKK and tortured them, using molten plastic to brand crosses on their faces.

'I was shocked and became very ill, mourning for my village. My family took me to hospital in Istanbul and I was there for four months. For thirty years I was a priest in that village. How can I start again? With a new congregation somewhere else? I couldn't do it. I cannot forget Hassana.

'Even now I don't feel well about it. My village burned, every house gone, my people dispersed. Some are sheltering here, four more families are at Deir ul-Zaferan; the others have gone to Istanbul. All want to emigrate now. They think there is nothing for them here. They are just waiting for their visas. Not since Ein Wardo has the situation been so desperate for us here.'

I had had my head down, taking notes as Fr. Tomas talked. It was only when I looked up that I saw his shoulders were heaving slightly and tears were streaming down his face. I put my hand gently on his shoulder.

The old priest was crying like an abandoned child.

Later, I asked Afrem what Fr. Tomas had meant when he referred to Ein Wardo.

According to Afrem, at the beginning of the First World War the Suriani saw the Armenians being led away by the Ottoman troops and heard the rumours of what was happening to them. They feared that they would be next, so they made preparations. They bought guns and stored wheat. They chose the most inaccessible of their mountain villages, Ein Wardo, and began to fortify it. They strengthened the walls of the church and secretly prepared barricades to fill the gaps between the houses.

When the Ottomans, backed by Kurd irregulars, began their attacks on the Suriani villages, the then Patriarch gave orders for all the villagers to retreat with their food and weapons to Ein Wardo. For three years the Suriani defended themselves there. Anyone outside the barricades was killed. Nearly every Suriani alive in eastern Turkey today is there because his parents or grandparents took shelter within those walls.

Afrem said that the village still stands, and that one of the defenders is still alive: a priest, ninety-four years old, who had been a child during the siege. He now lives with his son near Midyat. Tomorrow I hope to talk to him.

The Monastery of Mar Gabriel, 24 August

A bad start this morning.

Mas'ud, who has spent the last two days with his cousins in a village near Midyat, was due to return to the monastery early this morning. He did not show up until well after noon. When he did so, he looked white and shaken.

I asked what was wrong. He said that he had been stopped by the security police on his way through Midyat earlier that morning, and subjected to a lengthy interrogation, all on my behalf.

'The police asked me: "Where have you taken the English? Who has he talked to?" They said they had followed you from Ankara to Antakya, then on from Urfa to Diyarbakir, and that they were still watching now. Was that your route? Did you come from Ankara to Antakya to Urfa? You did not tell me that. I said you were just a tourist looking at old buildings, but they said they knew I was lying and that they knew you were a journalist.'

'It's OK,' I said, trying to reassure him. 'I have a press card. The Foreign Ministry must have got in touch with the police here and told them my itinerary. There's no problem.'

'Yes, there is a problem,' said Mas'ud.

'What do you mean?'

'I don't think you understand the situation here,' he said, barely suppressing his anger. 'Last spring I got a call at home. The man on the phone did not say who he was. He just warned me not to take journalists around. Soon after that I lent my car to another driver who wanted to take a foreign correspondent to Hakkari. He left the journalist there. On the way back someone shot the driver and stole my car.'

'The security police?'

Mas'ud shrugged and raised his open palms.

'I'm sorry,' I said lamely, feeling at once guilty and alarmingly out of my depth. 'I should have told you I had a press card. I had no idea you were in that position.'

'I always thought you were a journalist,' said Mas'ud.

'What can I say? I didn't realise your situation. I'm very sorry.'

'Don't be sorry. It's my job. But know you are playing a dangerous game,' he said. 'You don't understand the police here. You think they are like the English policemen we see on the television, the fat man with the blue hat, the little stick in his hand and the old bicycle. They are not like that, not at all like that. If you took my advice you would leave as soon as you can. It's too late to try and cross into Syria today. But tomorrow you must leave. Then I can go back home to my family in Diyarbakir.'

Before I left the Tur Abdin I still wanted to try to interview the old priest from Ein Wardo. An hour later, after Mas'ud had recovered his usual poise, we drove in to Midyat with Brother Yacoub, who had agreed to come and interpret.

We drove in silence through the burned-out landscape, the security I had felt inside the high walls of Mar Gabriel now thoroughly breached by what Mas'ud had said.

'The Archbishop used to make this journey every day,' said Yacoub at one point. 'His office was at the Bishop's House in Midyat. But since the troubles he stays in Mar Gabriel. Now the only people to make this journey are the children. By Turkish law they are obliged to come into the government school during term-time. Of course you know what happened to the truck on the road to Güngören? With the landmine?'

We neared the outskirts of the town and slowly crossed through the checkpoints, then past the sinister plainclothes police manning the crossroads at its centre. They all wore the same regulation dark sunglasses, with M-16 carbines strapped over their shoulders. Following Yacoub's instructions, we drove into the heart of the Midyat bazaar, and finally drew to a halt outside a shabby jeweller's shop.

'This business belongs to the old monk's family,' explained

Yacoub. 'They can tell us whether it would be possible to talk to him.'

Yacoub and I went into the shop; Mas'ud chose to stay outside and guard his car. The owner offered us seats and sent off his two grandsons, one to find out the whereabouts of the old monk, the other for bottles of Pepsi. Then he returned to serving his customers, a pair of elderly ladies upholstered, despite the heat, in velvet dresses with thick white scarves over their heads.

'Can you tell on sight who is Muslim and who is Christian?' I asked Yacoub.

'Only with the old people,' he replied. 'The old Christian ladies wear smaller headscarves which they tie in a particular way. Also they never wear green, the Muslim colour.'

One of the boys came back with the drinks. When Yacoub had taken a gulp, he continued: 'Years ago they say you used to be able to tell what religion someone was just by looking at what they wore: the Christians always had new clothes, while the Kurds had old broken ones.'

'Why was that?'

'In the villages the Christians had the best land; now the Kurdish *agahs* – the tribal chieftains – have just walked in and taken it from them, to distribute among their own people. They steal the crops of the Suriani from under their noses. There is nothing we can do. The government needs the support of the *agahs* if they are to win their fight with the PKK, so they never interfere. '

Yacoub finished his Pepsi and handed the can back to the boy. 'In the towns,' he continued, 'the Christians used to have all the jewellery shops; they were the tailors, shoemakers, leatherworkers. In the old days no Christian craftsman would employ a Muslim. But in the eighties, when most of the young Christians had already emigrated, the shop owners were forced to take on Muslim apprentices. Now those apprentices have opened their own shops. When I was at school fifteen years ago, perhaps 80 per cent of the shops were owned by the Suriani. Now it's less than 20 per cent. We still dominate the jewellery trade, but we are certainly not richer than the Kurds any more. If anything it's the reverse.'

Before long the door of the shop opened, and the second grandson walked in leading a doddering old man in baggy pantaloons. Yacoub greeted him and asked him some questions in Turoyo.

'Is this the old priest?' I asked.

'No,' replied Yacoub. 'This is Bedros, his son.'

'The old man must be pretty ancient.'

'He is. Bedros says his father is very deaf, and quite blind too, but we can certainly try to talk to him.'

We levered the old man into Mas'ud's car and drove through the labyrinth of Midyat's narrow bazaar alleys. Once we were out onto a rubble track in the outskirts, Bedros pointed out the silhouette of a monastery on the skyline, atop a hill overlooking the town.

'He says that this is where he lives,' translated Yacoub. 'It used to be the Monastery of Mar Obil and Mar Abrohom, but now there are no monks his family looks after the buildings and tries to stop them falling down.'

We drove into the old monastery cloister. Chickens and ducks pecked about the yard; piled up in front of the sculpted doorway leading into one of the two churches was a great mountain of straw. A family of long-haired Angora goats drank water from a disused fountain lying against the nave wall. The monastery had become a farmyard.

Bedros led the way into the house he had built amid what had once been the monastery kitchens. At the back of the living room, fast asleep under a gaudy poster of the Last Supper sat an ancient figure in a black cassock. He was slumped in a wooden chair, his head tilted forward, and over his face was lowered a wide-brimmed Homburg hat. As we walked in, the old man stirred and opened first one eye, then the other. The second eye was clouded blue.

Bedros walked up to the old priest, cupped his hands and bellowed into his father's ear. The old man bellowed back.

'What's he saying?' I asked Yacoub.

Yacoub smiled: 'Abouna Shabo says, "If they are not Christian I will not talk to them." '

Bedros reassured him, and explained what we had come for. An extremely loud Turoyo conversation ensued. Father and son were joined by Bedros's wife, who appeared from the kitchen and joined in the shouting match. At one point the old man lifted his shoe and pointed out to me a hole in its bottom, apparently to indicate that his daughter-in-law was not looking after him to his full satisfaction. But eventually he began to talk of the siege, and as he did so, Yacoub translated.

'It was Mar Hadbashabo who saved us!' shouted the old priest. 'The saint was wearing white clothes and attacking at the front of the Christians, throwing the Muslims back from the barricades of Ein Wardo. At evening time he stood on the church tower. We all saw him, even the Muslims, those sons of unmarried mothers! At first they tried to shoot him, thinking he was a priest, but the bullets went straight through him. Then they thought he was a *djinn*. Only towards the end of the siege, only after three years, did they realise he was a saint.'

'Let's go back to the beginning,' I said. 'What were relations with the Muslims like before the war?'

'They were not good,' said the old man. 'But before the war nobody was ever killed. In those days the Kurds were in the hills and the Christians were near the towns. We lived separately. But we were always fearful of what might happen, so as the war approached we began to sell our animals and buy guns. We had more than three thousand. They were old-fashioned matchlocks, ones that you had to light with a fuse, but they did the job. We melted down all our copper pots to make shot; the monks melted down their plate. We collected together a good stock of wheat. When the war broke out, and the Turks told the Kurds to go and massacre all the Christians, we were ready. By night all the Christian villagers came to Ein Wardo. They came from Midyat, Kefr Salah, Arnas, Bote, Kefr Zeh, Zaz Mzizah, Basa Brin. In the village there were about 160 houses. By the time everyone had gathered there were at least twenty families in every house.'

The old man broke off, turned to his son and began to berate him again.

'What's he saying now?' I asked.

'He's crying "Grapes, grapes," ' said Yacoub, grinning. 'He wants his son to bring him some fruit.'

119

Bedros's wife was sent off, scowling, to the kitchen. She returned with a huge bunch of ripe grapes. The old man lowered it into his toothless mouth and tore off the bottom three or four. He munched them noisily, and a broad smile spread across his face. When he had finished I asked about the siege.

'We built walls between the houses so that the village looked like a fort,' he continued. 'Then we dug tunnels so that we could go from house to house without getting shot by the Muslims. The strongpoint was the church, and on the roof we had a cannon that we had captured from the Turks in Midyat.

'They came after fourteen days: around twelve thousand Ottoman troops and perhaps thirteen thousand Kurds – irregulars who just wanted to join in the plunder. Any Christian left outside Ein Wardo was killed. Many were too slow and did not make it. In Arnas the Kurds captured thirty-five pretty girls. They locked them into the church, hoping to take them out and rape them one by one. But there was a deep well in the courtyard. All the girls chose to jump in rather than lose their virginity to the Muslims.'

'Did your supplies last for the whole siege?'

'The first summer we were not hungry. But by the middle of the winter things began to be difficult. We ran out of salt and people became ill for the lack of it. One group of about a hundred people tried to escape at night to get some salt from Midyat and Enhil. They were ambushed. Most of them got back, but fifteen people, including one of my brothers, never came back. That winter I lost my sister too. She went outside the barricades to fetch wood. The Muslims were hiding behind rocks. They captured her and cut her throat. That night I found her. Her head was separated from her body. I was twelve years old then.'

The old man's head dropped, and I thought for a minute that he, like Fr. Tomas the previous evening, was going to burst into tears. But after a minute's silence he recovered himself, and I asked if he had fought in the defence of Ein Wardo himself.

'They thought I was too young to hold a gun, but they let me collect stones to drop down the mountain slopes. I did my bit. There was plenty of opportunity. The first year the attack was very strong. Once I remember it was so strong that people ran away from the walls and began to retreat to the church, which was built with four very strong towers that could be held if everything else fell. But the monks, our leaders, threatened to shoot anyone who ran away, and in the end the defences held.

'That winter was very hard. One loaf of bread would go to each family per day, which meant that there was only one piece for each person. Many were wounded, but there was only one doctor; he did what he could, but most of the wounded had to rely on the old men who knew about roots and herbal remedies. But we never gave up. We had heard that the British had landed in Iraq, and we all believed they would come to rescue us. Of course nothing happened, but the hope of relief kept us from despair.'

'The Christians of the West have never done anything for us,' said Bedros, rolling a cigarette with his right hand, and spitting out the spare tobacco with a loud gob into the corner. 'The Turks help other Muslims if they are in trouble in Azerbaijan or in Bosnia, but the Christians of Europe have never shown any feelings for their brothers in the Tur Abdin.'

'The worst hunger was the following year,' continued the old priest, ignoring his son's interruption. 'During the siege no one could grow anything, so supplies were almost exhausted. I remember that second winter we were permanently hungry, and would eat anything: lizards, beetles, even the worms in the ground.

'But the Muslims were also growing hungry, and in 1917 disease – cholera I think – struck their camp. God willed it that we did not get the disease in Ein Wardo; somehow we were spared. The attacks grew less and less and gradually we became brave. At night we began to break out and attack their camp. Once we attacked the Ottoman barracks in Midyat.'

'You can still see the bulletholes,' said Yacoub.

'After three years,' continued Abouna Shabo, swiping at the bluebottles which were trying to settle on his face, 'they despaired of ever conquering us and said that we were being protected by our saints, Mar Gabriel, John the Arab and especially Mar Hadbashabo. Eventually a famous imam, Sheikh Fatullah of Ein Kaf, came to the Muslim army and said he would try to make peace between the two sides. The Muslims asked the Sheikh to say "Give up your guns," but the Sheikh, who was an honourable man, advised us not to surrender all our weapons.

'In the end we handed over three hundred of our guns. The Sheikh gave us his son as a hostage and said we should kill him if the Muslims broke their word. He then went on his donkey to Diyarbakir and took a written order from the Pasha-Commander that the soldiers and the Kurds should leave. I will never forget the sight of the Ottoman army taking down their tents and marching away down the valley towards Midyat.

'We gave the Sheikh back his son, saying we could not bear to kill the son of such a man, even if the Ottomans did break their word. Before the siege there were three Kurdish families living in Ein Wardo. When the fighting began we sent them away, but afterwards we welcomed them back. After that we lived together in peace and had no more trouble from the Muslims.'

'What do you mean, no more trouble?' said Bedros. 'Every day now we have trouble. How many Kurds live in the village now? Today they almost outnumber the Christians in Ein Wardo.'

'After the war, when I was a young man,' said Abouna Shabo, 'we were friends. But then we were in the majority, so they could give us no trouble. Now the Muslims have all the power and it is different. My son is right.'

'They give us very bad trouble,' said Bedros. 'In the last three years ten Christians have been killed in the villages around Ein Wardo. We cannot be friends like this.'

'Could we go and visit Ein Wardo?' I asked.

'It is too late today,' replied Bedros. 'It's not worth it. The Kurdish village guards will give you problems. It's after 3.30 already. Get home. Get behind the monastery walls.'

'These days feel just like those before 1914,' said the old priest, pulling himself slowly out of his chair and making his way, bent-backed, across the room. 'It feels like before a storm. You can see the black clouds, and the first drops are already falling.'

'Do you think there will be another massacre?' I asked.

'How many people are there left to kill?' said Abouna Shabo.

'There will not be a massacre,' said Bedros. 'Just a few killings every year. Priests will be kidnapped. Others will be kicked off their land.'

'All is in vain,' said Abouna Shabo, disappearing through the door. 'The English troops will not come!'

'And even if they did come,' said Bedros, showing us out, 'it would be too late now. We would not be here. How many years are left for us? Three years? Five? Ten?'

'Only God knows,' said the old priest. 'Only God knows.'

After Midyat, driving back through the wooden skeletons of the charred olive groves, Yacoub saw something hanging from a tree.

'Did you see that?' he said suddenly. 'In the branches.'

'What?'

'In the trees back there. I only caught a glimpse. It looked like a body.'

'Shouldn't we go back?'

'No,' said Mas'ud firmly. 'It is very dangerous. We must keep going.'

'Why?'

'If it was a corpse the PKK may still be about. They hang village guards by the roadside as an example to other collaborators. We must not go back.'

Mas'ud pressed his foot on the accelerator and the car lurched forward.

'I have heard of this before,' said Yacoub. 'The PKK stuff the collaborator's mouth with banknotes. It is to show that the village guards are taking Turkish money to betray their own people.'

Back at the monastery, Afrem was waiting for us. We told him what we had seen and he agreed that we were right to have pressed on, saying he would send out a search party in the morning. Then he took me aside.

'Listen, William,' he said. 'I have bad news for you. Soldiers were here all day wanting to speak to you. I told them you had already gone, but they did not believe me and waited for five hours. They left just forty minutes ago. They will come back tomorrow. I think you should leave as early as you can.'

'Don't worry,' I said, smiling. 'I'm going tomorrow.'

'It is for the best,' said Afrem gently.

HOTEL CLIFF, HASSAKE, SYRIA, 26 AUGUST

This morning, by the time I had got up, the monastery search party had already returned. They said that whatever Yacoub had seen the previous night, there was nothing there now. There was no body; the branches were empty. Yacoub, still convinced he had seen a corpse, suggested that the army could have removed it at dawn.

The previous night I had wanted to get out of the Tur Abdin as quickly as I could. But now the absence of a dead body swinging from the tree, and the reassuring clarity of the bright morning light, made me think I had perhaps been exaggerating the dangers, and I decided to try to see Ein Wardo before heading for the Syrian border. Yacoub, however, declined to come, saying the road to Ein Wardo had frequently been mined. It was up to me whether I wanted to risk it, but he was staying in the monastery. Nevertheless Mas'ud agreed to take me there as long as we left straight away. We said our goodbyes, and set off just after eight.

In Midyat, Mas'ud stopped to make enquiries in the bazaar. He had been anxious about landmines, but learned that two tractors had passed down the road from Ein Wardo the day before, and decided it would be safe to risk it. We passed the bullet-marked Ottoman barracks the Ein Wardo defenders had attacked in 1917, and headed off up the track.

As we drove the road climbed, and the narrow green valley grew hilly and arid. In the valley bottoms some narrow strips were still under plough, but the slopes were given over to sheep. At one point we passed a shepherd's stone sheiling and were chased for ten minutes by a huge Anatolian sheepdog with a collar spiked like a medieval instrument of torture. A few minutes after the dog had given up chasing us we rounded a bend in the road, and high above us Ein Wardo came into view.

It was easy to see why the Suriani had chosen it for their last line of defence. The village perched on top of a near-vertical moraine at the end of a valley; its slopes were so steep and the gradient so regular that they resembled a man-made *glacis*. At the top of the slope, a ring of stone houses formed a curtain wall as convincing as that of any Crusader castle. It was a perfect defensive position.

Dominating the village at one end of the slope was the church. At first, from a distance, you could see only the square steeple, topped with an ornamental cupola. But when you climbed the snaking path leading up to the village you were presented with a very different view. The four corners of the church were punctuated by massive thick-walled towers, each bantering upwards to a flat terrace. Each tower was pierced by three circuits of narrow loopholes and arrow-slits. A fortified church, it seemed, was the only kind of defence the Suriani could build in the years before the First World War without provoking the suspicion of the Ottoman authorities. All it lacked were crenellations or battlements at the top of the towers.

Leaving Mas'ud with his car at the entrance to the village, I clambered up the slope over a tumble of ruined houses, many still pitted with bullet or shrapnel holes. Compared with the ruinous look of much of the village, the church was still in a very good state of preservation. A series of outhouses (once perhaps the home of the priest) had collapsed and were now roofless, but the main fortification was still quite intact.

I wandered in, through a series of gatehouses each designed to expose any attacker to the full field of fire from the loopholes and wall-walks above. For an emergency measure, built in secret and disguised as a church, it was really an extremely competent piece of military architecture.

Within, the church was still in use. Lamps and fairy lights were festooned over the chancel arch, and the walls were cluttered with sacred images: icons of Eastern warrior saints; sentimental nineteenth-century oleographs of the Holy Family; brightly coloured textiles showing the Sacred Heart or a selection of weeping Madonnas.

As I sat at the back, a very old hunchbacked woman stumbled in, frantically crossing herself. She walked up to the altar and kissed an icon, then touched a cross painted on the apse wall. Turning back, she saw me and came straight up, chattering excitedly in Turoyo. From her imitation of a Maxim gun, it was clear that she was telling the story of the siege, but without Yacoub to interpret I couldn't understand what she was saying. She seemed unconcerned by my lack of comprehension, and pulling at my sleeve, led me up into the corkscrew staircase of one of the towers, chattering without ceasing as we climbed. From the terrace at the top you could see out over miles and miles of the surrounding hills and valleys, the slopes falling away steeply from the base of the towers.

So overcome was I by the beauty of the view that I did not at first see the bags of mortar and the trowels discreetly hidden in a corner of the roof terrace. It was only then that I noticed what I had missed from below, and what no one in Mar Gabriel had told me. The walls of all the towers had recently been reinforced and strengthened. New mortar had been applied to the walls, and the loopholes had been reconstructed. I felt sure it was more than a renovation. The fortress, the last refuge of the Suriani, was being quietly rebuilt, and was now nearly ready for an emergency.

The Suriani were expecting the worst; and the lessons of 1914 had not been forgotten.

Mas'ud and I drove back to Midyat in high spirits. We had got away with it: we hadn't hit a landmine, hadn't been kidnapped by the PKK, and had avoided being threatened by Kurdish village guards or hauled into a Turkish prison. Now we were finished. I had seen everything I wanted to see. I could get out of the war zone and cross the Syrian border; Mas'ud could return to his family. I had not realised the oppressiveness of the sense of imminent danger until now, when I felt its pall rising from us. It was a wonderful feeling: like coming up for air.

We whooped as we passed the shepherd's sheiling and were again chased by the enormous wolf-dog; we cheered and accelerated away down the bumpy potholed track, throwing up a thick dust-trail into which the slavering beast disappeared. As we crossed a ridge and saw Midyat laid out below us, we talked excitedly about what we would do that night, Mas'ud reeling off the enormous dinner his wife would prepare for him when he returned. He was still detailing the different kinds of Kurdish sweets with which he would end this meal, when an army Land-Rover suddenly pulled out from its hiding place behind a pile of discarded roadbuilding material and blocked the road in front of us. As Mas'ud screeched to a halt, only narrowly avoiding crashing into the Land-Rover's side, three soldiers appeared on top of the gravel and levelled their carbines at us.

We got out with our hands raised. The officer asked for our documents, and taking them from us, read out the details down his walkie-talkie. There was a crackle of static and some instructions. Putting our documents into his top pocket, he told us to get back into our car and follow him. The Land-Rover turned around and the soldiers jumped in, keeping their guns pointed in our direction.

At the crossroads in the town centre, the officer conferred with the plainclothes security police in their dark glasses. Two of them got into a waiting white Fiat and followed behind us. Sandwiched in this way, we were escorted out of town to a barbed-wire enclosure a mile or so on the far side of Midyat. Mas'ud looked accusingly at me, but neither of us spoke. I hid my notebooks under my seat. The officer jumped out and indicated that we should follow him. After a week in the company of the Suriani with their Turkish horror-stories, I half-imagined the Turks within to be preparing their thumbscrews and racks. To my alarm and disgust, I saw that my hands were shaking.

Inside, however, we found to our surprise that the Turkish

army could not have been much more polite had we been visiting dignitaries from Ankara. After a short wait in a corridor, we were escorted to the office of an army Captain. He turned out to be young and educated and bored, and seemed surprised and rather pleased to see us. Speaking in fluent French, he told us to sit down while the officer from the Land-Rover related the circumstances of our arrest and handed over our documents. When he had finished he saluted and left the room. The Captain took out a packet of cigarettes and offered it to us, calling at the same time for tea to be brought. Where was I from, he asked. Scotland? Did I have any Johnnie Walker in the car? He was from Istanbul, he said, and was looking forward to going back home on leave. He had had enough of this barbarous end of the country. He asked whether I had been to Istanbul, and I gabbled away nervously about the beauties of his home city. He briefly asked what I was doing in these parts, and I told him I was writing about Byzantine architecture. After twenty more minutes of general conversation, he dialled a number and spoke briefly to the person who answered. Then he apologised to us for the trouble he had caused us and said we were free to go.

Back in the car, Mas'ud leaned back in his seat and exhaled loudly.

'I don't believe it,' he said.

'If the police have been following us,' I said, 'they certainly didn't tell the army about it.'

'He was so friendly.'

'Let's go,' I said, 'before they change their mind.'

Mas'ud twisted the key in the ignition, turned the car around, and drove forward. He had nearly passed through the gates when from the building behind us there came a series of loud shouts. In the mirror we could see two armed recruits running frantically towards us, shouting for us to stop. I felt a lead weight sink to the pit of my stomach. The soldiers beckoned us back, and Mas'ud slowly reversed the car to the command post. We sat there without getting out, wondering what might be coming. There must have been a call from the secret police: who had I talked to? What had they said? Where were my notes?

Seconds later, the Captain came down the steps and walked over to the car.

'Messieurs,' he said gaily. 'Vous êtes idiots.'

So this was how it was going to be. Our eyes met.

'You've forgotten these,' he said.

In his hand he held my passport and Mas'ud's ID card.

'Bonne chance!' he said, smiling broadly and waving goodbye. 'Visit us again soon! Bon voyage!'

III

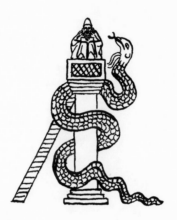

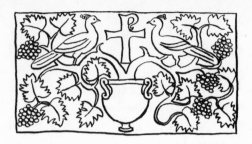

THE BARON HOTEL, ALEPPO, SYRIA, 28 AUGUST 1994

The Baron is a legendary place. Everyone from Agatha Christie to Kemal Ataturk has stayed here, while Monsieur T. E. Lawrence's unpaid bill of 8 June 1914 is still displayed in a glass cabinet in the sitting room. Downstairs, the decor, untouched since the 1920s, is so redolent of the Levant between the wars that you can almost hear the swish of flapper-dresses and baggy tropical suits echoing from the now chipped and silent dance-floor.

Despite the chaos of Syria's Ba'athist economy and the decay of many of its towns, the Baron is still, from the outside, rather a magnificent building: a stone-built Ottoman villa with a blind arcade of mock-Mameluke arches giving onto a wide first-floor terrace. At the top of the façade are sculpted the words *Baron's Hotel 1911, Mazloumian Frères*, in French, Armenian and Ottoman Turkish. Inside are high-beamed ceilings and brass chandeliers; a large notice dating from the early years of the French Mandate proclaims that the Baron is 'L'unique hôtel de 1ère classe à Alep: confort parfait, situation unique,' while another of the same period, decorated with a watercolour of Ctesiphon, announces that the Simplon–Orient Express can transport you in 'safety, rapidity and economy' from London to Baghdad in seven days (the original promise of six days, obviously over-optimistic, is crossed out).

Yet for all its charm, it would be dishonest to pretend that the Baron has not seen better days. The rooms – which look as though they haven't been painted since Leonard Woolley stayed here on his way to dig the Ziggurat of Ur in 1922 – are now shabby and unloved, with peeling wallpaper and potholed parquet floors. Moreover the *situation unique* – the shady cypresses, the gardens and bubbling canals which Lawrence writes of in his letters – have long since given way to lines of seedy hard-porn cinemas covered with lurid posters of nearly-naked American girls (this week *The Last Virgin in Las Vegas*) into which crowds of hungry-looking Arab boys pour each evening.

In the streets, jammed bumper-to-bumper, 1940s Pontiacs exhale a thick fog of black exhaust. The pollution wafts into the streetside restaurants and clings to the layers of grease dripping from the grilling doner kebabs. In between the *kebabji* and the blue-movie theatres lie the heavy-engineering shops and garages – *Sarkis Iskenian Caterpillar Parts, A. Sanossian Grinding: Vee Rubber Wambo Superstone* – belonging to the Armenian entrepreneurs who for the last forty years have dominated what is left of the once-vibrant Aleppo economy. If, like Lawrence, you tried to go shooting 'one hundred yards in front of the Baron', today you would be more likely to hit either a Bedu aficionado of the *Emmanuelle* films or some grimy-faced Armenian mechanic than the duck Lawrence was after.

Nevertheless, it is still easy to see why this hotel appealed so much to a former generation of English travellers. At eight this morning I woke up, momentarily confused as to where I was, and looked at the wall beside my bed. There hung an English coaching print and a framed portrait of a black retriever with a pheasant in its mouth emerging from a village stream beside a thatched cottage ('The most useful and adaptable of all the retrievers, with a formidable record of wins at county shows, the black retriever has a strong otter-like tail well suited for swimming'). It was then that the penny dropped. The inexplicably horrible food, the decaying neo-Gothic architecture, the deep baths and the uncomfortable beds: no wonder Lawrence and his contemporaries felt so much at home here – the Baron is the perfect replica of some particularly Spartan English public school, strangely displaced to the deserts of the Middle East.

And yet, despite its best efforts, I feel this place growing on me. I have always loved the fact that in Syria you can still walk on Roman roads that have not been resurfaced since the time of Diocletian, or stand on castle walls that have not been restored since Saladin stormed them. In the same way, perhaps I should be pleased that in the Baron you can sleep in sheets that have not been washed since T. E. Lawrence slept there, and even be bitten by the same colonies of bedbugs that once nibbled the great Ataturk.

As I sit here with a glass of whisky under an endearingly ludicrous picture of two top-hatted English coachmen, the troubles of Mar Gabriel feel a world away. But I must record how I got here from the roadblocks and minefields of the Tur Abdin.

After our arrest in Midyat, Mas'ud and I retraced our footsteps along the heavily guarded main roads to Mardin, and there, within sight of the Byzantine domes and cupolas of the monastery of Deir el-Zaferan, drove steeply downhill into the baking mud-steppe of Mesopotamia. From there we headed east again, along the Syrian border, on the main military road which leads through the plains towards the Iraqi frontier and Baghdad. Twin electrified border fences and a minefield flanked us immediately to the right; beyond stretched the plains of northern Syria. The smooth, wide military road was quite empty but for the occasional Turkish tank rumbling slowly in the opposite direction.

Delayed by our arrest and the interminable gauntlet of army checkpoints, we were in danger of failing to get to the border post before it closed for the day. But Mas'ud drove at breakneck speed, and after less than forty minutes the towers of the border town of Nisibis rose shimmering from the plain ahead. During late antiquity Nisibis passed back and forth between the Byzantines and the Sassanian Persians, finally being surrendered to the Persians in 363 A.D. Yet the town somehow managed to maintain an effervescent intellectual life despite its frontline position and the incessant skirmishes between its Persian garrison and that of the

Byzantine frontier post of Dara, less than forty miles to the west.

For after the Sassanian takeover of the city, Nisibis became the principal centre of Persia's large Nestorian Christian minority. Its university of eight hundred students came to rival that of Edessa. Indeed it was through Nisibis – along with the two other great Nestorian university cities, Jundishapur (near Teheran) and Merv (now in Uzbekistan) – that the Nestorians played an important part in bringing Greek philosophy, science and medicine first to the Persian and thence to the Islamic world. Moreover it was from the Nestorian school of Nisibis – via Moorish Cordoba – that many of the works of Aristotle and Plato eventually reached the new universities of medieval Europe.

As far as the Greeks were concerned, however, the loss of the town remained a continual slight to Byzantine pride; and the fact that it came to shelter a population of Christian heretics only made this worse. As a result the city figures surprisingly prominently in Byzantine letters, and John Moschos tells a story about Nisibis which, for all its piety, gives an intriguingly detailed and convincing picture of bazaar life in a Mesopotamian border town in the sixth century.

The anecdote concerns a Christian woman married to a 'pagan' (presumably Zoroastrian) soldier. The soldier had a small sum of capital which he wanted to invest. But his Christian wife (presumably a Nestorian) persuaded him to give it instead to the poor who waited in front of the five-arched portal of the Nisibis cathedral, promising that the god of the Christians would reward him many times over.

'Three months later, the couple's expenses exceeded their ability to pay. The man said to his wife: "Sister, the god of the Christians has not paid us back, and here we are, in need." In reply, the woman said, "He will repay. Go to where you handed over the money and he will return it right away." So her husband set off to the church at a run. When he came to the spot where he had given the coins to the poor, he went all round the church, expecting to find somebody who would give back to him what was owing. But all he found was the poor, still sitting there. While he was trying to decide which of them to speak to, he saw at his feet on the marble floor one large *miliarision* lying there, one of those which he himself had distributed. Bending down he picked it up and went back to his house. Then he said to his spouse: "Look – I just went to your church, and believe me, woman, I did not see the god of the Christians as you said I would. And he certainly did not give me anything, except this *miliarision* lying where I give fifty away." '

His wife told him to stop complaining and to go off and buy some food with the coin. Later the man reappeared with some bread, a flask of wine and a fresh fish. While his wife was cleaning the fish, she found inside a beautiful stone which she suggested he try to sell.

'He did not know what it was, for he was a simple man. But he took the stone and went to the moneychanger. It was evening, time for the changer to go home, but the soldier said, "Give me what you will," and the other replied, "Take five *miliarisia* for it." Believing that the merchant was making fun of him, the man said, "Would you give that much for it?" But the merchant thought the soldier was being sarcastic, so he said, "Well, take ten *miliarisia* then." Still thinking the merchant was making fun of him, the soldier remained silent, at which the other said, "All right – twenty *miliarisia*." As the soldier again kept silent and made no response, the merchant raised his offer to thirty, then to fifty *miliarisia*. By this time the soldier realised that the stone must be very valuable. Little by little the merchant raised his offer until it reached three hundred large *miliarisia*.'

Almost nothing appears to survive today of late antique Nisibis save the cathedral baptistry, dated by a Greek inscription to 359 A.D. Otherwise, Nisibis's muse has long departed, and as Mas'ud raced through the crowded bazaars, sending barrow-boys and pack-donkeys flying into ditches, there was no sign that the town had ever been more than what it was now: a dusty, flyblown frontier post, crawling with Turkish soldiers and gun-wielding security guards. We reached the crossing point – a tin hut and a coil of barbed wire standing beside a single, enigmatic line of Byzantine pillars – just five minutes before it closed. I embraced Mas'ud, wished him luck, and paid him double the amount we had agreed in Diyarbakir.

The Turkish border guards rifled through my rucksack, sniffing suspiciously at the mosquito repellant but, thankfully, ignoring the notebooks. Finally, at two minutes to three, in the sweltering heat of a Mesopotamian summer afternoon, I crossed the no-man's land into Syria.

Immediately the atmosphere changed. Ten years ago, on my first journey around the Near East, I remember my nervousness at leaving the then peaceable countryside of south-east Turkey for what I conceived to be the sinister terrorist state of Syria. Now the roles are reversed. Syria may still be a one-party police state, but it is a police state that leaves its citizens alone as long as they keep out of politics; certainly it feels like the Garden of Eden compared with the tension on the other side of the border. At the immigration shed, Kurdish and Turoyo were being spoken openly. On the roads there were no checkpoints, no tanks, no armoured personnel carriers and no burned-out car-skeletons. The taxi drivers seemed relaxed and happy to drive at night. No one spoke, in hushed voices, of 'troubles', of emptied villages or relatives who had 'disappeared'.

Indeed, at the Hotel Cliff in Hassake where I spent that first night (the name, disappointingly, turned out to be a reference to the Ottoman Caliph, not an ageing pop star), only the endless ranks of framed portraits of President Asad and his sinister son Basil (recently killed in a high-speed car crash) reminded one that Syria was still a Ba'athist dictatorship with a ubiquitous *mukhabarat* (secret police). The regime's claim to legitimacy still rests on the shaky foundations of a series of East European-style 'elections' that are so openly rigged they have become something of a national joke. I remember a story about them from my last visit. After one particularly dubious poll, a group of Asad's advisers is said to have gone to see the President with the results.

'There is good news, Mr President,' they said. 'You are more popular with the people of Syria than ever before. 99 per cent of the people voted for you. Only 1 per cent abstained. What more could you ask?'

'Just one thing,' Asad is said to have replied. 'Their names and addresses.'

The following morning I wandered around Hassake. Behind a modern gloss of avenues, roundabouts and streetlights lay a warren of mud-walled compounds, a timeless labyrinth that could have been built at virtually any time between the Tower of Babel and Operation Desert Storm.

It was in one of these compounds that I found George Joseph, a cousin of one of the monks at Mar Gabriel. George was a huge man with a thick black beard and an enormous paunch. He was very well educated – had picked up some sort of diploma in London – and now made his money running a taxi service and various dubious-sounding import/export businesses operating over the Iraqi and Turkish borders. When I introduced myself he shouted for tea, and quickly persuaded me to take his taxi to Aleppo. I had been planning to take the bus, at a fraction of the cost, but soon found myself convinced by George that his taxi was the only sensible choice.

While a flunkey went off to fill George's pick-up with petrol, we talked about the history of the old Nestorian university in Nisibis, and I asked whether there were any Nestorians still left in the area.

'There weren't any until the Gulf War,' replied George. 'But in 1991 fifty thousand Nestorian refugees fled here from western Iraq. They saw what had happened to the Kurds, and feared Saddam Hussein would use his poison gas on them next.'

'So where are they now?' I asked.

'Most have got away,' said George. 'Some got visas for the West; others have sneaked across the Turkish border. It is easier to get fake passports and visas in Turkey than here.' He broke into a sly grin. 'Smugglers and fakers are not so active in Syria,' he said. 'You have to be very good – very good indeed – to get away with that sort of business here.'

'And the Nestorians who are left?'

'There are about ten thousand of them, still incarcerated in a refugee camp ten miles from here, towards the Iraqi border. It's a horrible place. They're locked up in a barbed-wire pen with only two thousand devil-worshippers for company.'

'Devil-worshippers?'

'Yezidis,' said George. 'They're an Iraqi sect. Strictly speaking they're actually devil-propitiators, not devil-worshippers. They call Lucifer 'Malik Tawus', the Peacock Angel, and offer sacrifices to keep him happy. They believe Lucifer, the Devil, has been forgiven by God and reinstated as Chief Angel, supervising the day-to-day running of the word's affairs.'

'And how do they get on with the Nestorians?'

'Actually very well,' said George. 'Some people believe that the Yezidis were originally a sort of strange Gnostic offshoot of the Nestorian Church. I don't know whether that is true, but the Yezidi priests and the Christian bishops certainly make a point of visiting each other on their different feast days. '

Either way, I thought, it was a wonderfully exotic idea: respectably robed Nestorian bishops presenting their compliments to the Chief Priest of the devil-worshippers on the occasion of Satan's birthday. As George talked, I could not stop thinking about the extraordinary camp full of Yezidi devil-worshippers and Nestorians, the most ancient heterodox (and, in the eyes of many, heretical) Christian Church still in existence.

The Nestorians had initially disagreed with the Orthodox over the exact nature of Christ's humanity, maintaining that there were two entirely separate persons in the incarnate Christ, one human, the other divine, in opposition to the Orthodox belief that Christ was a single person, at once human *and* divine. Expelled from the Byzantine Empire in the fifth century, the Church had taken root with astonishing speed further to the east. By the seventh century Nestorian archbishops watched over cathedrals as far apart as Bahrain, Kerala, Kashgar, Lhasa and Sigan-Fu in north-west China. By 660 A.D. there were more than twenty Nestorian archbishops east of the Oxus, and Nestorian monasteries in most Chinese cities. Genghis Khan had a Nestorian guardian, and at one point the Mongol Khans very nearly converted to Nestorianism, which might well have made the Church the most powerful religious force in Asia. But instead, by the early years of the twentieth century a series of genocidal reverses had brought the Nestorians to the verge of extinction. This latest sad imprisonment in a wire pen in the desert was only the most recent in a long series of disasters for the Church that had once brought the secret of silk farming to Byzantium, Greek medicine to Islam, and which, most importantly of all, had helped transmit the forgotten philosophy of ancient Athens back to the West.

Separated from the rest of Christendom by their extreme isolation, the Nestorians have preserved many of the traditions of the early Church which have either disappeared altogether elsewhere, or else survived only in the most unrecognisable forms. Their legends – about the Holy Wood of the Tree of Life and the Holy Spices of the Tree of Knowledge – are fragments of fossilised early Christian folklore, while their eucharistic rite, the Anaphora of the Apostles Addai and Mari, is the oldest Christian liturgy still in use anywhere in the world.

Once, browsing in a library in Oxford, I remember stumbling across a rare copy of *The Book of Protection*, a volume of Nestorian charms and spells. It was a strange and wonderful collection of magical formulae which purported to have been handed down from the angels to Adam and thence to King Solomon. The spells – the Anathema of the Angel Gabriel for the Evil Eye, the Names on the Ring of King Solomon, the Anathema of Mar Shalita for the Evil Spirit, the Charm for the Cow which is Excited towards her Mistress – gave a vivid picture of an isolated and superstitious mountain people, surrounded by enemies and unknown dangers. They also emphasised the Nestorians' backwardness in the face of the artillery of their enemies – among them was a charm for Binding the Guns and the Engines of War:

> By the Power of the Voice of our Lord which cutteth
> the Flame of the Fire, I bind, expel, anathematise the
> bullets of the engines of war, and the balls of the guns
> of our wicked enemies away from him who beareth this
> charm. By the prayers of the Virgin, the Mother of Fire,
> may the stones which they fling with the machine and

with the guns not be moved, nor heated, nor come
forth from the mouth of our enemies' machines against
the one who beareth these charms, but let our enemy
be as dead as in the midst of the grave . . .

Yet this desperate primitiveness in war was apparently coupled
with an unwise enthusiasm for violent blood feuds with their
neighbours. Alarmed Anglican missionaries who tried to make
contact with the Nestorians in the nineteenth and early twentieth
century reported that they would go into battle against their tribal
enemies led by their bishop, wearing his purple episcopal trousers,
and that their priests would return bearing the severed ears of
their victims. On one occasion a dog-collared Anglican vicar was
invited to lunch by a Nestorian chieftain and had the temerity to
refuse, offering some lame excuses. 'It is my hope that you will
come and stay,' repeated the chieftain. 'If you do I shall be proud
to receive you; if you do not, my honour will make it needful for
me to shoot you.'

I told George how much I wanted to try to get into the camp
and talk to the Nestorian refugees. But even as I was speaking he
shook his head. It was impossible for outsiders to get in or out
of the camp, he said. It was surrounded by barbed wire, and the
only gateway bristled with *mukhabarat*. I would be wasting my
time even to try. The most I would achieve, he said, would be to get
arrested by President Asad's secret police, something he strongly
advised against. 'But you could always try to interview some Nestorians when you get back to England,' he suggested.

'What do you mean?'

'I believe there is a very large Nestorian community in . . . is
there somewhere in London called Ealing?'

'*Ealing?*'

'Yes, I think that's right,' said George. 'It was in Ealing that the
current Nestorian Patriarch was crowned. There should be far
more Nestorians in London than here. Ealing has the largest Nestorian community in Europe.'

Such are the humiliations of the travel writer in the late twentieth century: go to the ends of the earth to search for the most

142

exotic heretics in the world, and you find they have cornered the kebab business at the end of your street in London.

I threw my rucksack into the back of George's pick-up; we drove through the streets of Hassake and out into the cotton fields beyond. It was a bright late-summer day. A strong wind was blowing, and billowing clouds were gusting over the steppe. Unveiled Bedouin women were standing in lines in the fields, picking the white buds with babies strapped to their backs. Their faces were tattooed, and their headdresses were fringed with glinting silver coins. Their dresses were of deep purple velvet, belted at the waist.

We crossed the bridge over the Khabur River, and almost immediately we entered the desert. The road stretched straight ahead, its converging lines bisecting a flat horizon of dry and lifeless sand.

'My father was nearly killed on this road,' said George, breaking the silence.

'How?'

'It's a long story.'

'This is a long drive.'

'Well,' said George, 'in 1929 my father bought sixty thousand acres of desert near Hassake on the Khabur River. Until the Mandate, the area was deserted except for Bedouin. But the French offered land to anyone who would irrigate it and grow crops. My father was a younger son and inherited nothing from his father, so he took on the challenge. It was backbreaking work and he nearly went mad in the heat of the desert. But after five years of hard work, of watering and planting the land, he finally had a very successful harvest and made a big profit: fifty gold pounds. It was more than enough to pay off the money he had borrowed to buy the land. But he had a problem: he did not know how to get the gold from Hassake to Aleppo, as the road used to be famous for its brigands. But he knew it was probably less safe still among the Bedouin in Hassake, so he asked an Armenian driver with an old model-T Ford to take him the next time he went to Aleppo. The day came, and my father put the money under his girdle and set off with the Armenian.

'Halfway along the road, in the early evening, in the middle of the desert, they saw a very old Bedu. He was standing in the road, hitchhiking. My father said, "Poor man, let's pick him up," but the Armenian said he never took in strangers. They drove on, but then they began to feel guilty, for they knew the old man would be stuck in the desert all night. So they went back and picked him up. The Bedu was very grateful; he said, "*Salaam alekum*,' and sat smiling in the back.

'Then ten minutes later the old man pulled out two revolvers. He put one against the neck of my father, the other against the neck of the Armenian, and ordered that they stop the car. My father went mad: he was carrying on him every dinar he had earned for five years. So he begged the Bedu to be honourable and show mercy to two men who had tried to help him. But the Bedu merely sneered and said: "Undress." The Armenian undressed and turned out his pockets, but he had only a small amount of money. So the Bedu pointed a gun at my father and said that now he should undress. My father undressed very, very slowly. The Bedu began to get impatient. He said: "Hurry, hurry." My father took off his jacket, then his shirt, then his vest. "Hurry," said the Bedu. So my father took off his trousers, and as he did so the fifty gold pounds fell out and rolled onto the ground.

'The Bedu could hardly believe his eyes, and he jumped to catch the coins before they rolled off the embankment. As he did so my father kicked him in the face. The Bedu took off – into the hands of the Armenian. The Armenian held him while my father grabbed the guns. There they were in the road in the middle of the desert, two of them in their underpants, all of them scrabbling around trying to kill each other. The Bedu produced a knife, but the Armenian got him into an armlock with one hand and tried to strangle him with the other. All this time my father was punching the Bedu. He had lost all control: he had the strength of a madman. At first it was fear, then it was for revenge.

'After a while the man was overpowered, but not before all three of them were covered with blood. So the Armenian said: "We cannot leave this man here. Tomorrow he will be waiting for us to return, and he'll have forty other tribesmen with him.

144

We must kill him." But before my father had time to answer, the man fell down. He was stone dead.

'The Armenian said, "What did you do?" To which my father replied, "You killed him." "No," said the Armenian. "*You* killed him." They argued for a few minutes, then drove on in silence, leaving the dead Bedu by the road. They were very nervous. Neither of them had ever been in such a situation. After fifteen miles they came to a French patrol. The officer ordered them to stop and asked them what they were doing on the road so late. He could see how nervous they were, and became suspicious. So he ordered them out of the car, and as soon as they got out he saw the blood covering their shirts.

'The Armenian said, "It was his idea. He's just killed a Bedu hitchhiker." My father answered, "No, no – it was him." The Frenchman told both of them to be quiet. He put them in hand-cuffs and searched them. In the back of the car he found the Bedu's ID. "Was this the man you just killed?" he asked. Both men were silent. Then the policeman said: "Perhaps I should tell you that this is Ali ibn Mohammed, the most wanted brigand in the Near East. There is a reward of one hundred gold pounds for anyone who finds him, dead or alive." "Ali ibn Mohammed?" said my father and the Armenian, both looking at each other. "The most dangerous robber in Syria?" "It was me that killed him," said my father. "He's lying," said the Armenian, "I killed him." "No. I did . . ." '

'What happened?' I asked.

'They split the reward,' said George, smiling. 'In the end. After much argument.'

Towards late afternoon we saw in front of us a trickle of molten mercury: the Euphrates lit up by the sinking sun. It was pale and ghostly and shrouded by a thin halo of mist. To one side rose the hump of a prehistoric tell, and beside it a modern suspension bridge guarded by two sleeping Syrian army guards. We rolled over the bridge and onto the Aleppo highway.

The desert was now flecked with round, white Bedouin tents. Around them were flocks of thin sheep, each one throwing up its own faint slipstream of dust. Occasional villages of mud-brick rose from the sand, their shattered beehive domes clustered like a line of broken eggs in a punnet. Usually these villages seemed to be deserted, but some were still occupied, their ancient curves topped by television aerials and telephone wires.

As we drove on, the Bedouin encampments became more frequent. Then we came to a hillside covered in graves. The shanty towns and slums of Aleppo's outer suburbs opened up before us; and ahead rose the earthen drum of Aleppo's great citadel.

ALEPPO, 2 SEPTEMBER

Yesterday evening I fulfilled a promise I had made in Mar Gabriel.

Just before I arrived there, the Abbot had received from the printers in Istanbul a set of postcards. They reproduced some of the more remarkable illustrations from the medieval Syriac manuscripts in the Mar Gabriel library. The Abbot was very excited by his new pictures, and begged me to deliver a boxful to his Metropolitan in Aleppo.

Getting to see Metropolitan Ibrahim, however, proved more of a struggle than I had expected, if only because I made the mistake of accepting the offer of one of the Baron's own taxi drivers to take me there. The man was an Armenian which, I figured, would make him more likely to know his way around Christian Aleppo than a Muslim driver; but in the event all it actually meant was that he had a healthy thirst for Armenian cognac, a half-drunk bottle of which lay in his glove compartment, and from which he occasionally took a swig when we stopped at traffic lights. Thus fortified, he drove me at high speed around a bewildering variety of cathedrals, belonging in turn to the Chaldeans, Latins, Greek Orthodox and Greek Catholics, before finally admitting that he had no idea where the cathedral of the Syrian Orthodox was situated.

Eventually we pulled in at a rival taxi rank: 'Please,' I said to one of the drivers, 'I am looking for the Syrian Orthodox cathedral.'

TAXI DRIVER: You want cathedral? Which cathedral? We have many cathedral in Aleppo.

W.D.: I'm after the Surianis' cathedral.

TAXI DRIVER: Which Surianis? We have many Surianis in Aleppo. Syrian Catholics, Syrian Protestants, Syrian Orthodox...

W.D.: I want the Syrian *Orthodox*. I think I said that to begin with.

TAXI DRIVER: Which Orthodox? In Aleppo...

W.D. (*getting irritated*): Syrian Orthodox.

TAXI DRIVER (*surprised*): You want Syrian Orthodox?

W.D.: Yes.

TAXI DRIVER: Not Syrian Catholics?

W.D.: No.

TAXI DRIVER: Not Assyrian Orthodox?

W.D. (*explosive*): I WANT THE SYRIAN ORTHODOX CATHEDRAL.

TAXI DRIVER (*pensive*): Syrian Orthodox cathedral. (*Pause*) That I don't know.

Luckily, someone at the next stand did know, and after he had explained its whereabouts we set off again at terrifying speed, the Armenian driver attempting to mollify me with a display of his party trick, changing gear with his foot.

'Where you from?' he asked, changing down to second with his right foot while his right hand fumbled for the bottle in the glove compartment.

'Scotland.'

'I have been to New York and to L.A.'

'Holiday?'

'Little bit holiday.'

'What do you mean?'

'I went for operation. American hospitals very good. Last year I had car accident. Big problem...'

The Syrian Orthodox, it turned out, had cunningly secreted

their cathedral behind a filling station in the Suleymaniye district of the city; we had already passed it several times without noticing it. The Metropolitan's Palace was even more successfully hidden: it lay tucked in behind the back of the cathedral. I was met at the gates of the palace by a raven-robed flunkey and led up, past the long black cathedral Cadillac (emblazoned on its back window with a colour sticker of the Metropolitan's coat of arms) to a first-floor reception room. There I was shown to a gilt armchair beneath a huge photograph of a beaming President Asad, and a fractionally smaller portrait of the Syrian Orthodox Patriarch of Antioch.

After a few minutes the door was flung open and the small, round figure of Gregorios Yohanna Ibrahim walked in, backwards. In his hand he held a portable telephone into which he was talking animatedly, while at the same time waving goodbye to a young couple with his free hand. He turned a pirouette and advanced towards me, his free hand extended. As he did so he finished his telephone call, snapped shut the phone with a flick of his thumb, and popped it into his cassock pocket.

'Mr William?' he said. 'I've been expecting you. I received a letter from Mar Gabriel telling me you were coming. Come, let me show you something which will interest you.'

The Metropolitan took me over to a trestle-table at the side of the room, pausing only to sign a document that a bowing function-ary offered him. On the trestle lay some architect's plans.

'At the moment there are no functioning Syrian Orthodox mon-asteries in Syria,' he said, unrolling the blueprints. 'But now I'm going to rebuild Tel Ada. For many years this has been my dream. It was the monastery that the young St Symeon Stylites joined when he first left home. According to the great fifth-century Bishop Theodoret of Cyrrhus – you know his *History of the Monks of Syria*? I will lend you a copy – there were once 150 monks at Tel Ada, but it has been a ruin for nearly thirteen hundred years. Little is left. We bought the land from the farmer in 1987 and have just had our plans authorised by the authorities in Damascus. Look.' The Metropolitan pointed to a geometric shape at the centre of his blueprints. 'The church is to be based on St Symeon's church at Qala'at Semaan: it will be an open octagon and in the middle will be our stylite's pillar.'

'As a symbol?'

'No, no. It will be the real thing. It will have a stylite on top of it.'

'Are you being serious?'

'Perfectly serious.'

'But how are you going to find a stylite?'

'We have one already. Fr. Ephrem Kerim has volunteered to be our first pillar-dweller. He is in Ireland presently, at Maynooth, finishing his thesis. When he has his doctorate he wishes to mount a pillar.'

'I don't believe it,' I said.

'But it is true.'

'I thought stylites had died out hundreds of years ago.'

'No,' said the Metropolitan, shaking his head. 'According to my researches there were still stylites in Georgia in the eighteenth century. It's a bit of a gap, but hardly unbridgeable.'

'And your friend, Fr. Ephrem, is really prepared to spend the rest of his life perched up on . . .'

'He is determined to become as like St Symeon as he can,' said Mar Gregorios. 'But if he does find it too difficult, I know several keen young novices who will be happy to take it in turns to be stylites with him.'

'A kind of relay stylitism?'

'If you like.'

I frowned: 'But . . .'

'It is good to imitate the saints,' said the Metropolitan, anticipating my objections. 'They are an example to all of us.'

'Isn't it a bit exhibitionist to stand on a pillar?' I said.

'On the contrary,' said Mar Gregorios. 'For the stylites of old the opinion of this world was nothing. The saints became stylites for their own good, for the salvation of their own souls. For them the material world, their own bodies, were of no account. The spirit was all that mattered. To punish their bodies on columns gave emphasis to the world of the spirit.'

'Do you think you will become a stylite,' I asked.

'No,' replied the Metropolitan, smiling. 'I am too old.'

I gave him the parcel containing the postcards, and as he opened it he quizzed me about the situation in the Tur Abdin.

'It's very bad,' he said when I described what I had seen. 'The Turks . . . why do they do this? What have we ever done to them?' He shook his head. 'My father was from the Tur Abdin, my mother's family from Diyarbakir. After the massacres they were the only surviving children from both their families. All their brothers and sisters were killed. In 1921 my grandfather managed to get his children across the border to Qamishli; they crossed at night with a small group of friends. The French were here and my parents thought they would protect them. In Turkey there was still terrible insecurity – Kurdish tribesmen were still circling the country killing and enslaving any Christians they found. My mother's parents had crossed the year before and she was born here in Aleppo.

'So you are a refugee on both sides of your family?'

'I was born in Qamishli,' replied the Metropolitan. 'My father had been a landowner in the Tur Abdin, but of course after he came to Syria he had nothing: everything had to be left behind. So he worked the land of a rich Syrian family. Eventually he became their foreman. But despite this we have never thought of ourselves as refugees. Syria was where the Suriani had come from: the ruins and graves of our forefathers lie all around. We have always thought of ourselves as citizens, not refugees.'

'And do you think the Christians are safe in Syria today?'

'Christians are better off in Syria than anywhere else in the Middle East,' said Mar Gregorios emphatically. 'Other than Lebanon, this is the only country in the region where a Christian can really feel the equal of a Muslim – and Lebanon, of course, has many other problems. In Syria there is no enmity between Christian and Muslim. If Syria were not here, we would be finished. Really. It is a place of sanctuary, a haven for all the Christians: for the Nestorians and Chaldeans driven out of Iraq, the Syrian Orthodox and the Armenians driven out of Turkey, even some Palestinian Christians driven out of the Holy Land by the Israelis. Talk to people here: you will find that what I say is true.'

What Mar Gregorios said was indeed what I had been told ever since I had crossed the Syrian border. I heard more of the same at lunch today with Sally Mazloumian. Sally's husband, the great Krikor ('Coco') Mazloumian, owner and manager of the Baron for as long as anyone could remember, had died last year, leaving Sally widowed and shipwrecked in Syria with her family 'spread out across the world like United Nations: Aleppo, Geneva, New York . . .' Krikor had been succeeded as manager by his pipe-smoking, labrador-patting eldest son, the only member of the next Mazloumian generation to stay on in Syria. He was now known, like his father before him, simply as Baron Mazloumian.

The Mazloumians' house lay immediately beside the hotel, in the same compound. Gathered there, under the framed photographs of a succession of turn-of-the-century Mazloumians, were a dozen Aleppo Armenians, all of whose parents and grandparents had been survivors of the Armenian genocide, who had somehow escaped from the death-marches across the desert and found shelter in the narrow alleys of Aleppo. They had gathered, as they did every Sunday, to see Sally, to toast the memory of her late husband, and to raise their glasses to Armenia.

The elderly people sat back in the faded chintz armchairs and talked about old times. As they did so their stories came spilling out: the usual, familiar litany of indescribable Armenian tragedies: grandmothers raped, uncles beaten to death, aunts dying in the desert from thirst and starvation, all set against the counterpoint of how Syria provided refuge for the few straggling survivors.

'When the Ottoman army surrounded them, the Armenians of Zeitun defended themselves for two months,' said one man. He was old and grey, but his eyes were bright and animated as he told his story. 'Then the Catholicos from Sis came and persuaded them to surrender. He said: "I have promised that you will all give in your guns, and the army has promised you will be safe." My grandfather did not believe the word of Turks, so he and my father stayed in the redoubt. But his wife, who thought the Catholicos should be obeyed, took all my uncles and aunts and went back to their village. That night they were all clubbed to death . . .'

Everyone competed to tell their tales. 'There's not one Armenian family in Aleppo that hasn't got a better story than *Dr Zhivago*,' said Sally proudly. 'But don't expect any of them to give you a properly ordered account. They get much too excited.'

'My grandfather was saved by a friend,' said a well-dressed businessman with an American accent. 'Khachadurian was a shoemaker who made special boots for the Ottoman army. He was an Armenian, but he was important to the military so he was spared. They gathered the Armenians into a walled graveyard, but the shoemaker came in and started taking boys out. He said, "This is my son-in-law, this here is my nephew, that is my grandson. I need them all for my business. If you Turks want your boots you must let me have my workers." He saved thirty in all, so many that he could barely feed them all: my father had only one piece of bread each day, and that he had to share with his sister.'

Quite suddenly and unexpectedly the businessman began sobbing. His transatlantic self-assurance crumpled like a punctured balloon. He bowed his head. Sally said: 'It's all right, Sam. Don't continue. It's all right.'

'When the fighting started, my father fled to the mountains,' said an old widow, filling the silence. 'They had begun collecting Armenians for "deportation". Although he was only twelve, my father guessed what was happening. So he ran off up the hill above his house, barefoot in the snow. He was lucky: 90 per cent of the Armenians in the columns did not make it. There were forty-seven people in my father's family. They all died. Only he was left.'

Sam, the businessman with the American accent, lifted his head. 'I want to finish,' he said, dabbing his cheeks. 'I met Khachadurian in 1962 in Beirut. He was ninety years old, completely blind. My father was with me: he kissed Khachadurian's hand and told me to do the same. He said: "Without that man I would be dead now. And you would never have been born." '

'Both my parents walked to Aleppo,' chipped in another old man, as determined as the others to tell his story. 'My father was naked by the time he got here – his rags got so full of holes they just fell off. The Arabs clothed him. Later my parents found shelter in the Jewish Quarter, the Hayy el-Yehudi. Ten Armenian families put all their resources together and rented one room . . .'

'When my grandfather first came here all the Armenians were still poor,' said a younger woman, a musician, who had just returned from giving a concert in Yerevan. 'They had arrived penniless, but they worked night and day just to make sure that their children were educated.'

The massacres, everyone agreed, had changed the face of Aleppo: before the First World War there were only three hundred Armenian families in the town; by 1943 Armenian numbers had topped 400,000.

But as I had already learned, the Armenians were not alone. Between 1914 and 1924 similar waves of Suriani (and to a smaller extent Greek Orthodox) refugees followed in their wake. The influx turned Aleppo into a Noah's Ark, a place of shelter and safety for all the different Christian communities driven out of Anatolia by the Turks. The officials of the French Mandate welcomed the exiles, partly out of genuine sympathy for their plight, and partly in the hope that the Christian refugees would act as a break on the new Arab nationalism. Moreover, the French felt that the Christians would naturally be more enthusiastic supporters of their rule, and systematically gave them preferment in government jobs.

After Syria's independence in 1946, this inevitably led to a backlash. Although Michel Aflaq, one of the founders of the Ba'ath Party, was a Christian, as was Faris al-Khuri, a leading figure in the Syrian Nationalist movement who later became Prime Minister, anti-Christian feeling was widespread (and, in the post-colonial circumstances, understandable). There were attempts to make Islam the official religion of the country, and at one stage the imam of the Great Mosque in Damascus declared that as far as he was concerned, an Indonesian Muslim was closer to him than al-Khuri, his own (Christian) Prime Minister. The increasingly Islamic tone of the Syrian establishment led to perhaps a quarter of a million Christians leaving Syria throughout the 1960s; from Aleppo alone as many as 125,000 Armenians emigrated to Soviet Armenia. These refugees included the current Armenian President, Levon Ter Petrosyan.

The period of uncertainty for Syria's Christians came to an end with Asad's *coup d'état* in 1970. Asad was an Alawite, a member of a Muslim minority regarded by orthodox Sunni Muslims as heretical and disparagingly referred to as Nusayris (or Little Christians). Asad kept himself in power by forming what was in effect a coalition of Syria's many religious minorities – Shias, Druze, Yezidis, Christians and Alawites – through which he was able to counterbalance the weight of the Sunni majority. In Asad's Syria Christians have always done well: at the moment, apparently, five of Asad's seven closest advisers are Christians, including his principal speechwriter, as are as two of the sixteen cabinet ministers. Christians and Alawites together hold all the key positions in the armed forces and the *mukhabarat*. While the official population figures are distrusted by everyone I spoke to, the Christians themselves estimated that they now formed slightly less than 20 per cent of Syria's total population, and between 20 and 30 per cent of the population of Aleppo, giving that city one of the largest Christian populations anywhere in the Middle East.

The confidence of the Christians in Syria is something you can't help noticing the minute you arrive in the country. This is particularly so if, like myself, you cross the border at Nisibis: Qamishli, the town on the Syrian side of the frontier (and the place where Metropolitan Gregorios Yohanna Ibrahim was brought up) is 75 per cent Christian, and icons of Christ and images of his mother fill almost every shop and decorate every other car window – an extraordinary display after the furtive secrecy of Christianity in Turkey. Moreover Turoyo, the modern Aramaic of the Tur Abdin, is the first language of Qamishli. This makes it one of a handful of towns in the world where Jesus could expect to be understood if he came back tomorrow.

The only problem with all of this, as far as the Christians are concerned, is the creeping realisation that they are likely to expect another, perhaps far more savage, backlash when Asad dies or when his regime eventually crumbles. The Christians of Syria have watched with concern the Islamic movements which are gaining strength all over the Middle East, and the richer Christians have all invested in two passports (or so the gossip goes), just in case Syria turns nasty at some stage in the future.

'Fundamentalism is building up among the Muslims,' said a

pessimistic Armenian businessman I met while wandering in the Aleppo bazaars. 'Just look at the girls: now they all wear the *hijab*: only five years ago they were all uncovered. After Asad's death or resignation no one knows what will happen. As long as the bottle is closed with a firm cork all is well. But eventually the cork will come out. And then no one knows what will happen to us.'

In the meantime, while the Christians nervously sing Asad's praises, most of the Sunni majority continue to grumble about his repressive Ba'athist government and the ruthlessness of his secret police, although several Muslims I talked to did admit to a grudging admiration for their dictator's sheer shrewdness and tenacity. In the absence of any legal opposition, disaffected Syrians have taken refuge in a series of jokes at the expense of the Alawite ruling clique. The taxi driver who took me back from the Syrian Orthodox cathedral told me this Asad story as we crawled through the bazaars behind an ambling train of pack-mules:

'My cousin is a taxi driver in Damascus. One day he was waiting by some traffic lights when a limousine with clouded glass windows smashed into his rear. The back of the taxi was completely wrecked. My cousin is a hot-blooded man – we all are in my family – so he jumped out and began to harangue the occupants, calling them sons of unmarried mothers, brothers of incontinent camels, fathers of she-goats and so on. After two minutes of this, the rear window of the limousine lowered half an inch, and a visiting card was thrust through the crack. On it was written a single telephone number. My cousin started shouting, "What is the meaning of this?" but the window was wound up again and the limousine swerved around him and his concertina-ed taxi, leaving him shouting into space.

'My cousin was determined to get some compensation from the rich man who owned the car, so the following day he went to a phone box and rang the number that had been written on the card. He started by softening the man up with a few pleasantries, then went on to demand a new taxi, saying that fifteen people depended on the money he brought home, that his wife was sick and that his daughter was getting married the following year.

'There was no response to this, so my cousin began to get angry again, comparing the man to the vomit of an Israeli dog and the worms which wriggle in the belly of a wild pig. He had been speaking like this for five minutes when suddenly a quiet voice on the end of the line said: "Do you have any idea who you are talking to?"

'"No," replied my cousin.

'"You are speaking to Hafez al-Asad," said a sinister voice. "As you may be aware, I am the President of the Syrian Arab Republic."

'"I know who you are," said my cousin without hesitation, "but do you have any idea who *you* are talking to?"

'"No," said the voice, surprised.

'"Thank God for that," said my cousin, slamming down the phone and running back to his car as fast as he could, before the *mukhabarat* could trace the call and treat him to an extended stay at President Asad's pleasure.'

ALEPPO, 4 SEPTEMBER

I sat up last night reading the book lent to me by the Metropolitan, *The History of the Monks of Syria* by Theodoret, Bishop of Cyrrhus. Theodoret turns out to be a near contemporary of John Moschos, and if this book is anything to go by, even more eccentric in his tastes.

If Theodoret is to be believed, the greatest celebrities of his day were not singers or dancers or even charioteers, but saints and ascetics. St Symeon Stylites the Elder, whose pillar lay a few miles west of Aleppo, was a case in point.

'As his fame circulated everywhere,' wrote Theodoret, 'everyone hastened to him, so that with everyone arriving from every side and every road resembling a river, one can behold a sea of men standing together in that place. Not only inhabitants of our part of the world, but also Ismaelites, Persians, Armenians and men even more distant than these: inhabitants of the extreme west, Spaniards and Britons and the Gauls who live between them. Of Italy it is superfluous to speak. It is said that the man became so celebrated in the great city of Rome that at the entrance of all the workshops men have set up small representations of him, to provide thereby some protection and safety for themselves . . .'

Theodoret, as the principal chronicler of the great Byzantine ascetics, was effectively the leading celebrity biographer of his day, and his works were read as far away as Anglo-Saxon Canterbury. But his subjects – suspended in cages, walled up in hermitages, buried in cisterns – presented a rather different set of difficulties to the figures whose peccadilloes and appetites are so minutely examined by hack biographers today. For if Symeon was the most famous of Theodoret's celebrity subjects, he was by no means the most eccentric. There was, for example, Baradatus, who Theodoret congratulates for having devised 'new tests of endurance'. On a ridge above his hermitage he constructed out of wood 'a small chest that did not even match his body and in this he dwelt, obliged to stoop the whole time. It was not even fitted together with planks, but had openings like a lattice; and because of this he was neither safe from the assault of the rains nor free from the flames of the sun, but endured both.'

Eventually Baradatus's bishop persuaded him to come out of his latticed coffin, but far from going into ascetic retirement the hermit merely devised an even more unusual way to follow his calling. Baradatus decided that his new ploy was going to involve standing up all the time. But as this was a fairly common form of asceticism at the time (no less a figure than the youthful St John Chrysostom once pursued this method of self-punishment for two years without a break), Baradatus seems to have come to the conclusion that standing up for the rest of his life was, on its own, not going to be enough. He therefore decided to make things more difficult for himself. He covered his entire body 'with a tunic of skins – only around the nose and mouth did he leave a small opening for breath', so that in addition to having to stand all day he would also be baked alive in the sweltering Syrian midsummer heat: a sort of Byzantine boil-in-the-bag monk.

This was, however, tame stuff compared to one of Theodoret's heroes, Thalelaeus, who constructed a cage, then hung the contraption in the air. 'Sitting or rather suspended in this, he has spent ten years up till now. Since he has a very big body, not even sitting can he straighten his neck, but he always sits bent double with his forehead tightly pressed against his knees.'

When Theodoret went to visit this strange figure, he found him 'reaping the benefit of the divine gospels, gathering benefit therefrom with extreme concentration'. Only at this point does it seem to have occurred to Theodoret that this sort of behaviour was, perhaps, just a little strange. 'I questioned him out of desire to learn the reason for this novel mode of life,' wrote the Bishop. Thalelaeus had his answer ready: life, he said, was to be lived as uncomfortably as possible as an insurance policy against worse discomforts in the life to come: 'Burdened with many sins, and believing in the penalties that are threatened, I have devised this form of life, contriving moderate punishments for the body in order to reduce the mass of those awaited. For the latter are more grievous not only in quantity but also in quality, so if by these slight afflictions I lessen those awaited, great is the profit I shall derive therefrom.'

In most other societies, ascetics like this might perhaps be regarded with a certain amount of suspicion; but in Byzantium it seemed that every village wanted some self-torturing hermit to live among them, to bring them good luck, to cure them of diseases and demons, and to intercede for them both at the wordly palace of Constantinople and the more distant court of Heaven. Hermits were considered especially lucky to have around when they were dying: that way the village could claim the corpse, and add to its stock of sacred relics. If Theodoret is to be believed, hundreds of eager Byzantine peasants seem to have hung around dying saints, waiting to slice up the old men as soon as they dropped off their perches – quite literally in the case of stylites.

Theodoret records one such case, when word got out that a famous hermit named James of Cyrrhestica was reported to be dying. On a previous occasion when James had been seriously ill, Theodoret had had to exert all his episcopal authority to disperse a crowd of sickle-wielding relic-seekers. But a little while later, when James's condition suddenly worsened, Theodoret was away on business to Aleppo, and the people of Cyrrhus were forced to take the law into their own hands.

'As many [peasants] were coming from all sides to seize his body,' wrote Theodoret, 'when they heard what was happening, all the men of the town, both soldiers and civilians, hastened together [to where James lived, on a hilltop four miles to the west], some taking up military equipment, others using whatever weapons lay to hand. Forming up in close order, they fought by shooting arrows and slinging stones – not to wound, but simply to instil fear [in their rustic rivals]. Having thus driven off the local inhabitants, they placed the hermit on a litter while he was quite unconscious of what was happening – he was not even conscious of his hair being plucked out by the peasants [as a relic] – and set off [with the comatose hermit] to the city.'

As a result of a series of such pre-emptive swoops on dying ascetics, Cyrrhus became so clogged with relics that Theodoret lobbied to have it renamed Hagiopolis, the city of saints. On my map, the town's ruins lie forty-five miles to the north of Aleppo. Tomorrow I plan to drive out there, taking the Metropolitan's book with me, and see what is left of Theodoret's bishopric.

ALEPPO, 5 SEPTEMBER

There turned out to be no bus to Cyrrhus, so I decided to hitchhike instead. I woke early and filled a light pack with feta cheese, some flat bread and a bottle of weak Syrian beer. Then, taking a hotel taxi to the edge of town, I began to walk.

It was a beautifully cool and surprisingly cloudy day – a welcome change from the blazing skies and enervating heat that had followed me ever since Athos. Before long I came to a roadside stall run by a solitary Bedu. The stall was made of palm fronds and sold nothing but branches of ripe dates. I bought a sprig and when, half an hour later, I was picked up by a Kurdish truck driver, we ate the dates together, spitting the stones out of the windows.

As we headed north-west, the land grew slowly starker: the rich belt of walnut and pistachio trees that had shaded the roadsides on the northern edge of Aleppo gave way to more arid, mountainous territory. On small patches of arable land, teams of blinkered horses in harness pulled primitive wooden ploughs; peasant women in embroidered dresses and white kerchiefs scraped at the soil with picks while their daughters looked on, buckets in hand. Above them, on the edge of the slopes, you could see the ruins of deserted Byzantine watchtowers looking out over the thin soil that had once supported the rich vineyards whose dark Syrian wine was drunk in the taverns of late antique Antioch.

After many miles, on the slope of a hill opposite the road, I saw the ruins of what looked like a large Romanesque basilica sitting in the middle of a small grove of olive trees. It was roofless and deserted, but otherwise almost miraculously intact. Intrigued, I asked my Kurdish friend to drop me off. The truck drove away in a cloud of black exhaust, and in the sudden silence I set off on foot towards the ruins.

The basilica of Mushabbak sits in perfect isolation amid the olive groves, the last surviving witness to a period when these hills supported what must once have been a fairly dense Christian population. If a new wooden roof were raised over the nave, the floor were swept and the gables slightly repaired, the church would be ready for use tomorrow. But, like so many other churches across the Middle East, this astonishing basilica now acts as nothing more than a convenient sheep-pen: as I walked across the fields and through the olives, I could see a shepherd boy drawing water from a well to one side of the ruin. He poured the water into a trough which, as I drew nearer, I realised was actually the old church font. The boy salaamed, and led me inside.

A pair of ewes and four lambs were tethered in the side-chapel. Nearby stood a saddled donkey and a growling sheepdog. Two arcades of massively-built round arches rolled forward along the austere nave towards a gently curving apse; although totally bare of ornament or decoration, there was great beauty in the perfect harmony of the church's proportions. The building was clearly very early Byzantine, dating from around the late-fifth century, but its similarity to Romanesque work was extraordinary, and in its plan and style it almost exactly prefigured the French ecclesiastical architecture of the early twelfth century. In many ways it would not have looked out of place on an Auvergne hillside; yet for all that, its spirit was somehow very different.

When you think of French Romanesque – of Vézelay, Autun, Anzy-le-Duc or Moissac – you are left with an impression of teeming life: biting beasts entwined around capitals; tympana crowded with the twenty-four Elders of the Apocalypse busily fiddling on their viols; angels blowing the Last Trump; the dead resurrecting, emerging like uncurling crustaceans from their sarcophagi. The sculpture is playful, fantastic, anarchic, like those manuscript marginalia where the world is inverted and rabbits armed with crossbows hunt the hunters or chase the hounds.

But here, in this stone husk of Byzantine Syria, a more restrained and puritanical spirit was at work. A *chrismon* – a small equal-armed cross – was carved in a laurel wreath above the central keystone of the arch. Otherwise there was no decorative sculpture to break the stern purity of the stonework. The capitals were non-figurative, and were carelessly, almost accidentally decorated with palmettes and scroll volutes. There were no mouldings above the windows, and no acanthus-work above the doors or around the apsidal arch. Like the lifestyles embraced by Theodoret's ascetics, the guiding spirit of this church was almost fanatically austere.

This shared severity of outlook was no coincidence. For it was in such remote rural settlements that Theodoret's Syrian ascetics were most popular, most especially revered. In the towns, whose populations were better and more classically educated, opinion was sometimes divided about them: already in the fourth century the pagan orator Libanius thought of the monks as 'that black-robed tribe who eat more than elephants, sweeping across the country like a river in spate ravaging the temples and the great estates'. Libanius was clearly not alone in his feelings: in one of his sermons St John Chrysostom (a former pupil of Libanius who later turned against his pagan master) complained that 'wherever the people [of Antioch] gathered to gossip you could find one man boasting that he was the first to beat up a monk, another that he had been the first to track down his hut, a third that he had spurred the magistrate into action against the Holy Men, a fourth that he had dragged them through the streets and seen them locked up in jail.'

But in the farms and villages it was very different. There it was to the freelance and unordained holy men, and not to Imperial officials or the professional clergy, that the simple Byzantine peasants would turn when they were in trouble. As Theodoret once remarked, the holy men replaced the pagan gods: their shrines replaced the temples, and their feasts superseded the old pagan festivals. Theodoret's friend the cage-dwelling hermit Thalalaeus was an example of this. He moved into a still functioning pagan shrine and defeated all attempts to drive him out ('they were unable to move him since faith fenced him around and grace fought on his behalf'). Then he managed to convert the local people with the aid of some supernatural veterinary work: Theodoret himself interviewed some converts who 'declared that many miracles occur through his prayer, with not only men but also camels, asses and mules enjoying healing'. This healing of the village pack-animals seems to have tipped the balance: Thalalaeus had found his way into the farmers' hearts, and with the assistance of his new converts he 'destroyed the precinct of the demons and erected a great shrine to the triumphant martyrs, opposing to those falsely called gods, the Godly Dead'.

By their ability to endure physical suffering Byzantine holy men like Thalalaeus were believed to be able to wear away the curtain that separated the visible world from the divine; and by reaching through they gained direct access to God, something that was thought to be impossible for the ordinary believer. For by mortifying the flesh, it was believed that the holy men became transformed: 'If you will, you can become all flame,' said Abba Joseph in one of the stories of the desert fathers, holding up his hand to show fingers which had 'become like ten lamps of fire', radiant with the 'uncreated light of divinity', the same form of illumination that is shown surrounding the great saints in icons. In this heightened state the holy men were believed to be able to act as intercessors for their followers at the distant court of Heaven, and like the old gods had the power to give children to barren women, to cure the sick, and to divine the future.

But perhaps the holy men's most important task was to fight demons. The world was believed to be besieged by invisible agents of darkness, and to sin was not merely to err: it was to be overcome by these sinister forces. Demonic activity was a daily irritation, and was believed to intrude on the most ordinary, domestic activities. A recently discovered papyrus fragment tells the story of the break-up of the marriage of a young Byzantine couple, a prosperous baker and the daughter of a merchant: 'We were in time past maintaining a peaceful and seemly married life,' they wrote in their divorce petition, 'but we have suffered from a sinister and wicked demon which attacked us from we know not whence, with a view to our being divorced from one another.' In much the same vein John Moschos tells the story of a nunnery in Lycia which was attacked by a troop of demons; as a result 'five of the virgins conspired to run away from the monastery and find themselves husbands'.

Like the Muslim *djinns* which superseded them, Byzantine demons lurked especially in old temples and remote hillsides such as that around my isolated basilica: the *Life* of an Anatolian holy man named Theodore of Sykeon tells how a group of farmers digging into a mound of earth on a distant hillside inadvertently released a great swarm of demons that took possession not only of them, but of their neighbours and their animals; only a holy man like Theodore was able to drive the evil spirits back into their lair and seal them in. Monks and holy men were thought of as 'prize-fighters' against the Devil's minions, and only with their help – and their amulets, relics and remedies – could demons be fought or defeated. Across the east Mediterranean that tradition still continues: to this day Christian monks are believed to be powerful exorcists, a talent they share with their Islamic counterparts, the Muslim Sufi mystics.

I thought of this as I walked along the empty country road, hoping for a lift to Cyrrhus. It was two hours before I had any luck. My saviour was Monsieur Alouf, an old francophile Arab with an astonishing resemblance to Omar Sharif. No one lived at Cyrrhus any more, he said as we drove off, but he knew the way as there was the shrine of a famous saint, Nebi (prophet) Uri, on the edge of the ruins. He was not busy today, added M. Alouf. If I wanted, for a small price he could drive me all the way there. He named a reasonable figure and I accepted his offer.

We headed north along a narrow hill road. The further we drove, the more olives came to dominate the thin soil. As we crossed a narrow ridge, a great panorama of silver-grey trees unfolded before us, chequering the hills in a regimented gridiron. On some south-facing slopes, a few peasant families were beginning the olive harvest. Rickety wooden ladders were being propped against the gnarled old olive trees while sheets were laid out on the ground; tethered donkeys stood about nearby, their empty saddlebags ready to receive the harvest. Nearby, groups of baggy-trousered harvesters loaded olive sacks onto waiting horsecarts.

We passed a waterfall in which some small children were splashing about, then crossed a pair of beautiful hump-backed Byzantine bridges. One of these, I knew, had been commissioned by Theodoret himself. We were on the edge of our destination.

The sheer remoteness of the place was surprising, but in retrospect this was something I should have expected. In his private letters, Theodoret was always complaining about the provincial character of his bishopric. Brought up in a well-to-do family in metropolitan Antioch, he often found life in distant Cyrrhus frustrating. He begged his correspondents for gossip from Constantinople, and complained that there was not a decent baker anywhere in his bishopric. In one particularly revealing letter, he calls Cyrrhus 'a little city' whose ugliness he claimed to have 'covered over' by lavish spending. In another, addressed to his friend the sophist Isocasius, he writes of his excitement when a skilled woodworker arrived in town. In Antioch no one would have noticed such an unexceptional occurrence, but in Cyrrhus everyone in authority – the Governor, the General, Theodoret himself – wanted to employ him, and Theodoret promises to send the carpenter on to his friend as soon as he has finished with him.

After three miles of increasingly precipitous mountain slopes, the shattered ruins of Cyrrhus rose quite suddenly from the olive groves. A jumble of broken buildings – the arc of a theatre, fragments of arcaded public buildings, a few random columns and pillar bases – littered the ground. Few buildings stood higher than a couple of courses. But dominating everything, crowning the horizon on a precipitous rock in the centre of the ruins, rose the jagged silhouette of the citadel which had been rebuilt and refortified by Justinian as a defence against the Persians.

M. Alouf dropped me off by the honey-coloured skeleton of one of the Byzantine gateways, and I climbed up towards the fort, following the line of the basalt-black town walls. Basking lizards scuttled between the stones. Although it was now midday it was still cool; grey clouds billowed over the citadel and a fresh breeze was blowing. Halfway up the hill I came across a great stumbling tortoise crunching amid the stones as he began, with infinite slowness, to dig in for the winter with a slow-motion breaststroke of legs and ebony claws. The weather was turning: summer was drawing to a close.

Alone of the buildings of the city, the citadel stood intact: the great round corner bastions and the square turrets of the wall-walk that connected them still rose in several places to their original height. I clambered up onto the parapet, sending loose rubble rolling down the hill behind me, and sat there munching my bread and cheese, looking down over the broken remnants of Theodoret's city.

In the middle, a little to the north of the citadel, you could see the outline of Theodoret's cathedral, the great church of Saints Cosmas and Damian, a long apsidal-ended basilica standing out clearly from amid the square foundations of the city's smaller secular buildings. To one side of the cathedral stood what must have been the bishop's palace. It was to this building, I thought, that Theodoret would have returned from one of his interviews, thrilled that some wiry old hermit had let him break down the sealed door of his cell, or that some famously bad-tempered stylite had granted him permission to place a ladder against his pillar and climb up for a chat. On the other side of the cathedral, linked to the south wall of the apse, stood the foundations of a small annexe, probably a shrine. I wondered, as I headed off down the hill, whether it was here that the hermit James had eventually ended up, despite all his efforts to resist Theodoret's attempts to add him to the Cyrrhus relic collection.

Outside the walls, at the opposite end of the town to the cathedral, rose the silhouette of a late antique martyrium. It had a six-sided pyramidal roof and its stone was of a wonderfully rich colour, like the crust on Cornish clotted cream. Sometime in the thirteenth or fourteenth century A.D. this elegant classical building had been walled around and converted into the shrine of a Sufi saint. The shrine was still functioning, and it was there that I had agreed to meet M. Alouf.

I found him sitting cross-legged on a carpet in the prayer hall of the small mosque that had been built beneath the tower. He was talking to the Sheikh who looked after the shrine, a limping old man with a stick, baggy *sharwal* trousers and a thin grey beard; his *keffiyeh* was wound into a turban with its end trailing down the back of his neck. From the ceiling immediately above the Sheikh dangled a bunch of dried yellow flowers. I asked my friend what they were there for.

'The Sheikh says they are to stop anyone ever again putting the evil eye on the mosque,' said Alouf.

'Someone has put it on before?' I asked.

'Sadly yes,' replied the Sheikh. 'Before we put those up, two thieves came and stole all the carpets, the clock, the fan and the loudspeaker from the mosque. Come and see.'

He led us through a door into the vaulted burial chamber of the tomb. Cuckoo-like, the cenotaph of the Muslim saint had been placed immediately above the spot where the original Roman occupant must have been laid.

'This is where the sick people come to spend the night,' said the Sheikh. 'In the morning they are cured, thanks to Nebi Uri. It is a

holy place but those thieves dug down here. They thought they
would find money, but all they did was to desecrate the grave. Afterwards I said to Nebi Uri, "You must take more care of yourself,"
and I struck his tomb twice with my stick to show that I meant it.'

'You talk to the saint?' I asked.

'Of course,' said the Sheikh, laughing indulgently, as if I were
questioning him about something so obvious that only a foreigner
could possibly ask it. 'Every day.'

'How?'

'He comes to me in dreams,' said the Sheikh. 'He gives me
advice and instructions: "Don't leave my shrine, look after it,
make it nice." '

'What does he look like?'

'He has a round face, a thick black beard . . .'

'And his clothes?'

'I don't know: I see only his face,' said the Sheikh. 'Twenty
years I have been Sheikh here. And before me my father, and
before him his father.'

'For many generations?'

'Many. I am Abdul Mesin, my father was Maamo, his father
Sheikho, Sheikho was the son of Misto, Misto was the son of
Maamo, son of Ishan . . . Before that I don't remember. It is far
away.'

'Tell me about Nebi Uri,' I said.

'You don't know about Nebi Uri?' asked M. Alouf, surprised.
'But he is revered by Christians also. Many Christians –
Armenians, Suriani, Catholics – come here to pay their respects.
Nebi Uri is in your Bible as well as our Koran, I think.'

'He is?'

'He was the leader of the Prophet David's army,' said the Sheikh.
'David had him killed so that he could marry Nebi Uri's beautiful
wife. Two angels, Mikhail and Jibrael, appeared and asked David
why he needed an extra wife when he already had ninety-nine
others. You know this story?'

'Yes. I think we Christians know Nebi Uri as Uriah the Hittite.'

It was an unlikely tangle of tales: a medieval Muslim saint
buried in a much older Byzantine tomb tower had somehow been

confused with the Biblical and Koranic Uriah; perhaps the saint's name *was* Uriah, and over the passage of time his identity had been merged with that of his scriptural namesake. More intriguing still was the fact that in this city, long famed for the shrines of its Christian saints, the Muslim Sufi tradition had directly carried on from where Theodoret's Christian holy men had left off. Just as the Muslim form of prayer, with its bowings and prostrations, appears to derive from the older Syriac Christian tradition that I had seen performed at Mar Gabriel, and just as the architecture of the earliest minarets unmistakably derives from the square late-antique Syrian church towers, so the roots of Islamic mysticism and Sufism lie with the Byzantine holy men and desert fathers who preceded them across the Near East.

Today the West often views Islam as a civilisation very different from and indeed innately hostile to Christianity. Only when you travel in Christianity's Eastern homelands do you realise how closely the two religions are really linked. For the former grew directly out of the latter and still, to this day, embodies many aspects and practices of the early Christian world now lost in Christianity's modern Western incarnation. When the early Byzantines were first confronted by the Prophet's armies, they assumed that Islam was merely a heretical form of Christianity, and in many ways they were not so far wrong: Islam accepts much of the Old and New Testaments, and venerates both Jesus and the ancient Jewish prophets.

Certainly if John Moschos were to come back today it is likely that he would find much more that was familiar in the practices of a modern Muslim Sufi than he would with those of, say, a contemporary American Evangelical. Yet this simple truth has been lost by our tendency to think of Christianity as a Western religion rather than the Oriental faith it actually is. Moreover the modern demonisation of Islam in the West, and the recent growth of Muslim fundamentalism (itself in many ways a reaction to the West's repeated humiliation of the Muslim world), have led to an atmosphere where few are aware of, or indeed wish to be aware of, the profound kinship of Christianity and Islam.

It is this as much as anything else that has made the delicate position of the contemporary Eastern Christians – awkwardly caught between their co-religionists in the West and their strong cultural links with their Muslim compatriots – increasingly untenable in recent years. Hence the vital importance of the syncretism which still exists at shrines like that of Nebi Uri. Such popular syncretism – Christians worshipping at Muslim shrines and vice versa – was once much more general across the Middle East, but now survives only in a few oases of relative religious tolerance. The practice emphasises an important truth about the close affinity of the two great religions easily forgotten as the Eastern Christians – the last surviving bridge between Islam and Western Christianity – emigrate in reaction to the increasing hostility of the Islamic establishment.

'Very many Christians still come here,' continued the Sheikh, breaking into my thoughts. 'Mainly they are sick people who want to come and get healing. We had one Christian girl last week. She was sick for many months – her head was bad – and Nebi Uri appeared to her in a dream. So she came here and spent the night on the tomb. The next day she was healed. Last Friday she returned with a sheep, all covered with flowers and ribbons and with its horns dyed with henna. After prayers they cut its throat. Then they cooked it and everyone ate it.'

'Does this happen often?'

'Every week. I say some prayers over the animal, then afterwards the people slaughter it themselves, just over there by the wall.'

'And it's always sheep?'

'No,' said M. Alouf. 'Usually it is, but sometimes people slaughter a young camel, an ox-calf or a young goat. Whatever it is, it must be a good animal – not a dog – and it must be young and healthy. It must not be ill or pregnant.'

'Afterwards,' said the Sheikh, 'they drag the animal round the grave three times and pour some of the blood over Nebi Uri's grave and onto the doorway leading into the chamber. It is to thank Nebi Uri for fulfilling their wish.'

'Before they come,' explained Alouf, 'they will always have

promised such-and-such an animal to Nebi Uri if he performs some favour for them. So when he does what they want they must fulfil their promise.'

'We believe that if they give a different – or less good – animal or do not come at all, then Nebi Uri will punish them,' said the Sheikh.

'How?'

'The punishment can take many forms,' said M. Alouf. 'He can give an illness or cause a *djinn* to take possession of the person. There are many forms of misfortune he can visit on the man who breaks his vow.'

'Once a man who had died was brought here to be buried. They left him by the well outside to wash him. But some time before he had made a promise to Nebi Uri and not honoured it. So when they brought him here the spring dried up and they could not wash the corpse. Nebi Uri did not want him near him. He had rejected him and the man had to be buried elsewhere. The next day water reappeared in the well.'

'If a saint rejects a dead man it is the worst thing that can happen,' said Alouf. 'We regard that as a very great insult to the honour of a family.'

'But if a man is generous and gives a good sheep to fulfil his vow,' said the Sheikh, 'then we believe that that person will ride that sheep at the Day of Judgement. The sheep will carry him into Paradise.'

'And the Christians believe this too?'

'There is no difference between ourselves and the Christians on this matter,' said the Sheikh, 'except that sometimes the Christians make the sign of Christ over the forehead of the person whom they want Nebi Uri to cure.'

As we were talking the Sheikh had led us up a flight of monolithic stairs onto the vaulted and arcaded terrace on the roof of the Byzantine mausoleum. Each side of the hexagon was broken by a great arch, from which sprung the pyramid above us. Through one of the arches I looked out over the rustling trees of the tomb compound. At the gate of the shrine a tractor was unloading a trailer-full of Kurdish workers. The old men were streaming inside for Friday prayers while the children waited with their mothers by the well-head outside.

The Sheikh stood facing south, raised his hands to his ears and called the *azan*. His soft and gentle voice, undistorted by amplification, drifted out over the ruins of Theodoret's cathedral, over the olive trees and the shattered graves of the myriad saints and martyrs of Hagiopolis, to the lavender-blue hills of the Kurd Dagh beyond.

ALEPPO, 9 SEPTEMBER

This morning, my last in Aleppo, I stumbled by accident upon the most unexpected survival from Byzantium that I have yet come across on this trip. Hidden away in a church in the grimy backstreets of the city, like a rare fossil secreted in some obscure quarry-face, there survives, apparently unpolluted by changes in fashion, an ancient form of plainsong that appears to be the direct ancestor of Gregorian chant. If so, extraordinary as it seems, it may represent one of the principal roots of the entire Western tradition of sacred music.

It was Metropolitan Mar Gregorios who first put me onto the trail. During our meeting he had mentioned in passing that among the different groups that had taken shelter in the winding bazaars of Aleppo were the Urfalees: the descendants of the Syrian Christians of Urfa, ancient Edessa. In what I had read of Urfa's recent history, and from what I had picked up when I visited the town last month, I had understood that the town's Syrian Ortho-dox community had suffered the same fate as its unfortunate Armenians. But apparently this was not the case. Although a great many of the Urfa Suriani were indeed massacred during the First World War, there were still enough left in 1924, when Ataturk retook the town from the French, to make the Turkish leader worried about Urfa's ethnic purity. He therefore ordered the immediate expulsion of all those Christians who had so far failed to succumb to the Ottomans' bayonets.

The Urfalees had left Edessa in a succession of great wagon-caravans, and somewhat to their own surprise, made it safely across the Syrian border. There they were escorted by the French Mandate officials to a field full of tents on the outskirts of Aleppo. They are there still, although as with the refugee camps of the Palestinians constructed twenty-three years later, the tents have given way to a jumble of ragged concrete buildings. Mar Gregorios had told me that one last survivor of the original exodus was still alive, and he arranged a meeting.

I found Malfono Namek's flat up a steep staircase off the narrow, grubby lanes that now make up the Hayy el-Surian, the Quarter of the Syrian Orthodox. Malfono [Teacher] Namek had a thin, ascetic face, a small toothbrush moustache and an alert owl-like expression. He wore a 1930s pinstripe suit, like those worn by bootleggers in Al Capone films. After we had drunk tea, I asked Malfono Namek whether – as he must have been very young at the time – he could remember anything of the Urfa he had left in 1924.

'Anything?' said Malfono Namek. 'I can remember everything! I even remember what we were reading in school the day the order to leave came through from Istanbul. If I went back to Urfa today I would know my quarter, my street, my house! It is still my town, even though I have been in Syria for seventy years now.'

The old man thumped the table: 'I would go back tomorrow,' he said. 'But of course the opportunity has never come.'

'How old were you when you had to move?'

'I was twelve. We were each allowed to take one suit of clothes, a couple of blankets and food for one week. Everything else – churches, convents, lands, schools, possessions, money – it all had to be left behind. I remember well: it was wintertime so I wore *shalwar* and a thick jacket. I remember saying goodbye to our Turkish friends and leaving the house and . . .'

He frowned: 'When I think of this I feel so angry . . . It was the Turkish government's fault. Many of our Turkish neighbours

172

were very sad to see us go. They were very sorry for us. You know I still have one friend left alive in Urfa? We write to each other. It is seventy years since we last saw each other, but still we correspond. It was the Turkish government: they called us *gavour* [infidels] and said we had to go. It was they who hated the Christians, not the people of Urfa.'

I asked if, at the time, he had realised what was happening.

'No, not at all!' said Malfono Namek. To my astonishment he threw back his head and laughed. 'At the time I was far too excited. We left in wagons for Ain al-Arab, where we were to catch a train. I was very happy: I had never seen a train. And when we arrived I was very pleased. I had never even imagined such a big and magnificent town existed anywhere on earth. Aleppo was much bigger than Urfa. It had such splendid buildings, and gas street-lighting at night. I saw carriages for the first time, and automobiles: at that time there were maybe ten or fifteen cars in the streets of Aleppo, while none had ever been seen in Urfa. Instead of streetlights, we had been used to carrying paraffin lamps from house to house. For a boy of twelve it was very exciting.'

The old man shook his head. 'The disillusion came later, when we found there was nothing for us except tents. It was February and very cold and there was nothing to eat. I was unhappy in our tent. There was no money, no light, no water. I could not understand the language. All of a sudden we felt strangers ... It took many years for us to feel at home here. In fact it was only recently that we Urfalees finally got a proper church of our own.'

'You don't pray with the other Suriani?'

'No, no,' said Malfono Namek. 'We have to have our own church as we have our own liturgical practices, and because our chant is very different from – and much older than – the music of the other Suriani.'

When I questioned him further, he said that the people of Urfa had scrupulously preserved the traditional chants of ancient Edessa, and in particular the hymns composed by St Ephrem the Syrian, the greatest of the town's saints. An Italian musicologist was currently in Aleppo, he said, studying the Urfalees' chants; if I accompanied him to vespers in the Urfalees' church, Gianmaria

Malacrida would probably be there and I could talk to him afterwards.

The old man put on a Homburg hat and, reaching for his stick, led me slowly down the stairs. Together we walked through the lanes of Aleppo, Malfono Namek chivalrously tipping the brim of his Homburg whenever we passed one of his friends. The streets were narrow and medieval-looking which, when we came to it, made the brash new Urfalee church of St George look more surprising still. It stood out like an office block in a Georgian crescent, all pre-stressed concrete and gleaming modernity, as different from the austere classical chapels of the Tur Abdin as could be imagined. Inside it was worse still: jarring Technicolor icons hung from the brightly-lit walls; at the back of the altar, behind the priest, a barrage of fairy lights winked like a neon advertisement in Piccadilly Circus.

But for all the flash modernity of the setting, the singing was still astounding. A cortège of elderly priests conducted the service, accompanied by a string of echoing laments of almost unearthly beauty, sinuous alleluias which floated with the gentle indecision of falling feathers down arpeggios of dying cadences before losing themselves in a soft black hole of basso profundo. At the elevation, the altar boys rattled *flabellae*, ecclesiastical fans which are often depicted on Pictish and Irish cross-slabs, but which died out in the West before the Norman Conquest, and have survived in use only in the Eastern Churches.

When the service had drawn to a close, the congregation – pious ladies with rigid perms and lacy white veils, old men in light tropical suits – poured outside. On the steps Malfono Namek introduced me to Gianmaria Malacrida. Malfono explained that I had recently been in Urfa, and I said I was interested in the Italian's theory that the Urfalees had managed to preserve the chants of late antique Edessa.

'It's a very difficult subject,' said Gianmaria, offering me a cigarette and lighting up himself. 'I've been working on the music of Urfa for seven years now, and it may take that long again before I manage to prove anything conclusively.'

The three of us walked round the corner to Gianmaria's flat.

It was bare and almost empty of furniture, but its shelves groaned with weighty reference books, stacks of notebooks and lines of neatly catalogued cassette tapes.

'What I don't understand,' I said, 'is how you can ever know that what we heard tonight is unchanged since the Byzantine period.'

'We don't know for sure,' replied Gianmaria. 'Up to now there have been no specialised studies of the Urfalees' music, and before my coming here the music was never written down. But it does appear to be a very early and very conservative tradition. There is no hard evidence, but it is difficult to believe that the form of this music has been substantially changed over the ages: sacred traditions change very, very slowly, if at all, over the centuries. Yesterday I was listening to the tapes I made seven years ago when I first started working on this. Although nothing is written down, since then there has not been one change – not one note has been added or omitted.'

'And if there have been no changes made to this music, what does that mean?'

'In manuscripts of the hymns of St Ephrem of Edessa – some of the very first Christian hymns ever composed – Ephrem writes in about 370 A.D. that he took his melodies and rhythms from Gnostic songs composed by the Edessan heretic Bardaisan. He says that their 'sweet rhythms still beguiled the hearts of men' – in other words that they were still popular and everyone in Edessa knew the tunes. Ephrem merely added new words – and orthodox sentiments – of his own. So if there has been no change to those melodies over the centuries, they should, in principle, be those composed by Bardaisan.'

'In the third century A.D.?'

'Bardaisan died in 220, so they could be earlier still, late second century.'

'And how does this compare with the oldest texts of Western music?'

'There is no agreement on which is the oldest Western text. There are four contenders, all of them very early forms of Gregorian chant. The most likely is Ambrosian, the chant of Milan; but there's also Romano Antiquo, the chant of Rome; Mozarabic, that of Spain; and Gallican, early French plainchant. They all represent very ancient forms of music, almost certainly dating back to the fifth century in the case of Ambrosian, but we have no musical notation written down for any of them before the tenth century A.D.'

'But their melodies could be as old as those of Urfa?'

'In principle,' said Gianmaria. 'But in practice that is extremely unlikely.'

'Why?'

'Because the earliest forms of Western plainchant all have markedly Eastern characteristics.'

'In other words they look like imports?'

'Exactly. And there is firm documentary evidence, in the church of Milan at least, that this new Western chant was deliberately modelled on older Syrian practice: St Ambrose's biographer writes that the hymns and psalms of the church of Milan "should be sung in the Syrian manner" because it was so popular.'

All this fitted in very well with what I knew from my own reading. Certainly there was no doubt that Syrian music was regarded with reverence throughout the Byzantine world. There are references in the sources to bands of Syrian monks bursting into song in Haghia Sophia, astounding the Sunday congregation with their strange litanies to the crucified Christ. Moreover the greatest of all Byzantine composers, St Romanos the Melodist, was a Syrian from Emesa (modern Homs), just to the south of Aleppo. His hymns and antiphons took Justinian's Constantinople by storm, but they have been shown to be heavily indebted to those of St Ephrem of Edessa. Furthermore, St Hilary of Poitiers, who first introduced the hymn to Europe – and likewise drew heavily on St Ephrem's Edessan hymns for his models – seems to have first heard the new form when he was exiled from Gaul to Asia Minor by the Emperor Constantius.

'So is it possible that what we heard tonight may be the most ancient form of Christian music still being sung anywhere in the world?'

'That's what I am investigating. Coptic and Eastern Chaldean chants are also very old. They may have affinities with certain types of very ancient Jewish synagogue chants, particularly those preserved by the Jews of the Yemen. If so, elements in their tradition may predate the Urfalees' music. But from what we know of the sources, the chants of ancient Edessa should be the oldest original chants in the Christian tradition. What we heard tonight shows every sign of being the unadulterated music of late antique Edessa. If that is so – and it's a big if – then you could certainly argue that it may well be the most ancient Christian chant still in existence, yes.'

'And so the ultimate origin of the Western Gregorian tradition, and everything else that followed – the root from which Palestrina, Allegri and Victoria all grew . . . ?'

Gianmaria stubbed out his cigarette. 'That's speculation,' he said. Then he shrugged his shoulders and smiled. 'Wait until my research is published.'

THE CONVENT OF SEIDNAYA, 11 SEPTEMBER

A series of lifts – a truck, a pick-up and finally a tractor – brought me to the ruined Byzantine town of Serjilla in time for lunch. I sat at the brow of the hill munching the sandwiches they had packed for me at the Baron, looking down over the extraordinary expanse of late antique buildings spread out across the valley below.

It was the sort of classical townscape that you normally see only in Roman and Byzantine mosaics. There were houses, a church, an inn, a set of baths, a couple of villas facing onto their own courtyards, and a scattering of farm buildings, with the pitched rooflines of still more pedimented and colonnaded buildings visible over the brow of the hill. Elsewhere such late classical towns are represented only by bald archaeological sites: tidied lines of bleached pillars, crumbling metopes and fallen architraves. But here, through a strange accident of fate, more intact domestic

Byzantine buildings lay clustered at my feet in this obscure valley than survive today in all three of the greatest Byzantine metropolises – Constantinople, Antioch and Alexandria – put together.

The perfection of preservation here is extraordinary. Outside some of the houses you can still see olive presses – round basins with a stone funnel leading into a lower tub for the pressed oil – standing as if ready for this year's olive harvest. The colonnade of the inn still provides shade from the sun; the town meeting house, with its pedimented roof and tabernacled windows, still exudes an air of pompous provincial pride, as if the Byzantine gentlemen farmers who lived here were only out in the fields, overseeing their labourers, and would be back in the evening to discuss some weighty matter of village politics.

The view before me was almost exactly as it would have been when John Moschos passed through these hills on his way to Antioch at the end of the sixth century. Looking inside one villa, peering under the superbly carved entablature of a doorway, I could see in the darkness that the first-floor ceiling was still totally intact: in two thousand years, the earthquakes and upheavals that had levelled Antioch had left not one crack in this structure. Only the total absence of furniture and wooden fittings hinted at what had happened to this fine late antique townhouse; and after the perfection of the view from the top of the hill, I was almost disappointed not to find tables and chairs in the kitchens, nor plates of fruit waiting on the dressers, as they do in the mosaics at Antakya.

On the lower slope of the hillside, behind the town baths, lay an empty Byzantine sarcophagus. Its heavy granite cover was half broken off and there seemed to be no one about, so I hid my heavy rucksack inside it, out of sight under the remaining half of the covering slab, and set off across the low hills towards the neighbouring town of al-Barra.

It was a cool, bright autumn afternoon and thick clouds were racing overhead, casting quick-moving shadows over the massif. The hills were rolling and stony, and on the summits square Byzantine watchtowers rose vertically from the scree. Descending into al-Barra I found myself facing a small, square fifth-century

church. It had a triple-arched portal, with each doorway sur-
mounted`by a finely carved tympanum. The doorways led into a
tiny interior, only three bays long. The capitals were covered with
vine-scroll interlace, each leaf raised by drilling away the stone
behind it, as with an engraving; between the fronds small equal-
armed Greek crosses nested like birds among the grapes and the
vine tendrils.

I clambered up onto a wall and from that height saw what was
invisible from the ground: that littered throughout the olive groves
was another complete Byzantine ghost town, the stone skeletons
of towers, vaults, and half-collapsed townhouses rising everywhere
from the soft loam. At the edge of the trees, to the east, some of
the largest and airiest of the villas were still inhabited. From my
vantage point I could see a Syrian woman in a patterned headscarf
peeping out of a late Roman window in one of the largest houses.
A washing line ran from the final pillar on her colonnade to the
handle of a massive Roman sarcophagus to one side; on it, children's clothes were hanging out to dry in the afternoon sun.
Nearby, hens were perching on another fallen pillar which had
been hollowed out to make a drinking trough. But the villagers
clearly disdained to live in the slightly less grand villas that lay on
the lower ground, a little deeper into the groves; after all, these
houses had only four or five main rooms, which did not leave
enough space for the stabling of horses, asses, goats and sheep;
nor, as I discovered when I made a closer inspection, did they
have any baths with hypocaust systems, so useful for keeping
bantams in.

Carrying on through the trees, I began to climb over a small
drystone wall that separated the land of two farmers; only when
I was halfway over did I notice that the wall was made up of a
pile of discarded doorjambs, carved tympana and inscribed lintels,
an almost ridiculous richness of fine Byzantine sculpture piled up
between the trees. Only in Syria, I thought, could a currency
of this richness be so debased in value by the embarrassment
of its profusion that it could be used for so humble a purpose as
walling.

A little beyond this wall, across the ruins of the town's old marketplace, lay a pyramid. It rested on a squat cube of warm honey-coloured limestone. At the corners of the cube four stumpy pilasters rose to a quadrant of richly curlicued Corinthian capitals. Bands of deeply cut acanthus ran along all four sides of the cube, the swirling leaf-patterns broken by a series of medallions. These turned out to contain the *chi-rho* monogram that Constantine turned into the symbol of his new Christian Empire. The apparently pagan pyramid was in fact a very unusual early-fifth-century Christian monument.

Inside the half-light of the tomb chamber lay five great sarcophagi. Unusually, the lids still sealed the caskets shut; the sleepers slept on undisturbed. In the centre, flanked on either side by two smaller caskets, lay the great sarcophagus of what was clearly the family patriarch: a ton of polished porphyry, unornamented but for a massive *chi-rho* monogram contained within a laurel wreath. The sheer baroque bulk of the sarcophagus somehow suggested a portly landowner, a big-bellied, bucolic figure, dangling grapes into his open mouth as he reclined on his couch.

The pyramid lay in front of the ruins of a magnificent villa, three storeys high. The way the pyramid was located in relation to the house implied that it must have been the dynastic mausoleum of the family who had lived there, not dissimilar to the arrangement – centuries later, in a very different world – at Castle Howard.

Now the villa was deserted except for a single tethered donkey belonging to one of the olive harvesters. But as I wandered around its collapsing and deserted rooms I wondered about the family that had lived here. Who had built this small palace? The provincial governor? A local landowner? A prominent senator, returning to his home town for burial after a life of politicking in the capital? The house and its adjacent tomb indicated the existence of an entire world – that of the provincial Byzantine aristocracy – which is passed over in the written sources. In the tenth century there are the writings of the misanthropist Cecaumenus, a grumpy provincial squire who advised his readers to avoid the court, lock up their daughters and keep their wives far from any visitors; but from the early Byzantine period there is relatively little to illuminate the life of the landowning class in the eastern provinces, except when such a figure forms the background for a saint's miracle story or emerges briefly from obscurity to lead a rebellion or champion some obscure heresy.

The sheer magnificent solidity of the family sarcophagi, the confidence and certainty of the workmanship and the conservative nature of the design seemed to hint at a world far removed from the nervy credulity of Theodoret's monks suspended in their cages and raised on their pillars. They also emphasised the degree of continuity between the late classical and the early Byzantine world, a continuity that is easily forgotten when reading the chroniclers' narratives of interminable palace coups, mutinous Gothic generals and collapsing frontiers.

For this ostensibly Christian monument is only barely converted from paganism, and the thinnest veneer of Christianity rests uneasily on what is unashamedly a pagan classical pyramid. Looking at the great porphyry caskets, I wondered whether the calm certainty of the mausoleum was a sham – a brave attempt to maintain classical values in a world where the surface of ancient life was being betrayed at every turn: in the new-fangled clothes that were being worn, in the beliefs that were held, in the strange chants of the Syrian monks and the prophecies of the stylites. Or did it in fact represent the reality? Did the people in these sarcophagi still lead a version of the old life of the late classical landowner: their youth spent in the law school at Beirut or the School of Libanius at Antioch; a period as a provincial official posted to Hippo or Harran; or perhaps a spell in the army on the Rhine frontier, peering over the cold battlements of Cologne or Trier to catch a glimpse of a Gothic raider padding across the ice into Roman territory; then the return to the home estate and the comforts of the richest and most civilised part of the Empire, with winters of hunting and feasting, the occasional marriage party of a neighbouring landowner or a trip to the theatre at Apamea; of afternoons wallowing in the baths at Serjilla and evenings spent reading Homer by the light of an oil lamp. Wandering through the Byzantine villa, through a succession of cool, high-ceilinged rooms, the stone still fitted perfectly, joint by joint, a classical pediment on every window frame, I felt sure that more of the ancient world had survived for longer in the Byzantine East than any of the surviving sources – including John Moschos – now indicate.

Lost in my Byzantine thoughts, I hadn't noticed that it had turned chilly. A faint yellow-gilt pallor now hung over the olive groves, and the oblique late-afternoon light threw long shadows among the trees. Worried that I had already spent too long in al-Barra, I set off at a brisk pace on the road back to Serjilla to pick up my rucksack before darkness fell. As I walked I wondered what had happened to these strange, deserted Byzantine towns. They certainly had not been burned and destroyed by raiding parties of Persians or Arabs; their marvellous preservation showed that. So what did happen?

No one is sure, but the results of a number of recent digs appear to have convinced archaeologists that the entire Levantine coast underwent some form of major economic and demographic crisis towards the end of the sixth century, a full half century *before* the Arab conquest. Plagues, political upheavals, the Persian wars and the raids of desert nomads were responsible for the gradual erosion of urban life and its replacement by a landscape of small villages and monasteries. Some of the larger secular estates and their estate villages might have survived for a while (including that, perhaps, of the entombed aristocrat of al-Barra), but in most places the ancient Levantine trading towns – places like Palmyra, Bosra and Jerash – disappeared forever, forgotten by the world until the Scottish painter David Roberts popularised their ruins, turning them into neat idylls, perfectly tailored to the tastes of nineteenth-century European romantics. While the ancient classical trading towns were falling into decay, in the countryside the ever-growing cohorts of monks and hermits were gradually settling in and taking over the abandoned forts, forums and pagan temples.

Certainly in the pages of John Moschos the three great metropolises – Antioch, Alexandria and Constantinople – still appear to be thriving: there are, for example, stories about labourers rebuilding public edifices in Antioch. But elsewhere in the eastern

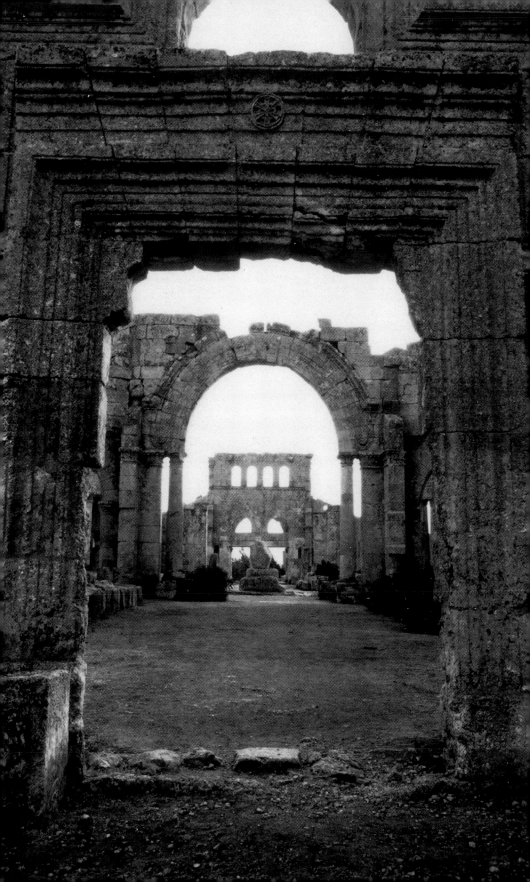

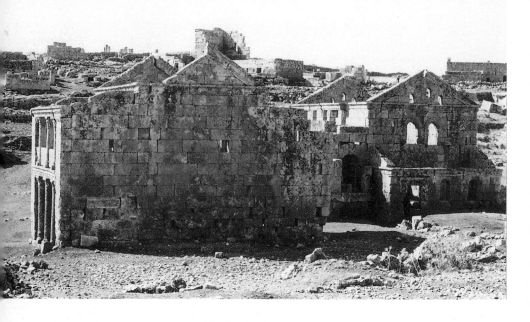

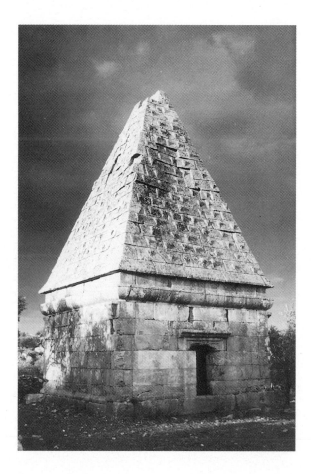

Previous page Qala'at Semaan, the Basilica of St Symeon Stylites, Syria.

Above Deserted Byzantine buildings, Serjilla, Syria,

Left Late antique pyramid tomb, al-Barra, Syria.

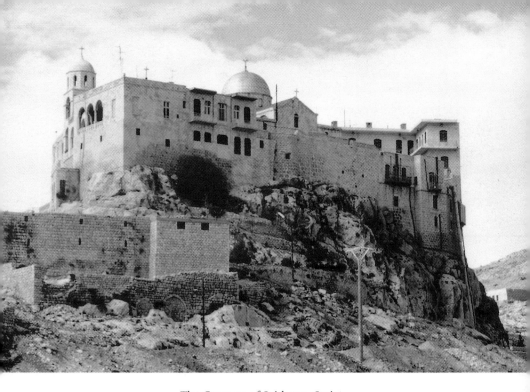

The Convent of Seidnaya, Syria.

Drive-in Armageddon, Beirut.

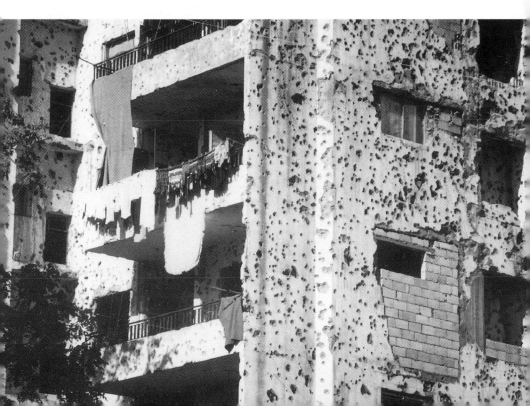

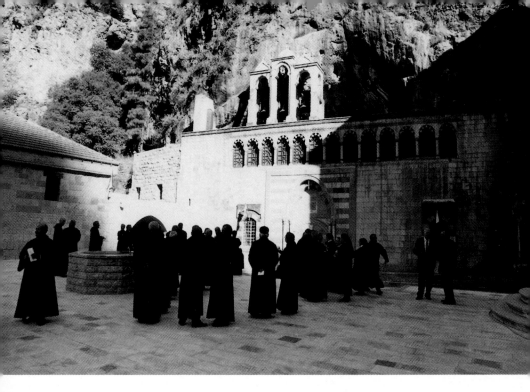

The Monastery of Koshaya, Qadisha Valley, Lebanon.

Sculpture from the Temple of the Sun, Ba'albek.

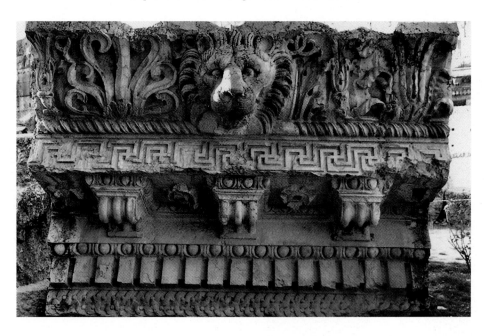

provinces there are only very occasional glimpses of the old classical civic life, with its theatres, schools, brothels, markets and circuses. We hear, for example, about an actor from Tarsus who cohabits with two concubines and 'performs deeds truly worthy of the demons who urged him on', implying that the Tarsus theatre was still functioning healthily. At the same time we know that the ancient trading city of Apamea still had a functioning hippodrome, for Moschos tells us how a former champion charioteer from the town went on to become a monk in Egypt, where he was later captured and enslaved by desert nomads.

Moreover, *The Spiritual Meadow* contains occasional references to merchants and trade, which implies that international commerce – the prerequisite for true urban life – had not yet completely died. At Ascalon Moschos hears about a merchant whose ship has sunk and so is thrown into prison, while his wife is forced to prostitute herself in order to pay his debts. On another occasion he tells of a gem engraver travelling by sea; he hears from his cabin boy that the crew is about to murder him for his boxes of precious gems, so he throws the entire hoard overboard.

But these stories are exceptions. Far more common are tales set against a background of small villages or remote estates, or else in the distant wilderness where hermits can live alone for years undisturbed by anyone – so much so that their deaths can go unremarked for decades. In one particularly macabre tale, a community of monks see mysterious lights at night at the top of the mountain high above their monastery. When daybreak comes they send up a party to investigate, who find that the source of the strange celestial aura is a small cave. Inside they discover an anchorite in a hair shirt. One of the monks embraces the ascetic, only to realise that he is dead. Although his body is miraculously well preserved, a note written by the dying monk indicates that he had 'departed this life' more than seventeen years previously.

The degree to which monasteries, with their mystical and otherworldly outlook, came to dominate the culture of the region is demonstrated by a set of gospels illuminated in the sixth century at the lost monastery of Beth Zagba, believed by Byzantinists to lie somewhere in the hills around Serjilla. In the illustrations of the Rabula Gospels, the angels are as real as the saints, who in turn are drawn to look like local monks: gaunt rustics caught in mid-argument, hands wildly gesticulating, their expression masked beneath thick growths of beard. In the most famous picture, of the Ascension, Christ hovers in his fiery chariot only just out of reach of the apostles. No dramatic gulf separates his divine world from that of his followers; he is the same size as them, has similar features and wears similar clothes. No barrier separates the natural from the supernatural.

Another illustration, that of Christ Enthroned, takes this immediacy even further. Christ is shown in majesty, on a golden throne studded with huge cabochon jewels. But around him, flanking him on either side, are not the expected crowd of seraphim and cherubim but a crowd of rough-robed Syrian monks. They are hooded and cowled in their sober brown sackcloth, hair grey, eyes staring, gospel books clutched to their chests as if they were clustered around the abbot in the chapter house or refectory. There is none of the chill remoteness of much late Byzantine art; here the superhuman is considered tangible and everyday, the divine imminent and directly accessible.

This sort of mystical abstraction is a world away from the practical late Roman farmers of Serjilla or the pyramid-dynasty of al-Barra. And yet if recent scholarship is correct, it seems increasingly likely that the two worlds – those of the gentrified landed estates and the isolated wild-eyed illuminator monks – coexisted side by side in these hills, and that the transition both from the pagan-classical to the Byzantine-Christian, and then, three centuries later, from the Byzantine-Christian to the medieval-Islamic, was a far more gradual process than the traditional accounts of violent change and invasion would allow.

In the Middle East, the reality of continuity has always been masked by a surface impression of cataclysm.

Returning in the dusk to Serjilla, I narrowly avoided being torn limb from limb by a pack of enormous sheepdogs. I had just rescued my pack from its sarcophagus and was returning up the hill when the beasts came howling out of the shadows, closing in on me with great leaps and bounds. With only seconds to spare, I managed to scramble up the fallen wall of a tumbledown Byzantine farmhouse, and stood there perched on a projecting gable like a stylite on his pillar. Pulling my rucksack up after me, I looked down to see three wolf-dogs growling below me, mouths open, each exhibiting a truly Baskervillian set of fangs. It was little comfort to think that sheepdogs also seem to have been a hazard of the region in Byzantine times: the unattractive anti-Semitic monastic rabble-rouser Barsauma survived an attack by dogs during his youth, which according to his biographer was understood to presage his future sainthood.

Eventually, just when I was beginning to think that I was going to have to spend the night up on my perch, the shepherd – a small fifteen-year-old boy – came up. He scattered the three dogs as easily as if they were poodles with a torrent of abuse and a hail of small pebbles. At my request he escorted me out of the ruins and onto the track before returning to his flock and the night-shelter of the old Serjilla bath house.

Quickening my pace, and mouthing prayers that I would not pass any more shepherds or their dogs, I headed back to the main road, and just managed to catch the last bus of the day before darkness fell. It was heading south.

A two-hour drive brought me to Homs. At the time of John Moschos, Homs was known as Emesa, and was home to figures as diverse as, on the one hand, Romanos the Melodist, and on the other, St Symeon the Fool, who used to defecate in the centre of the marketplace and complained that the girls of Emesa were 'as licentious as any in Syria'. Homs was famous for its taverns, jugglers, mimers, prostitutes, dancing girls and beggars, as well as for the overheated libido of its clergy: Deacon John of Emesa, the Casanova of the Byzantine Church, was notorious for his habit of making love to all the most beautiful married women in his congregation. Homs was also the place where the early Anglo-Saxon pilgrim St Willibald was imprisoned for several months on his way to Jerusalem. It is still one of the principal Christian towns in Syria, but today is famous only for the stupidity of its inhabitants: contemporary Homsis play the same role in Syrian jokes as the Polish do in those of America, the Irish in Britain, and Kerrymen in Ireland. I decided against staying the night in the city and headed on instead to the convent of Seidnaya, the most important of the three Byzantine monasteries still functioning in Syria.

On the rattling country bus I sat beside an old Arab farmer. Discovering where I was going, he regaled me with stories of the exploits of a figure he called Malik Jylan of Rum. It was only later, when I read about the myth of the monastery's foundation by the Emperor Justinian, that I realised that my companion had been telling me a version of the same story: of how the Emperor – Malik Jylan in Arabic – out on a hunting expedition, had chased a stag up a rocky eminence. Just as he was about to draw his bow, the stag changed into the Virgin Mary. The Virgin commanded him to build a convent on the site, which, she said, had previously been hallowed by Noah himself, who planted a vine there soon after the Flood. According to my friend on the bus, if I understood him correctly, the Emperor then installed his own sister as the first abbess. The origin of the legend would appear to be etymological: in Aramaic Seidnaya means both 'our lady' and 'a hunting place'.

The road wound steeply up into the hills, and the bus stopped in village after village. By the time it dropped me off in the dark at the bottom of the hill leading up to the monastery it was after nine o'clock, and I was worried that the abbey gates would have closed for the night. Exhausted, I trudged uphill towards the lights of the convent, which sat, more like a crusader castle than a shrine, on a spur of rock at the very top of the village. In the cold and the darkness I was anxiously aware that the last bus had just departed and that the small village around the foot of the rock contained no hotel or lodging house.

The gateway of the convent was reached up a steep flight of stairs; and at the top, to my relief, I found that the door was open. Walking into an empty courtyard, my feet echoing on the flagstones, I wondered where the nuns had gone. Then I heard the distant sound of Orthodox chant drifting from the church and headed towards it.

Two nuns in black veils were chanting at a lectern, while a priest, hidden behind the iconostasis, echoed their chants in a deep reverberating bass. The church was no older than the early nineteenth century, despite some medieval masonry low down in the walls of the nave. But its atmosphere was as authentically Byzantine as any I had seen on Athos. The only light came from a few flickering lamps attached to steel chandeliers suspended from the ceiling on gold chains. As the candle-light waxed and waned with the draught, the frescoes in the domes and semi domes flashed momentarily into view then disappeared again into the shadows.

When the travel writer Colin Thubron visited the convent in 1966, he claimed to have witnessed a miracle: to have seen the face of the icon of Notre Dame de Seidnaya stream with tears. In the same church I too witnessed a miracle, or something that today would certainly be regarded as a miracle in almost any other country in the Middle East. For the congregation seemed to consist not of Christians but almost entirely of heavily bearded Muslim men. As the priest circled the altar with his thurible, filling the sanctuary with great clouds of incense, the men bobbed up and down on their prayer mats as if in the middle of Friday prayers in a great mosque. Their women, some dressed in full black *chador*, mouthed prayers from the shadows of the exo-narthex. A few, closely watching the Christian women, went up to the icons hanging from the pillars of the church, kissed them, then lit candles and placed them in the candelabra in front of the images. As I watched from the rear of the church I could see the faces of the women reflected in the illuminated gilt of the icons.

Towards the end of the service, the priest reappeared with a golden stole over his cassock and circled the length of the church with his thurible, gently and almost apologetically stepping over the prostrate Muslims blocking his way, treading as carefully as if they were precious Iznik vases. While I had seen Muslims and Christians praying together on the island of Buyuk Ada, off Istanbul, this was something quite different: a degree of tolerance – in both congregations – unimaginable today almost anywhere else in the Near East. Yet it was, of course, the old way: the Eastern Christians and the Muslims have lived side by side for nearly one and a half millennia, and have only been able to do so due to a degree of mutual tolerance and shared customs unimaginable in the solidly Christian West.

How easy it is today to think of the West as the home of freedom of thought and liberty of worship, and to forget how, as recently as the seventeenth century, Huguenot exiles escaping religious persecution in Europe would write admiringly of the policy of religious tolerance practised across the Ottoman Empire. The same broad tolerance that had given homes to hundreds of thousands of penniless Jews, expelled by bigoted Catholic kings from Spain and Portugal, protected the Eastern Christians in their ancient homelands, despite the Crusades and the continual hostility of the Christian West. Only in the twentieth century has that traditional tolerance been replaced by a new hardening in Islamic attitudes; and only recently has the syncretism of Cyrrhus and Seidnaya become a precious rarity.

As vespers drew to a close the pilgrims began to file quietly out, and I was left alone at the back of the church with my rucksack. As I was standing there I was approached by a young nun in a knitted black balaclava; it was shaped a little like the Sutton Hoo helmet, with a long tailpiece which trailed down the back of her neck. Sister Tecla had intelligent black eyes and a bold, confident gaze; she spoke fluent English with a slight French accent. She asked me where I was from, and after I had told her I remarked on the number of Muslims in the congregation. Was it at all unusual, I asked.

'The Muslims come here because they want babies,' said the nun simply. 'Our Lady has shown her power and healed many of the Muslims. Those people started to talk about her and now more Muslims come here than Christians. If they ask for her she will be there.'

As we were speaking, we were approached by a Muslim couple. The woman was veiled – only her mouth was visible through the black wraps; her husband, a burly man who wore his beard without a moustache, looked remarkably like the wilder sort of Hezbollah commander featured in news bulletins from southern Lebanon. But whatever his politics, he carried in one hand a heavy tin of olive oil and in the other a large plastic basin full of fresh loaves, and he gave both to the nun, bowing his head as shyly as a schoolboy and retreating backwards in obvious embarrassment.

'They come in the evening,' continued the nun. 'They make vows and then the women spend the night. They sleep on a blanket in front of the holy icon of Our Lady painted by St Luke. Sometimes the women eat the wick of a lamp that has burned in front of the image, or maybe drink the holy oil. Then in the morning they drink from the spring in the courtyard. Nine months later they have babies.'

'And it works?'

'I have seen it with my own eyes,' said Sister Tecla. 'One Muslim woman from Jordan had been waiting for a baby for twenty-five years. She was beyond the normal age of childbearing, but someone told her about the Virgin of Seidnaya. She came here and spent two nights in front of the icon. She was so desperate she ate the wicks of nearly twenty lamps.'

'What happened?'

'She came back the following year,' said Sister Tecla, 'with triplets.'

The nun led me up the south aisle of the church, and down a corridor into the chapel which sheltered the icons. At the doorway she removed her shoes and indicated that I should do likewise. I placed them with my rucksack, beside the great mountain of footwear already deposited in the antechamber and Sister Tecla led me into the muffled sanctuary. It was darker even than the church, with no windows to admit the faint light of the moon and stars which had cast a silvery light over the high altar during vespers. Here only the twinkling of a hundred lamps lit the interior, allowing us to avoid tripping over a pair of Muslims prostrated on their prayer carpets near the entrance.

'And you have no objection to so many Muslims coming here and praying in your church?' I whispered.

'We are all children of God,' said Sister Tecla. 'The All Holy One brings us all together.'

She kissed an icon of the warrior saints Sergius and Bacchus, then turned back to face me. 'Sometimes the Muslims promise to christen a child born through the Mother of God's intervention. This happens less frequently than it used to, but of course we like it when it does. Others make their children Muslims, but when they are old enough they bring them here to help us in some way, perhaps with cleaning the church or in the kitchens.'

The shrine of the icon was thick with the low murmur of prayer and chanting; those pilgrims who were talking to each other did so in hushed voices. Behind me a Syrian paratrooper in full khaki fatigues entered the shrine, having first deposited his heavy boots by the entrance. He advanced towards the icons on his knees, crossing himself all the while and murmuring prayers to the Virgin. Here, you felt instinctively, rather than in the church, was the centre of the convent's devotion.

In the lamplight, smoke-blackened icons were everywhere, some of them very fine. There was a Beheading of John the Baptist, from which pious pilgrims had scratched out the face of the executioner; there were several of the Panaghia, including one in which the Madonna was shown with thin, almond-shaped eyes as if she was a Persian princess; there was a fine image of the Dormition, the composition of which, intriguingly enough, seemed to be derived from the Ascension in the Rabula Gospels. But the most famous of the images of Our Lady of Seidnaya, the sacred icon supposed to have been painted by St Luke, was invisible, so cluttered was it with knotted silk ribbons, scribbled petitions and silver plaques representing the parts of the bodies of the pilgrims which had been healed through the Virgin's prayers.

As Sister Tecla led the way from the shrine she said, 'Come: I will take you to the guest rooms. You must eat before you go to bed.' Up to that point neither of us had broached the subject of where I was to spend the night.

In the guest rooms I was shown to a divan, while a servant

took my rucksack to my cell. Sister Tecla poured me a small cup of bitter Arab coffee from a thermos flask, then sent the servant to the kitchens for some food. It arrived a few minutes later, brought by a young novice: a plate of thin soup and some feta cheese accompanied by flat pitta bread. Sister Tecla sat opposite me as I ate, and I asked her about an unexpected photograph which was framed on the wall beside my table.

'These are our Syrian cosmonauts,' she said, pointing to a picture of three men in space suits clutching their helmets under their arms rather as stage ghosts hold their heads. 'They spent a month together on the Soviet space station Mir.'

'But why is the picture here?' I asked.

'It was given to us by the cosmonauts after they returned to Syria.'

'They came here?'

'Of course. All three are Muslims, but they visited Seidnaya before they went, to pray for good luck. As soon as they had returned safely they came here again.'

'To tell the nuns about their adventures?'

'No, no,' said Sister Tecla, looking at me as one might at a rather dim ten-year-old. 'They came to thank the Virgin and give us presents: this picture and a sheep.'

'A sheep?'

'A sheep.'

'As . . . as a pet?'

'No, no,' said Sister Tecla, frowning again. 'The cosmonauts came here to cut the sheep's throat, of course.' She gave me another withering look. 'It was a sacrifice to the Virgin,' she said, 'to thank her for their safe return from outer space.'

IV

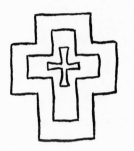

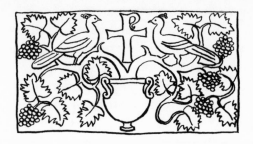

HOTEL CAVALIER, BEIRUT, LEBANON, 23 SEPTEMBER
1994

After a fortnight of glorious indolence staying with friends in a
diplomatic suburb of Damascus, I was woken this morning by the
sound of Bing, their Filipino manservant, blow-drying my now
spotlessly clean rucksack.

Slowly the daunting prospect of the day ahead began to take
shape: leaving the soft beds, the cool blue swimming pool and my
hospitable hosts – all for the uncertainties of the Lebanon, a
country which for the last two decades has been virtually a syn-
onym for anarchy.

To an earlier generation, Lebanon brought to mind images of
skiing amid the cedars and sunbathing on the lido at Byblos,
followed by flighty evenings in the casinos of Jounieh. But for
those of us who grew up during the eighties, Beirut is of course
associated with a rather different set of images: grainy front-page
pictures of the massed Palestinian corpses at Sabra and Chatila;
Don McCullin's photographs of the fire-blackened ruins of the
lunatic asylum the Israelis bombarded with phosphorus; television
pictures of the hostages; the impacting shells of the bloody militia
wars – the PLO versus the Phalange, the Phalange versus Amal,
Amal versus Hezbollah, Hezbollah versus the PLO. None of these
made one in a particular hurry to rush to see the country for
oneself.

For two weeks this diary has lain unwritten, unread, under a pile of freshly washed and immaculately ironed clothes. Since I last opened it in Seidnaya, the days have been filled neither with writing nor research; instead I have spent an unscheduled fortnight on the carousel of Syria's diplomatic whirl: a *soirée* at the Greek Ambassador's (dancing until 2.30 in the morning); a vast dinner with an Armenian entrepreneur; trips in the Land-Rover to an old ruin or a new restaurant; swimming; lunch in a palace in the old city; drinks with a Damascene aesthete amid his collection of icons. After the tensions of Turkey and the Spartan eccentricities of Seidnaya and the Baron it was a welcome – in fact an almost unbelievably wonderful – change. The only real irritation in the entire period was the incessant noise of building in the apartment above that of my hosts, where a *mukhabarat* general was about to move in and where the builders were busy installing marble floors, mirrored ceilings and pink bathtubs with gilt taps the shape of flying swans – apparently the sort of kitsch accessories that make secret policemen feel at home.

But now I was ready to move on, and the more I heard about Lebanon the more fascinated I became by the prospect of that strange country. Over drinks, people would tell the most bizarre stories about the war and its aftermath: the time the victorious Palestinian militias exhumed the Christian dead from the cemetery at Damour, scattering a couple of hundred cadavers and skeletons around the streets, all of them still dressed in the frock-coats and Sunday suits in which they were buried a century earlier; stories of Beirut's cockerels, that appeared to be suffering from a form of post-traumatic stress syndrome (they start crowing at midnight, only to fall silent at dawn); the renowned Lebanese vineyard of Château Musar, that only lost one vintage during the entire war – in 1984, when the front line between the Christian and Muslim militias ran between the vines and the winery.

Most of all, however, I was becoming fascinated by the Maronites. They sounded very different from any of the other Christian communities I have so far come across on my journey. Although they do not appear in *The Spiritual Meadow*, the Maronites started off as a cult around a Byzantine hermit who was a near-contemporary of John Moschos. Indeed St Maron's ascetic tendencies were so extreme that he earned a place in Theodoret's compendium of eremitical eccentricity, *The History of the Monks of Syria*. In this, their first appearance in history, the Maronites started as they meant to continue: on St Maron's death a 'bitter war' broke out among his followers and their neighbours over the saint's body: 'one of the adjacent [Maronite] villages that was well populated came out in a mass, drove off the others and seized this thrice-desired treasure'.

Later, the Maronites' somewhat eccentric theology came to be deemed heretical by the official Byzantine Church. The details of this are wonderfully Byzantine: Monothelitism, the particular brand of Christology then favoured by the Maronites, had originally been promoted by the Emperor Heraclius as a compromise definition of the person of Christ which would be acceptable to both Orthodox and Monophysites and so unite the divided Empire; inevitably, however, it was rejected by both parties, leaving the unfortunate Maronites, the only community to accept the definition, to be branded as heretics and persecuted accordingly. This was largely due to the influence of John Moschos's travelling companion Sophronius, who in his old age became a rigorously Orthodox Patriarch of Jerusalem, and set himself up as the most bitter opponent of Monothelitism.

To escape further Byzantine harassment, the Maronites were gradually forced to emigrate from their low-lying Syrian heartlands into the impenetrable fastness of Mount Lebanon. There, amid the cliffs and narrow passes, they were able to defend themselves against all their enemies, both Christian and Muslim, until centuries later, at the time of the Crusades, they came into communion with Rome and managed to form an alliance with the Franks. It was an alliance that very loosely, in one form or another, was to continue up to the twentieth century: in 1920, out of the Syrian territories they inherited from the Ottoman Empire at the end of the First World War, the French created a 'State of Greater Lebanon' specifically for the Maronites and at the Maronites' explicit request.

In return the Maronites attempted – and indeed still attempt

– to be more French than the French. The Maronite upper classes speak French as their first language and usually refuse to speak Arabic except to servants and tradesmen. Most of them have French Christian names. They send their children to Paris for as much of their education as they can afford. Moreover they adamantly deny their Syrian roots, and in the course of this century have invented an almost entirely mythical Phoenician (i.e. semi-European) origin for themselves, while visualising Lebanon as a sort of Near Eastern outpost of France, a country which they still refer to as 'the nourishing mother'.

Most commentators have tended to attribute the balance of responsibility for the outbreak of the civil war to the Maronites' intransigence, their unapologetic Christian supremacism, their contempt for their Muslim neighbours, and their point-blank refusal to share Lebanon with the landless Palestinian refugees ejected from their homes at the creation of Israel in 1948.

Under the terms of the 1943 Lebanese National Pact, supreme power – in the form of the Presidency – was placed in the hands of the Maronites as a reflection of the Christians' numerical superiority. But by the 1970s the Maronites were no longer the largest single religious group in Lebanon, being outnumbered by both Sunni and Shia Muslim communities. Despite this, the Maronites adamantly refused to discuss any reform that would share power more equally between the different groupings. Instead, they began to arm themselves and to prepare for war.

When the civil war finally broke out, the Maronites were ready. Modelling themselves on the Crusaders, they went into battle with crosses sewn onto their uniforms and icons of the Virgin glued to their rifle butts. Their militias were given neo-medieval names like the Knights of the Virgin, the Youth of St Maron and the Wood of the Cross. Yet for all these chivalrous titles, the Maronite militias were responsible for more than their fair share of the war's worst atrocities: the notorious massacres at Sabra and Chatila, where at least six hundred (and perhaps as many as two thousand) Palestinian civilians were butchered, was the work of the Maronites' Phalange militia, albeit under Israeli supervision.

The Maronite clergy did little to restrain their flock. Expatriate

Maronite priests such as the parish priest of Our Lady of Mount Lebanon, Beverly Hills, exhorted their congregations to donate money to arm the militias, while the Maronites' enemies accused even the supposedly cloistered Maronite monks of involving themselves in arms dealing. Referring to the large sums said to have been raised by the monks for the war effort, the Druze leader Kemal Jumblatt observed that 'the tonsured heads of Lebanese monks give off a golden halo.'

Certainly, as in Byzantine times, the monks involved themselves closely in politics, tending to support the more extreme ultra-nationalist Maronite militias. Most popular of all in the monasteries were the sinister Guardians of the Cedars, whose symbol was a sword-cum-cross amid flames, and whose particular speciality was cutting the ears off their dead Muslim opponents, then displaying them as trophies. The monastic support given to this group continued, despite the Guardians holding a press conference to applaud the Sabra and Chatila massacres and adopting the macabre slogan 'It is the duty of every Lebanese to kill at least one Palestinian.' The monks were, however, prepared to give their support to other suitably extreme figures: on one occasion Fr. Boulos Naaman, the Superior of the Maronite Order of Monks, went so far as to compare one of the most vicious and bloodthirsty Phalangist leaders, Bashir Gemayel, to 'Christ, with complete understanding of his Christian mission'.

The civil war left between 100,000 and 150,000 dead, and no one came out of it well; but the Maronites certainly emerged with their reputation for ruthlessness, brutality and political incompetence enormously enhanced. They also came out of it fatally weakened. By the final stage of the war, which set Christian against Christian, a third of a million Maronites – over a quarter of the entire Christian community in Lebanon – had fled the Middle East for good, joining the haemorrhage of Christians leaving virtually every country of the region.

After lamenting the demise of a succession of Christian communities in the Middle East which failed adequately to defend themselves, it may seem perverse to criticise the only one that has taken serious action in an attempt to hold its own; but even the other Eastern Christians seem to regard the Maronites as some-thing of an embarrassment in their determination to cling on to their privileges whatever the cost. They certainly sounded very different from the defeated and depressed Armenians and Syriacs I had met in Turkey, or the timid, discreet and low-key Christians of Syria.

If nothing else, I told myself, Lebanon was certainly going to be a change.

By ten o'clock Bing had ironed my jacket and arranged the taxi that was to take me over the mountains to Beirut. I ate a last cooked breakfast (when will I next smell bacon and eggs?) and had just finished packing when the windows shook and, with a noise like a revving chainsaw, the Beirut taxi drove up outside the front gate. It was a souped-up American Thunderbird, the size of small tank, with chrome fenders and a sunshade jutting out above the windscreen. It was driven by a Lebanese spiv in Ray-Bans and a leather jacket. I embraced my anxious hosts, then, with another roar, we were off.

Ten minutes took us out of Damascus, and soon the Thunder-bird was burning into the scrub beyond. A further forty minutes and we were heading up into the foothills of Mount Lebanon. A convoy of T-72 tanks crunched down the highway in the opposite direction; President Asad waved goodbye from a hoarding. The road wound steeply upwards, corkscrewing through pine trees and slopes of gorse, and suddenly we were there: the Syrian frontier post – a rambling collection of concrete huts huddled among the pines – lay a little above us at the summit of the mountain.

The border formalities on the Syrian side were surprisingly quick and efficient, easier indeed than it used to be to pass from one European country to another. The guards collected our pass-ports from the car, like waiters in a drive-in McDonald's, then brought them back again a minute later, stamped with their exit visas. We drove on through a no-man's land, past the skeletons of three burnt-out cars – although, rather disappointingly after all I had read about the war, these looked as if they had crashed rather than suffered the strafing of Israeli F-16s. To our right rose a slope of conifers from which wafted the acrid scent of pine resin. We turned a corner and there, amid the trees, recently rebuilt, lay the Lebanese frontier post. Outside it flapped the Lebanese tricolour, overlaid with the Cedar of Lebanon.

Entering Lebanon was rather more problematic than leaving Syria. Six mustachioed beefcakes in camouflage jumpsuits kept us waiting for two hours in the cold while a busload of Libyans begged and pleaded to be let in. The border hut was a grim, seedy bunker, the guards were bored, and none of the Libyans had visas. But eventually, after much twiddling of thumbs, the Libyans gave up and got forlornly back into their bus. Our passports were stamped and the chief official wished us 'Bienvenu au Liban.'

The Thunderbird roared back into life, and at some speed we set off downhill into the green basin of the Bekaa Valley. From above, it seemed as beautiful and bucolic as the Valley of Kashmir: rivers, water meadows, green fields, long lines of poplars and beech avenues all turning yellow in the early autumn cold. It looked the picture of pastoral innocence; nothing about the Bekaa indicated it to be the seedbed of one of the world's largest opium harvests and home to some of the Middle East's most formidable drug barons.

As we twisted down the mountain slope, however, the impression of a gentle pastoral oasis quickly disappeared. Rubbish – cartons, old tyres, cans, crisp packets, binliners – lay like a carpet across the ground, as if there had been no refuse collections for twenty years. Disused carrier bags caught in the barbed wire and furred the hedgerows with white polythene. Wrecked buildings dotted the roadside, neither repaired nor demolished since the end of the war three years earlier. The power lines had everywhere been hijacked by pirate operators, and from every pylon a cat's-cradle of wires tangled their way through a hundred illegal connections to the houses lining the roadside.

One of the root causes of the outbreak of the Lebanese civil war is often said to have been the weakness of the country's central government and its inability to control an overheated economy of unregulated libertarian capitalism: no one paid taxes, therefore there was no government spending, therefore no public services were provided. To all intents and purposes there was no state, and everything, for better or worse, was left to the initiative of the individual. In this respect nothing has changed; indeed it looks as if any semblance of central government control has now broken down completely.

One aspect of this is the role still played in Lebanon by the Syrians. Although we had left Syria ten miles behind us, Syrian troops in clumsy, ill-fitting khaki uniforms – very different from the chic designer camouflage of the Lebanese army – still manned checkpoints at intervals along the road. Syrian *mukhabarat* Range-Rovers, their windows blacked out with friezes of Asad posters, stood parked beside pillboxes painted the colours of the Syrian flag. On the concrete crash-barriers beside these Syrian pockets, the otherwise ubiquitous posters of the Lebanese Prime Minister, Rafiq Hariri – all jowls and double chins like some corpulent Italian waiter – were replaced by the Asad family iconography familiar from Syria: Asad in his paratrooper's fatigues, Asad the general with his peaked cap, Asad the statesman in international pinstripe, Asad's dead son Basil in his trademark reflector shades.

Sometimes the hagiography became more whimsical: on one Syrian pillbox, Asad and Basil were transformed into the idiom of Haight Ashbury flower children, their scowling faces hanging from the stalks of bright, naively-painted sunflowers. At other times the iconography of the different power-brokers in Lebanon was strangely intermingled, so that pin-ups of Asad, Basil, Hariri and a brace of turbaned Iranian mullahs (popular among the Shia of the Bekaa) would all appear together on a single crash-barrier, sometimes in the unlikely company of a leggy Lebanese *chanteuse* or some sequined Egyptian movie starlet.

Perhaps strangest of all were the unlikely lines of hoardings that rose above the forbidding ruins lining the highway: a smiling Claudia Schiffer stretched out leopard-like in Salvatore Ferragamo next to a yellow sandstone French colonial villa so riddled with great round shrapnel-holes it resembled an outsized slice of

Emmental; the Marlboro cowboy with his ten-gallon hat and herd of steers beaming out over an apocalyptic wasteland of shattered tower blocks; a metal tube of Bodymist – *un beau corps sans effort* – set against a carbon-black skeleton of twisted metal that had once been a filling station.

From the bottom of the Bekaa we crawled sluggishly up a narrow ridge, a single lane of traffic moving slowly behind a pair of massive Syrian tank-transporters until, at the top, we found ourselves looking down from an unexpected eminence, through a fug of smog, over the ruins of Beirut to the shattered mirror of the Mediterranean beyond. The Thunderbird's outsized bonnet swung over the hogsback of the ridge, and we were off: down we twisted, through a series of S-bends, under the ruins, past the posters: *Salvatore Ferragamo Pour Hiver 94*; an Ottoman villa pock-marked with small-arms fire; *Valentino: En Exclusivité*; a Bible-black hearse parked outside a church; *Martini: Right Here, Right Now*; two decapitated palm trees; *Calvin by Calvin Klein*; a dead tank; *Cool Budweiser – On Tap*; a bombed-out hospital; *Lucky Strike*; a cluster of skyscrapers so pockmarked with shrapnel they looked like a mouthful of severely rotten teeth; *Versatile by Versace . . .*

It was like a morality tale, spiralling downwards through one of the world's greatest monuments to human frailty, a huge vortex of greed and envy, resentment and intolerance, hatred and materialism, a five-mile-long slalom of shellholes and designer labels, heavy artillery and glossy boutiques. Like a modern updating of a Byzantine Apocalypse, it was the confusion that was most hell-like: Ayatollah Khomenei, hands raised in blessing, shared a billboard with a bottle of American after-shave; below, huge American cars – Thunderbirds, Chevrolets, Corvettes – roared past building sites where monstrous machines, thickly carapaced like metal-clad cockroaches, moved earth, demolished ruins, dug holes. Occasionally there was an explosion and a small mushroom-cloud of dust as a doomed tower block crashed to the earth, nudged by one of the grunting metal beetles below.

As we corkscrewed down towards the coastal plain the temperature rose and a thick fug of pollution hovered among the ruined buildings like a pall of gunsmoke. Here and there rose a scattering of kitsch new neo-Baroque villas with red roofs and marble balustrades: the product, presumably, of looting, arms or drug-trade money, for precious few legitimate fortunes have been made in this country during the last two decades. But as we drove deeper and deeper into the shattered city, such signs of prosperity became rarer: we headed on, faster now, on a potholed freeway, hotter and hotter, fuggier and fuggier, more polluted, more wrecked.

Yet for all this destruction, in some places the shrapnel marks were strangely beautiful, like a Kandinsky abstract: a perfect peppering of dots and dashes. It was a tribute to the arms dealers' art: a hail of metal perfectly distributed across a plaster canvas. Even the hideous ruins of the sixties blocks had a strange fascin-ation. Some appeared as if newly built; only the puncture-mark of a massive shellhole through the lateral wall of an apartment indicated what had happened to its interior and its occupants. Others were utterly wrecked: a single wall remained like a grave-stone to mark the whereabouts of an entire tower block; at a distance, an oblique exclamation of concrete and a tangle of metal rods – the building's top storey – would remain where it had landed in the aftermath of the blast or the collapse. Strangest of all were those blocks where the collapsed concrete stories were now folded down on top of each other, like a pile of neatly pressed shirts that had been left hanging off the edge of an ironing board, thick layers of tons of pre-stressed concrete curved over the edge of a hundred-foot drop like soft folds of fine cotton.

Despite the mess, astonishingly, the great majority of the wrecked apartments were still inhabited. In some whose walls were so eroded by shrapnel that they resembled pieces of chronically worm-eaten wood, I would notice washing hanging out to dry or perhaps a shadowy figure taking the air on a half-collapsed bal-cony. As twilight fell over the ruined city, pale and ghostly lights began to come on in one after another of the apparently aban-doned blocks. The ruins, it seemed, were vertical shanty-towns, makeshift billets for impoverished Shia labourers or homeless Palestinians, all rushing to fill the vacuum left by the rehoused rich. Most had patched up their flats with pieces of corrugated iron or slashes of black plastic sheeting; but many others, perhaps the newest arrivals, had not. As we drove past, I found I could look into the illuminated interiors of these people's flats, for they were missing walls or had such huge shellholes that entire suites of rooms were opened up for public inspection like some sort of outsized Advent calender. In one flat I saw a man getting dressed, nonchalantly pulling on his jeans. It was an unremarkable, everyday scene, except that the wall of his apartment had entirely disappeared, so that he was framed by the black concrete superstructure around him, lit up like a cinema screen in a dark auditorium.

As we drove on, past the Green Line which for ten years marked the battlefront between Muslim West Beirut and the Christian East, we left the very worst destruction behind us. But the vision got stranger still. For roughly twenty-five years between 1950 and 1975 – the darkest period in Lebanese architectural history – Beirut's developers laboured to convert an Ottoman jewel of rare beauty into the most hideous high-rise city in the entire Mediterranean. Then for the fifteen years after that, from 1975 to 1990, the Lebanese – with a little help from their friends and neighbours – did their best to tear it all down again, using an impromptu mixture of suction bombs, phosphorus shells, rocket-propelled grenades and Israeli napalm. Yet somehow neither the uncommon ugliness of the post-war development nor the spectacular pockmarked legacy of the bloodbath that succeeded it were quite as surprising as the almost surreal lines of glass-fronted and spotlit couture shops that have recently reopened amid the craters, and which now line the bombed-out boulevards of Hamra, their windows full of the latest creations by the fashion houses of Milan and Paris.

The tanks and checkpoints, the shrapnel-marked ruins and collapsing, shell-smashed skyscrapers – all these things, featured in a hundred television documentaries, were expected, and seemed somehow obvious from the first moment of arrival. The real revelations on the final stage of the journey into Beirut – particularly after two months in the rural hinterland of eastern Turkey and

205

northern Syria – were the glitzy American limousines queuing at the lights, and the new ice-cream parlours that have sprung up by the gun emplacements. *This?* I thought, after a twenty-year civil war: *This?* Armageddon I expected; but Armani I did not.

Then, quite suddenly, we were through the city and on the seafront, and everything was all right again, as if the war had never happened and the city had never been besieged and destroyed. The houses on the corniche seemed for some reason relatively untouched by the bombardments, and the silhouettes of the seafront palm trees stood undamaged against the darkening sky. There were girls in shorts and boys in jeans and semi-circles of old men on stools sucking hookahs. Dusk was falling now and many people were promenading, taking the air before it grew dark: chic women with Hermès shoulderbags strutted through the traffic, mobile phones held to their ears; little boys in baseball caps raced their bikes along the pavements; couples strolled hand in hand, or dropped into the seaside cafés.

I told my driver to pull in by a newsstand where copies of European newspapers and magazines were on sale. On the top rack, amid the latest issue of American *Vogue*, the London *Tatler* and a French edition of *Hello!*, a line of *Cosmopolitans* were on sale, one emblazoned with the banner headline: ARE YOU GETTING ENOUGH?

I got back into the car and we drove to the Hotel Cavalier in Muslim West Beirut. There I checked into a room and spent the next few hours in the bar recovering from the journey with the help of several glasses of cold Stella Artois and one of the most optimistic documents I have ever read. Its title: *Lebanon: The Promised Land of Tourism*.

At nine that night I was still sitting in an alcove of the smoky hotel bar reading *The Promised Land of Tourism*. It really was the most remarkable publication. 'Lebanon is the ideal country,' it maintained, 'for those who desire to enjoy their holiday surrounded by a gay nature, between kind and hospitable people and in the solemn scenery of mountains or on the shores of the blue Mediterranean. It is also an ideal country for those who want to pass their holidays in picturesque cities, staying in touristic localities where feasts and manifestations of all kinds are held.'

It was these manifestations that worried me. What sort of manifestations? Massacres? Gang rape? The mass exhumation of corpses? Undaunted, the anonymous writer of *The Promised Land of Tourism* continued in the same vein: 'Among the countries that are proposed to the choice of the modern tourist, Lebanon, better than any other, allows one to make, apart from the first properly said voyage, a second voyage, equally touching and even richer in spiritual treasures – "a voyage in time". Actually, nobody by visiting Lebanon has the chance of feeling lonely! The hospitality of Lebanon has already become proverbial the world over . . .'

Too right, I thought, as Brian Keenan and John McCarthy had discovered. And after all, who could possibly feel lonely when chained to Terry Waite, with the additional diversion of a truckload of grimly bearded Hezbollah for company?

'For,' continued the brochure, 'when the Lebanese utters the famous phrase "*ahlan wa sahlan*" ("welcome") he squeezes it from his heart and uses his tongue only as a tool for expressing it. No wonder the fame of that worldwide saying that Lebanon is the Home of Goodwill! When you leave this Promised Land you will be carrying a gift that no one shall contest, which no custom officer will dare to charge you for . . .'

What was coming next, I wondered? What was this unique duty-free item that it was possible to smuggle through the Lebanese customs? A crate of raw opium? A trunkful of powdered heroin? A ton of Semtex? None of these, apparently:

'. . . that gift, that will lie in the depth of your heart, is a feeling of all pervading gratitude and majesty, a deep rooted human feeling which only great civilisations can offer to their guests.'

I was still wading through great drifts of this slush when I looked up and to my surprise saw across the bar a friend whom I had met and very much liked on a previous assignment in the West Bank. Juan Carlos Gumucio is a huge, Bolivian-born journalist, formerly with Associated Press and *The Times*, now representing *El Pais*. Juan Carlos (or J.C., as he is known) is a heavily built, densely bearded giant with a great mop of wiry hair and a barrel for a belly. He has enormous hands, a loud laugh, and is utterly fearless: apart from Robert Fisk, he was the only Western journalist who dared to stay in Beirut to cover the dramas of the hostage crisis rather than fleeing before the Hezbollah kidnap-gangs. He has survived, so he believes, partly because no one thinks of the Bolivians as an enemy, partly because no one believes the Bolivian government would be able to afford a ransom, and partly because with his swarthy appearance and thick mat of facial hair he is visually indistinguishable from a Hezbollah commander.

Juan Carlos had flown in from Amman an hour before, and rather than going to his room he had made straight for the bar where he was already demolishing a string of double vodkas and tearing into an outsized *shwarma*. He bought me a drink and after we had exchanged gossip about mutual friends in London and Jerusalem, I showed him *Lebanon: Promised Land of Tourism*, through which he flicked with a growing smile.

'The Lebanese!' he chuckled through a mouthful of kebab. 'They're worse than the Greeks!'

While he read, I asked him what it was like living on in Beirut when all the other journalists had either fled or been taken hostage. 'Weren't you constantly terrified you would get kidnapped?' I asked, thinking of how shaken I had been by Beirut in peacetime. 'Imagine spending seven years in a basement, chained to a radiator.'

'I've been married three times,' replied J.C. without looking up from the brochure. 'It's not so different.' Suddenly he became animated: 'Willy! Look at this!'

He pointed to the back of the brochure. There, hidden away in the final pages, was a series of great double-spreads advertising nightclubs, 'massage parlours' and escort agencies. Busty Russian blondes wielded whips and fiddled with suspender belts; thick-lipped and slim-waisted Filipinas did their best to reveal charms only partially masked by the skimpiest of bikinis.

'The new Lebanon!' he said. 'There hasn't been anything like this here since 1971! *Habibi*' – he was talking to the barman now – '*Habibi*! Get me a phone this minute!'

While the barman went off to find the mobile, J.C. turned to me. 'How this country has changed!' he said. 'When I first came here twenty years ago all anyone knew about Bolivia was that it was the country of Che Guevara. Now all they know is that it is the only other country in the world that makes quite so much money through narcotics.'

The phone arrived and J.C. dialled the number emblazoned below a picture of five smiling brunettes in matching pink leotards. After only three attempts he got through (quite a stroke of luck in a country whose telephone network was fairly recently so bombed-out that it became totally inoperable).

'Hello?' said J.C. 'Hello? Who is that? OK, *habibi*, listen. This is Juan Carlos speaking. I'm a big oil magnate from Texas and I want to know if you can provide me with – how to put it? – an escort service. No, I'm not coming anywhere: you send her to me. No: I'm not going to wait . . .'

He slammed the phone down. 'Damn it! Fucking "Greensleeves"! They've put me on hold.'

With the eye of a connoisseur, J.C. flicked through the pages of the brochure, finally settling on a pouting black girl lying back on a tigerskin, one long ebony leg raised in the air, the other placed so that her big toe rested on the tiger's outstretched tongue; below was the caption: 'I'm Pussy Cat and you're my Tiger. Come on big boy: make my day.'

Juan Carlos picked up the phone again. 'Right,' he said. '*That* looks like what we're after.'

After four or five attempts, he again got through.

'Hello? That's the manager? OK, listen here *habibi*. This is Juan Carlos. I'm a big diamond millionaire from Amsterdam. I've just had a long flight and need some . . . attention. Can you provide me with some pretty female company tonight, please? Yes: Pussy Cat would do nicely. HOW MUCH? Is that dollars or Lebanese pounds? You must be joking. Look, *habibi*, inflation isn't that bad: I could fly in my girlfriend for less. I'll be back in touch. Thank you very much.'

He put the phone down and turned to me.

'Unbelievable. I can't believe what's happened while I've been away. And to think I was planning on leaving this country . . .'

It took a while to track down the two men who, I felt, would be best able to make some sense for me of the complexities of Lebanon. Both were the authors of exceptional books on the recent conflict. One was a historian, Kemal Salibi of the American University of Beirut, author of *A House of Many Mansions*, a brilliant debunking of the myths in Lebanese history which had led to and exacerbated the conflict. The other was the great award-winning foreign correspondent Robert Fisk of the *Independent*, author of *Pity the Nation*, much the best account of the 1982 Israeli invasion yet published.

Professor Salibi was easily accessible, but Fisk proved a more difficult man to pin down. He has always tended to keep aloof from his journalistic colleagues, and even Juan Carlos, who appears frequently in *Pity the Nation*, had not seen him for months and did not have an up-to-date number for him. He could give me no better lead than suggesting I try ringing the *Independent* foreign desk. Amazingly, the *Independent* also had no address for him, apparently part of the elaborate security precautions Fisk practises which have so far saved him from assassination or kidnapping. The paper did, however, have the number of a satellite phone in New York which, they said, would somehow beam through to Fisk in Beirut.

So it was that I finally got hold of Fisk – who turned out to be living less than half a mile from my hotel – via tens of thousands of miles of cables to New York then back again to Beirut bounced off some satellite. By this route I offered to take him out to lunch. He accepted, suggesting an Italian place in a Druze area near the seafront.

I had arranged to see Professor Salibi that same morning in his office at `the American University, which lay only a short walk away from my hotel, and I walked over there after breakfast.

For an institution whose campus had been under siege for a year, whose main hall had been destroyed by a car bomb, whose acting president and librarian had both been kidnapped by Islamic Jihad, another of whose presidents had been killed and many of whose students had been maimed, murdered and wounded, the American University of Beirut looked remarkably like any other university the world over. The Pizza Hut at the gates was full of undergraduates lounging around, making eyes at each other and spooning mountains of ice-cream into each other's mouths. Noticeboards in the porter's lodge advertised student raves along-side the rather more staid option of a forthcoming piano recital. Undergraduates, late for lectures, ran across lawns that had recently supported batteries of anti-aircraft guns. Lecturers, books in hand, walked along the cinder paths chatting to pretty female students whose fathers and brothers had, only months earlier, no doubt been blazing away at each other in the alleys outside.

Salibi had just finished teaching a small class of history students when I walked into his rooms; a sketch map of the Middle East was still chalked up on the blackboard above his seat. We shook hands and I said how surprised I was to see the university looking so normal after all it had gone through in the war. The Professor smiled. 'Thankfully we are a very forgetful culture,' he said, pulling out a chair and indicating that I should sit. 'Those who committed the worst crimes and atrocities have long been forgiven. Few people in Lebanon can afford to bear grudges for too long. Who remembers Sabra and Chatila? At the time it was terrible: who could ever forgive mass murder like that? But twelve years later even the unfortunate Palestinians have probably forgotten and forgiven.'

I asked the Professor how the war had affected him personally.

'I was driven out of the city altogether,' he replied with a smile.

'By the shelling?'

'No, no. I survived the bombardment. I was driven out by a death threat from the Hezbollah. I had to go to Amman. That's where I put together *A House of Many Mansions*. It was written from memory, without a single reference book. You see, I lost all my books in the bombardment.'

'Your house was destroyed?'

'We suffered twenty-six direct hits. I was in the basement at the time. It was a lovely old Ottoman house, built by my great-grandfather: very beautiful. But by the time it was finished the house was uninhabitable.'

The Professor offered me coffee, and as he fussed around with the kettle he talked quite calmly about the destruction of everything he had owned, as if describing some minor inconvenience: a blown fuse, or a broken lightbulb.

'We heard the shelling start and I said it would be a rough night. So we all began to move into the basement, taking all our things with us. Then the three windows above where the children were playing collapsed inwards: glass flew everywhere, but somehow no one was hurt. We ran downstairs after that, with a bottle of whisky and a candle.

'Whenever a shell fell the candle would be blown out. It was very frightening: so frightening that I thought I couldn't go on. After a while you begin to feel sure that the next shell will get you, that you can't possibly survive. You just hope it won't be too painful. Then oblivion sets in. There's a mechanism in the human mind which obliterates terrible memories. I sometimes wonder now whether it really happened.'

'It can't have left you with very warm feelings towards the Palestinians.'

'It wasn't the Palestinians who shelled us,' said the Professor. 'It was the Maronites, the Phalange. Like many Christians who found themselves on the wrong side of the Green Line, I carried on living in Muslim West Beirut where I always had lived. I was unharmed until Amin Gemayel turned his guns on us and began randomly shelling West Beirut. I never approved of the Phalange. They were intolerable. They considered that Lebanese of Christian origin should have rights which Lebanese of non-Christian origin did not have. In a sense it was a racist doctrine. Luckily their policies ended in the failure they richly deserved.'

'So you think the Christians lost the war?'

'There is a widespread feeling that they did. The Phalange wanted one of two things: either to have political control over the whole of Lebanon, or to retreat to the north and partition the country so that they could at least have control over a Christian enclave. They lost both those battles. They couldn't retain unconditional control over the whole country, nor could they create a canton all to themselves. On the other hand they emerged from the war with their share of power virtually undiminished, and in one way came out unequivocally the winners.'

'What do you mean?'

'Before the war the whole idea of Lebanon was in question. It was adamantly rejected by almost everyone except the Maronites, who were believed to have cooked up the idea in collusion with the French. But the war changed all that. There is now hardly a single person in this country who does not have a strong sense of Lebanese identity. They might be Lebanese with Hezbollah sympathies, or Lebanese who want to cooperate with Syria, or Lebanese who think that to cooperate with Syria is anathema. But they have no doubt of their Lebanese identity. So in a way you could say that the Christians won their point.'

'And yet despite this,' I said, 'the Christians are apparently still emigrating from here *en masse*.'

'True. But the reason they are leaving is no longer because they are threatened, or because their country is going to disappear. It is because – how to put it? – they are weary. There is a feeling of *fin de race* amongst Christians all over the Middle East, a feeling that fourteen centuries of having all the time to be smart, to be ahead of the others, is long enough. The Arab Christians tend to be intelligent, well qualified, highly educated people. Now they just want to go somewhere else, make some money and relax. I can understand it. There is discrimination – sometimes very subtle – against them in almost all Middle Eastern countries. Sometimes when I am with Arab scholars there will be sly digs against Arabs who are not Muslims, doubts about how Arab they are, how patriotic they may be.'

'And do you think it really matters if the Christians do leave?'

'It is a very serious matter,' said Salibi. 'Each time a Christian goes, no other Christian comes to fill his place, and that is a very bad thing for the Arab world. It is the Christian Arabs who keep the Arab world "Arab" rather than "Muslim". It is the Christian Arabs who show that Arabs and Muslims are two different things, that not all Muslims are Arabs and not all Arabs are Muslims. You see, many Muslims regard Arab history as having little meaning by itself, outside the context of Islam. In that sense we are the Arab world's guarantee of secularism.'

Salibi leant forward on his desk. 'Since the nineteenth century the Christian Arabs have played a vital role in defining a secular Arab cultural identity. It is no coincidence that most of the founders of secular Arab nationalism were Christians: Michel Aflaq, who founded the Ba'ath Party; George Antonius, who wrote *The Arab Awakening*. If the Christian Arabs continue to emigrate, the Arabs will be in a much more difficult position to defend the Arab world against Islamism.'

'But isn't that battle already being lost?'

'Everyone is very frightened by the spread of fundamentalism,' said the Professor. 'And of course it is unsettling to read about what is happening in Algeria and Upper Egypt. But this is not the end of history.'

He smiled. 'The battle,' he said, 'is not over yet.'

It was raining heavily when I left the university, and Beirut's streets were suddenly awash. The water sluiced down the steep incline of the roads and the cars slewed through the streets, horns blowing, up to their gunwales in water.

'It's the fault of the Syrians,' explained the taxi driver. 'When they resurfaced the roads after the war they covered over the drains by mistake.'

Now the only drain was the sea, and the water – in some places nearly a foot deep – was flowing fast downhill towards the corniche. Getting from the car to the door of the restaurant was an operation that really required fishing waders.

Fisk was already at his table, an unexpectedly boyish figure with a coif of springy hair swept back over his high forehead; only the odd grey strand betrayed the fact that he was actually in his late forties.

'See out there?' he said by way of introduction. 'During the siege Israeli shells used to land all the way along that stretch of road.'

'So you had to forgo the pleasures of pasta during the siege?'

'No, no,' replied Fisk. 'They kept the place open and I used to come here regularly. Always have. Its got a wonderful view – though of course during the hostage crisis I tended to keep my back to the window so I wouldn't be seen by the kidnappers.'

For all his slightly self-conscious bravado, Fisk proved an unexpectedly kind and avuncular figure. Throughout lunch he freely offered advice and was generous with his contacts, flicking through his address book to pass on the phone numbers of war-lords and archbishops, patriarchs, torturers and mass murderers. Nevertheless no amount of kindness could disguise the fact that Fisk was clearly a chronic war junkie, suffering from all the usual side-effects of an addiction to bombs, kidnapping, loud explosions and unhealthy quantities of adrenalin. This first became obvious when, at the end of the *antipasto*, I asked about the possibility of interviewing one of the Phalangist commanders.

'Well,' he said, puffing at a huge cigar he had just ordered at my expense from the *maître d'*, 'it's not easy. Most are dead: assassinated. The rest are in jail, or in Geagea's case about to go there.'

'Who's Geagea?'

'One of the Phalangist leaders implicated in the massacres at Sabra and Chatila. He's going on trial after Christmas.'

'For the massacres?'

'No, no. For blowing up a church.'

'But I thought the Phalangists were all Christian.'

'They are.'

'So why would they blow up a church?'

'It was Geagea's way of warning the Pope not to visit Lebanon. He thought it would be too dangerous for His Holiness.'

'So there are no senior Maronite militia leaders left for me to talk to?'

'Well, I suppose there's still General Lahad of the SLA.'

'The SLA?'

'The South Lebanon Army: the Israelis' puppet Maronite militia in the zone they've occupied in the south of Lebanon.'

'And you think I could get to see him?'

'Piece of cake,' said Fisk, embarking on a lengthy explanation on how I could make contact with the SLA. This involved going to some obscure scrapyard in the suburbs of Beirut and asking for a man called Haddad.

'Don't talk to anyone else. Leave your name and details. Three days later go back. If Haddad gives you the go-ahead – fine. Have you got a map?'

I nodded and reached in my bag for the map of Lebanon I'd bought in the hotel. It was a simplified tourist chart dotted here and there with optimistic little pictures of the country's principal archaeological monuments.

'Well,' said Fisk, wrinkling his nose as he examined my chart, 'for a start you'll need a better map than this. But this will have to do for the time being. Drive south along this road through the Chouf. Then take a left along this little road here. Leave your car there, at that spot: you see? I'll mark it with an X. Get out – very slowly, no sudden movement, they'll have their snipers trained on you already – and walk the final five hundred yards to the SLA checkpoint with your hands on your head. You'll be all right. As long as your name is on the list, that is.'

'It doesn't sound very safe.'

'I would do it – no problem. I went to the SLA headquarters in Marjayoun last month, as a matter of fact. There are Hezbollah all round, of course. They might take a potshot at you, but they generally don't shoot unmarked cars. At least not normally. It's not as if you'd be travelling in an Israeli army convoy, ha ha.'

'Ha ha.' I shuddered at Fisk's idea of an easy assignment and privately made up my mind to forget interviewing Lahad, and to keep well away from the SLA.

Over coffee (for me) and vintage cognac (for Fisk) I mentioned that I had just been to see Salibi and that we had talked about the problems of the Arab Christians.

'The Arab Christians' principal problem is that the West is Christian,' said Fisk, 'and in one way or another since 1948 the West has humiliated the Muslims of the Middle East over and over again. The Christians simply cannot divorce themselves from the West, however many times they tell their Muslim neighbours that Christianity is really an Eastern religion.'

According to Fisk it was nevertheless a myth that the Lebanese civil war was in essence a clash of civilisations, Christian against Muslim. It was, he said, more a case of the Maronites against everyone else.

'The Maronites brought the war down on their own heads. The first event of the civil war was a massacre of Palestinians by a group of Phalangists trying to win power. The Greek Orthodox always realised that the different communities in Lebanon would have to learn to coexist, but the Maronites never came to terms with this. They are a very immature community politically, very stupid, and always letting themselves be used – first by the French, then by the Israelis, now by the Syrians. The Maronites have always really wanted a francophone Lebanon that they can dominate, totally separated from the Arab world, with the Muslims reduced to some sort of folkloric survival tolerated to please the tourists. Is it any wonder that the Hezbollah headbangers now want to kill them all?'

'But all the same, quite a lot of the war did seem to have a Christian–Muslim clash behind it, didn't it?'

'In the course of the war the Phalange attacked the local Armenians and the Greek Orthodox – who themselves quite often fought with the Druze against the Maronites – as well as the Christian Palestinians and other Maronites. Then, at other points, the fighting was almost entirely Muslim against Muslim: in the Camp Wars from 1985 to 1988 it was Shiites against Sunni Palestinians. It's a ridiculous oversimplification – in fact a total misunderstanding – to see the war as a simple Christian–Muslim struggle.'

It had stopped raining as suddenly as it had started and the sun was now shining brightly. So after I had paid the bill, Fisk offered to take me on a tour of his favourite ruins. This didn't turn out to be the sightseeing trip around the archaeological remains of ancient Beirut that I had been expecting. Instead it was a nostalgia tour through the scenes of Fisk's civil war glory days, carefully avoiding any part of the city which still had a house with its roof intact, a window *in situ*, or whose façade was not thoroughly honeycombed with shrapnel holes.

'Look,' said Fisk, nodding excitedly from the back seat of our taxi at a ruinous building opposite. 'Classic sniper's nest.'

'There?' I asked, pointing to a window on the third floor.

'Never *ever* point in Lebanon,' hissed Fisk. 'You'll get yourself killed *very* quickly if you break basic rules like that.'

'What . . .'

'People will think you're an informer, and shoot you. And me too if I'm with you.'

'I'm so sorry . . .'

'But you had the right window. Look again. What do you see?'

'A pile of old sacks?'

'Sandbags, with a crate in between.' Fisk was in his element now, like an overexcited trainspotter let loose in the sidings at Crewe. 'That crate is where the sniper would have rested his rifle. During the war that line of buildings would have had corridors knocked through the houses so snipers could move from one house to another without venturing onto the street. Of course, all that is over now,' he added, with what seemed a touch of sadness.

We drove on, Fisk pointing out sites of interest: 'See that spot? That's where a mine went off, killing a Lebanese journalist. Friend of mine. Horrible business. Blood everywhere. Couldn't even identify the body afterwards . . . And over there, see? That's where Terry Anderson was kidnapped. He was taken off screaming down that road. Didn't get released for years . . . And there: that was the French Embassy. '

'God. What happened to it?'

'Car bomb, shells and everything else. But it's still there, sort of. Which is more than you can say about the American Embassy. It used to stand there.' Fisk nodded at a huge empty lot. 'It was bombed by Islamic Jihad. They finally pulled down what was left last week.'

We drove on, and soon came to a warren of narrow streets. Garbage lay uncollected all around, and every building was badly peppered with shrapnel. It looked as if pretty well everything had gone off here: small-arms fire, mortars, howitzers, aerial bombardment, suction bombs, rocket-propelled grenades, car bombs, the lot.

'Gives you an idea what Beirut used to be like,' sighed Fisk, 'before they started messing around trying to clean it all up.'

'Why are there so many pin-ups of the Ayatollah Khomeni everywhere?'

'This used to be the Jewish area of Beirut. That was the synagogue. But the Shiites have taken it over now. You don't want to come here on your own.'

'What happened to the Jews?'

'After the creation of Israel they stayed on. But after the 1982 Israeli invasion and the siege of Beirut, Jews came to be seen as legitimate targets, so they had to, er . . . leave.'

From the opposite direction a huge armoured personnel carrier rumbled toward us. It was followed by an army truck full of heavily armed Lebanese troops in their camouflage jumpsuits. We pulled in behind the charred carcass of an old Citroën to let them through.

'These patrols go through to make sure there are no armed militia men around,' said Fisk. 'There are, of course, hundreds of them, but they keep out of sight. In fact there's not a family here without a stash of Kalashnikovs and couple of mortars hidden away in their back yard. But they keep them tucked away and the army don't poke around too much. It's an unspoken agreement.'

Fisk gave instructions to the driver and we headed into a great wide square, desolate and empty but for a bronze statue at its centre.

'This was the Place des Martyrs. It was like Dresden until they pulled it all down. Shame, really. In the old days there was almost total silence in this area. No traffic. No people. Just the gentle *crack, crack* of snipers. Wonderful.'

219

We got out and walked over to the statue. Like everything else in the vicinity it was thoroughly peppered with shrapnel and small-arms fire.

'They're going to leave the statue as a memorial,' said Fisk, 'but everything else is going to go. They're planning to bulldoze it all into the sea.'

He explained about the plans to redevelop the area: the Downtown Project. It all sounded very Levantine. If I understood correctly, the monopoly to redevelop the entire centre of the city had just been awarded by the President to a company called Solidere, in which the President happened to be a major shareholder.

We walked over to the corner of the square, where a roofless Maronite church stood looking onto the wasteland.

'Follow me,' said Fisk, 'and don't stand on the piles of rubble. You never know where there might be a landmine or a UXB.'

'UXB?'

'Unexploded bomb. Hundreds of them all over Beirut. And landmines. Scattered like confetti all over the shop.'

Following closely in Fisk's footsteps, I was led up to a platform. From it you could look down into a deep hole, thirty feet below. At the bottom, amid the puddles and the rubbish, lay a jumbled pile of old Roman pillars.

'That,' said Fisk, gesturing at it dismissively, 'is all that's left of five hundred years of classical Beirut.'

'It's not much, is it?' I said.

'No,' said Fisk. 'Mind you, had the war continued much longer, modern Beirut wouldn't have looked so different.'

He pointed to the edge of the square. There stood the wreck of what had once been a neo-classical public building dating from the early years of the French Mandate. All that remained was a line of pillars; even the pediment had been completely blown off. The wreck was indistinguishable from the ruins of a classical temple.

'See what I mean?' said Fisk.

Few ancient cities give off less historical resonance than Beirut. Its post-war high-rise hellscape immediately conjures up some terrible Apocalyptic vision of the future, but the city's past casts few shadows over the shellshocked present. Everything old has been swept away or blown up. There is nothing on which the historical imagination can find purchase. It is difficult enough to imagine the city as the elegant Ottoman port it must have been only eighty years ago; the ancient classical past now seems hopelessly distant, almost impossible to visualise.

Nevertheless, in the early Byzantine period the Metropolis of Berytus was one of the principal cities in the Empire: as an intellectual centre it was the site of the Empire's leading law school, while as a centre of commerce it was one of the most prosperous trading ports in the eastern Mediterranean, a major focus of Byzantine silk manufacture and export. Its harbour would rarely have been empty, and during the sailing season – from April to October – would have been cluttered with galleys from Gaul and barques from as far afield as Alexandria, Athens and Carthage.

In Byzantine times a law degree took five or six years to complete, and was a course of study open only to the children of the very rich. Libanius of Antioch mentions one law student, a certain Heliodorus, who was 'a retailer of fish sauce', but such cases were most uncommon: the law students who congregated in Beirut accompanied by their armies of household slaves and concubines were the children of senators, provincial governors and landowners from across the Empire. They came because a Beirut degree was the quickest way to rapid advancement in the Imperial Civil Service, the Byzantine equivalent of a diploma from Insead or Harvard Business School. Indeed Libanius complains loudly and angrily that modern parents were more interested in the prospects of quick promotion afforded by a Beirut law degree than in the more rounded (and old-fashioned) education in rhetoric he offered at Antioch. It is the same cry professors of Classics can be heard uttering today as their brightest students desert them for vocational degrees in economics or the law.

One of the most curious aspects of the history of the east Mediterranean is the way that the character of its cities often seems to remain strangely constant, despite the long series of cataclysmic invasions, genocides and exchanges of population that make up their history. Jerusalem, for example, has always been a centre of religious fanaticism, whether inhabited by Jews, Byzantines, Arabs or Crusaders. In the same way Beirut has always had a reputation for hedonism, sharpened, then as now, by occasional outbreaks of aggressive fundamentalism.

That it was so in the Byzantine period is demonstrated by the fifth-century *Life* of the Monophysite Bishop Severus of Antioch, written by his friend and companion, Zacharias the Rector. The two friends began their secondary studies in Alexandria, where Zacharias comments with a shudder on the number of professors involved in occult activities: many of the senior members of the faculty were apparently in the habit of secretly visiting a clandestine temple of Menuthis packed full of wooden idols of cats, dogs and monkeys.

At Beirut, where the pair went to finish their legal studies sometime in the 480s, things were little better. Though there appeared to be fewer pagans around than in Alexandria, the rich students indulged in all manner of pleasures repugnant to a puritanical Christian like Zacharias: there was a theatre and a circus, while in the evening there were dice games and drinking with dancing girls and prostitutes. This hedonism caused a reaction among the more pious students, rather in the way the excesses of Beirut's wild and salacious nightlife during the 1960s and seventies provoked, a decade later, the puritanism of Islamic Jihad. In response to the law students' orgiastic behaviour, the more zealous of the Christian activists formed religious brotherhoods, urging Zacharias and Severus to attend church every evening, to avoid the theatre and to follow the famous advice of St Jerome that 'he who has bathed in Christ [i.e. been baptised] does not need a second bath': giving the lead, the head of the brotherhood apparently used to wash only once a year.

As in Alexandria, there were scandals involving the occult. The lodgings of the chief suspect were searched, his grimoires confiscated, his magical books burned and his friends denounced to the bishop. One of the accused, Chrysaorius of Tralles, then tried to escape. He rented a ship, loaded it with his books of spells, his concubine and children; they set sail, but soon sank (as ships carrying magicians have a tendency to do in pious Byzantine literature: there are several similar stories involving wicked pagans and magicians coming to damp ends on the high seas in the pages of *The Spiritual Meadow*).

John Moschos seems to have passed fairly quickly up the coast of what was then Byzantine Phoenicia. Indeed he mentions only three places within the boundaries of modern Lebanon: Tyre, Porphyreon and Ba'albek. Byzantine Beirut he does not refer to at all, perhaps because by the late sixth century the city was in serious decline. This was partly the result of the bankruptcy of the local silk industry, when many of the silk merchants were forced to migrate to Persia in search of work, and partly due to a severe earthquake in 551 – the last of a series of ominous tremors throughout the early sixth century – which brought down many of the city's buildings. Indeed the evidence of another contemporary traveller, the Italian pilgrim Antonius Martyr, seems to indicate that in 570 'the school of letters' (presumably the law school) had completely ceased to function, and the only place on the Lebanese coast where Antonius saw any prosperity was Beirut's great rival, Tyre. There he reported that the city's looms were still operating, while its brothels were apparently packed to bursting.

I had asked Professor Salibi about rumours I had heard in Damascus, that the remains of Byzantine Beirut had been turning up during demolition work for the Downtown Project. He in turn had put me in touch with Leila Badr, one of archaeologists at the American University who had been involved in the digging.

Dr Badr confirmed that in the rescue excavations which had taken place during the demolitions, the diggers had indeed struck Byzantine levels and managed to uncover long stretches of the Byzantine, Roman and Phoenician town walls, all of which followed roughly the same course. There was not a great deal to see, but it was an important discovery: previously no one had known the boundaries of the ancient town. Some badly preserved fragments of Byzantine floor mosaics had also been found, but these had been sent away for conservation and I wouldn't be able to see them. But, said Dr Badr, there were some other recently-discovered Byzantine remains that I should definitely try to look at.

Apparently just before the Israeli invasion, in early 1982, workmen digging in the sand dunes on the coast at Jiyyeh, twenty miles to the south of Beirut, had stumbled upon a series of well-preserved Byzantine monastic ruins: churches, hostels, halls and agricultural buildings. Inside was a collection of the most remarkable mosaics, many with dated Greek inscriptions. These identified the site as the Byzantine port of Porphyreon, one the three Lebanese cities visited by Moschos.

Moschos tells two stories about the port. One concerns the companion of his friend, the hermit Abba Zosimos the Cilician, who was bitten by a snake and 'died immediately with blood flowing from all his members'. The other is the tale of Procopius the lawyer, who is away in Jerusalem when he hears that the plague has broken out in his home town. Terrified for the safety of his children, he goes to see the renowned Byzantine holy man Abba Zachaios, and tells him of his fear.

> When [Abba Zachaios] heard this, he turned towards the east and continued reaching up to heaven for about two hours without saying a word. Then he turned towards me and said: 'Take heart and do not be distraught: your children shall not die in the plague. In fact two days from now, the plague shall abate.' And indeed it came about as the elder foretold.

The recent excavations apparently confirmed Moschos's report that Porphyreon was a major port in the late sixth century. It was probably as large as its rival Beirut, and specialised in olive oil production and textile manufacture, and also, as was indicated by its name, in the making of purple dye. Despite the economic crisis plaguing Antioch and much of the rest of the Levantine coast,

Porphyreon was clearly still a very prosperous place, and its monastic buildings had once been magnificent.

Almost all the antiquities discovered in Lebanon during the civil war were exported illegally and sold on the black market in Europe and America. At one point things got so bad that in Tyre militiamen were blowing open sarcophagi with dynamite to get at the grave-goods within. But by good fortune Jiyyeh fell within the sphere of influence of Walid Jumblatt, the Druze leader. Jumblatt was a history scholar before turning politician, and almost alone of Lebanese warlords had a sense of the past and understood the importance of a country's archaeological heritage. Dr Badr told me that Jumblatt had kept the mosaics safe during the war, and had recently brought them out and placed them in his palace at Beit ed-Din in the Chouf. The only problem, she said, was that I would need Jumblatt's permission if I was to get in to see them.

Following Dr Badr's instructions, I duly set off in a taxi to the offices of Jumblatt's Progressive Socialist Party. This organisation was, by all accounts, neither progressive nor socialist; rather it was a sort of glorified feudal support group through which Lebanon's Druze were enabled to pledge their allegiance to their tribal chieftain, W. Jumblatt. The office was a suitably rackety-looking place, riddled with the regulation Beirut bulletholes, but I climbed the dingy stairs and at the top almost ran into Jumblatt and his squad of bodyguards.

Jumblatt had the appearance less of a ruthless warlord than of a left-wing Sorbonne sociology don from the barricades of 1968. He was an unexpectedly tall and commanding figure in his late forties, balding, with a large nose and a droopy Mexican moustache. He wore a black leather jacket and tight black jeans, and he spoke fluent English.

It turned out that I had been very lucky. Jumblatt was leaving for France in less than an hour, but agreed to see me for five minutes before he left. Armed Druze flunkies frisked me then ushered me into a study. After twenty minutes Jumblatt walked in and asked how he could help. I explained what I wanted, and he immediately gave his permission.

'Go ahead. Tell my men at the gate that you are my guest. They will show you the mosaics.' Then he added, 'It's so rare to see English writers in Beirut these days. You know Charles Glass?'

'Very well.'

'How is he? Still alive?'

'Becoming rather a playboy in his old age, by all accounts.'

'The Hezbollah should never have let him escape from his captivity,' he said. 'You know he was kidnapped on his way to see me? What about David Gilmour? The last time I was in London he took me to lunch at the Travellers' Club. What's he doing now?'

'He's just written a book on Lord Curzon.'

'David always was an unreconstructed imperialist,' said Jumblatt. 'But tell me,' he asked politely, 'what are you writing about?'

I explained that I was researching a book about the Middle Eastern Christians, and Jumblatt raised his eyebrows: during the war he had been one of the most formidable enemies of the Christian militias. Despite the fact that the Christian forces were supported by both Israel and the Americans, Jumblatt's forces had managed to drive the Christian militias out of the Druze heartlands in the Chouf, and in the process had gained a reputation for savage tenacity. The Druze, it was well known, seldom took prisoners.

'The Maronites have always been their own worst enemies,' said Jumblatt. 'They have always wanted to dominate Lebanon as if it were an entirely Christian state. They have never been prepared to give the majority their rights, to share power or in any way to bring about democratic reforms.'

'I understand you were no friend of the Phalangists during the war.'

'The Phalange was a fascist organisation founded by Pierre Gemayel after a visit to Nazi Germany in 1936,' he said, with indisputable historical accuracy. 'When they started committing atrocities – slitting the throats of three hundred Muslims at roadblocks on Black Saturday in 1975, or massacring the Palestinians in the camp at Tel el-Za'atar a year later – we had to respond. Coexistence is only possible if the Maronites resist their more extreme right-wing tendencies.'

'So are you pessimistic about the future?'

'Lebanon is an artificial creation,' replied Jumblatt. 'It was created by the French in 1920. Economically and politically speaking it has no future on its own. We need the Arabs. We are the gateway to the Arab world: that is our natural environment. We are not some part of the French dominions, or the Vatican, or whatever it is the Maronites want. If they accept this, then maybe this peace will hold.'

One of Jumblatt's aides came in to say that his car was ready to take him to the airport. Jumblatt pulled himself out of his chair. 'I will miss my plane,' he said. 'I'm sorry. I hope you get to see your mosaics.'

As we walked down the stairs together Jumblatt made some remark about the civil war, and I asked him whether he thought that in retrospect it could have been avoided altogether.

'If the Maronites had been less intransigent,' he said, shrugging his shoulders. 'Then maybe . . . But the ifs of history: if Cleopatra's nose had been one inch longer,' he said, 'would Antony have lost the battle of Actium?'

The road to the Chouf led through the squalid southern suburbs of Beirut. Thirty years ago, this road bordered Ouzayeh Beach. It was once the Ipanema of Beirut, the favourite playground of *le tout Beirut*. Now it is Hezbollah territory, and a vast meandering shanty-slum of tin sheds and breezeblock huts, cheap restaurants and rundown bakeries lines the strip between the road and the now almost invisible beach.

On the central reservation, running between the two lanes of the road, rose a series of giant hoardings depicting the hugely enlarged features of a line of Iranian mullahs. Each cleric stared out blankly through heavy Joe-90 spectacles, under a tightly wrapped and immaculately starched white turban: as strange and surreal a sight as a line of giant Andy Warhol Marilyns raised above a motorway. Interspersed between the mullahs, much smaller and crudely nailed onto a low picket of wooden posts, stretched a line of idealised portraits of smiling, bearded *shaheedin*, the Hezbollah 'martyrs' who had died fighting the Israelis in occupied southern Lebanon. To indicate the heavenly bliss currently being enjoyed by these fighters, their heads were sometimes shown floating on clouds of white cumulus. Other hoardings showed the Dome of the Rock in Jerusalem, inscribed with a series of fearsome invocations to Free Palestine and Crush the Zionist Entity, along with other varieties of the sort of bloodcurdling threats, promises and admonitions which Shia fundamentalists like to read as they drive into town to do their shopping.

It had turned wet and windy, and each time the taxi dived into one of the deep brown puddles that filled the potholes in the road, an explosion of muddy water splashed over the bonnet and windscreen. As we bounced along, past tumbledown garages, scrapyards and tyre shops, I could see thickly bearded Hezbollah men pottering around with spanners under the bonnets of battered, shrapnel-shattered Datsuns or war-weary Volvos; others were holding pots of paint and paintbrushes with which they dabbed on splashes of colour here and there in an attempt to distract attention from the dents and bulletholes that dotted their cars' chassis. I remarked to the taxi driver, Nouri Suleiman, that I had expected somewhat higher-calibre weapons than sprayguns from these men.

'Guns are not so useful now we are at peace,' he replied. 'At the end of the war a new M-16 used to cost $1,000. Now you can buy one for $100. A pistol used to be $500. Now it's down to $150.'

'So a pistol is now more expensive than an M-16?'

'That's because people still like to have small guns,' replied Nouri.

'Why?'

'They're useful. You can't hide an M-16, but it's easy to hide a pistol. Put it in your pocket or a briefcase. No problem.'

From the back of his glove compartment he whipped out a small snub-nosed pistol and showed it to me: 'You see? Easy to hide. No problem.'

We drove on through the uncontrolled ribbon of Beirut's rambling southern suburbs, past the sad, huddled slums belonging to the landless Shias and the barbed wire and collapsing shanties of various miserable-looking Palestinian refugee camps. Half an hour later we arrived at the outskirts of Damour, the Christian town that had suffered most severely in the civil war. First it was attacked and pillaged by the Palestinians in revenge for Maronite atrocities against them in Beirut. Most of the inhabitants escaped by sea, but 350 remained in their homes. When Arafat's gunmen stormed into the town on 20 January 1976, the Fatah guerrillas machine-gunned the men, raped the women and dynamited the houses. It was then that the Palestinians, apparently dissatisfied at having had the chance to wreak revenge on so few living Maronites, hit upon the idea of exhuming their dead and scattering the cadavers around the ruins of the town they had just desecrated. Later on, the town was captured and destroyed a second time, on this occasion by the Israelis, before being resettled on their departure by the Druze. Jumblatt now keeps his principal office in Damour. But there are no Christians living here any more.

We drove quickly through what was left of the town: a few houses, all riddled with bullet and shrapnel holes; the odd ruin of a sixties bungalow, now overgrown with vines and creepers; a scrappy plantation of banana palms; a few old Druze men sitting around on their covered verandahs looking out into the drizzle in their white *keffiyehs* and baggy black *charwal* pantaloons. We then took a left turn and began winding upwards into the steep, thickly-wooded slopes that led into the Chouf.

It was raining hard now, and the gleaming road was slippery with fallen leaves. Cars coming down from Beit ed-Din sluiced past us, windscreen wipers on full. Low cloud obscured the tops of the mountain peaks rising above us; below, the valleys fell away in a steep precipice of abandoned cultivation terraces and balding beech trees, their few remaining leaves turning bright autumnal yellow. For the final twenty minutes of the journey, as on the way into Beirut, we found ourselves crawling uphill behind another pair of the ubiquitous Syrian tank-transporters, each weighed down with its cargo of two Soviet T-72 battle tanks. Looking at the map, I realised that the Israeli Occupation Zone, the current front line between the armies of the Jewish state and the local Hezbollah guerrillas, lay only twelve miles to the south.

At the top of the mountain, in Deir el-Qamar, the driver stopped to fill up with petrol and to let his battered radiator cool down. Deir el-Qamar was a fine medieval town and, uniquely in Lebanon, had been well preserved, thanks to Walid Jumblatt's interest in conservation. It was built of warm honey-coloured sandstone and was full of old Ottoman khans and churches, lovely even in the rain. As I sat in a café, warming my hands around a glass of tea, I caught sight of a Maronite priest in black cloak and biretta hurrying along the road outside, a bent figure scurrying under the shelter of a wide umbrella. I had understood that the Christians of the Chouf, like those of Damour, had been driven out of the area during the fighting. Surprised, I chased after the priest and invited him into the café to join me. Clearly as amazed to see me as I was to see him, Père Abbé Marcel abi-Khalil accepted.

The old priest shook his wet umbrella and folded it up. 'Before the fighting,' he said, 'Deir el-Qamar was half Christian and half Druze. The Chouf was traditionally a Druze area, but the Maronites began to migrate here from the north in the eighteenth century. By 1975, before the fighting, there must have been five thousand Christians living here, maybe twice that number in summer.'

He sipped his tea. 'Then there was the War of the Mountains,' he said, 'and all the Christians left. Today there are no more than one thousand of us living here.'

'So some Christians have returned?'

'Yes. They've started trickling back. Jumblatt is giving them a little money to help them start again. He is a good man. He has suffered himself – his father was assassinated – so he knows what it is to suffer loss. He wants to heal the wounds.'

'I'm surprised to hear a Maronite say that.'

'In 1860 the Druze and the Christians fought each other, but from then until the war we lived happily side by side. In our school we used to have 150 Christians and 350 Druze.'

'Druze? In a Christian school?'

'*Mais oui*,' said Fr. Marcel. 'The fathers taught everyone, what-ever their religion.'

'So what went wrong during the war?'

'It was Geagea and his Phalange. Before he came to the Chouf, we had lived together peacefully for generations. But while the Israelis were here in 1982, Geagea's men fought against the Druze in the Chouf and in Sidon. Geagea treated the Druze very badly. He made many murders. The Israelis pretended not to see and let Geagea do what he wanted. As a result, when they withdrew, everyone attacked the Christians. We were besieged and for three months there was nothing to eat: only grass. The Red Cross sent food but the Druze ate it on the way. In the end the Syrians supported Jumblatt and Geagea lost his war. Because of what he did, the Christians were expelled from both here and Sidon. We have a saying: "Where Geagea sets foot, no Christian remains." With a champion like him, we need no other enemies.'

'Did you meet Geagea?'

'*Bien sûr*,' said the priest. 'I hid him in the school for two months. It was in 1983, after he lost his little war. Personally I did not like him. In fact he almost made me embarrassed to be a Christian. When he left – walking over the mountain, by foot, in disguise – I was glad. He created only trouble for us.'

The driver came into the café and said that the car was ready. Fr. Marcel swallowed the last of his tea and we both stood up.

'Now Geagea has gone and the war is over, it is better in the Chouf,' said the priest as we walked outside. He raised his umbrella. 'The Druze have even begun coming to church again.'

'The Druze come to your church?'

'They always have. We have a miraculous picture. When they need babies or are ill or in difficulties they come here. They give oil and incense and are healed.'

He shook my hands warmly. 'In this part of the world,' he said, 'for all our difficulties, religion has not just torn people apart. It has often brought them together. It is important to remember that.'

The great early-nineteenth-century palace of Beit ed-Din lay a short distance away, on the opposite side of the valley. Its double gates were bolted shut, and in front stood three Druze guards, all armed with Kalashnikovs. They were warming their hands around a spluttering brazier, with their guns slung casually from the shoulders of their damp greatcoats. The driver got out and talked to them, saying that I was a friend of Jumblatt. They immediately bowed and pushed open the gates.

Through the gatehouse, in the fading light, the palace felt like a Cambridge college out of term time: echoing, empty courtyards led one into another, damp with fallen leaves and swept by sudden gusts of rain. In the centre of the principal courtyard lay a low black marble monument to Kemal Jumblatt, Walid's assassinated father. The guard led me past it, and turning on his flashlight, conducted me down, through a narrow warren of dark passageways, into the drafty vaulted basements that had once been the palace stables and dungeons.

The guard fumbled for a switch. Suddenly the great arcaded underpass was lit up by racks of powerful spotlights. I had been expecting a modest collection of interesting new finds, but nothing had prepared me for the wonderful quantity of Byzantine artwork Jumblatt had managed to save. There, laid out on the walls and on the floor, in room after vaulted room, unstudied by scholars, unknown to the outside world, lay what is without doubt the most magnificent collection of Byzantine floor mosaics to survive to the present day outside the city of Byzantium itself: more than thirty large, room-sized mosaics dating from the mid-sixth century, and as many smaller fragments. It was a truly extraordinary abundance of fine late antique art, certainly one of the very greatest Byzantine finds to have come to light this century.

The Porphyreon mosaic-makers appear to have been influenced less by Imperial fashions in the capital – where, judging by the floors in the Great Palace, gory hunting and gladiatorial scenes were *de rigueur* – than by work from contemporary monastic sites in Byzantine Palestine. They too used relatively large tesserae and show a preference for geometric subjects over figurative ones. Most of the mosaics are filled with intricate patterns: *trompe l'oeuil* based on interlocking cross-shapes, hypnotic swirls of peltas, chevrons, swastikas and key patterns. Some of these interlace patterns resemble similar designs on fragments of floor mosaic from the Byzantine monastery of St Stephen, just outside the Damascus Gate in Jerusalem. Others contain tangles of vine-scroll ornament closely paralleled by a lovely mosaic that decorated the great Armenian monastery which once stood a short distance from St Stephen. One of the mosaics in the basement depicts a mallard and two ducks resting on a lilypond in a style very close to the mosaic of the River Nile at Tabgha on the Sea of Galilee. The link to Palestine is therefore striking, and it seems entirely possible that the same *atelier* of mosaic-makers served both northern Palestine and what is now southern Lebanon.

The somewhat austere choice of subject-matter almost certainly represents a conscious reaction against the sort of voluptuous late Roman pavements discovered outside Antioch and Carthage. On these mosaics plump, disrobed goddesses sport with hoary satyrs, while gods and demi-gods, Hercules and Dionysus, lie befuddled on their couches, overflowing rhytons raised in the air as they engage in riotous drinking contests: hardly the sort of scheme to appeal to ascetic early Christian monks. What is perhaps more unexpected is that the Porphyreon mosaics also represent a striking contrast to the worldly triumphalism of the Imperial panels at Ravenna, where the apse walls of San Vitale are filled with magnificent depictions of Byzantine court ceremonial: long lines of Justinian's world-weary bishops and sycophantic courtiers, flanked by Theodora's urbane and gossipy ladies with their gold and pearls and silks.

Instead there is something decidedly puritanical in the spirit of Porphyreon, a spirit which mirrors the often austere monastic outlook of John Moschos. Indeed they are products of the same world. Several of the mosaics have inscriptions which reveal them to date from exactly the period Moschos was collecting material for *The Spiritual Meadow*. One inscription shows that the mosaic – a series of interlocking lozenges containing bears, storks, stags and a gazelle – was commissioned as a memorial 'for the rest of the soul of Elias' in December 594/595 A.D. In other words it is quite possible that both John Moschos and the men from Porphyreon that he mentions in *The Spiritual Meadow* – Procopius the lawyer and Abba Zosimos the Cilician – could have seen some of these mosaics being made, and may even have walked over their gleaming, newly-laid tesserae.

Yet the feature that is perhaps most interesting about the work at Porphyreon is the mosaic-makers' strong preference for the geometric over the figurative. Of sixty-three mosaics, only three depict the human figure: one shows a female saint holding a cloth; another shows a saint (presumably John the Baptist) standing in water and holding a staff; while the third is a personification of Ktisis ('Creation'), shown holding a spear and surrounded by a group of animals – bulls, bears, leopards and a lion. The sixty other mosaics are all, without exception, aniconic and non-figurative.

This is important, for it emphasises quite how far taste was already moving away from the humanism, gaiety and decadence of the late classical world towards the cold and inward-looking intensity of early medieval Byzantium. This was a spirit which was to lead directly to the violent iconoclasm of the eighth and ninth centuries: only fifty years after the completion of the Elias mosaic, the Byzantine Emperor Leo III ordered the smashing of all icons and figurative *ars sacra* across the Christian Empire.

Nor was Byzantium the only force to be affected by this change of feeling: one of the Porphyreon mosaics, dated 500, was laid at exactly the period that an Arab trader from Mecca was touring the Levant, talking to and disputing with Byzantine monks, and formulating his own – thoroughly disapproving – ideas about the depiction of living creatures. The prohibition on reproducing the human form that Mohammed was later to impose on all Muslims still affects a billion people today, and it is fascinating to see the roots of that unease – a feeling that to depict man, to erect graven images, was somehow pagan and obscene – clearly apparent in these mosaics. Certainly the exuberance and vivacity of late antique and early Christian work – the crowding of living forms, of horse-men and their quarry, leaping lions, fleeing gazelles, the Emperor and his consorts, even the querulous saints and the prophets of the Ravenna baptistries – have already given way to a cold, carpet-like abstraction. The birds in the vine tendrils are still and silent and two-dimensional; a chill has descended, and left the mosaics frozen, arrested. There is no movement, no noise. The Bacchic riot of Antioch and the courtly trumpets of Ravenna have been stilled.

I spent two hours in the dungeons of the palace, closely examining the mosaics, astonished by their stern beauty and their fantastically intricate and abstract detailing. Porphyreon was clearly still a prosperous place at a period when most of the other trading ports of the Levant were already in fast decline, and presumably this prosperity was linked to the olive-oil mills that the archaeologists dug up in their rescue excavations. After all, oil was a very valuable commodity, needed by cities around the Mediterranean for both cooking and lamplight, and its price was clearly marked up considerably in the process. St Augustine, used to the cheap oil of his rural North African childhood, could not believe the cost of lamp oil when he arrived in Rome for the first time, and complained bitterly about the expense it imposed on reading at night. But as the rich spread of mosaic-work around me demonstrated, the merchants of Porphyreon had used their profits well.

Carried away by the thrill of being one of the first ever to see these mosaics, I lost all sense of time. But quite suddenly, I was brought back to reality by the sound of a loud explosion outside. The noise echoed around the vaults for several seconds before finally dying away.

'What was that?' I asked the guard.

'It is nothing,' he replied casually, sucking on his cigarette. 'Just the planes of the Israelis.'

'A sonic boom?'

'They make the noise deliberately,' he said. 'Once, twice a day.'

'Why?'

'Just to remind us,' said the guard. 'Just to remind us that they are still there. Just to remind us what they can still do.'

Everyone I talked to seemed to agree. If I wanted to understand the Maronites there was one place I had to go: Bsharre.

In the cliffs below the town, deep in the Qannubin gorge, the first Maronite hermits had taken shelter when they were driven out of Syria by Byzantine persecution in the sixth century. Fourteen hundred years later, at the end of the nineteenth century, the town produced the Maronites' most famous poet and writer: Kahlil Gibran, author of *The Prophet*. This at any rate was what Maronites told me about Bsharre, and what I read in my trusty *Lebanon: Promised Land of Tourism*.

Non-Maronites also said that I should go to Bsharre, but for rather different reasons. They seemed to regard the town as a sort of Maronite Heart of Darkness, pointing out that Bsharre was the home of the notorious Samir Geagea, and the place from which he drew his most loyal and bloodthirsty troops. If Geagea was the man who for the final stages of the war led the Phalange militiamen who committed mass murder at Sabra and Chatila (as well as slightly smaller and less notorious massacres at three other Palestinian camps, Karantina, Tel el-Za'atar and Ein Helweh), and who gunned down two of his principal Maronite rivals in their beds, then many of the men who actually performed these atrocities could no doubt now be found sipping mint tea in Bsharre's cafés and bars.

The unusual proportion of psychotics in Bsharre's population seemed to be emphasised by another story I was told. It concerned what happened when, on his death bed, Kahlil Gibran left Bsharre all the royalties from *The Prophet*, then running at an astonishing $1 million annually. The gift did not have the beneficial effect he presumably hoped for. Instead the two rival Maronite clans that dominate Bsharre, the Kayruz and the Tawq, broke into open warfare over the division of the money. For many months the town was plunged into its own miniature civil war, with bombings, assassinations, murders and exchanges of heavy mortar-fire. According to my informants, it was that battle over the profits of a book of mystic poetry, not the words of gentle counsel offered by Gibran, that represented the true face of this town at the heart of the Maronite world.

One Maronite academic friend of mine, now a don at Oxford, also warned me about the primitive behaviour of the people of Bsharre. A couple of years ago he had been sitting on the verandah of a bar in the town, watching the sun going down and drinking a glass of beer with a colleague. Suddenly, from a balcony immediately behind him, a double-barrelled anti-aircraft gun opened up, firing volley after volley into the air. Assuming some sort of air raid was in progress, my friend took shelter behind a nearby wall. But when, after five minutes, no aircraft appeared and the gun continued firing, he darted along the road, climbed up the stairs and knocked on the door of the flat to try to find out what was going on.

'Are you crazy?' he said when the door was opened. 'What the hell do you think you're doing?'

'I'm sorry,' replied the man with the anti-aircraft gun. 'I've just heard that my daughter in Australia has had a baby boy. It is my first grandson. I am so happy.'

As there appeared to be no functioning public transport in Lebanon, to get to Bsharre I was forced to again hire the services of Nouri Suleiman, the extremely expensive taxi driver who took me to Beit ed-Din. Nouri is a septuagenarian former swimming champion who has been taking people around Lebanon since he won the Lebanese national lottery in the 1950s; he spent the money on a new Mercedes which, he tells me proudly, he is still driving forty years later.

But before I could leave to visit this town which, according to *Lebanon: Promised Land of Tourism*, 'still rings with the soothing sound of Gibran's peaceful words', I had a morning appointment to keep in Beirut. Fisk had told me that the opposition to the bulldozing of what little remained of historic Beirut – the so-called Downtown Project – was being coordinated by one Yvonne, Lady Cochrane, who had memorably described the President's ambitious plans for Beirut's redevelopment as 'the dream of a retarded adolescent'. Lady Cochrane was apparently the head of a family of old Beirut grandees who had come by her very unLevantine name when she married a former Irish Honorary Consul in Beirut, now long since dead.

I suppose I had guessed that Lady Cochrane was not going to be living in poverty in some poky flat when, on the telephone, she gave her address as Palais Sursock in Rue Sursock. But even so I had not expected the vision that confronted me when Nouri's taxi dropped me in front of Lady Cochrane's gates.

In the middle of the drive-in Apocalypse that is post-war Beirut, surrounded by the usual outcrops of half-collapsed sixties blocks – conical termite heaps of compacted, crumpled concrete – there stood an astonishing vision: a perfect Italian Baroque palace, enclosed within its own walled garden. Everything was beautifully kept, with wide terraced lawns framed by a pair of date palms looking down over the smart Christian district of Ashrafiyeh to the blue wash of the Mediterranean far below. A double marble staircase led up to the front door; only the broken balustrade – which appeared to have received a glancing hit from a mortar or a rocket-propelled grenade – indicated that the war had touched this small oasis at all.

I was let in by a servant and conducted to the library. On the wall hung a fine portrait of a seventeenth-century Greek merchant flanked by a series of superb oils of Ottoman townscapes: domes and caïques and wooden palaces on the Bosphorus. Shelves groaned with old leather-bound books; on one side a seventeenth-century escritoire was covered with the latest magazines from London and Paris.

After maybe ten minutes there came the sound of brisk footsteps and a petite but stylish woman walked in, hand extended. She was strikingly beautiful. In the half-light of the library I took her for about forty; only in the course of her conversation did it become clear that she must have been at least seventy, and possibly a good deal older than that.

'Do forgive me,' she said in an old-fashioned upper-class accent, the 'r's slurred almost into 'w's. 'I've been with the lawyer. We're having the most trying time with the Greek Orthodox Bishop next door. He's behaving like a total gangster. All the institutions in Lebanon have collapsed, and the Church is unfortunately no exception. Last year this bishop helped himself to the funds of the Greek Orthodox hospital donated by my family for the benefit of the poor. Now he is now trying to pinch a strip of my garden. You see, the boundary wall was destroyed in the Syrian bombardment.'

'You were bombarded here?'

'Several times.'

'Who by? I thought this part of Beirut escaped the worst of the war.'

'The first time, in '75, it was by the Palestinians. Then there was a second, more serious bombardment by the Syrians in '76. I was the other side of Beirut when it began again: couldn't get across the Green Line. Eventually I found someone who was prepared to bribe the Syrians, brave the shells and take me across. I arrived to find that the house had been appallingly battered. My son was here giving out water from the well in our garden to queues of people from the street. The Syrians had cut the water supply.'

'But the house was still standing?'

'Just about. This room was blown out by a phosphorus bomb. Came back to find the place looking like a surrealist picture. That entire wall had disappeared, but the bookcase was still standing, upright against the sky.'

Lady Cochrane arched her eyebrows: 'Next door the chandelier was blown apart in the blast, the mirrorwork ceiling was destroyed and my late husband's remarkable collection of fifteenth-century Chinese bowls was smashed.'

She stood up and led the way to the door into the hall. 'I suppose we were very lucky that none of the shells cut the main load-bearing pillars, otherwise the whole thing would have collapsed. But by pure good fortune most of them went straight through: down the passage, into the dining room and out the other side into the garden. Ruined my borders. Holes everywhere.'

'And you carried on living here, despite everything?'

'Oh yes. We lived in the shell for seven years. You can get used to anything. In time.'

'And you didn't rebuild?'

'There didn't seem much point while the shelling was continuing. It was 1985 before we felt it was worth trying to begin restoring the house.'

Lady Cochrane led the way into the main hall, an astonishing piece of mid-nineteenth-century Lebanese architecture enclosed by a quadrant of Saracenic arches. At the far end she pointed to an empty space on the wall; a shadow and a copper picture-hanger indicated where a large canvas had once hung.

'We had to sell the Guercino to the Met,' she said. 'It was painted for one of my ancestors, but the Syrians were shelling and we were left with no money at all. Couldn't even pay the servants. I panicked and sold it for a fraction of its worth.'

'And this?' I asked, pointing to a Venetian canalscape. 'Canaletto?'

'No,' she said. 'It's Guardi. But it's nice, isn't it?'

Outside the door of the sitting room my hostess paused by a small Baroque table with finely carved ball-and-claw feet. On it were displayed a few lumps of twisted metal.

'And these,' I said. 'Giacometti?'

'No, no,' said Lady Cochrane. 'Those are shells. All of that lot landed inside the house. Those ones on the left are mortars: used to come whizzing through the house six at a time. Made a terrible racket. We keep them just to remind us what we went through.'

We sat at a table and Lady Cochrane called for coffee. She then talked about her views on the redevelopment of Beirut: how the town had once been a green Ottoman garden city and should now be trying to return to that ideal rather than aiming at a sort of Middle Eastern version of Hong Kong, all high-rise blocks and plate glass. The brutalist architecture, she believed, was partly responsible for the brutalisation of Lebanon.

'In the past rich and poor had their own green space,' she said. 'A workman had something to look forward to: a peaceful evening sitting with his family round a small fountain surrounded by sweet-smelling herbs. Now he comes back to a concrete box in a slum. His children are screaming, the television is blaring. It's no wonder the Lebanese turned somewhat irritable and aggressive during the 1970s.'

A servant padded in with a tray of coffee. Lady Cochrane poured me a cup. In the background a telephone rang and a minute later the servant reappeared and whispered into his mistress's ear. She smiled a broad smile

'Good, good,' she said. 'That was my lawyer. He's rung to say the Bishop has just received the order to stop building in my garden. But you see, that Bishop is a splendid example. The Lebanese who are even remotely civilised are now reduced to a tiny minority. Before the civil war there was an artistic life: painters, musicians, actors. Now there is a terrible exodus of brains and honest people – the best Lebanese, Christian and Muslim, have all left, or are in the process of leaving. Among the Maronites 300,000 – a third of the total community – fled the Middle East in the course of the war. We're left with the bottom of the barrel.'

'Are you a Maronite?'

'I'm Greek Orthodox,' said Lady Cochrane. 'My family were Byzantines from Constantinople: the name Sursock is a corruption of Kyrie Isaac, Lord Isaac. They left at the fall of the city in 1453 and settled near J'bail.'

I asked how much responsibility she thought the Maronites had to bear for what had happened to Lebanon.

'The Maronites presided over both the birth and the death of Lebanon,' said Lady Cochrane. 'Without them, Lebanon would never have existed. With them behaving as they have a tendency to do, it can't go on. Of course, the war brought out the worst in everyone. The Muslims all turned into terrorists and the Christians into mafiosi: kidnapping and robbing people, protection rackets and so on. At the beginning they were so brave and honourable: we willingly gave them money, and even our own sons. But by the end we refused: it was just people like Geagea. Gangsters.'

'I'm off to Geagea territory – Bsharre – this afternoon.'

'Well, you be careful,' said Lady Cochrane briskly.

'What do you mean?'

'During the war my son Alfred went up there to see some friends. On the road, he was stopped by the Marada militia. They put a gun to his head and tied him to a tree. When Alfred was at Eton he.quickly learned how to get out of beatings, and this experience came in very handy on this occasion. They said they were going to execute him. He kept telling them he was great friends with the Franjiehs – the ex-President's family who commanded the militia – and said that he was going to spend the weekend with them. Of course he had no such plans, but the lie eventually did the trick. Most of the militia men did not believe him, but Alfred kept going on about his important Maronite friends and eventually one of them got cold feet. The others were saying, "Let's just shoot him and ask questions afterwards," but the one with cold feet said, "No, we must telephone the Franjiehs and check what he's saying." So they did.

'Luckily they got the former President, Suleiman Franjieh. He was a little surprised to hear that Alfred thought he had been invited for the weekend, but he told the militiamen to release Alfred immediately nonetheless. The next day Robert Franjieh, the President's son, rang up here. He and Alfred had known each other since they were in playpens together: it's a very small world here in Lebanon. Robert said: "I'm so sorry, Alfred. Rotten luck. Won't you come to lunch?"'

'And what was Alfred's reply?'

'He said, "Thanks a lot, Robert, but not today. I'm afraid I'm a little busy."'

Oddly enough, before I left England a journalist friend had given me Robert Franjieh's number. Intrigued by Lady Cochrane's story, before I left Beirut for Bsharre I gave him a ring and received an invitation to lunch later in the week. Unlike Alfred, I accepted.

The main road north from Beirut hugged the coast. The cliffs of the mountains rose steeply to our right while a ribbon of new seafront high-rise blocks towered to the left. We headed past the harbour with its phalanx of bulldozers pushing great piles of rubble and tangles of reinforced concrete into the sea, then crawled slowly through a long traffic jam past the casinos, nightclubs and restaurants of Jounieh. A little to the north we passed along a small stretch of six-lane motorway elaborately decorated with strange road-markings and numbers. As none of Lebanon's roads normally have any markings at all (or, indeed, traffic lights, signposts or lighting for that matter), I was baffled by the complex network of characters and symbols, and asked Nouri what they were.

'They were for the planes, sir.'

'I'm sorry?'

'Aeroplanes, sir. During the war, when Beirut airport was on the front line, the air force moved here. This side was the main runway, while the other lane was where the planes were parked.'

Just after Jebail, once famous across the Mediterranean for its orgiastic worship of Astarte, we turned inland, driving up into a dark and narrow river valley, barren but for a thin covering of thorn and gorse. The gradient became steeper. Soon the valley had grown into a great gash, slicing through the landscape with near-vertical cliffs rising on either side of us; on some small ledges, cowering under the weight of strata, you could see the old rock chapels of the early Maronite hermits, some of which – the more accessible ones – had later been dignified with simple façades. Others, stranded high above the abyss and apparently reachable only by rope, gaped out of the cliff-face like yawning mouths.

It was a strange, tortured geology that played around us: the ancient beds of rock were ripped, twisted and contorted like a body turning on a rack. The further we climbed, the deeper the gorge below us sunk until we found ourselves winding along on a narrow road above a dark drop. There were no crash-barriers. Occasionally a small village with a stone chapel would appear, clinging to the ledges between us and the chasm, but as we rose these became more infrequent and increasingly primitive. It grew chilly, and before long we passed the snowline: at first just a soft dusting of snow caught in the shade of the ridges and the old cultivation terraces, then, as we climbed, a thicker covering burying the pavements and masking the slates on the roofs. Our pace dropped to a crawl.

Then, on a remote turning, several miles from the nearest house, we suddenly came upon a roadblock. It was manned by a picket of cold Syrian paratroopers; to one side stood a pair of plainclothes *mukhabarat*. Nouri wound down his window and answered a long series of questions put to him by the secret policemen. Eventually we were waved through, and I asked him what he had been questioned about.

'They asked who you were. Then they asked me about myself.'

'What did you tell them?'

'I said I am Nouri Suleiman, sportsman and swimming champion. I told them I swam the English Channel twice and said that they could ask anyone in Beirut: everyone there knew what I had done. The Syrian said he was a sportsman too. Then I told him that in 1953 I drove Frank Sinatra and Ava Gardner to Ba'albek.'

'What did he say to that?'

'He said: "Who's Frank Sinatra?" '

We drove on in the fading winter light, still snaking upwards, higher and higher into the Qadisha Valley. At some bends in the road, silhouetted against the snow, we passed shrines to the Virgin, each one topped with a small wire cross. No one was about and a chill wind was blowing, yet candles were burning outside most of these shrines, lit by figures unseen and casting flickering shadows over the statues within.

The snow was lying thickly over everything now and the villages we passed through were strangely silent, with closed shutters and empty streets. They had all been summer resorts for the Beirut rich, said Nouri, but the rich had left the country and no one came up here any more. The towns had been out of season for nearly twenty years.

Bsharre sat at the end of the valley, strung out along the edge of the chasm. After two decades of war there was only one hotel left in what had once been Lebanon's premier skiing resort. It was shuttered and darkened; only after ten minutes of hammering did we manage to rouse the caretaker. He let us in, then disappeared, leaving us in total darkness while he went off with his torch to get the diesel generator going. After the lights had eventually flickered on we were taken upstairs by the disbelieving owner. He said he had not had any visitors for a month, and no foreign guests for four years.

At first the hotel was almost unbearably cold, but within half an hour Mr Ch'baat had built a blazing log fire in the grate downstairs, while his wife prepared some hot soup for Nouri and myself. I went to bed soon afterwards with my diary, two hot-water bottles and half a bottle of whisky. I drank it propped up in bed, fully clothed, under two feet of blankets and eiderdowns.

BSHARRE, 5 OCTOBER

Light streaming in through the curtainless windows woke me early this morning. It had dawned a bright, clear winter's day. Pulling on my jacket, I walked out onto the balcony to take in the view.

Our arrival in the dark had given no hint of Bsharre's astonishing position. It was huddled on a narrow ledge between high snow peaks and the dark abyss of the Qadisha Valley. Stone houses with red roofs stretched out along the edge of the cliff in either direction, broken occasionally by the twin towers of a Maronite church. All the churches and chapels were built in the same French colonial mock-Gothic style; indeed the whole town had an inescapably French feel, like some remote Auvergne spa in the depths of winter. Only the extraordinary drama of the geology placed the scene firmly in Asia rather than Europe.

I drank a cup of thick Turkish coffee by the fire in the dining room. Then, leaving a note for Nouri to come and pick me up at the bottom of the valley later that afternoon, I set off on foot for Qadisha, the sacred valley of the Maronites.

The streets of Bsharre were clogged with the snow that had fallen during the night, and the town's traders were out in force, clearing the pavements outside their shops. I followed the road

245

out of town around the edge of the precipice, past the tail of the gorge. To one side stood an orchard, its trees heavy with hard, cold apples. There I left the road and clambered down a steep track. It corkscrewed sharply downwards along the face of the cliff, curling around the jagged contours of the precipice in a series of dizzy hairpin bends. Halfway down I found three woodcutters smoking cigarettes on a treetrunk by the side of the road; pointing down the valley towards the sea they gave me directions to the old patriarchate. It lay four miles down the gorge, they said. All I had to do was to follow the river along the bottom of the valley; sooner or later it would lead me to my destination.

The bottom of the valley was cold and damp in the way that only places never reached by the sun can be cold and damp. The rock of the cliff-face blossomed with a thick beard of moss and strange grey lichens. An untended herd of long-haired goats were nibbling the grass in a small water-meadow by the river; high above, the fire-blackened caves of early medieval hermits hung like swallows' nests beneath overhangs in the rock.

The track passed between the muddy brown river and the rock-face, with a tangle of snow-covered thorns and creepers, vines and aerial roots hanging between the two and occasionally brushing my face as I passed. Every so often the terracing on the far side of the valley would be broken by the platform of a house, but always these were shuttered up and deserted. After a mile or so I passed the carcass of a small goat. Its front half was perfectly preserved, but its back had been eaten away, perhaps by a dog or a large bird of prey. Blood stained the slush all around it. The valley was dark and damp and eerily quiet. The sheer cliff-faces loomed on either side. I quickened my pace.

Eventually, after a four-mile walk, I came to a makeshift sign on which had been crudely scribbled an arrow and the message: SILENCE! PRIÈRE! I left the track in the direction indicated and followed a small path that led up to the right, through a thicket of firs and poplars. There, just a hundred yards from the track, in the shadow of a large fig tree, stood the old Maronite Patriarchate. It was partly built into the face of the cliff and sur-rounded by a scattering of modest stone buildings: a range of cells, a church, some workshops, a kitchen building and a bell tower. Like everything else in the valley it was shuttered, silent and strangely sinister. The only sign of life was a single outsized lizard which shot into a crack in the wall as I climbed up the steps to the cells.

This then was the cold heart of the Maronite world: an abbey said to have been founded by the fourth-century Byzantine Emperor Theodosius the Great, then for a thousand years the hidden Patriarchate of a persecuted (and in Byzantine eyes heretical) Church. Suitably inaccessible for a church on the defensive, Qanubbin's remoteness came to be an obstacle as the Maronites' power grew throughout the eighteenth century, and in 1820 it lost its primacy to the abbey at Bkerke on the cliffs above Beirut. It was finally deserted in the early years of the twentieth century. It is still a sacred site to the Maronites, yet no one seems to come here now, and its doors are all locked and bolted, perhaps to prevent one of the Maronites' many enemies from desecrating their most holy relics.

Disconsolate at finding everything shut up after so long a walk, I rattled irritably on the various doors around the compound. Just as I was about to give up, I noticed a narrow flight of stairs running up the outside wall of a chapel, and found that from the top step I could reach a window whose shutters had been left open. Pulling myself up, I balanced on the window frame and looked down into the unlit interior.

Inside it was pitch dark, but for the faint illumination of the light admitted by the one window. As my eyes adjusted to the gloom I began to be able to make out a vaulted semi-subterranean chamber, around whose walls were scattered some large objects of ecclesiastical lumber. After the long walk down the cliffs and through the valley I felt I had an obligation to be inquisitive. So, mouthing a prayer, I jumped down into the night-blackness of the crypt.

I fell through the darkness for fifteen feet and landed badly on the mud floor. When I had got my breath back I groped around the walls, but there were no light switches, and the doors turned out to be locked rather than bolted. I could not open them and so remained trapped in the darkness, a darkness which grew still more intense when, with a creak, a gust of wind blew one of the two shutters of my window closed.

Slowly, however, my eyes got used even to this deep gloom, and I felt my way over to an object that turned out to be a large metal candle-stand. It contained a bed of waxy sand where a line of votive candles had guttered. Next to the stand was a broken white cross; and beyond that, in the centre of the room, a low rectangular chest on four squat legs. It was flanked on either side by two brass-topped candle-holders on wooden stands. The chest had a glass top and looked rather like an old-fashioned museum display-case, except that it was much lower. I went over and, wiping away a thin lint of cobwebs, peered through the glass to see if I could make out what was contained within.

Near the far end of the case were laid out some clerical vestments of finely patterned lace, above which had been placed a glinting stole of cloth-of-gold. The lace was slightly crumpled, and bringing my face closer to the glass I noticed what looked like a stick poking out from the bottom. Then I realised it was a leg bone, and it finally dawned on me what I was looking at.

At the top of the glass coffin, through a gauze veil, I found myself staring at the mummified face of a long-dead Maronite Patriarch. He was still crowned with his gilded mitre, and his gaunt face was turned slightly on its side, so that his features caught the light from the window. His skin had the consistency of old leather. It was hard and cracked, pitted with small tears and holes, yet every feature was still perfectly preserved: the high cheekbones, the left ear flat and shrivelled like an old buckle, the lips thin and slightly parted, revealing an unsettling line of grinning white teeth.

Then, distantly, from far away in Bsharre, I heard a peal of bells calling the angelus. The noise woke me from my daze and reminded me how imminent was the coming night. I stumbled over to the wall and found to my relief that the stone was pitted with enough cracks and hand-holds to allow me to climb out of the crypt. Two minutes later I emerged blinking into the open. Already it was late afternoon and I had, I calculated, less than an hour to get up the cliff and out into the valley before darkness fell. Wiping the cobwebs from my hands on my trouser legs, I willed myself not to run, but soon found myself stumbling rapidly down the bank to the track.

At first I jogged back along the path, anxious to get up the cliff and out of the valley before the onset of darkness. But after a quarter of an hour I was exhausted, and decided to take a rest on an old treetrunk beside the road.

As I sat there scribbling what I had just seen into my notebook, I heard a branch break behind me. Turning around with a start I saw a bearded old man in rough, dark robes staring at me from a grove of trees a short distance away. We stood looking at each other in silence for a second before, in a low voice, he said: '*Qui est là?*'

I introduced myself and asked him who he was.

'*Je suis le père eremite,*' he said, adding after a pause, '*Le dernier eremite dans Liban. Peut-être le dernier eremite dans le Prochain Orient.*' A proud smile flashed momentarily across his face as he said this. '*Et vous? Vous êtes Chrétien? Catholique?*'

I nodded, and he beckoned me over. He held my hand and peered closely into my eyes. He was old and frail, with long fingers and very white skin, but he had a tremendously gentle face.

'*Venez,*' he said, and led the way up a narrow path overhung with trees and covered with pine needles and acorns. He pulled aside a rough wicket gate and led me towards his hermitage, a small stone hut built against the rockface and enclosing an old cave chapel. To one side stood a small but carefully tended olive grove.

'My predecessor planted those trees in the time of the Ottomans,' said the hermit.

He opened the door of the chapel and indicated that I should go in. Inside it was very cold, but candles flickered against the sanctuary icons, giving off a little reflected light.

'For thirty-five, forty years there were no hermits at all,' said the old man. 'Now I am the only one.'

'When did you begin?'

'At the end of May 1982, on the day of Pentecost. Before that I was the Superior of the Monastery of St Antony at Koshaya, a little down the valley. But I asked for a dispensation from my duties as Abbot so I could become a hermit.'

'Why?'

'It is a vocation. To be a hermit is the summit of the Christian life. Not everyone can do it. For me it was very difficult to separate from my brothers, to give up meat, to live on my own. Most of all it is difficult to pray the Maronite liturgies for hermits – the ancient hermit liturgies of Antioch – which ordain long prayers to perform every day.'

'Very long?'

'Well over eight hours every day. The hermit should be occupied all day with prayer and spiritual reading. According to the Rule of St Antony he is allowed only small breaks to tend his grapes and olives and vegetables. This life is not for everyone.'

'Does it get easier?'

'Every day is difficult. It is the same for all hermits. As you get closer to God your enemy attacks you more. Those who are content to live in sin do not suffer from the temptations of the Devil so badly as those who try to live with God. For a hermit temptation follows you all your life. But after a while you do feel you are making progress. You do feel you are drawing closer to God.'

I asked why it was necessary to leave a monastery to achieve this, what benefit there was in isolation. In answer, the hermit pointed to a small icon of St Antony hanging on the chapel wall. 'The desert fathers had a saying, that just as it is impossible to see your face in troubled waters, so also the soul: unless it is clear of alien thoughts and distractions it is not possible to pray to God in contemplation. It is like two lovers. If they want to discuss their love they want to be alone. They do not want to sit in the middle of a crowd.'

'Is it a happy life?'

The old man considered for a second before answering. 'Yes. It is happy, but only because it is so difficult. That is why the satisfaction is so great when you succeed. The desert fathers had another saying. They said that being a hermit was like building a fire. At first it smokes and your eyes water, but later you get the desired result: after the smoke disperses, the light and the heat comes. So with hermits. In the beginning there is a struggle and a lot of work for those who wish to come near to God and to light the divine fire within themselves. At first they feel lonely and depressed. But after that there is the indescribable joy of feeling the presence of the Lord.'

He paused and looked at me. Then he said: 'Of course there is smoke in every life: misunderstandings, difficulties. Everyone must carry the cross, not a cross made of wood, but the troubles of every day. Some people pretend they have no difficulties, but it is not true. Everyone has their troubles.'

I thought of the troubles which had resounded all around the valley in which the hermit lived, and I asked him whether the war had impinged on his life at all.

'No,' said the hermit. 'It did not come here. This is the Valley of the Saints. It is protected by God. I was never worried. Even though the Christians made many mistakes, I was not frightened. I knew we were still protected.'

'Do you worry that so many Maronites have emigrated now? That they are now a minority in Lebanon?'

'The others will come back, I hope. But that is politics. It is not my world. Whatever happens I will stay. I am a prisoner of God. I cannot leave this place.'

Worried by the fading light, I said goodbye to the hermit and stumbled down the path to the track at the bottom. I walked along it in the gathering darkness until I saw a pair of headlights coming slowly towards me. It was Nouri, worried that I had got lost. Only after I got in and we were heading back towards Bsharre did I realise that I had never learned the hermit's name.

BSHARRE, 9 OCTOBER

The Qanubbin Gorge was once famous for producing saints. Now it is more remarkable for the number of Christian warlords and mafiosi that spring from its soil.

Bsharre claims Geagea; Zghorta, twenty miles further down the gorge, produced the Franjiehs, one of the most powerful clan of warlords in all Lebanon. Geagea is now awaiting trial, but the Franjiehs still live in great style in their feudal stronghold, where they mourn the memory of the greatest of their clansmen, Suleiman 'the Sphinx' Franjieh, mafia godfather, reputed mass murderer and one-time President of Lebanon.

Tales of Suleiman Franjieh's enormities fill the annals of modern Lebanon. There are references to his boasting of the number of men he had personally killed (seven hundred according to one version), and to his policy of getting one of his toughs ostentatiously to shoot dead a Tripoli Muslim every month just to remind the townsmen who it was that controlled northern Lebanon. His most famous outrage took place as part of a vendetta with a rival Maronite clan, the Douaihys, who in his view were beginning to encroach on his political territory. The climax of this dispute saw Franjieh's gunmen massacring the Douaihy family while they were attending a requiem mass a short distance from Zghorta; witnesses claimed that Suleiman was himself one of the gunmen. Different versions of the story circulate, but all agree that a full-scale shoot-out took place during the funeral, with the gunmen of the rival clans blazing away at each other from behind pillars and inside confessionals; that several priests conducting the service were caught in the crossfire and killed; and that the Douaihy clan came off much the worst with at least twelve (and possibly as many as twenty) dead. Certainly at the end of it, warrants were issued for the arrest of forty-five Franjieh toughs, and Suleiman was forced to flee. He went to Syria, where he was sheltered by friends in the Alawi mountains. Their name was Asad, and Suleiman came to be specially friendly with one of them, a young air force officer named Hafez. Twelve years later, in 1970, long after Suleiman had been granted a pardon and allowed to return to Lebanon, Hafez al-Asad seized power in Damascus in a *coup d'état*.

By chance, the same year saw Suleiman elected to the Presidency of Lebanon. His election was reputedly pulled off only when his gunmen, smuggled into the parliament building with the complicity of a sympathetic policeman, enforced a vote in his favour by producing revolvers and turning them on the Speaker. In characteristic style, Suleiman Franjieh used his appointment to fill the Cabinet with his friends and relatives: the Mayor of Zghorta was suddenly promoted from organising flower shows to being Director of the Ministry of Information; Iskander Ghanem, a close personal friend, became Commander-in-Chief of the Army; while Tony Franjieh, Suleiman's eldest son, became the Minister of Posts and Telecommunications. Later, on the outbreak of war, Tony was put in charge of the Franjiehs' personal Marada Militia, where he behaved with characteristic brutality: on one occasion three hundred Muslims were massacred in one day in the Matn region in revenge for four Maronites found slain. Tony continued in this way until, in typical Maronite fashion, he died as he had lived, dispatched by two rival Maronite leaders, Bashir Gemayel and Samir Geagea, in a night raid on the Franjieh summer palace.

The story of the raid was remarkable, and revealed more clearly than anything the medieval feudal reality behind the civilised twentieth-century veneer of Lebanese politics. Just as Jumblatt's Progressive Socialist Party was really only a mechanism for the Druze to support their feudal lords, the Jumblatts, so the dispute between Gemayel, Geagea and Tony Franjieh, ostensibly a struggle for power between two rival Christian militias – the Gemayel-Geagea Phalange, which wanted to partition Lebanon into sectarian cantons, and the Franjiehs' Marada Militia which wished to keep it whole – in fact had its true roots in something more primitive still: a century-old blood feud between Bsharre, Geagea's home town, and Ehden and Zghorta, the Franjieh strongholds forty miles to the west.

The feud was explained to me by Mr Ch'baat at the hotel this morning when he joined me for breakfast. 'Some time about one hundred years ago,' he said, 'a Geagea woman from Bsharre was breast-feeding her child in a village on the coast. Two horsemen from Ehden stopped by her house, and she gave them water and fed their horses. Rather than saying thank you, they killed her dog and threw it in the well. Then they tore the baby in two and shot the mother. When they heard this in Bsharre the priest began to ring the bells. The people gathered by the church and discussed what they should do. Eventually they hit on a plan.'

'What was that?' I asked.

'They walked down to Ehden. They burned the town. Then they killed lots of people.' Ch'baat nodded his head approvingly. 'Since then the two towns have been enemies. There is a saying in Lebanon: "The enemy of my grandfather can never be my friend."'

When I said I was going to visit Ehden that morning, Ch'baat raised his eyebrows. 'Be careful, then. In Bsharre we shoot you in the face, but in Ehden they shoot you in the back. We have a proverb: "You can eat in Ehden, but make sure you sleep in Bsharre. Sleep in Ehden, and they will shoot you while you are asleep."'

Yet by all accounts, this was exactly what Gemayel and Geagea had done to Tony Franjieh on the night of their commando raid on Ehden. On 13 June 1978 Geagea amassed a thousand of his Phalange troops at Jounieh and drove up into the mountains at night. Another force of around two hundred came down from Bsharre. In all around 1,200 Phalangists were involved, all heavily armed with machine guns, cannons and rockets, moving in two convoys of open-topped jeeps.

The diversionary force from Bsharre attacked first, just before four a.m., ambushing and killing the militia men woken by the first sounds of battle. This drew the defenders away from the centre of Ehden, leaving the Franjiehs' Summer Palace undefended. And it was on the Summer Palace, where Tony Franjieh lay sleeping, that Geagea directed the main Phalangist force. He led it into battle himself.

The attack was over in less than a quarter of an hour. Quickly overcoming the few remaining guards, Geagea's force surrounded the building. There was a brief exchange of fire, during which Franjieh managed to wound Geagea severely in the shoulder, but the matter was quickly settled with a grenade. By the time the raiders withdrew, Tony Franjieh and his entire immediate family had been killed.

I pointed out to Ch'baat that rousing a man from his bed and killing him and his family in their pyjamas hardly seemed to square with Bsharre's honourable tradition of shooting people awake and in the face, but he simply shrugged his shoulders. 'Geagea is a very honourable and very holy man,' he said. 'We are very proud of him in Bsharre.'

I listed some more of the crimes I had heard Geagea accused of: as well as the killing of Tony Franjieh, the equally cowardly night murder of another Christian rival, Dany Chamoun and his wife and two small sons (twenty-seven bullets were pumped into the two children); the bombing of the church in Jounieh (apparently an attempt either to keep the Pope away or to persuade the international community that the Christians of Lebanon were being oppressed and terrorised by wicked Muslim extremists); the mass murder and terrorising of the Druze of the Chouf.

'You must not believe what people say about Samir Geagea,' said Ch'baat.

'But you can hardly call him holy.'

'Certainly yes,' he said, quite serious. 'He went to mass every day and prayed by his bed every night. He had a church built wherever he was, wherever he fought. Every Christmas his troops expected money as a present, but instead he gave them prayer books and rosaries. Of course he went to confession every week. He never went into battle without his cross. In his office, he always had a picture of the Virgin and a cross: never any picture of Che Guevara or anything like that.'

We left Bsharre at ten in the morning and took a winding mountain road down towards the north-west. It was a spectacular drive, snaking through the snowy hills and Alpine meadows towards the coastal plain and the blue haze of the coastline. Only the constant punctuation of Syrian army checkpoints hinted at the area's recent history of conflict.

At Ehden a line of Syrian tanks was drawn up outside the French-built colonial post office with its Moorish arcade. I asked

Nouri to take me to the scene of the attack, and we pulled up behind a middle-aged man at the outer gates of the Summer Palace to ask exact directions. He offered to conduct us himself. It was only when he got in that I noticed what it was that he was carrying: not an umbrella as I had at first thought, but a pump-action shotgun.

'Are you a security guard or something?' I asked, alarmed.

'No,' replied the man. 'I was going out shooting.'

'Shooting what?'

'Cats.'

'Cats?'

'Cats. I hate cats.'

'Why?'

'Because,' said the man, 'I like dogs. I like powerful dogs. I have two dobermans at home.'

He reflected on this for a second.

'Cats,' he added, 'are vermin.'

Driving into the gates of the Franjiehs' Summer Palace, the doberman-lover directed us away from the main palace to a small bungalow that stood in the grounds.

'This is where Tony was sleeping when they attacked,' he said.

'Were you here at the time?' I asked.

'No, I was in London. It was midsummer. Geagea only got away with the murder because everyone was away. There were a thousand of them and no one was here to protect Tony. A couple of guards, nothing more.'

The man spat on the ground and pointed over to the gatehouse of the compound. 'They left their jeeps over there and came the final distance on foot. Geagea and his boss, Bashir Gemayel, were standing over there directing everything. Tony heard something and woke up in time to get to the kitchen and shoot six of them dead – and wound Geagea – before they blew him up with a grenade. Without their grenades they would never have been able to kill him.'

The man fiddled angrily with the safety catch of his shotgun. 'They were cowards. After they killed Tony, they walked into the house and shot his wife, his daughter, the maid, even the dog. I didn't think a human being could do that. The girl was three years old; like an angel. Afterwards they found thirty bullets in her body and head. What kind of person could do that?'

'Wasn't there any resistance?'

'Of course. When they heard the shooting, our people came rushing out of their houses to see what was happening. At the same time some reinforcements arrived from Zghorta. Many of the Phalangists were killed, even though most of our people were just armed with knives and shotguns. When they saw that Geagea was wounded the Phalange just ran away. Like cowards. They left their jeeps and machine guns and just ran. We were still hunting them down in the hills days afterwards.'

The man led me over to the bungalow and pointed out the bulletholes around what he said had been the child's bedroom.

'Most of them must have been taking drugs. Something like this no one can do if they are normal. You can kill someone who is three years old? No. No one can do this. Only an animal. But if you take drugs you can. Maybe. Maybe then.'

After all I had heard of the firepower of the different Christian warlords in the mountains, I carried on down to Zghorta half expecting that my lunch with the Franjiehs would be held in some sort of castellated mafia fortress. I could not have been more wrong.

The surviving Franjiehs turned out to live in an elegant new neo-colonial villa, built sometime in the 1970s and surrounded by a thicket of rich green palms. I was conducted inside by an old retainer and left to wait amid the polychrome Moorish arches of a reception room. The walls were decorated with fans of Ottoman daggers and muskets, mounted fragments of Byzantine mosaic and fine Turkish kilims. Along the side of the room were lines of chairs, enough to sit maybe thirty or forty retainers coming to pay their respect to their feudal lord.

No less surprising, when they finally appeared, were the

Franjiehs themselves. Despite quite recently possessing a sizeable private army, indulging in bloody feuds and running one of the most powerful mafia-type networks in Lebanon, nothing said or done by my hosts indicated that they were anything but good-natured, wealthy provincial landowners of the sort you might be pleased to meet anywhere around the Mediterranean. Tony's younger brother Robert, my host, turned out to be gentle and artistic. I had been told by our mutual friend that he was a very different figure from his late father: a reluctant politician, he had voluntarily handed over control of the family's Marada Militia to his nephew, Tony's surviving son. Nevertheless I had certainly not expected such an intelligent and sympathetic figure. Nor was there anything at all sinister about his mother, the late Suleiman Franjieh's elderly widow. I sat next to her at lunch. She was bubbly and apparently sweet-natured, as were her two middle-aged daughters. As we sat around a huge table and course after course of *mezze* were produced by a stream of bowing servants, Mme Franjieh made polite small talk about her visit to England.

'Oh, Monsieur William,' she said in a strong French accent as she poured me some *arak*, 'when I was a little girl in Alexandria all I wanted to hear was the sound of your Big Ben. So famous, so *célèbre* – le Ding of Big Ben: we schoolgirls talked of little else. Now of course they have mended it, and it is not the same. They tried to arrange it but what could they do? When my late husband was President we went to visit Bristol and le Longleat: so beautiful. We have nothing like this in Liban or in Egypt. And your Royal family. Oh! *La Reine d'Angleterre*: so serene. How can her son write this book and say the bad thing about the *Duc d'Edinbourg*? I used to like the Prince Charles, but now . . .'

The highlight of Mme Franjieh's life – judging by the number of times her conversation returned to the subject – was the time she and her husband attended the Shah of Iran's famous *levée* at Persepolis in 1970, ostensibly to mark the twenty-fifth centenary of the founding of the Persian Empire by Cyrus the Great.

'The Shah! Such a charming man. So handsome! Such manners! So many charming people were there at the Shah's party: la Princesse Anne (what elegance!), Monsieur Tito (so big a man!), Monsieur Bhutto and his beautiful wife, Mrs Asad (*maladroite et très silencieuse*), Mrs Sadat (never stopped talking) ... In those days the politicians were more sophisticated, I think. This Clinton – he is like a performing monkey, *non*? He has not got down from his tree. Of course, as I was brought up in Alexandria so I was used to cosmopolitan society. Oh! In my youth in Alexandria: everyone was there: *les Grecs! Les Juifs! Les Anglais!* The dances! The beautiful hotels! The Cecil, The Windsor, Le Metropole ... *Une glace au chocolat* at the Groppi! Oh! Of course in those days children respected their parents. We always waited for our parents to finish their ice before we began ours. *Qu'est-ce que tu veux, Maman? Oui Maman! Non Maman!* But these days. The young. Other than my darling Robert, Robert who is martyred by his mother, isn't that right, *mon petit?*'

Afterwards, when Mme Franjieh had stopped talking, the ladies departed for their siesta. I was left alone chatting with Robert.

'I was at university when the war broke out,' he said at one stage, breaking into the small talk. 'I was studying to be an architect. All I wanted to do was to start my life. Then suddenly this strange mentality developed: everything became polarised into Christian versus Muslim. All my life I had never asked anyone whether he was a Christian or not. Then quite suddenly you had to give up half your life: half your friends, half the places you knew. I still have more Muslim friends than Christian ones. When the war broke out, I suddenly could not see them, could not speak to them.

'It was amazing to see how the hysteria evolved. In 1969 you began to see lines of friends from a street in Zghorta being drilled: lines of old butchers and grocers learning how to hold a rifle or fire a mortar. Perhaps one guy from the town had been in the army, and he would be there instructing all the old farmers.'

'It must all seem very distant now.'

'No,' said Robert. 'The war lives on. Everything in my life – everything in Lebanon – has been marked by that boundary: everything is either before or after the war. It has changed and brutalised everything. When I was young, if someone died from cancer or an accident, people would stop talking about it when I came into the room. Now I see friends talking about death in front of their children as if they were talking about bread or wine. During the war most people in this country ceased to make an effort, to work or to study: they knew they could be dead the next day, so they lived for the moment. It is the same today. In fact it may be the only thing people *have* learned from the war.'

He sipped his coffee. 'To be honest with you, I don't like to think about the war. I try to forget it, but you can't, of course, not finally, not unless you're insane. I just thank God every day that we can still appreciate, you know, the simple things: flowers, streams, beautiful weather . . .'

Robert was so obviously intelligent and reasonable that I longed to ask him what he thought about his father's mafia activities, but the subject never arose, and it seemed impossible to think of a way of phrasing the question without causing grave offence. But Robert did eventually touch on the murder of his brother Tony.

'I cannot forgive those who were responsible,' he said. 'The other day I was at a dinner party. There were about one hundred people. Suddenly at the other end of the room I saw Solange Gemayel, Bashir's widow. I tried to avoid her, but she saw me across the party and came running across the room. She said: "It is reconciliation time." Why? She does not represent anything. I do not represent anything. Neither of us are politicians. Why reconcile? It would just hurt more. I don't want to be hurt again.'

'What did you do?'

'Out of respect for the guy who was giving the party I could not make a scandal. I had to shake her hand. But I hope I never see her again. Or any of her family. How can you ever forgive the family who shot your brother and his little daughter in cold blood?'

There was one last thing I hoped to do before I left Lebanon and headed south to the Holy Land. I wanted to talk to some of the Christian Palestinian refugees expelled from their ancestral homes at the creation of Israel in 1948. Lebanon's Christian Palestinians were the group which more than any other must have found itself caught in the crossfire during the civil war. As Christians, one might imagine that the Palestinians would have seen them as potential traitors; as Palestinians, the Lebanese Christians would have regarded them as 'terrorists' and vermin, fit only to be exterminated in the most brutal fashion possible. Corralled into their squalid and indefensible camps, the Palestinians suffered more than any other group in the civil war; and in such a situation the friendless Palestinian Christians must presumably have suffered worst of all. Special refugee camps had apparently been set up in Beirut to house this awkward group, and Nouri said he had some contacts who could get me into one of them.

We drove back to the capital by a different route in order to visit the ancient city of Ba'albek, one of John Moschos's stopping points as he passed up the coast of Byzantine Phoenicia. From Bsharre we headed south-east over the high rocky ridges of Mount Lebanon, then corkscrewed down into soft green fields of the northern Bekaa. Despite the fertility of the soil and the estimated ten thousand tons of hashish it produces every year, quite apart from unspecified amounts of raw opium, the Bekaa looked much poorer than anywhere else in Lebanon. Peasants in rags were selling boxes of battered-looking apples by the roadside, and in the fields the untidy brown hessian tents of nomadic Bedouin flapped in the wind. The houses that dotted the roadside were little more than crude concrete boxes, with sacking for windows. Plastic bags and drifts of uncollected rubbish billowed across the valley, past the Syrian army radar station and out into the unseen opium fields beyond.

The poverty of the Shiite farmers of the Bekaa made them

especially fertile soil for the new fundamentalist ideas of the Iranian Revolution. When the Ayatollah's Revolutionary Guards took up station here – with tacit Syrian approval – at the end of the civil war, they quickly evicted the (overwhelmingly Christian) Lebanese army from their barracks in Ba'albek and raised the flag of the Islamic Republic of Iran over the ruins of the Roman Temple of the Sun at the centre of the town. From that point on, Ba'albek became a centre of Iranian-backed anti-Christian militancy.

The Iranians opened a two-storey propaganda office and strewed the Bekaa with posters denouncing the Israeli and American 'imperialists' and their Maronite 'lackeys', while exhorting all good Lebanese Muslims to find salvation through Islamic martyrdom. The Revolutionary Guards and their Shiite Lebanese allies together staged assaults on the Maronite villages in the northern Bekaa while their mullahs recorded viciously anti-Christian sermons to be broadcast on the Iranian-financed Ba'albek Television, the Shia equivalent of the fundamentalist American gospel channels. It was probably in Ba'albek that the suicide bombings which destroyed the American Embassy and military headquarters in Beirut were planned, and it was certainly to Ba'albek that many of the Western hostages were taken and held. Although the hostage crisis is now officially over, only a month ago a group of Danish diplomats were caught indiscreetly taking pictures of themselves in front of the Ba'albek Hezbollah headquarters. They were detained by the Hezbollah for a tense fortnight before a flurry of frantic diplomatic activity finally gained their release.

Though no one in the Bekaa probably realised it, the Shia mullahs were in many ways repeating history when they chose Ba'albek as the centre of their operations. For in late antiquity Ba'albek was also a centre of anti-Christian activity, this time as a beacon of unreconstructed paganism. At the beginning of the fifth century, St John Chrysostom tried to stamp out the militant idol-worshippers of Lebanon by sending a task force of his monks to destroy the area's temples. According to Theodoret, 'Hearing that some of the inhabitants of Phoenicia were addicted to the worship of demons, John selected some ascetics who were filled with fervent zeal and sent them to destroy the idolatrous temples, inducing some ladies of great opulence to defray the monks' expenses; and [in due course] the temples of the demons were thrown down from their very foundations.'

Not in Ba'albek, however. For 150 years later, in the 550s, the Emperor Justinian was forced to again order the destruction of Ba'albek's great Temple of the Sun, which was clearly functioning as busily as it had in the great days of pagan Rome. Justinian sent orders that all pagans must accept baptism, under penalty of confiscation and exile, and to make sure that the temple was not rebuilt, he ordered that many of its largest pillars be shipped to Constantinople, there to be re-erected at the centre of the Emperor's new basilica of Haghia Sophia.

Even these extreme measures did not mean the end of paganism in Ba'albek. In 578 A.D., the year John Moschos set off on his travels, it was learned that the pagans of the town – still apparently the majority of the population – were again actively persecuting their Christian neighbours. The Emperor Tiberius Constantine duly ordered that five pagan priests were to be burned along with their idolatrous writings, and commanded that the remaining pagans of the town be brutally punished by the army. One source talks of there being no fewer than seven purges of pagans during the course of the sixth century, yet none of these measures seems to have had the slightest effect. Ba'albek was still active as a cult centre at the death of the Emperor Maurice in 602 A.D., and continued to flourish as a pagan centre well into the early Islamic period.

Certainly when Moschos visited Ba'albek sometime in the early years of the seventh century, it still had a reputation as a redoubt of impiety. Moschos includes in *The Spiritual Meadow* a story about a blasphemous (and presumably pagan) actor from the city.

> This actor, Gaianas, used to perform in the theatre an act in which he blasphemed against the Holy Mother of God. The Mother of God appeared before him saying: 'What evil have I done to you that you should revile me before so many people and blaspheme against me?'

He rose up and, far from mending his ways, proceeded to blaspheme against her even more than before. Three times she appeared to him with the same reproach and admonition. As he did not mend his ways in the slightest degree, but rather blasphemed the more, she appeared to him once when he was sleeping at midday and said nothing at all. All she did was to sever his two hands and feet with her finger. When he awoke he found that his hands and feet were so afflicted that he just lay there like a treetrunk.

Gaianas apparently spent the rest of his days being carried on a stretcher from town to town across the length of Byzantine Phoenicia warning others not to fall into the same errors as himself. John Moschos points out with some relish, however, that despite his contrition, the Virgin did not see fit to restore his faculties to him.

As we neared Ba'albek, signs of Iranian influence visibly increased. On the roadsides we began to pass the same hoardings of turbaned Iranian mullahs I had seen in Beirut's southern suburbs. Other tableaux, painted in the gaudy primary colours of Egyptian film posters, showed Kalashnikov-wielding Shi'ite fighters blazing away at Israeli troops in southern Lebanon; some of these posters were topped with small pennants decorated with the insignia of the Hezbollah, the pro-Iranian Party of God. The men trudging along the road began to display bushy, moustacheless Islamic beards while their womenfolk became more and more heavily shrouded in layers of thick black *chador*. At every crossroads we were approached by small boys in white cotton robes shaking collecting tins and soliciting donations for the Hezbollah's war against the Israeli occupying forces in the south of the country.

On the outskirts of the town we passed the Galerie Balkajian, a ritzy new Armenian (Christian) furniture shop. It enthusiastically trumpeted its unlikely loyalty to Shia Islam by filling the entire exterior of its warehouse with the iconography of the Islamic Revolution, centred on a huge mural of the Ayatollah Khomeini glaring down over the Dome of the Rock. Beyond the warehouse, the magnificent ruins of some of the most spectacular Roman buildings ever constructed rose above the dusty rundown houses of the modern town. Nervous of Ba'albek's reputation for violence, Nouri opted to stay in the street guarding his precious Mercedes while I went off alone to look at the ruins of the Temple of the Sun.

Like the decor of modern Maronite drawing rooms, the emphasis in the temple's decoration seemed to be on opulence rather than good taste: as you wandered around, you kept thinking: 'How much did this cost?' The temple was a monument to decorative excess: whole gardens of acanthus tendrils and palmettes voluted over the stonework; imperial lion-masks – unembarrassed lumps of high classical kitsch – roared out over the great baroque orgy of the ruins. The columns, each eight feet thick, were taller than any elsewhere in the classical world; each capital was larger than a fully-grown man, and covered with enough different leaf forms to fill a greenhouse at Kew. It was an exuberant, theatrical monument, designed more for ostentation than religiosity, and it undoubtedly achieved its aim. Flanked on either side by snow peaks, sheltered by a windbreak of cypress, it was a wonderfully flash piece of Roman showmanship, and showed that an unrestrained love of glitz is nothing new in this part of the world.

I knew from my reading that the Byzantines had built a fine basilica in the middle of the temple as part of one their periodic attempts to suppress the town's militant population of pagans. Yet despite the temple's generally excellent state of preservation, I looked in vain for any sign of Byzantine work. I have since learned from archaeologists in Beirut that the reason for this was not so much a pagan wrecking campaign as a piece of French colonial *dirigisme*. Apparently when French archaeologists dug the ruins in the 1930s they removed the Byzantine basilica, assuming, with typically Gallic certainty, that posterity would find their reconstruction of a pagan classical altar more interesting than the Byzantine basilica that succeeded it.

I sat in the small Temple of Jupiter, watching a handful of Lebanese tourists circle the ruins. There was a couple with a pushchair, a few modest Shia women in dark headscarves and a carload of noisy Maronite babes in tight hip-hugging jeans, thick lashings of mascara and great bouffant beehives of back-combed hair. Despite the recent kidnapping of the Danish diplomats and Nouri's nervousness, the visitors seemed relaxed and happy as they clambered around the pillars taking photographs of each other, giggling and smiling, determined to make the most of their day out from Beirut.

Then, quite suddenly, a burst of automatic fire echoed over the ruins. A few seconds later there were two more loud bursts of rapid fire followed by a massive explosion on the hillside above the town. As I watched a great brown mushroom cloud of dust and smoke exploded into the air from a ridge half a mile from the temple. I immediately took shelter behind a capital, but to my embarrassment none of the Lebanese jumped or even looked twice at the menacing plume of the explosion. One businessman filming his family with a camcorder swung briefly around to record the cloud of smoke, then swept back to pan over the pediments of the temple and his smiling wife and baby. He saw me picking myself up, dusting the dirt from my jeans, and smiled. 'It is only the Hezbollah,' he said. 'Probably they are just training. Almost certainly they are just training.'

Nouri was waiting, as arranged, in the lobby of the Cavalier at nine this morning. With him was his friend Abed, another taxi driver who said he had good contacts in the Palestinian camps. Abed said he could take me to some Christian Palestinians and suggested we try the Mar Elias refugee camp, not far from the notorious massacre site of Chatila.

The camp was a very different place to the squalid shanty towns I knew from the West Bank. Rather than rotting behind some high-tension razor-wire fence, it lay instead behind a line of smart boutiques – Valentino, Lagerfeld and Benetton – their exquisitely dressed dummies frozen in strange sartorial contortions behind the spotlit plate glass of the shop fronts. No clear boundaries separated the camp from the surrounding houses. Only the extreme, visible poverty of its residents and the density of shrapnel holes pockmarking the façades of the buildings marked it out from its unexpectedly prosperous surroundings.

Abed parked his battered old Mercedes just outside the camp and led me confidently through the narrow warren of breezeblock houses. Mar Elias, he explained, had been one of the luckiest camps in the war. Sure, it had been intermittently shelled by the Israelis, who had used phosphorus and even cluster bombs on the refugees' shacks, but unlike some neighbouring camps it had never been completely flattened by Israeli carpet bombing or Phalange bulldozers, nor had it ever suffered a major massacre like nearby Chatila, Sabra or Karantina. Its residents were very poor, of course, and suffered the same disabilities that hamstring all Palestinians in Lebanon – banned from all but menial jobs, forbidden from buying property or travelling freely, refused access to state schools – but, relatively speaking, they had been lucky. Moreover they were not in any immediate danger of eviction. Lebanese politicians were currently threatening to tear down the Palestinians' camps elsewhere in Beirut and dump the refugees out of sight somewhere on the front line in southern Lebanon. But Mar Elias was built on Greek Orthodox Church land, and if there was no obvious hope of the Palestinians ever being allowed to go back to their homes and farms in what was now northern Israel, then at least they were not in any immediate danger of being expelled from their makeshift camp in Beirut.

As Abed led me through the fetid lanes of the camp, he bumped into a friend, a burly man in a leather jacket. Abed shook his hand then embraced him, kissing him on either cheek in the Palestinian manner. He asked a question in Arabic and his friend pointed out a nearby three-storey house.

'He says that all the residents of that house are Palestinian Christians,' said Abed after the man had gone. 'Let's see if anyone is at home.'

'Who was that?' I asked as we climbed the stairs.

'Abu Nidal.'

'*The* Abu Nidal? The hijacker and bomber?'

'No, not the man himself,' said Abed casually. 'His representative here. He runs the Mar Elias branch of Abu Nidal's Fatah Revolutionary Council '

We knocked on a door at the top of the stairs, and after a minute it was opened by a Palestinian woman in a knotted kerchief. Abed talked to her, and after sizing us up to see whether she believed what he said, and conferring with someone inside, she opened the door to let us in.

'*Salaam alekum*,' she said. 'Welcome.'

Inside, we found the room full of Palestinian women. Our host was called Sarah Daou, and we had dropped in on the morning she happened to be entertaining her mother, Samira, and her pretty teenage sister Ghada. Her two small daughters, Rana and Rasha, fetched us a pair of plastic chairs, while Sarah went off to the kitchen to make us coffee. It was a bare, simple flat, small and undecorated except for a framed picture of the Virgin and a cheap Japanese wall clock; but it was spotlessly clean.

None of the family spoke English, so Abed acted as interpreter. Soon we were hearing a recital of the depressing, but familiar, Palestinian story of loss and dispossession.

'Since the time of Saladin my family had owned several hundred acres of land in the village of Kafr Bir'im,' said Samira, Sarah's mother. She was a large, cheerful middle-aged woman with a wide smile, but her face was heavily lined and there was a weariness in her voice as she told her story. 'The village was north of Acre, near the border with Lebanon. I was only five when we fled, but I remember that Kafr Bir'im was a very beautiful place.'

She made a sweeping upward gesture with the palm of her hand, as if trying to brush away the vision rising before her.

'My father was working in Haifa at the time of the catastrophe,' she said. 'I was at a Sisters of Charity school. I very well remember when the planes were bombing and a house nearby was destroyed. We were all very frightened. We had no idea what was happening or what to do.

'My father was about twenty-five at that time. He was a butcher and worked for a Jewish company in Haifa. He had a very good relationship with his Jewish employer. The man said, "If you are

268

frightened, send your family to Lebanon. Stay here and work for us. Then when the war is over go and collect them." But my father was too afraid. Everyone knew what had happened to the Palestinians massacred by the Jewish terrorists at Deir Yassin, and he was worried that maybe the border would close and he would be separated from us. Then the Jews began firing their mortars into the Arab areas of Haifa and our building was completely destroyed. Luckily, by some miracle, none of us were in at the time, but it made up my father's mind.

'His employer gave him a month's leave and lent us his van. That was how we left Palestine, with my father driving a Jewish van to exile in southern Lebanon. My father's mother-in-law, my grandmother, was a Maronite from that region, so he drove us straight to her house. By that stage the Israelis controlled much of the road, but they did not bother us because we had a Jewish truck. Sometimes the Israeli planes were flying just above us, but they probably thought we were Jews because of the Hebrew writing on the van and they did not bomb us. We were very lucky, but we made one big mistake: we didn't bring anything with us, because we thought the war would only last two weeks, a month maybe. We left everything behind. The only thing of any value that we had with us was my mother's gold earrings. How were we to know the Israelis would never let any of us return to our homes? Later, when the Israeli planes destroyed Kafr Bir'im – they bombed every house in the village – everything we owned, everything we had worked for, was destroyed. Only the church was left standing. Our land was divided between new Jewish settlements, and given to people from Poland and America.'

At that moment, from outside, there came the unmistakable *clack-clack-clack* of automatic gunfire. After my humiliation the day before in Ba'albek, I stayed rooted to the spot and tried to look as if I regularly sat inside Palestinian refugee camps listening to the ominous sound of approaching machine-gun fire. This time, however, I was clearly not alone in being anxious. Everyone immediately got up from their seats and went over to the windows to see what was happening.

'It's outside the camp,' said Sarah.

'Its probably just the Syrian army firing into the air,' said her mother. 'Probably celebrating someone's birthday.'

'The cars are moving normally on the roads,' said Abed, looking over towards where his car was parked.

'Maybe it's an assassination,' said Ghada, our hostess's sister. 'Maybe someone has killed Arafat and now the people are firing into the air to celebrate.'

'Maybe it's the anniversary of the beginning of the *intifada*.'

'Wrong month.'

'Maybe they are celebrating Mr William's visit,' suggested Abed.

'Is this dangerous?' I asked Abed. 'Should we go?'

'It's safer to stay,' he said. 'At least until we know what the problem is.'

Sarah and Ghada stayed by the window, peering nervously in the direction from which the firing was still coming, but their mother, clearly used to such alarms after a life spent in besieged camps, returned wearily to her seat and continued her narrative.

'We stayed all that year in southern Lebanon in my grandmother's house. It was very primitive, and my father couldn't find work because he was a Palestinian. The Lebanese wouldn't even let him drive the van, and eventually he had to sell it. After the nice school in Haifa I hated the life on the farm. My grandmother's house was very small. My uncle was living there with his family, so there were already eight people in the house even before we arrived. It was unbearable: there was no space, no privacy. All the small children were quarrelling all the time. I remember always being hungry. Often we slept without eating. We suffered a lot.

'After a year, when it became clear we would not be allowed back home for some time, we got a tent in the Baas refugee camp near Sidon. The camp had originally been built for the Armenians when they fled to Lebanon in 1916, but they had since become rich and moved out. I remember it was very cold, and when it rained the tent leaked. At night when we were all in the tent there was no room to move, and my brothers had to sleep with their legs outside the tent because they could not fit them inside.

'After some time, in 1953, my father got a job as a UN bus driver between south Lebanon and Beirut. But he never really recovered from losing everything. He hated the tents and he missed his village and his old life in Palestine. He would have given anything to return, but he knew that all his friends who had tried to sneak across the border to their old villages had been shot dead by the Israelis. They gunned down any Arab they saw crossing the border, calling them terrorists. So he had no choice but to stay in the tent. Sometimes he would just sit there looking at the keys of his house in Kafr Bir'im and the title deeds the British had given his father to prove the ownership of our land. He got ill and very depressed. It was as if something had broken inside him. He died in 1956. He was only thirty-four years old.'

'Soon after that the UN transferred all the Christians to the Dbayyeh in East Beirut, leaving Baas to the Muslims. At Baas all the children had been going to a UNRWA [United Nations Relief and Works Agency] school. It was very good and things seemed to be getting better. But with my father's death and the transfer to Beirut, all my brothers and sisters had to leave school and begin work. My brothers got work on building sites; as they were Palestinians they could not get work permits, so they were paid only the lowest day-rates. My sisters and I cleaned houses. When I was a little girl in Kafr Bir'im we used to have three household servants and many workers and tenants. Now we had sunk to begging for the most menial work that was available.'

Outside the rattle of machine guns was getting louder and louder, as more and more guns joined in the shooting. At the window Samira's daughters were still nervously discussing what the cause was. As the traffic was moving freely on the roads they still thought that it must be some sort of celebration rather than fighting or an attack on the camp, but they were unable to think of any event which was due to be celebrated. From the window they shouted out to neighbouring families who were also looking nervously out towards the shooting, exchanging ideas about its possible causes.

'Maybe it is to celebrate the heroes of the October [1973 Arab–Israeli] War?' suggested Sarah, repeating the theory favoured by the family in the apartment immediately above theirs.

'Wrong date,' said Ghada.

'Asad's birthday?'

'That was earlier this month. The sixth is Asad's birthday.'

'What about Basil?'

Inside, Samira shrugged off the din and the chatter of her daughters. She had got into the swing of her story and was anxious to continue.

'So were you still in Dbayyeh camp when the civil war broke out?' I asked.

'Yes,' said Samira. 'We were very nervous. You see, Dbayyeh was in the Christian half of the city, and the Phalange attacked and captured it in January 1976. In some of the other camps they captured – Tel el-Za'atar, Maslakh and Karantina – they shot the inhabitants, even the women and children, and bulldozed the camp. But in Dbayyeh – perhaps because it was Christian – they merely sent in their secret police, and tortured only those they thought were Fatah activists.'

'So the Phalange did not hurt you personally?'

'At first we were unharmed. Then one afternoon in early February they came for my husband.'

'You didn't say when you were married.'

'I was married in 1958, when I was seventeen. My husband was a boy from another big Kafr Bir'im family. We had been married eighteen years and had six children when the Phalange captured the camp. I will never forget the day they came for him. They took him at four o'clock, accusing him of being in the PLO. As soon as they took him I managed to get a message to some Lebanese relations of my grandmother who had contacts in the Phalange. They made calls and within four hours he was back here. But what they had done to him in that time!'

'What do you mean?' I asked.

Samira looked down and began to speak in a low voice. 'They had beaten him with metal bars,' she said. 'They used electricity. They burned cigarette butts into him. They broke both his legs, smashed his kneecaps and snapped one of his arms. Also his chestbone. All in four hours!'

'But he survived?'

'When my relative intervened the Phalange were ready to kill

272

him. My relative told the truth: he said that my husband was also a Maronite. The Phalange did not know there were any Palestinian Maronites. After they released him we had him rushed across the Green Line to the American University Hospital.' She added proudly, 'They sent an ambulance. Because he was an employee.'

'He was a doctor?'

'No,' replied Samira, a little crestfallen. 'In Lebanon a Palestinian could not hold such a job. He was a cleaner at the hospital.'

'How long did he take to recover?'

'For four months he was in emergency,' she said. 'After that I made the decision that we would stay in Muslim West Beirut and not return to the east, the Christian half. Before I left Dbayyeh I said to the guards: "I am a Christian like you. But if you treat us like this I will cross to the other side and be protected by the Musulmen." '

'And did they protect you?'

'Yes. The Muslims treated us very well: much better than the Christians. We stayed the rest of the war in West Beirut, but I never heard anyone mention the fact that we were Christians. The Muslims I know are better Christians than most Christians. Jesus Christ said that we should love and care for each other, but the Phalange were very cruel. What the Phalange did was the work of the Devil.'

'The Phalange made me ashamed to be a Christian,' said Ghada, turning her head away from the window for a second. 'The Muslims were much kinder to us. I hated myself for being a Christian when I saw the kindness they showed us.'

'My father was a Maronite,' said Sarah, 'but still I do not like them. The Maronites have no feelings.'

'When we crossed the Green Line we lost everything for a second time,' continued her mother. 'The Phalange wouldn't let us take anything. Like my mother I had only my jewellery. We left all the contents of our house: the TV, the furniture, our utensils.'

'So you were destitute all over again?'

'Not entirely. The PLO gave us a flat on the seafront in Raoche. It belonged to a Christian family who had fled to West Beirut and was partly furnished. Again we began to rebuild our lives. But in 1982 the Israelis invaded and the Israeli warships began shelling Beirut. As our flat was on the seafront it was very exposed. For fifteen days we were being shelled and bombed from both the land and the sea. It was terrifying. Most of all I was frightened for my children, that somehow I would survive and they would be killed. We stayed all that time in a shelter at the bottom of the apartment block, lying on the floor. There were fifty-five apartments in the building, fifty-five families, maybe 250 people. But the Israelis had invented a special kind of bomb which did not explode until it hit the basement, so even there down under the ground we knew we were not safe.

'One day they used one of these [suction] bombs on the building next to ours. It was completely destroyed. The four hundred families in the basement – maybe a thousand people – were all crushed to death. We had several relations in there, from my father's family. They were from al-Bassa, the next village to Kafr Bir'im. Apparently there was a rumour that Arafat was in the basement of that building. Of course it wasn't true, but what did the Israelis care? At about the same time some other cousins of ours were in a building that was shelled by phosphorus. They were killed too, but with phosphorus it is a very slow death. It burns very slowly from your skin down to your bone.'

I knew a little about the Israelis' phosphorus bombing of civilian areas of Beirut from Robert Fisk's book *Pity the Nation*. In a book filled with horrors, the worst moment of all is Fisk's description of a visit to a maternity hospital shortly after this phosphorus bombardment had taken place. There he met a nurse. After the bombardment had ended she had had to put several burning babies into a big bucket of water in order to put out the flames. When she took them out half an hour later, they were still burning. Even in the freezing cold of the mortuary they smouldered. The following morning the doctor took the tiny corpses out of the mortuary for burial. To her horror, they again burst into flames. I shuddered at the memory of this, but Samira was still continuing with her story.

'After fifteen days,' she said, 'a rocket from one of the Israeli ships hit our building. There was an earsplitting sound and the whole

tower moved. It felt worse than an earthquake, but luckily the building did not catch fire. Nevertheless when we ventured out of the
shelter we discovered that our apartment had been completely
destroyed, and we still had to leave. That night when the bombing
had stopped we ran down to Hamra Street, where we were given
shelter in another basement belonging to some relations.

'Soon after that the Israelis entered West Beirut and the bombing stopped. I saw them the next day when I went to buy bread.
Here were the people who had taken my home, who had farmed
my land, who broke my father, murdered my relatives and then
bombed my apartment. Yet many of them were just little boys. I
looked at them and thought: these are the people I hate?' She
paused, then added: 'If you are a Christian you have to learn to
forgive your enemies. It is not for me to judge them.'

'But doesn't what has happened to you make you question your
faith?' I asked. 'Don't you ever wonder how God could allow the
sort of horrors you have witnessed?'

'It's not God's fault,' said Samira. 'Its the fault of people. I
thank God that he has protected us.'

'What do you mean? You've had a horrific time.'

'We are still in good shape. I don't want money or luxury. I
haven't lost any of my children. That's what matters to me. We
are still alive and still together.'

'But you are still in exile.'

'Of course,' she said. 'After all I have suffered from the Israelis
and the Lebanese I would like to go home even if it meant I was
naked and starving. Even after forty-seven years I still feel a
stranger in this country, feel that I don't belong. Even if I had
lived a hundred years here I would still like to go back to Palestine,
go back to Kafr Bir'im where no one can tell me that I'm a refugee
and that I don't belong.'

'And do you think you will?'

Her daughter Ghada cut in from her watch by the window: 'Of
course not,' she said. 'We would all like to go home. That goes
without saying. But after Arafat's surrender, what hope is left?'

But Samira just shook her head and smiled: 'It is in the hands
of God,' she said. 'We shall see.'

V

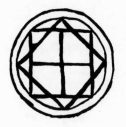

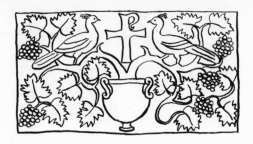

The Monastery of Mar Saba, Israeli-occupied West Bank, 24 October 1994

Again I inhabit a bare cell with white walls and a blue dado. Again, through the window, I hear the quiet rumour of hushed monkish talk, the occasional peal of bells, the purposeful rustle of habits. On the balcony next to mine a black-robed figure with a short beard, long hair and a tall cylindrical hat – Fr. Gregori, the monastery cook – is watering his pots of basil and tending his orange trees. Nearby a myna bird chatters in a cage. It could be Athos, and indeed an old oleograph of the Holy Mountain is framed on the wall of a corridor outside; but one glance at the bare rock wall of the cliff-face opposite my cell places this monastery firmly in the wilderness of Judaea, far from the cooling waters of the Aegean.

This is the desert where John Moschos took his vows and where he spent most of his monastic life, and tales of the monks of these bare hills fill most of the pages of *The Spiritual Meadow*. Having read so much about these Judaean desert fathers it is strange finally to see the austere landscape that forms the background to their exploits. It is stranger still to find many of their superstitions, fears and prejudices alive in the conversation of the monks who still inhabit this, the last of the ancient monasteries of the Holy Land to survive as a functioning community. But the stories of devils and demons, visions and miracles which sometimes seemed ludicrously outlandish when I first read them under a grey London sky sounded quite plausible last night, when told in the starlight looking out onto a cliff-face honeycombed with the cells of long-dead hermits and holy men.

'Look at it!' said Fr. Theophanes, the monastery's tall, gaunt Guest Master, waving a hand at the dark rocky gorge beneath us. 'There it is: the Valley of Doom. The Valley of Dreadful Judgement.'

Below us the monastic buildings of Mar Saba fell away in a ripple of chapels, cells and oratories, each successive layer hanging like a wasps' nest from a ledge on the rockface. Opposite, the top of the cliff wall had turned an almost unnatural shade of red in the last of the evening light. The rock was pitted with caves, each formerly the cell of a Byzantine monk. All were now deserted.

'It's very beautiful,' I said.

'Beautiful?' said Fr. Theophanes, rustling his robes in horror. 'Beautiful? See down there at the bottom? The river? Nowadays it's just the sewage from Jerusalem. But on Judgement Day that's where the River of Blood is going to flow. It's going to be full of Freemasons, whores and heretics: Protestants, Schismatics, Jews, Catholics . . . More ouzo?'

'Please.'

The monk paused to pour another thimbleful of spirit into a small glass. When I had gulped it down, he continued with his Apocalypse. 'At the head of the damned will be a troop composed of all the Popes of Rome, followed by their deputies, the Vice-Presidents of the Freemasons . . .'

'You're saying the Pope is a Freemason?'

'A Freemason? He is the President of the Freemasons. Everyone knows this. Each morning he worships the Devil in the form of a naked woman with the head of a goat.'

'Actually, I'm a Catholic.'

'Then,' said Theophanes, 'unless you convert to Orthodoxy, you too will follow your Pope down that valley, through the scorching fire. We will watch you from this balcony,' he added, 'but of course it will then be too late to save you.'

I smiled, but Fr. Theophanes was in full swing and clearly in no mood for joking. 'No one can truly know what that day will be like.' He shook his head gravely. 'But some of our Orthodox fathers have had visions. Fire – fire that will never end, terrible, terrible fire – will come from the throne of Christ, just like it does on the icons. The saints – those who are to be saved, in other words the Orthodox Church – will fly in the air to meet Christ. But sinners and all non-Orthodox will be separated from the Elect. The damned will be pushed and prodded by devils down through the fire, down from the Valley of Josephat, past here – in fact exactly the route those Israeli hikers took today – down, down to the Mouth of Hell.'

'Is that nearby?'

'Certainly,' said Theophanes, stroking his beard. 'The Mouth of Hell will open up near the Dead Sea.'

'That is in the Bible?'

'Of course,' said Theophanes. 'Everything I am telling you is true.'

I had arrived at the Great Lavra of Mar Saba earlier that afternoon. From Beirut the distance is less than three hundred miles, but this being the Middle East it took a six-hundred-mile detour via Damascus and Amman – three and half days' non-stop travel – to get here. I finally crossed the Jordan into Palestine at noon yesterday.

The West Bank, and with it East Jerusalem, were captured by Israel from the Jordanians following Israel's great victory in the 1967 Six Day War. To create a buffer zone between the Jewish state and its hostile Arab neighbours East Jerusalem was annexed, while the West Bank was placed under Israeli military occupation. In defiance of international law both areas have since been subject to a campaign of colonisation: around 150 exclusively Jewish settlements have been established in the conquered territory, between them containing some 280,000 Israeli settlers (including the 130,000 settlers living in East Jerusalem). The military authorities have also appropriated 80 per cent of the West Bank's water, most of which is now piped south to Israel.

The Palestinian *intifada* made this great tract of land familiar territory, images of which were broadcast nightly into the world's sitting rooms, the backdrop to countless scenes of stone-throwing Palestinians confronting the Israeli army. Despite the stumbling peace process and the handing over of some Arab towns to Yasser Arafat's Palestinian Authority, the area, like Bosnia or Rwanda, still seems inexorably linked to violence, refugee camps and army patrols.

What is therefore so surprising when you first leave the small Jericho oasis and your taxi climbs through this great expanse of rolling hill country, past the Bedouin encampments with their brindling sheep and chickens, is the astonishing, unexpected beauty of the West Bank's dry, stony hills. Many of the valleys appear at first to be empty: dry hills whose pale rocks are scattered like lumps of feta cheese amongst the scrub-gorse. But as you wind your way down the slopes, under the weak light of a winter sky, forms begin to take shape: the stone roof of a steading hidden by a small cypress grove, the domes of an abandoned caravanserai, the minaret of a ruined mosque, the gently rolling slopes topped by newly harvested olive groves. It is a familiar Mediterranean picture; the same carefully polled olive slopes form the background to a hundred Tuscan paintings, and nearly a millennium before that, to the landscape mosaics of the Ummayad Mosque in Damascus.

The ancient Palestinian villages that you pass are built of honey-coloured limestone which changes tone according to the colour of the sky. Shepherd boys lead their flocks out into the valleys; old men in full Arab *jellaba* and *keffiyeh* suck hubble-bubbles in the shade of vine trellising; from cafés you can smell the charcoal scent of cooking kebabs and the hot, sweet odour of Turkish coffee. At first sight, the modern West Bank is still much closer to David Roberts's prints of mid-nineteenth-century Palestine than to the harrowing television images of refugees and razor wire.

Yet beautiful as it is, the signs of conflict are still there. In some valley bottoms where there should be cornfields, there are UN camps, home to those Palestinians expelled from their ancestral homes at the birth of Israel in 1948: huge, shockingly dirty shanty towns surrounded by army watchtowers and floodlights. Above them squat newly built Israeli settlements, modern suburban housing estates made up of ranks of detached whitewashed bungalows, with long lines of solar panels glinting on their roofs. Two different peoples, separated by thick tangles of razor wire and a small matter of legal status: the settlers have guns, vote in elections, enjoy Israeli civil justice and can join the army; the Palestinians under Israeli occupation are forbidden to own weapons of any sort, cannot vote in Israeli elections and are subject to the arbitrary and dismissive verdicts of military courts.

The largest of the Israeli settlements is Ma'ale Adumim, a ring of concrete blockhouses, cranes and half-completed apartment blocks, recently built over the site once occupied by the great Byzantine monastery of St Martyrius. It is currently home to thirty thousand Israelis – mostly new emigrants from Russia, Canada and the United States – yet despite the peace process the Israelis have announced plans to double the town's population over the next decade. Around the settlement's perimeter stretches an electrified razor-wire fence. Above it cluster blocks of identical eggbox houses: Milton Keynes transported into the landscape of a medieval Italian fresco.

Just beyond Ma'ale Adumim the road splits. The main branch heads on to Jerusalem. The smaller branch – potholed and neglected – winds off to the south. We bumped along this track for a few miles before arriving at a ledge overlooking the cliffs of the Valley of Kedron, a deep, arid canyon of wind-eroded chalk-like rock. At the top of the far side of this ravine stood a domed Greek Orthodox church, enclosed by a towering wall. Before I did anything else in Palestine – and certainly before I headed on to Mar Saba for the night – I knew I had first to make a pilgrimage to this shrine.

The driver parked the car in front of the gatehouse and I pulled at the bell rope; there was a distant ringing, but no one appeared. I rang the bell a second time, and soon afterwards the wimpled head of a nun peered suspiciously down over the parapet and asked in Greek what I wanted. I explained why I had come. After a few minutes there was a rattling of bolts and the great black gate swung open.

At the far side of the courtyard stood a gleaming new basilica with an octagonal dome, a bell tower and a red-tiled roof; around its edge ran the arcade of a cloister. The nun led me to a small cupola in the centre of the courtyard, and taking a huge bunch of keys from her pocket, unlocked a door. Then she lifted a storm lantern from a niche, lit it and led me down a flight of ancient stairs. From the dark below seeped a dank smell of musty air tinct with the sweet scent of burning oil-lamps.

As we sank deeper underground, masonry gave way to the living rock of a cave wall, and we entered a wide, echoing underground cavern. A pair of recesses at the far side of the cave were illuminated by the dim, flickering light of a cluster of lamps placed in front of two gilt icons each depicting a heavily bearded Byzantine saint. Another group of lamps flickered at the bottom of the stairs, under an ancient icon of the Magi. To one side of it stood a huge pile of skulls.

'This was the cave where the three wise men hid from King Herod,' whispered the nun, holding the storm lantern aloft. 'St Theodosius saw the cave in a vision and founded his monastery in this place to honour the Magi.'

'And the skulls?'

'They belong to the monks that were slaughtered by the Persians when they burned the abbey.'

'When did that happen?'

'Not so long ago,' she said. 'Around 614 A.D.'

The nun held the storm lantern above the charnel so that the light picked out the sword-gashes cleaving the crania of the topmost skulls.

'What you have come to see lies over there,' she said, pointing at the lamplit recesses on the far side of the cave.

I walked over towards the lamps. As I drew nearer I could see that they rested on a pair of Byzantine grave-slabs, both of which had been propped up some time in the last century by a pair of small neo-classical pillars. On both the tomb-slabs had been carved in shallow relief an intricate design of equal-armed Byzantine crosses, some set in diamonds, others in circles. Between the crosses were carved inscriptions in clear Byzantine Greek. That on the left read 'Sophronius'; that on the right bore the name of John Moschos.

'St John Moschos died in Constantinople,' said the nun, 'but his dying wish was that he should be brought back here to the Lavra of St Theodosius. He regarded this as his home: this was where he was first tonsured, and where he spent most of his life. But the Holy Land was still occupied by the Persians and it was not until much later that St Sophronius was able to fulfil his promise to bring back John Moschos's body and to rebuild the monastery.'

'And the monks?'

'Before the slaughter there were seven hundred elders here. It was the most celebrated monastery in the Holy Land. There was a hospital for lepers and a rest house for pilgrims; also an inner monastery for those driven insane by the rigours of their asceticism. There were four separate churches. Monks came here from as far away as Cappadocia and Armenia . . . But after the Persians the monastery never recovered. It has never had as many monks ever again.'

'And now? How many of there are you today?'

'What do you mean? There is only me. I am the last. A priest is supposed to come from Jerusalem once a week to celebrate the liturgy, but he is old and sometimes he forgets.'

The nun bent forward and kissed the icon of Moschos. 'I will leave you,' she said. 'If you have come all the way to see the grave of St John Moschos you will want to be alone with him. Bring the lantern with you when you have finished.'

Holding the lamp aloft, I looked around the crypt and paused for a second before the macabre pile of skulls. I had read so much about the monks of St Theodosius in the pages of *The Spiritual Meadow* that I felt I must know some of the men who had been slaughtered by the Persians, men whose anonymous bleached bones now lay piled in front of me. They were characters like Brother George the Cappadocian, 'who was pasturing swine in

285

Phasaelis when two lions came to seize a pig'; rather than running off 'he seized a staff and chased them as far as holy Jordan'. Then there was Moschos's friend Patrick, 'the native of Sebastea in Armenia, who was of very great age, claiming to be one hundred and thirteen'. He had once been an abbot, but 'being very humble and much given to silence' had relinquished his position and 'placed himself under obedience, saying that it was only for great men to shepherd the spiritual sheep'. What had been the fate, I wondered, of another of Moschos's companions, Brother Christopher the Roman? Every night he deprived himself of sleep, performing a hundred prostrations on each of the steps that led down into the cave-crypt, never stopping until the bell rang for matins. I could certainly guess what happened to Brother Julian the Arab. He had made the pilgrimage to the pillar of St Symeon Stylites the Younger on the Mons Mirabilis outside Antioch, several weeks' journey from Judaea; but being completely blind, of all the brethren he must have been the least likely to have escaped the massacre.

Indeed, of the monks of St Theodosius mentioned by Moschos, only two definitely did avoid the Persians' swords. These were 'two brothers [at the monastery] who had sworn an oath that they would never be separated from each other, either in life or death. While they were in the community, one of the brothers was attacked by a yearning to possess a woman. Unable to withstand this yearning, he said to his brother: "Release me brother, for I am driven by desire and I want to go back into the world." But the brother did not want to release him from his vow, so he went to the city with him. The first brother went into a brothel whilst the other stood outside, throwing dust from the ground onto his own head. When his brother who had gone into the bordello came out, having done the deed, the other said to him, "My brother, what have you gained by this sin? Let us go back to our cloister." But the first replied, "I cannot go back into the wilderness again. You go. I am staying in the world."'

Unable to change his mind, the second brother stayed with him, and the pair found work on a construction site on the outskirts of Jerusalem, where a new monastery was being built. 'The brother who visited the brothel would take both their wages and go off to the city each weekend where he would squander their earnings in riotous living. But the other brother never complained. Instead he would fast all day long, performing his work in profound silence, not speaking to anybody.' The other workmen on the building site soon realised that something odd was going on and eventually told the Abbot, Abba Abraham. The Abbot soon winkled out the whole story.

'"It is because of my brother," said the good monk, "that I put up with all this, in the hope that God will look on my affliction and save my friend." When the godly Abraham heard this, he replied: "The Lord has granted you the soul of your brother too." He dismissed the good brother, and behold! Outside the Abbot's cell, there was his fallen brother, crying: "My brother, take me into the wilderness so I can be saved!" He immediately took him and went to a cave near the holy Jordan where he walled him up. After a little while, the sinful brother, having made great spiritual progress in things that are God's, departed this life. The other brother, still faithful to his oath, remained in the cave, and eventually he too died there.'

I stood before the grave of John Moschos, the man whose writings had brought me on this journey, and in whose footsteps I was travelling. On top of the slab rested a modern icon of the man, shown old and grey with a scroll in one hand and a quill in the other. So, I thought, this was where he started off, and where, after all his travels through the width and breadth of the Byzantine Levant, he ended up.

Prompted by the example of the nun, despite having half dropped the habit, I began to pray there, and the prayers came with surprising ease. I prayed for the people who had helped me on the journey, the monks who had showed me the manuscript on Mount Athos, the frightened Suriani of Mar Gabriel, the Armenians of Aleppo and the Palestinian Christians in the camp at Mar Elias. And then I did what I suppose I had come to do: I sought the blessing of John Moschos for the rest of the trip, and particularly asked for his protection in the badlands of Upper Egypt, the most dangerous part of the journey.

Then I rose, climbed the stairs, and emerged blinking into the bright light of the Judaean midday.

The Monastery of Mar Saba lies ten miles from that of St Theodosius, a little to the north of the Dead Sea. Around St Theodosius the soil is still grudgingly fertile, and the olive trees stand out against the terraces cut into the hard white hillsides. But as you drive east, the cultivation recedes. The soil becomes thinner, the valleys deeper, and the villages poorer. The taxi driver warned me that we were entering Hamas territory, and hung a Palestinian *keffiyeh* over half of the windscreen to make sure we would not be mistaken for Israeli settlers and stoned by the local *shabab*.

Passing the last village, we entered the desert; the *locus horrendae et vastae solitudinis* of the Bible. Below us the barren shale hills fell away towards the lowest point on earth, the Dead Sea, a quivering drop of mercury in the far distance. Straight ahead, in the distance a pair of small rectangular Byzantine watchtowers rose vertically against the lip of a deep *wadi*. In the forty miles of landscape visible from the hilltop, those two towers were the only buildings in sight.

It was only when we passed underneath the machicolation of the nearest tower that we caught our first glimpse of the great monastery that lay hidden in the lee of the sheer cliff-face below. It was the most extraordinary sight. The two towers are linked by a jagged wall which sweeps audaciously down in a near-vertical plunge to enclose the monastery's great spread of turquoise domes and cupolas, balconies and cave-cells, staircases and platforms, all propped up on narrow artificial ledges by great ranks of heavy, stepped buttresses. Despite its massive rocky solidity, the monastery's implausible position on a cliff-face in the midst of the wilderness somehow gives the whole place a fantastic, almost visionary appearance, like one of those castles in children's fairy tales capable of vanishing in the blink of an eye.

At the time of John Moschos, the wastes of Judaea had become so densely filled with monks and monasteries that, according to one chronicler, 'the desert had become a city'. Yet of the 150 monasteries founded during the Byzantine rule, only six are still lived in, and of those only one, Mar Saba, still supports enough monks to really qualify as a living monastery. It has been occupied continuously since its foundation in the late fifth century: since the two-week hiatus following the massacre of the monks by the Persians in 614 A.D. – the same raid that devastated St Theodosius – divine office has been sung in the rock chapel of St Sabas every morning for the last 1,380 years. As in St Theodosius, the skulls of the hundreds of monks killed by the Persians, along with those subsequently murdered by marauding Bedouin, have been carefully kept in the abbey church, stacked in neat rows as nonchalantly as other churches might stack their hymn books.

Mar Saba, I quickly discovered, remains the most austere of monasteries. The monks rise at two in the morning and sing the office for five hours, until dawn begins to break over the iconostasis of the abbey church. The fathers then rest until eleven, when they eat their one meal of the day: bread (baked once a week, palatable enough for three days but increasingly hard and stale thereafter), thin soup, boiled vegetables and strong feta cheese. They do not eat meat, and allow themselves fish and oil (for dressing the vegetables) only on Sundays and feast days. After their meal they retire to their caves and cells for the rest of the day, emerging only to sing vespers and compline at the appointed times.

If Mar Saba is now remarkable mainly for the terrible severity of its asceticism, it was once famous for its scholarship, and despite the monastery's extreme isolation it was nevertheless one of the intellectual and philosophical powerhouses of Byzantium. When the Anglo-Saxon pilgrim St Willibald visited it in the early eighth century he remarked on the fact that all the monks were busy copying out manuscripts and composing hymns and poems. The monastery's library, now kept in the Greek Orthodox Patriarchal Palace in Jerusalem, is almost unrivalled amongst medieval collections in the esoteric breadth of its interests and the number of languages represented; it is also evidence of the extraordinary quality of the copying and calligraphy produced in the Mar Saba scriptorium.

Here Cyril of Scythopolis wrote his *History of the Monks of Palestine*, an unusually critical and intelligent work of hagiography. Mar Saba's hymnography, the work among others of Romanos the Melodist, was, according to the great Byzantine scholar Brehier, 'the most original manifestation of the poetic genius of the medieval Greeks'. Moreover it was in a cell in Mar Saba that St John Damascene wrote his great *Fount of Knowledge*, probably the most sophisticated and encyclopedic work of theology produced anywhere in Christendom until the time of Thomas Aquinas; indeed, Aquinas drew heavily on John's theology, and wrote that he read a few pages of John Damascene's work every day of his adult life. But the scope of the monastery's manuscript collection, and the erudition of John Damascene, is perhaps most dramatically demonstrated by one of his more unusual productions, the *Romance of Barlaam and Joasaph*, an Indian tale of the Buddha reworked in Christian form; it was later translated from Greek into Latin and widely circulated in the West. But you would never guess any of this from talking to Mar Saba's current inhabitants.

'So, you're a writer, are you?' asked Fr. Theophanes when he brought me my supper on a tray after vespers that evening. 'I've stopped reading books myself.'

'Oh yes?'

'The Divine Liturgy contains all the writing I need. Once you've read the Word of God everything else becomes very dull.'

'They say books are like food,' pointed out Fr. Evdokimos, the Deputy Archimandrite. 'They feed your brain.'

'But Father,' said Theophanes quietly, 'monks should try to eat as little as possible.'

It was nearly dark. We were sitting out on the terrace, watching the last of the light begin to fade from the sky. As we talked, Theophanes took out a box of matches and began to light a pair of battered old paraffin storm lanterns: there is no electricity in Mar Saba.

'Look at those clouds in the east,' said Fr. Evdokimos. 'There may be rain tomorrow. What do you think, Theophanes?'

'The rains here in Palestine are not like the rains of Greece,' replied the other monk. 'There we get big rains – proper cloudbursts.' He smiled happily at the memory. 'Ah, the rains of Greece,' he said. 'They are a reminder of the Deluge.'

'What did you do in Greece before you became a monk?' I asked Theophanes.

'I was a policeman, in Athens,' he replied, looking up from the lanterns, whose wicks he was engaged in trimming. 'I came here for the first time on a pilgrimage. As soon as I saw this monastery I recognised it as my true home. I went back to Athens, handed in my resignation and said goodbye to my mother. A week later I was back here. Since then I've never left.'

'Never?'

'I went back only once. For forty days.'

'Was that difficult?'

'My mother cried sometimes. But otherwise, no. Things change very quickly. I hardly recognised my old city. My people had suddenly become rich from your European Community. There were so many new buildings. New buildings and new crimes.'

'And you don't miss anything of your old life?'

'What is there to miss? I have everything here.'

'But this must have been quite a change from your previous work.'

'Not so different,' replied the monk. 'Now I am the policeman of my soul. Demons are very like criminals. Both are very stupid. Both are damned.'

The lanterns were alight now, and the flickering of their flames threw shadows over the terrace and across the face of Fr. Theophanes.

'You believe in demons?' I asked.

'Of course. They are in the Bible.'

'Sometimes, when we are praying, the demons make strange noises,' added Fr. Evdokimos, who had been sitting quietly in the corner, stroking his beard. 'At first I thought it was just the animals of the desert. But then I noticed the noises came most loudly when I was praying. It is the demons trying to distract us.'

'Each demon has its own personality,' said Theophanes. 'They live in the desert and come to the cities to make men into criminals and Roman Catholics.'

'They can work miracles and make false prophecies,' said Evdokimos.

'They are worse than criminals,' said Theophanes. 'But here, within the walls of Mar Saba, we are protected.'

'What do you mean?'

'St Sabas is alive here. He protects his monastery. I have experienced it myself.'

'How?'

'Three years ago on a windy night in winter I was praying in my cave. I had not lit a lamp so my cell was pitch black. As I prayed I heard footsteps coming up the corridor. It was the noise of a monk walking: I could hear the rustling of his habit. The footsteps came closer and closer and then stopped outside my room. I waited for the monk to speak, but nothing happened.

'Suddenly I heard very clearly the noise of many feet tripping down the stairs from the opposite direction. They were like madmen, jumping down the steps very quickly – loud, irregular footsteps: there were maybe nine or ten of them, all running. I thought: the Bedouin have climbed the walls and broken in and now they want to kill us all. I froze behind my door, but nothing happened. Five minutes passed. Still they didn't come in. So very slowly I opened the door and went out.

'It was a full moon that night. I could see clearly that the corridor was empty. There was silence in the monastery. I walked up to the courtyard and at that moment I saw Fr. Evdokimos's light moving from the latrines to his room. So I went up and said: "Father – there are thieves in the monastery." He asked: "You are sure?" I said I was. "All right," he said, "we'll look together." So we both took sticks and for an hour we went all around. We searched in the church, in the towers, inside the deepest caves. Nothing: the door was secure and no one had come in over the wall.'

'It was only later,' said Fr. Evdokimos, 'when we discussed the matter with the Archimandrite, that we understood what had happened. The first set of footsteps were those of St Sabas. The rabble were demons coming to turn Fr. Theophanes into a Freemason. St Sabas knew what they were planning, so he stood in front of Fr. Theophanes's door to guard it. Then he chased the demons away.'

'The Devil will capture everyone if he gets the chance,' said Theophanes gravely. 'But the saints protect us. In this monastery I feel secure, although it is in the middle of the desert, with Bedouin all around us. We are protected.'

It was late, and the monks began to drift off to their cells carrying their lanterns. Theophanes showed me to mine and promised to wake me for matins at two.

All night, it seemed, bells were pealing. At one o'clock a monk began to knock the wooden *simandron* to call the brethren from their beds; he rang it again at one-thirty and at five to two. At two I was treated to a full-scale bell-ringing display: the bells in the campanile assisted by a selection of handbells, one rung very loudly at the door of my cell by Fr. Theophanes. But as soon as silence had returned I fell asleep again, and it was nearly four a.m before I finally pulled myself out of bed. It was pitch dark and very cold. I dressed by the light of the lantern, then picked my way down through the empty stairways and corridors of Mar Saba, towards the deep swell and eddy of monastic chant.

In the church all the lamps were lit, casting a dim glow over the basilica. The monastic *kyries* echoed around the dome. Only the occasional creak of a misericord gave away the position of the singers; the monks themselves were invisible in their black robes as they roosted in the choirstalls. Every so often a breeze would swing one of the chandeliers, rotating it slightly so that shadows raced around the church, the returning flash of candlelight picking out the highlights in the frescoes: the wings of angels and the long white beards of the desert fathers. The chant eddied out across the narrow valley, echoed and amplified by the domes and cupolas. As I sat at the back, I kept thinking that the very same sound would have been heard by John Moschos over fourteen hundred years ago.

Towards six o'clock first light began to filter in, gently illuminating the Christ Pantocrator in the dome. Half an hour later, with the sun now rising over the desert, I began to be able to pick out the monks themselves, black bearded, black robed, hooded and veiled in their stalls. What I had initially taken to be a low table near the lectern turned out to be Fr. Evdokimos, kneeling, bent forward on the ground in a long prostration before the iconostasis.

One by one the monks glided from the church, each stopping to kiss images of the saints on the frescoes and icons as they went. I returned to my bed and slept until noon, when Fr. Theophanes woke me with a tray of food: a lump of strong-smelling feta cheese, some coarse monastic bread and, sitting proudly on its own on a white plate, a small round chocolate.

'It is the feast of St Methodius the Stylite,' said Fr. Theophanes gravely. 'This is for you to celebrate it with.'

I spent the afternoon in my cell reading John Moschos's stories of the monks of the Judaean desert. Together, the stories in *The Spiritual Meadow* form a detailed picture of one of the strangest periods in the region's history. For around two hundred years the deserts of the Holy Land were filled not only with 150 fully functioning monasteries, but also with countless cave-dwelling hermits and great herds of 'grazers', nomadic monks who, according to Moschos, 'wander in the desert as if they were wild animals: like birds they fly about the hills; they forage like goats. Their daily round is inflexible, always predictable, for they feed on roots, the natural products of the earth.'

Today it seems inexplicable that so many people – many of them highly educated – from across the width of the civilised Byzantine world would give up everything and travel for thousands of miles to live a life of extreme hardship in the discomfort of the desert; yet to the Byzantine mind nothing could have been more logical. In one of Moschos's stories, a stranger visits the renowned holy man Abba Olympios in his monastery in the heat and humidity of the Jordan Valley. 'How can you stay in this place with its burning heat and so many insects?' he asks. The holy man gives a simple answer: 'I put up with the insects to escape from what scripture calls "the worm that sleeps not". Likewise, I endure the burning heat for fear of the eternal fire. The one is temporary, but of the other there is no end.'

Yet this was not the whole story. While Moschos never underestimates the hardship involved in the life of the desert fathers, he is also well aware of its joys. Indeed one of the principal themes of his writing is that by living in utter simplicity and holiness, the monks were returning to the conditions of the Garden of Eden, in harmony with both the natural world and its Creator. This is particularly true of the grazers, who like Adam ate without planting and were supposed to have command over the wild animals. 'With Christ,' wrote the early Christian traveller Sulpicius Severus, 'every brute beast is wise, and every savage creature gentle.' The close relationship of beasts and saints was not a new theme in monastic literature: the early Coptic *Life* of St Pachomius, for example, tells how the saint summoned crocodiles to ferry him across the Nile, rather as today one might call a cab from a taxi rank. Moreover *The Paradise of the Fathers*, one of Moschos's principal literary models, contains a number of stories on this theme:

'There was an old man who dwelt by the Jordan practising asceticism. One day he went into a cave to escape from the heat, and there he found a lion. It began to gnash its teeth at him and to roar. So the old man said to it, "Why are you annoyed? There is room here to take me and to take you also. If you do not wish to abide with me, arise and go!" And the lion did not carry him off but instead went out.'

Moschos first introduces this theme in a story told by Abba Agathonicos, the Abbot of Castellium, once the sister monastery to Mar Saba, now a ruin five miles further down the Kedron Valley:

'One day,' Abba Agathonicos tells Moschos, 'I went down to Rouba to visit Abba Poemon the Grazer. When I found him, I told him the thoughts which troubled me. When night fell he left me in a cave. It was winter and that night it got very cold indeed. I was freezing. When the elder came at dawn, he said to me: "What is the matter, child? I did not feel the cold." This amazed me, for he was naked. I asked him of his charity to tell me how he did not feel the cold. He said: "A lion came down and lay beside me; he kept me warm."'

But perhaps the most memorable fable of the Eden-like closeness of monks and beasts in the desert is Moschos's famous tale of St Gerasimos and the lion. Centuries later in the West, the story was mistakenly grafted onto the life of St Jerome, apparently through the ignorance of Latin-speaking pilgrims. In the Eastern Church, however, the tale has remained correctly attributed to St Gerasimos, and is still one of the most popular Orthodox saints' tales. Moreover, it is one of the few of Moschos's tales to have entered the repertoire of Byzantine art, and is occasionally found frescoed on Orthodox monastery walls: in Athos, for example, I saw several scenes from the story painted in the porch of the abbey church of the Monastery of Xenophontos. The story is set in St Gerasimos's monastery, 'about a mile from the Holy Jordan'.

'When [Sophronius and I] were visiting the monastery,' writes Moschos, 'the residents told us that St Gerasimos was walking one day by the banks of the Holy Jordan when he met a lion, roaring mightily because of the pain in its paw. The point of a reed was deeply embedded in it, causing inflammation. When the lion saw the elder, it came to him and showed him the foot, whimpering and begging some healing from him. When the elder saw the lion in such distress, he sat down and, taking the paw, he lanced it. The point was removed and also much pus. He cleansed the wound well, bound it up and dismissed the beast. But the healed lion would not leave the elder. It followed him like a disciple wherever he went. The elder was amazed at the gentle disposition of the beast and, from then on, he began feeding it, throwing it bread and boiled vegetables.

'Now the *lavra* had an ass which was used to fetch water for the needs of the elders, for they drink the water of the Holy Jordan which lies about one mile away from the monastery. The fathers used to hand the ass over to the lion, to pasture it on the banks of the Jordan. One day when the ass was being taken to pasture by the lion, it went away some distance from its keeper. Some camel-drivers on their way from Arabia found the ass and took it away to their country. Having lost the ass, the lion came back to the *lavra* and approached Abba Gerasimos, very downcast and dismayed. The Abba thought the lion had devoured the ass. He said to it: "Where is the ass?" The beast stood silent, very like a man. The elder said to it: "Have you eaten it? From now on [as a punishment] you will perform the same duties the ass performed." From then on, at the elder's command, the lion used to carry the saddlepack containing four earthenware vessels and bring water.

'[Many months later] the camel-driver who had taken the ass came back to the Holy City with the animal loaded up with the grain he hoped to sell there. Having crossed the Holy Jordan, he suddenly found himself face to face with the lion. When he saw the beast, he left his camels and took to his heels. Recognising the ass, the lion ran to it, seized its leading rein in its mouth just as it had been trained to do, and led away not only the ass, but also the three camels. It brought them to the elder, rejoicing and roaring. The elder now realised that the lion had been falsely accused. He named the lion Jordanes and it lived with the elder in the *lavra*, never leaving his side for five years.

'When Abba Gerasimos departed to the Lord and was buried by the fathers, by the providence of God the lion could not be found. A little later the lion returned, searching for the elder, roaring mightily. When Abba Sabbatios and the rest of the fathers saw it, they stroked its mane and said to it: "The elder has gone away to the Lord and left us," yet even saying this did not succeed in silencing its cries and lamentations. Then Abba Sabbatios said to it: "Since you do not believe us, come with me and I will show you where Gerasimos lies." He took the lion and led it to where they had buried the elder, half a mile from the church. Abba Sabbatios said to the lion: "See, this is where our friend is," and he knelt down. When the lion saw how he prostrated himself, it began beating its head against the ground and roaring. Then it promptly [rolled over and] died, there on the elder's grave.'

Over the days that followed I explored many of the caves, cells and chapels which honeycomb the cliffs within the great boundary walls of Mar Saba. Earthquakes and Bedouin raids have led to much rebuilding over the centuries, but if you look hard enough, many fragments of the Byzantine monastery known to John Moschos still survive. The great cave chapel 'Built by God' stands as bare and austere as it would have done in the early Byzantine period. The only obvious additions are some late-medieval icons, a line of eighteenth-century choirstalls and the four hundred stacked skulls of the monks slaughtered in the seventh-century Persian invasion. In another grotto, the Retreat of St Sabas, the floor is still covered with the fragmentary tesserae of a simple geometric mosaic dating from the late sixth century. But the most interesting chapel of all is that built around the tomb and hermitage of St John Damascene.

John Damascene is probably the most important figure ever to have taken the habit at Mar Saba. He was the grandson of the last Byzantine Governor of Damascus, a Syrian Arab Christian named Mansour ibn Sargun. Ibn Sargun was responsible for surrendering the city to the Muslim General Khalid ibn Walid in 635, just three years after the death of Mohammed. Despite the change from Christian to Islamic rule, the family remained powerful. John's father, Sergios ibn Mansour, rose to become a senior figure in the financial administration of the early Ummayad Caliphate, whose accounts, significantly enough, continued for many decades to be kept in Greek. Because of this John grew up as a close companion of the future Caliph al-Yazid, and the two youths' drinking bouts in the streets of Damascus were the subject of much horrified gossip in the new Islamic capital. In due course John assumed his father's post in the administration, and he remained throughout his life a favourite of the Caliph. This relationship made him one of the very first Arab Christians capable of acting as a bridge between Christianity and Islam, even if, like so many who attempt to bring together two diverging cultures, he eventually ended up being regarded with suspicion by both: dismissed from his administrative job after Caliph Yazid's death and falsely accused of collusion with the Byzantine Emperor, he was nevertheless regarded with great mistrust in the Byzantine capital, where he was dubbed *Sarakenophron*, or Saracen-Minded.

John was in an excellent position to write the first ever informed treatise on Islam by a Christian, and when he retired to Mar Saba he dedicated his declining years to writing doctrinal homilies and working on his great masterpiece, a refutation of heresies entitled *The Fount of Knowledge*. The book contains an extremely precise and detailed critique of Islam, which, intriguingly, John regards as a form of Christian heresy related to Arianism (after all, like Islam, Arianism denied the divinity of Christ). It never seems to have occurred to John that Islam might be a separate religion, and although he looked on it with considerable suspicion, he nevertheless applauds the way Islam converted the Arabs from idolatry, and writes with admiration of its single-minded emphasis on the unity of God.

If a theologian of the stature of John Damascene was able to regard Islam as a new – if heretical – form of Christianity, it helps to explain how Islam was able to convert so much of the Middle Eastern population in so short a time, even if Christianity remained the majority religion until the time of the Crusades. Islam was as much a product of the intellectual ferment of late antiquity as Gnosticism, Arianism and Monophysitism, and like those heresies it had its greatest success in areas disgruntled with Byzantine rule. Many Syrians expressed opposition to Byzantium and its ruthless attempt to impose its rigid imperial theology by converting *en masse* to the heterodox Christian doctrine of Monophysitism; later they greeted the conquering Arab armies as liberators and many converted again, this time to Islam. No doubt they regarded the Arabs' new creed as a small step from Monophysitism; after all, the two faiths started from a similar position: that God could not become fully human without somehow compromising his divinity.

Whatever the reason for its success, Islam certainly appealed to the former Monophysites, and within a century of the Arab conquest Syria was a mainly Muslim country. By contrast, the inhabitants of Palestine, who had done well out of Byzantine patronage of the Holy Places, never showed much interest in converting either to Monophysitism or to Islam, and Jerusalem remained a predominantly Orthodox Christian city until the Crusaders conquered it in 1099.

In Damascene's own lifetime, however, the most influential part of *The Fount of Knowledge* was not the section on Islam, but his attack on the heresy of Iconoclasm. For at the same time as John was becoming a monk, Byzantium was being engulfed by a wave of image-smashing. All the icons in the Empire were ordered to be destroyed, and their painting was henceforth banned. The reason for this may well have been the rise of Islam and the profound soul-searching which the loss of the Levant provoked in Byzantium. Many came to the conclusion that God was angry with the Byzantines for their idolatry, and thus gave the iconoclastic Muslims success in their wars.

Just as John's public life demonstrates the astonishing political tolerance of the Ummayad Caliphate in its willingness to employ a Christian in a senior administrative role, despite almost continuous hostilities with the rest of the Christian World, so his retirement demonstrates the surprising degree of intellectual freedom it permitted. For under the Ummayads John was able to do what no Byzantine was permitted to attempt: to write and distribute a systematic defence of images, in which he provided the fundamental theological counterblast to iconoclasm. John argued that although no man has seen God at any time, nevertheless, since Christ deigned to take upon himself the human form, it was necessary to worship the human face of God in the sacred icon. Moreover he demonstrated that not only was their cult based on reason, but that it was sanctioned by ancient precedent:

> Paintings are the books of the illiterate. They instruct those who look at them with a silent voice and sanctify life ... Since not everyone knows how to read, or has the leisure for reading, the Fathers of the Church saw fit that the Incarnate Christ be represented by images,

like deeds of prowess, to serve as reminders. Often when we are not thinking of the Lord's passion, we see the image of the crucifixion, and being reminded of that salutary passion, we fall to our knees and revere . . . If I have no books I go to church, pricked as by spines by my thoughts; the flower of painting makes me look, charms my eyes as does a flowering meadow and softly distils the glory of God in my soul.

This afternoon, after I had woken from a siesta, Theophanes took me to John Damascene's old cell. We walked along the narrow staircases and winding paths that connect the different platforms of the monastery. Eventually we came to a small chapel backing onto the rock wall. 'This chapel was where St John's body used to lie,' said Theophanes, 'before your Pope's Crusaders came and stole him.'

'Where is he now?'

'In Venice,' said Theophanes. 'One of the world capitals of body-snatching and criminal Freemasonry.'

Inside the chapel hung a line of icons, and over the spot where the tomb used to lie, a fresco showing the death of St John Damascene, an icon clutched firmly to his breast. Below this a narrow wooden staircase led down into a tiny cave, its ceiling cut so low as to make standing virtually impossible.

'St John spent thirty years in that place,' said Theophanes. 'Although he could not stand he hardly ever went out of it. He believed he had become too proud because of his high position in the court in Damascus, so he chose this cave in which to live as a monk. He said it was very humbling – very good for the soul – to live in such a place for many years.'

'After an *hour* in there you must feel like a hunchback,' I said.

'Better hunchbacked than damned,' replied the monk.

While Theophanes stood by the empty tomb, contemplating, no doubt, the damnation of the Papist body-snatchers, I clambered down the wooden stairs into the gloom of the saint's cave. On either side two stone benches had been cut from the rock, while ahead stood a low shelf that had once acted as the saint's writing

301

desk. Beyond was a small shrine: at the far end of the cave stretched a recess, four feet high, six feet deep, which John Damascene had used as a bed. A small Byzantine icon of the Madonna hung from the wall; otherwise the cell was almost impossibly austere.

It seemed strange that a book of such breathtaking sophistication as *The Fount of Knowledge* could be produced in so astonishingly crude and primitive a cave. It was certainly an unlikely setting for the writing of one of the most important tracts ever to be penned in defence of artistic freedom. What Damascene wrote in this cave was largely responsible for saving Byzantium from the ban against sacred art that has always been a part of Islam and Judaism. Without Damascene's work, Byzantine *ars sacra* would never again have been permitted, Greek painters might never have been able to pass on their secrets to Giotto and the Sienese, and the course of the Renaissance, if it had happened at all, would have been very different.

Sometime in the late 1960s, soon after the Israeli conquest of the West Bank, the number of monks at Mar Saba fell for the first time below twenty. At this time the Abbot of the monastery had been persuaded by the Greek Orthodox Patriarch in Jerusalem to cease trying to be self-sufficient. He should sell Mar Saba's ancient lands to the Israeli government, advised the Patriarch; the Orthodox hierarchy would invest the money and in return send to the monastery all the cheese and fish the monks could possibly need. The Abbot acceded to the Patriarch's wishes, and ever since then the monks' food has been brought in by van from Jerusalem once a week. The van was due on the last day of my stay at Mar Saba, and Fr. Theophanes promised to arrange that it should take me back to Jerusalem on its return journey.

There were still many Byzantine remains in the valley below the monastery that I had not seen, and I woke early on my final morning, in the hope of seeing some of the more distant cells and grottoes before I was collected later that afternoon.

I was let out by Fr. Cosmas, the gatekeeper, who slid back the heavy medieval bolts of the gate behind me. Outside I found the old path down the cliff-face into the valley. It led off from the top of the cliff beside the Byzantine tower built by the Empress Eudoxia; it had once been home to a small convent of nuns, but was now abandoned and quite deserted. I picked my way down the hairpin bends, stopping to pluck a sprig of wild rosemary from a bush and squeeze it between my thumb and forefinger. As I was standing there, a dun-coloured desert fox darted from its shelter in an abandoned cell and shot off behind a bend in the *wadi*.

At the bottom of the valley I forded the dark waters of the heavily polluted river. It was a steep climb up the other side of the valley, but the reward was a breathtaking view of the monastery. Indeed it was only from the opposite lip of the chasm that the full strangeness of Mar Saba's position became apparent: the great tumble of lavender domes and egg-shaped cupolas were perched precariously on the narrowest of ledges and overhangs. All this was enclosed by the near-vertical wall built soon after the Persian massacre whose massive strength had, for nearly 1,400 years, successfully protected the monks from human and natural calamities.

Looking down the steep slope on which I was standing, I saw that the rockface was pockmarked by the entrances to monks' cells, all of which were now deserted. Some of these cells were little more than burrows; others, perched on ledges above the gorge, were relatively sophisticated conical beehives, intriguingly similar in design to the cells of the Celtic monks of the same period preserved in the more remote corners of Ireland, such as the coastal island of Skellig Michael. Like their Irish counterparts, these cells were drystone, built without mortar, and rose to steeply pitched gables; like the cells of Skellig Michael they were usually bare and unornamented but for an arched prayer niche on the east wall; like them they had the same low entrance capped with a monolithic lintel.

There were also other quite distinct cell-types. Some were partially-walled-up caves. A few were elaborate multi-storeyed affairs

303

containing cisterns, living quarters and oratories; like the *kelli* of modern Athos, these were clearly designed not for single hermits but for the use of small groups of monks: perhaps a superior and four or five of his disciples, or a party from some distant and distinct ethnic group – say Georgians or Armenians – who wished to keep together. In some of the chapels and oratories attached to these more elaborate cells there were still traces of mosaic floorings and even fragments of simple geometric frescoes on the walls: floral patterns created by overlapping circles, or designs of intermeshing crosses.

Different as they were, all the monks' cells in the valley had two things in common. One was that nearly all had been attacked at some stage by treasure hunters who had dug great holes in their floors, presumably in search of buried coins or precious chalices. The other was the prayer niche, a small arched cut in the eastern wall of the cell indicating the proper direction for prayer. As I passed from cell to cell, I realised that the prayer niche must be another of those features of the early Christian world which has been lost to modern Western Christianity, yet which is still preserved in Islam. No mosque is complete without its *mihrab* pointing in the direction of Mecca; yet how many Western churches today contain prayer niches? Certainly all are still orientated towards the east, but the idea of a niche emphasising this fact is now quite forgotten. Just as St John Damascene's life stressed the close relationship between Christianity and early Islam – a kinship and proximity that is now forgotten by both faiths – so the prayer niches contained in the cells around Damascene's old monastery seemed to emphasise how much Islam inherited from the Byzantine world.

As at Cyrrhus, I was left pondering the probability that if John Moschos came back today, he would be likely to find as much that was familiar in the practices of Islam – with its fasting, prostrations, prayer niches and open prayer halls, as well as its emphasis on the wandering holy man – as in those of modern Western Christendom. In an age when Islam and Christianity are again said to be 'clashing civilisations', supposedly 'irreconcilable and necessarily hostile', it is important to remember Islam's very considerable debt to the early Christian world, and the degree to which it has faithfully preserved elements of our own early Christian heritage long forgotten by ourselves.

Fr. Theophanes brought me my lunch on a tray and announced that the van would soon be ready to carry me to Jerusalem. He stood by as I ate, like a *maître d'hôte* waiting to see a diner's reaction to some especially delicate soufflé. This precipitated something of an etiquette problem.

Lunch at Mar Saba was never a very ritzy affair at the best of times, but towards the end of the week, when the bread baked days earlier had hardened to the texture of pumice, and the feta cheese had begun to smell increasingly like dead goat, eating Fr. Theophanes's offerings became something of a penitential exercise, and sounding sincere in one's appreciation of the monks' culinary abilities was a task that needed advanced acting skills. I looked at the lump of rock-bread and the festering cheese, and tried to think of something nice to say about them. Then I had a flash of inspiration.

'Mmm,' I said, taking a sip from the glass. 'Delicious water, Fr. Theophanes.'

This, oddly enough, went down very well.

'The water here is very sweet.' The monk allowed himself a brief smile.

'Very sweet, Fr. Theophanes.'

'During this summer we had a drought. Our cisterns were beginning to run dry. August went by. Then September. One after another our cisterns gave up. We were like the Children of Israel in the wilderness. But St Sabas takes care of us. We are never without some drinking water. We always have the spring.'

'The spring?'

'The spring of St Sabas. He prayed and it came. You do not know the story?'

'Tell it to me.'

'In the days of St Sabas more and more monks were joining the *lavra* to be with the saint. Eventually the number of brethren grew to seven hundred, and there was not enough water to go around. So St Sabas prayed. For thirty days and thirty nights he prayed on the roof of his cell, refusing to eat in the hope that our Lord would look down with mercy on his people. Finally, at the end of the thirty days and thirty nights, it happened to be a full moon. St Sabas went onto the roof for the last time to beg the Lord for mercy. He began to pray when all of a sudden he heard the beating of a wild ass's hooves in the valley below. He looked out and saw the animal. It was charging down the valley as if sent by the Angel Gabriel himself. Then it stopped, looked around and began digging deep into the gravel. It dug for twenty minutes, then it bent down and began to drink.

'St Sabas spent the night giving thanks to the Lord. The following morning he climbed down the cliff. At the bottom, just as he expected, he found that the ass had revealed a spring of living water. It was a constant supply that never ever fails. Even today. And incidentally it tastes very good in ouzo. This is one of the compensations that St Sabas gives us for our sufferings.'

'What are the others?' I asked.

'There are many,' he said. 'But the most remarkable is this: after we leave our mortal frame, our bodies never grow stiff.'

'I'm sorry?'

'After we are dead we never get stiff. We never suffer from . . . how do you say . . . ?'

'Corruption? Decomposition?'

'That's right: decomposition.' Fr. Theophanes rolled the word around his mouth as if savouring the notion of mortal decay. 'But the monks of this monastery, instead of giving off a foul stench of decay, emit a sweet fragrance. Like the scent of precious myrrh.'

I must have looked sceptical, for Theophanes added: 'It is true. Many scientists have visited the monastery and declared themselves baffled. Anyway,' he said, changing the subject, 'what were you doing in the valley this morning?'

I told him, and remarked on the number of cells which appeared to have been desecrated by treasure hunters.

'It is the Bedouin,' replied Theophanes. 'They are always looking for buried gold. Sometimes they ring the bell of the monastery and ask for incense from the cave of St Sabas to help them find their gold.'

'How does that help?'

'Sometimes they find gold in caves or old ruins, but they dare not take it in case it is guarded by a *djinn*. They go to their sheikhs, but they can do nothing, so the sheikhs tell them to come here. The Muslims believe that if they get incense from here they can burn it and the holy fumes will scare away the *djinn*.'

'Do you give them incense?' I asked.

'No. It would be blasphemous to use a holy substance for such a purpose. But sometimes I wonder . . .'

'What do you mean?'

'Well . . . Once a man from Bethlehem came here. He was a taxi driver, named Mohammed. I knew him a little because he sometimes brought monks or pilgrims to us. Anyway, one day he rang the bell and asked for incense, saying that he had found some gold in a pot: it had been turned up by a plough on the land belonging to his family. He said his family were worried in case it was guarded by an evil *djinn*. I said no, he could not have it. Now he is dead. Sometimes I wonder whether I should have said yes.'

'What do you mean, "Now he is dead"?'

'He left here, went home and broke open the pot. Straight away he went crazy. He got iller and iller, skinnier and skinnier. Before, he was a strong man. But slowly he became like a skeleton. Bones, a little skin, nothing more. Finally, three months ago, he died.' Theophanes shook his head. 'The Muslims think the *djinns* are different from demons, but this is just a trick of the Devil. There is no such thing as *djinns*: just devils in disguise. Now this man's soul will go to Hell.'

Theophanes crossed himself, from right to left in the Orthodox manner: 'He lost the gold and he lost his soul. Now he will burn like a Freemason.'

'Fr. Theophanes,' I asked, my curiosity finally getting the better of me, 'I don't understand why you are so worried by the Free-masons.'

'Because they are the legions of the Anti-Christ. The storm-troopers of the Whore of Babylon.'

'I always thought Freemasons just held coffee mornings and whist drives and that sort of thing.'

'Wheest drives?' said Theophanes, pronouncing the word as if it were some sort of Satanic ritual. 'Probably this wheest drive also. But their main activity is to worship the Devil. There are many steps,' he said, nodding knowingly. 'But the last, the final step, is to meet with the Devil and have homosexual relations with him. After this he makes you Pope or sometimes President of the United States.'

'President of the United States . . . ?'

'Certainly. This has been proved. All the Presidents of the United States have been Freemasons. Except Kennedy. And you know what happened to him . . .'

Theophanes was still raving about the Freemasons, and the way they had masterminded the Ecumenical movement and invented the supermarket barcode, when a young novice knocked on the door to tell us that the Patriarchate van was ready to take me to Jerusalem. Theophanes helped carry my luggage to the gate.

'Be careful,' he said, as we stood by the great blue door. 'These are the Last Days. They are near their goal. They are everywhere now. Always be on your guard.'

'Goodbye, Fr.Theophanes,' I said. 'Thank you for everything.'

'They say this may be the last Pope.'

'Yes?'

'Some Holy Fathers have said this. Then the Arabs will be in Rome and the Whore of Babylon will be in the Vatican.'

'And the Freemasons?'

'These people. Who knows what they will do . . .' Theophanes frowned. 'Anyway,' he said, 'you must visit us again.'

'Thank you.'

'Maybe you will have converted to Orthodoxy by then?'
I smiled.
'I will pray for you. While there is still time. Maybe you can be saved.'

Taking a huge key from a gaoler's ring, the monk undid the bolts of the low gate in the monastery wall. 'Think about it seriously,' he said as he let me out. 'Remember, you will be among the damned if you don't.'

The heavy metal door swung closed behind me. Outside, a dust storm was just beginning.

ARARAT STREET, THE ARMENIAN QUARTER, OLD CITY OF JERUSALEM, 4 NOVEMBER

The Armenian Quarter is the most secretive of the divisions of the Old City of Jerusalem. The Muslim, Christian and Jewish Quarters all look outwards; wandering down their cobbles it is impossible not to get sucked into their flea-markets and junk shops, cafés and restaurants. The Armenian Quarter is very different. It is easy to pass it by without realising its existence. It is a city within a city, entered through its own gate and bounded by its own high, butter-coloured wall.

The gatehouse gives onto a warren of tunnels and passageways. Off one of these I have been given an old groin-vaulted room smelling of dust and old age, with a faint whiff of medieval church. In the streets around my room, hidden behind anxiously twitching lace curtains, lives a displaced population, distinct from their neighbours in language, religion, history and culture.

At the time of John Moschos, Jerusalem contained many such communities: large groups of Georgians and Armenians, Syrians and Galatians, Italians and even some Franks, most of whom had initially come to Jerusalem on pilgrimage and stayed on. Although the city is still full of small church missions, usually staffed by clerics on temporary postings, the Armenian Quarter is the last substantial community of permanent Christian exiles resident in Jerusalem.

The surprise isn't that the others have disappeared. It is that the Armenians have managed to remain. For despite the reference in the psalms to 'the peace of Jerusalem', the Holy City has probably seen more rapine and pillage, more regularly, than any comparable patch of ground on the planet. Here the Israelites battled with the Jesubites, Canaanites, Philistines, Assyrians, Babylonians, Persians, Greeks and Romans; here the Arabs eventually succeeded them only to lose control successively to the Crusaders, the Turks, the British and the Israelis. In Jerusalem every street corner has its own martyr or monument, saint or shrine. Its soil is drenched in blood spilt in the name of religion; its mental hospitals are full of whole hagiarchies of lunatics claiming to be David, Isaiah, Jesus, St Paul or Mohammed.

Yet amid this conflict between competing truths and rival certainties, the Armenian quarter is a startling example of peaceful continuity. In the third century A.D., the Armenians were the first nation to convert to Christianity, and they quickly became enthusiastic pilgrims to the Holy Places. Palestine may have been a dangerous spot to visit, but it was usually paradise compared to the Armenians' anarchic homeland. By the time of John Moschos there were over seventy Armenian churches in the city.

The Jerusalem Armenians became adept at living under foreign rule. In the eighth century, when Jerusalem was ruled by the Arab Abbasid dynasty, the Armenians managed to arrange it so that two of the Caliphs had Armenian mothers; in 1099, when the Crusaders captured the town, the first two queens of Jerusalem were also Armenian. Later, when Saladin reconquered the city for Islam, the Armenians played their cards with such skill that they were the only Christians who avoided being expelled or carried off into slavery.

After 1915, following the genocide of perhaps a million and a half Armenians at the hands of the Young Turks, the Jerusalem Armenian Quarter became a place of refuge for many of the ragged

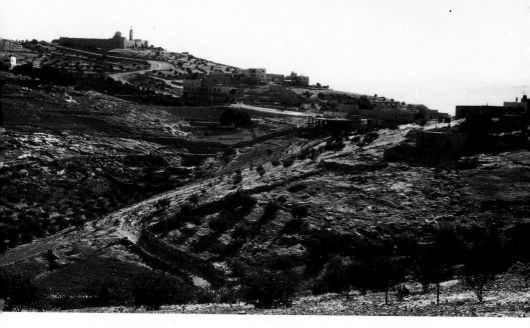

John Moschos's home monastery, Mar Theodosius, near Bethlehem.

The watchtowers of Mar Saba in the wilderness of Judaea.

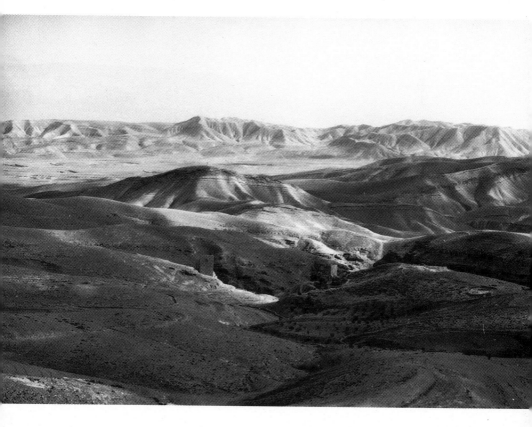

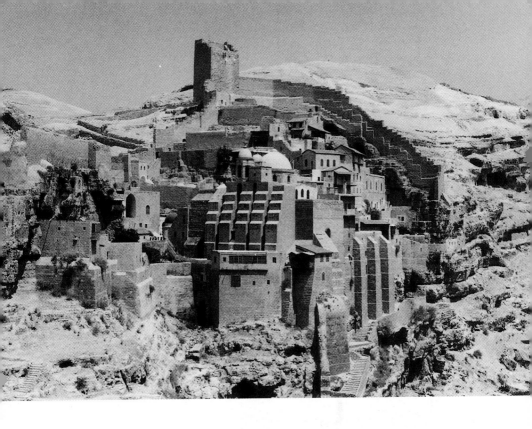

Above The Monastery of Mar
Saba.

Right Fr. Theophanes, Guest
Master of Mar Saba, at the
monastery gate.

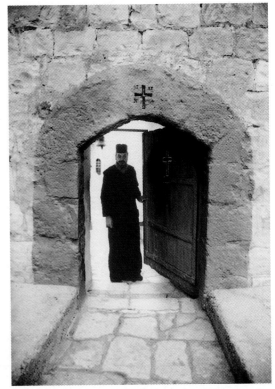

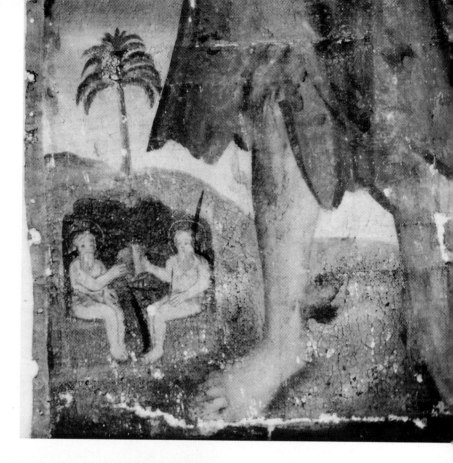

Above St Paul and St Antony breaking bread. Detail of icon at the Monastery of St Antony, Egypt.

Left The same scene carved on a Pictish symbol-stone, St Vigeans, Dundee.

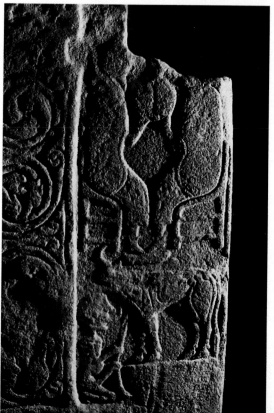

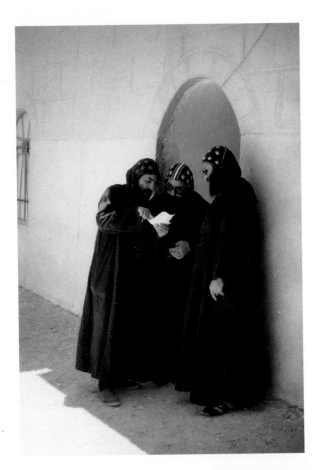

Left Fr. Dioscorus discusses the latest sighting of St Antony, Monastery of St Antony, Egypt.

Below The desert between Asyut and the Great Kharga Oasis.

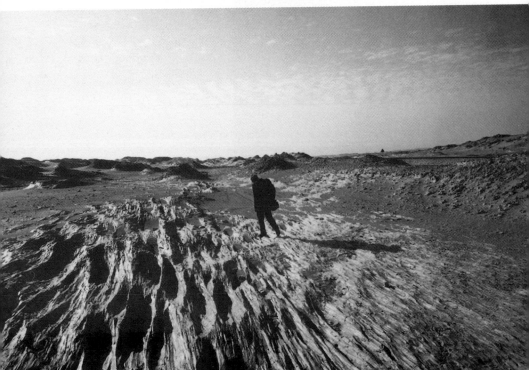

survivors. Within a couple of years the number of inhabitants in the quarter doubled, and the descendants of these people still make up about half the population of the quarter today.

Having lived through the rule of tyrants such as the hideous Mameluke Sultan, Baybars of Egypt (an ex-slave so ugly that he was once returned to the market by a horrified buyer), it might be expected that the Jerusalem Armenians might consider the current Israeli dominion over the Old City as a relatively benign period in their history; after all, the Jews and Armenians have much in common, sharing a history of wandering, trade, persecution and suffering. But it is not quite as simple as that.

A short distance from my room, in a cloister overhung with pot plants, vines and flowering shrubs, I found the rooms of Bishop Hagop Sarkissian, a friend from previous visits. Bishop Hagop is a gentle amateur antiquary who has renovated many of the medieval chapels in the quarter. His enthusiasm for Armenian architecture has overflowed into his rooms, which are now cluttered with small wooden models of Armenian churches, painstakingly reconstructed from old prints and daguerreotypes.

Bishop Hagop is a small, quiet figure with a lavender-blue cassock and a grey goatee beard. He is generally a gossipy, high-spirited man, but he has a penchant – understandably common among Armenians – for telling depressing stories about the genocide. Hagop's mother was the only one of fifty family members to survive the 1915 massacre of her people; his father, a renowned botanist and ethnographer, was one of the few Armenian intellectuals to escape the Young Turks' purges, and only did so by walking five hundred miles through Anatolia and the Levant disguised as a Turkish woman in full *chador*. Before he died in Jerusalem from the shock of the experience, he managed to finish writing what is arguably the best eyewitness account of the whole Armenian genocide.

As we sat in his rooms sipping fiery Armenian cognac, the Bishop talked angrily about a decision taken by Israeli television some time previously. A documentary film on the Armenian genocide scheduled for prime-time viewing had been mysteriously cancelled at the last minute. There had been a furious response not only from the Armenians but from many Israeli liberals, yet the television executives refused to alter their position.

'The Israelis are always insisting on the uniqueness of their Holocaust,' said Hagop. 'Now it seems they want our genocide to be forgotten. It is as if they want a monopoly on suffering.' The old man shook his head: 'In a million little ways, the Israelis make life difficult for us. Many of my people believe they want to squeeze us out.'

'That is a pretty strong accusation,' I said. On my previous visits the Bishop seemed far too absorbed in the Armenian past to worry much about contemporary politics. So I was surprised when, after downing another glass of cognac, he began to pour out his worries about the future.

'Many right-wing Israelis now say that Jerusalem should belong to the Jews only,' he said, lifting his glass to his lips again. 'These people say that Jerusalem is their eternal capital, and that we are trespassing in their city.'

The Armenians, he said, had been shaken a couple of years earlier when fundamentalist Jewish settlers of the Ateret Cohanim (Garland of the Temple Priests) had used a succession of Panamanian cover-companies to sub-let and take over the St John's Hospice near the Holy Sepulchre in the very heart of the Christian Quarter. The Armenians were more shaken still when it emerged that the settlers had been given $2 million of government funds to effect their purchase.

Under an Israeli Supreme Court ruling, non-Jews are excluded from the Jewish Quarter, and all Arabs resident there in 1967 were evicted from it. At the same time, on 10 June 1967, the entire Maghariba (Moors') district was demolished to create a plaza around the Wailing Wall. The area dated back to the fourteenth century, and included a mosque and shrine of Sheikh A'id; but despite their antiquity the 135 buildings in the district were bull-dozed and the 650 Palestinians who lived there were expelled from their homes. Yet while all the two thousand Jews who had lost property there in 1948 had their land restored, none of the thirty thousand Palestinians evicted from the Christian suburbs of West Jerusalem in 1948 were allowed to return to their old homes, nor was any reverse law promulgated to prevent Jews from settling in the Christian, Armenian and Muslim Quarters of the Old City; indeed, funds from the Israeli Housing Ministry are available to finance such colonisation, on the grounds that Jews have a right to settle anywhere in their Holy City.

By Easter 1990, when the St John's Hospice was seized, more than forty properties in the Muslim Quarter had already been acquired by the Ateret Cohanim and other radical settler groups, but the takeover of the hospice was the first attempt by settlers to move into the Christian Quarter. The move quickly snowballed into a major international controversy.

According to a report in the London *Sunday Telegraph*, a Greek priest who had forced his way inside the hospice to try to stop the looting of the property asked a settler to hand him a picture of the Last Supper. The Israeli broke the frame over his knee and trampled the canvas into the floor.

Following this incident, the octogenarian Orthodox Patriarch, the owner of the hospice, led a Maundy Thursday protest march to the property. During the demonstration one of the Greek monks attempted to remove a Star of David which the settlers had just erected over a cross carved above the hospice doorway. As he reached for the star, the Israeli policemen assigned to guard the settlers pushed the elderly Patriarch onto the ground, hit him, then pepper-gassed both him and his monastic entourage. Television cameras recorded the entire incident, setting off a further chain of international protests.

According to Hagop, the settlers were now stepping up their efforts to buy Armenian land in the Old City. Every month, he said, the Armenian Patriarchate received dozens of enquiries from middlemen acting for settlers willing to pay very high prices for a toehold in the Armenian Quarter. Others applied directly. Ariel Sharon, architect of Israel's invasion of Lebanon, had allegedly offered nearly $3.5 million for an empty parking lot and some houses backing onto it.

'We refused, of course,' said Hagop. 'But these people are fanatics. They will never give up.' The Bishop frowned. 'I am seriously worried for our future. We have been here for 1,600 years, yet we cannot be sure what will happen tomorrow. The Israelis claim that they are champions of religious freedom, but behind that smokescreen they make it impossible for our community to flourish. They have not granted one building permit to us since 1967, and they destroy any building we construct illegally. It took four years for us to get a telephone for our infirmary, while a Shin Bet [Israeli Secret Police] informer I know got one within a week. They neglect our streets. The Jewish Quarter is properly maintained, but the streets in the other quarters are subsiding because the old Ottoman-period drainage system is collapsing. It's worst of all in the Muslim Quarter. The people there believe the Israelis want to make their houses uninhabitable so that they have to leave; then the buildings can be acquired by settlers.'

The Bishop snorted: 'They even use their tax system to put our shopkeepers out of business, charging them totally arbitrary tax demands. In 1967 we had eighty or ninety shops in the Old City, now – what? – maybe ten are left, possibly less. All the rest have been bankrupted by tax officials who refuse to believe their accounts. In several cases shopkeepers got demands for more than the entire value of their businesses.'

I suggested to the Bishop that maybe he was getting just a little paranoid. The old man shook his head. 'In the course of the furore over the St John's Hospice it emerged that the Israeli government had allocated 7.5 million shekhels [£2.5 million] to buy more Christian and Muslim buildings in the Old City. That figure is not disputed. It is not my imagination. There is a concerted government policy to Judaise the Old City. We are an obstacle to that policy. Sooner or later they will find a way of getting around the obstacle we represent.'

The Bishop poured another glass of cognac for me. 'In my lifetime I have seen my community wither like a diseased tree. The Armenian community used to contain millionaires. Now the young Armenians in my choir look up to their contemporaries who manage to get jobs as waiters in Israeli restaurants. The most ambitious and talented young people are emigrating, to America mainly. They know there is no future for them here. But it's not just the young. Whole families are going.'

When Bishop Hagop had been a young man, he said, there were over ten thousand Armenians in Palestine. Now fewer than two thousand were left. The whole community structure had shrunk. In the old days there had been five Armenian clubs and a theatre group; there had been plays, concerts, gatherings, dances. Now the quarter was a quiet place; those with energy and ability had left and made new lives for themselves in Boston and New York. A shadow had fallen over the Armenian Quarter; the place seemed to be shrinking in on itself.

On my way back to my rooms later that evening I fell into conversation with some Armenian teenagers. To my surprise they echoed the Bishop's despair.

'There is nothing for us here,' said one girl. 'Nothing. If Armenian boys are lucky they will end up washing dishes, or working on a construction site. For us there is even less choice. No non-Jew can get a decent job.'

Another of the teenagers, Krikor, said that the month before there had been a stabbing incident and the Israeli police had randomly arrested him and five hundred other non-Jewish boys. He had been taken to a police station, beaten up and made to stand all day in the sun without water. During the *intifada* that sort of thing had become almost routine.

The girls agreed. One said how, only a week before, she had been beckoned over to a car belonging to an Orthodox Jew which was parked outside the main gate to the quarter. Thinking the man was lost and needed directions, she had bent down to talk to him. The man spat in her face and drove off. She was tired of all this, she said. She wanted to emigrate to Boston, where she had distant cousins.

'The Israelis rule us, but we are not Israeli citizens,' she said. 'We have no votes. We have no influence.'

'They make us feel like a piece of filth they would like to flush down their lavatories,' added Krikor, 'that we are somehow too dirty to be in this town.'

'All of us want to leave,' said the girl. 'Everyday life is just too difficult in Jerusalem. They make *everything* a struggle for us.'

The Armenians were not alone. In the days that followed, as I walked around the Christian Quarter talking to the Palestinian Christians, I found that the inhabitants of the Old City were overwhelmingly gloomy about the long-term prospects of a Christian presence surviving in Jerusalem. Rightly or wrongly, the Palestinians all seemed to believe that there was a concerted campaign to drive them out, or at any rate to make their life so difficult that the majority would opt to leave of their own volition. In 1922, 52 per cent of the population of the Old City of Jerusalem had been Christian; now they made up just under 2.5 per cent of the population of the municipality. There were now more Jerusalem-born Christians in Sydney than in Jerusalem. The Old City ceased to be dominated by Christians in the 1940s; now everyone agreed that it would probably soon have no permanent Christian presence at all.

All this is part of the most dramatic decline in a Christian population to have taken place anywhere in the modern Middle East, with the single exception of Turkish Anatolia. There the progressive campaign of massacres and deportations, culminating in the 1915 Armenian genocide and the 1922 Greco-Turkish transfer of population, left only a few thousand Christians where at the turn of the century there had been around four million. In Palestine the decline of the Christian population over the course of this century has been more gradual, but no less overwhelming.

In 1922, twenty-six years before the creation of the State of Israel, Christians made up around 10 per cent of the population of British Mandate Palestine. The Christians were wealthier and better educated than their Muslim counterparts, owned almost all the newspapers and filled a disproportionate number of senior jobs in the Mandate Civil Service. While numerically they dominated the Old City of Jerusalem – as indeed they had done almost continuously since the fourth century A.D. – their leaders and merchants had already moved out from the narrow streets around the Holy Sepulchre and the Via Dolorosa to build fine villas for themselves in the West Jerusalem suburbs of Talbieh, Kattamon and Bak'a – now home to the better-off Israeli businessmen and Knesset MPs.

The exodus of the Palestinian Christians began in 1948, during the war which followed the withdrawal of British troops from Palestine. In the fighting some fifty-five thousand Palestinian Christians – around 60 per cent of the total community – fled or were driven from their homes, along with around 650,000 Muslim Palestinians. After the Israeli conquest and occupation of the West Bank during the Six Day War, a second exodus took place: between 1967 and 1992 around 40 per cent of the Christians then in the Occupied Territories – a further nineteen thousand men, women and children – left their homes to look for better lives elsewhere.

The great majority of Palestinian Christians now live abroad, in exile: only 170,000 are left inside Israel and the West Bank, compared with the 400,000 living outside the Holy Land, either in squalid refugee camps in Lebanon or elsewhere. The Christians now make up less than a quarter of 1 per cent of the population of Israel and the West Bank. Moreover their emigration rate remains very high, double that of the Muslim Palestinians, not because the Christians suffer any worse indignities than the Muslims, but because being better educated they find it far easier to emigrate and get jobs abroad. So far, the stumbling peace process has done little to stop this flood of emigrants. A recent survey by Bethlehem University showed that around a fifth of those Palestinian Christians still remaining in their ancestral homeland hope to emigrate in the near future.

All this matters very much. Without the local Christian population, the most important shrines in the Christian world will be left as museum pieces, preserved only for the curiosity of tourists. Christianity will no longer exist in the Holy Land as a living faith; a vast vacuum will exist in the very heart of Christendom. As the Archbishop of Canterbury recently warned, the area, 'once centre of a strong Christian presence', risks becoming 'a theme park' devoid of Christians 'within fifteen years'.

The future looks particularly bleak for Christian Jerusalem as

Jewish settler organisations focus their energies on the Holy City. Rings of Israeli settlements are springing up all around East Jerusalem, while within the Old City radical settler groups continue to try to buy up land within the Muslim, Christian and Armenian Quarters of the Old City. Within ten years of the Israeli conquest of East Jerusalem, 37,065 acres of Arab land had been confiscated and settled; today only 13.5 per cent of East Jerusalem remains in Palestinian hands. Less assertive but equally insistent is the Muslim claim to the place they call Al-Quds (the Holy City), as King Hussein and Yasser Arafat compete for the right to protect the Muslim Holy Places. Between these two competing claims, the Christians' stake in Jerusalem seems increasingly irrelevant.

The various Churches in Jerusalem are more than aware of the seriousness of their situation. Traditionally, the forty-seven Christian denominations represented in the Holy City were famous for their pointless and petty squabbling: year after year newspapers across the globe would celebrate Easter with some light Paschal story about the Greek Orthodox feuding with the Roman Catholics over the cleaning of such-and-such a window sill in the Holy Sepulchre or the Church of the Nativity in Bethlehem. But since 1989 the Patriarchs and Archbishops of the major Churches have come together – possibly for the first time since the First Crusade in 1095 – to issue an annual joint statement 'to make known to the people of the world the conditions of life of our people here in the Holy Land who experience constant deprivation of their fundamental rights . . . [and to] express our deep concern and alarm for the growing feeling of insecurity and fear among our people and Churches . . . [which constitutes] a serious threat to the future of Christianity and its rights in the Holy Land'.

Yet despite the apparent hopelessness of the Christian position, the leaders of the Eastern Churches remain surprisingly defiant. Yesterday morning, armed with a letter from Fr. Theophanes, I was granted a brief audience with the Greek Orthodox Patriarch of Jerusalem, Diodoros I. A hover of black-robed archbishops and metropolitans conducted me into a tall, vaulted reception room. Portraits of centuries of Orthodox Patriarchs stared down impassively from the walls. In the centre of the room, slumped over a large red velvet throne, sat Diodoros, the present holder of the office once occupied by Sophronius. Now very old, he was still a large, powerfully built man with a white beard tumbling down his Patriarchal robes; as he sat on his great gilt throne he resembled an elderly lion with a long grey mane.

'This land,' he boomed, 'this Holy Land, is watered with the blood of the martyrs. It has never been easy for the Christians who live here, and these present times are no different. During the *intifada* we condemned the suppression of our flock. We intervened to get prisoners released. We took food to our people when they were under curfew. We share the aspirations and agonies suffered by our people. The Holy Land has never been a place for quiet contemplation, somewhere peaceful like Mount Athos. Here we have a mission, a mission we have to try and keep going.'

I asked the Patriarch whether he thought the end of the Christian presence in Jerusalem appeared to be imminent, and whether his mission was not now drawing to a close.

'In Byzantine times when we Greeks ruled the Holy Land, this city was entirely Christian,' said Diodoros. 'Of course you cannot compare the present situation with then: our numbers are now very few. But then you do not judge a light by the size of its container.'

The Patriarch rearranged himself on his throne and clutched a miniature icon in a gold setting, suspended on a chain around his neck. 'Even a small oil lamp,' he said, 'can give light to a big room.'

JERUSALEM, 10 NOVEMBER

The Patriarch was right: for the three hundred years of Byzantine rule in Palestine, Jerusalem had been a Christian city; indeed in many ways it was the capital of Christianity. For the barbarians of Dark Age Europe as for the Byzantines themselves, Jerusalem was thought of as the navel of the world, and well into the late medieval period world maps like the Hereford Mappa Mundi depicted the city in the very centre of the earth.

Bishops across Christendom looked to Jerusalem for instruction on how to conduct their Holy Week services and how to order their liturgical calenders; European pilgrims, such as the Spanish nun Egeria, sent back almost ludicrously detailed accounts of the city's liturgical practices to their correspondents, 'knowing how pleased Your Charity would be to learn what is the ritual observed day by day in the Holy Places'. When Pope Gregory I wished to cement an alliance with the Lombards, he sent their Queen a flask of oil from the shrine of the Holy Cross at Jerusalem. Jerusalem was the Holy City, and the eyes of the Christian world were firmly fixed upon it.

All this was a dramatic departure from the situation at the end of the Pagan Empire. Not only had the Romans looked on Palestine as an obscure province wedged between the far richer and more civilised lands of Egypt and Syria, since its destruction by Titus in 70 A.D., Jerusalem had sunk to little more than an anonymous garrison town. As late as 310 A.D. it was possible for the Roman Governor of Palestine, based in Caesarea Maritima (south of modern Haifa), to express ignorance as to the whereabouts of Jerusalem; interrogating a Christian suspect who said he came from the town, the Governor Formilianus replied by asking, 'Jerusalem? Where is that?'

The accession of the Emperor Constantine and the adoption of Christianity as the official religion of the Roman Empire changed all this for ever; overnight the obscure province became the Holy Land, pampered and patronised by a string of emperors, their wives and courtiers. Within a few years of Constantine's Edict of Milan in 313, announcing the official toleration of Christianity, the Emperor's mother Helena had personally travelled to Jerusalem and conducted a series of excavations to locate the Holy Places – even if, as Sir Steven Runciman laconically noted, her discoveries of such relics as the wood of the Holy Cross, were made 'with miraculous aid seldom now vouchsafed to archaeologists'. On the site pinpointed by his mother as that of the Crucifixion and Resurrection, Constantine ordered the building of 'not only the finest basilica in the world, but one where everything shall be of such quality that all the most beautiful buildings of every city may be surpassed by this'. Constantine also commissioned huge basilicas in Bethlehem, at the site of the Nativity, and on the Mount of Olives.

Others soon followed his lead. The Empress Eudoxia, the headstrong wife of the Emperor Theodosius II (builder of the great Land Walls of Constantinople) lived in Jerusalem for sixteen years and spent one and a half million pieces of gold on building projects, at a time when two gold pieces was enough to keep most people in some style for at least a year. Her donations included the Patriarchal Palace, repairs to the city's fortifications, a new loop of wall enclosing Mount Zion within the city limits, and the church and monastery of St Stephen, the place where Sophronius later said the last liturgy before the Holy City fell to the armies of Islam. Eudoxia also built a leper hospital near Herodion on the West Bank, and a tower in the wilderness of Judaea to protect the monks there from the raids of desert nomads. Meanwhile, in nearby Bethlehem, St Jerome had gathered under his wings a gaggle of wealthy Roman matrons. These included an heiress named Paula who 'gave up all her worldly goods' before her pilgrimage to Palestine, yet who still had enough spare change left over to build two monasteries and a hospice, as well as supporting a multitude of monks and paupers, including of course St Jerome himself.

Even the ascetics, living in poverty in the caves and ravines of Judaea, were often from the smartest Imperial families. The monk Photius, for example, was actually the stepson of Justinian's greatest general, Count Belisarius. According to Procopius, Photius escaped from the Empress Theodora's secret torture chambers, into which he had been thrown when he threatened to divulge details of various sexual shenanigans amongst Theodora's ladies in the court at Constantinople. Eluding Theodora's secret police, Photius managed to flee to Palestine, seeking refuge as a monk in the desert somewhere outside Jerusalem.

The wealth and social standing of many of the pious pilgrims who settled in the town is also hinted at by John Moschos. He records a story originally told to him by Amma Damiana the Solitary, mother of his friend the Bishop of Petra. Amma Damiana was related to the Imperial family, and in the story she tells how she persuaded one of her smart Imperial cousins to accept the charity of a poor woman.

'In the days before I was enclosed [as a nun],' said Amma Damiana, 'I used to go to the Church of Saint Cosmas and Saint Damian [in Jerusalem] and spend the whole night there. Every evening there came an old woman, a native of Phrygian Galatia [modern central Turkey], and she gave two *lepta* [small coins] to everybody who was in the church; she often gave me these alms. One day a kinswoman of mine – and of the most faithful Emperor Maurice – came to pray at the Holy City and remained there a year. Soon after her arrival I went to the Church of Cosmas and Damian, taking her with me. While we were in the oratory, I said to my kinswoman: "Look, my lady; when an old woman comes distributing two coins to each person, please swallow your pride and accept them." With obvious distaste, she said: "Do I have to accept them?" "Yes," I said. "Take them, for the woman is great in the eyes of God. She fasts all week long, and whatever she is able to gain by this discipline she distributes to those who are found in the church. Take the coins and give them to somebody else. Do not refuse the sacrifice of this old woman."

'As we were speaking in this way, the old woman came in and began her almsgiving. In silence and with serenity she came and gave me some coins. Then she gave some to my kinswoman too, saying: "Take these, and eat." When she had gone, we realised that God had revealed to the poor old woman that I had suggested to my relation that she give the money away. My kinswoman therefore sent a servant of hers to get vegetables with the two coins. These she ate, and she affirmed before God that they were as sweet as honey.'

The flow of money into the Holy Land brought by the Empire's richest families caused new trades to flourish. Religious tourism, then as now, must have brought in much business for innkeepers and tour guides; certainly by the sixth century there was already a set tour 'circuit', and guide books (some furnished with maps) were available to help the pilgrims understand what they were seeing. Another flourishing cottage industry was the trade in relics. Palestine had something of a monopoly in Old Testament bones, and a good share of New Testament mementoes as well. The relics of Joseph and Samuel, Zachariah and Habakkuk, Gamaliel and St Stephen were all exported during this period, as were the chains of St Peter, the nails which fastened Christ to the Cross and a painting of the Virgin Mary by St Luke. A local Jewess used to display the robe of the Virgin Mary, while the priests of Bethlehem would, for a fee, show pilgrims the bones of the children slaughtered by King Herod, or at least those they had not already sold to the churches and reliquaries of the capital. Famous relics were very expensive – Theodosius II paid a fortune in gold coin as well as a huge gold cross for the relics of St Stephen – but even the most humble pilgrim would be able to afford second-division relics such as casts of Christ's footprints, oil from the lamps at Golgotha and dust upon which the feet of Christ had trod. For the inventive Byzantine entrepreneur, the relic trade must have been an almost inexhaustible source of income.

The Church had much more power here than anywhere else in the Empire. When the local Samaritan population broke out in revolt in 529 A.D., the Emperor Justinian sent to suppress it not a general but 'a monk of high rank named Photion'. Photion fulfilled his duties with somewhat unmonastic zeal, 'fighting against them and conquering them, putting many of them to torture, driving others into exile, and generally inspiring great fear'. According to some sources, more than a hundred thousand Samaritans lost their lives in Photion's purges.

But Jerusalem, like Palestine as a whole, was not just full of clerics, monks and credulous pilgrims; laymen always outnumbered clerics, a fact that caused the always irascible St Jerome some irritation. Writing to his friend Paulinus of Nola, who was planning a trip to Jerusalem, Jerome warned that he should not expect a city of saints: 'It is a crowded place, with the whole variety of people you find in such centres: prostitutes, actors, soldiers, mimes and buffoons. Such a throng of both sexes that you might wish to avoid in part elsewhere you are forced to suffer here in its entirety.' St Basil's younger brother, the choleric Cappadocian Gregory of Nyssa, was equally unhappy at the moral character of the inhabitants of Jerusalem. He wrote home in a fury that 'if God's grace were more plentiful in the vicinity of Jerusalem than elsewhere, then the people who live there would not make sin so much their custom. But in fact there is no sort of shameful practice in which they do not indulge: cheating, adultery, theft, idolatry, poisoning, quarrels and murder are everyday occurrences . . . What proof is there then, in a place where things like that occur, of the abundance of God's grace?'

Indeed the monks themselves could be pretty unruly. They had to be permanently banned from Gaza when they insisted on disrupting night spectacles at the theatre and various festivals they considered 'pagan'. In Chalcedon, on the Asian shore of the Bosphorus opposite Byzantium, when the monks protested about the staging of Olympic Games, the local bishop reminded the leader of the protesters that he was a monk and should therefore 'go and sit in a cell and keep quiet'; but in Palestine the monks were much more numerous and were clearly made of sterner stuff. On one occasion troops had to be used to restore order after the Palestinian monks rose in revolt against a Bishop of Jerusalem they considered heretical. Things got even more out of control during the reign of the heretical Emperor Valens: when the monks demonstrated violently against a bishop he had installed, the Emperor deported large numbers of them, condemning them to the Imperial mines and quarries in the deserts of Upper Egypt.

Sometimes the monks did get away with it, however. Under an oppressive and bigoted late Roman law, the Jews were forbidden to enter Jerusalem except once a year on the Jewish festival of Sukkoth, when they were permitted to come and weep over the ruins of their Temple. In 438 A.D. these regulations were relaxed by the Empress Eudoxia, an act which electrified the Jewish diaspora but outraged the more fundamentalist monks. As the Jews gathered in unprecedented numbers on Temple Mount, the Syrian monk Barsauma led one of the most horrific anti-Semitic pogroms of the period, attacking and killing many of the Jewish pilgrims. Barsauma protested that he and his followers had not been directly involved and that the Jews had been killed by 'missiles coming, as it were, from Heaven'. But the surviving Jews had evidence that this was not true, for they had managed to seize eighteen of Barsauma's followers, and brought them to the Empress for trial. But even the Empress could do nothing in the face of the monastic mob Barsauma was able to muster: cheerleaders in the crowd threatened to burn her, and set up a chant of 'The Cross has conquered'; 'the voice of the people spread and swelled for a long time, like the roar of a wave of the sea, so that the inhabitants of the city trembled because of the noise of the shouting.' Barsauma was never brought to justice, and indeed was later canonised by the Syrian Orthodox Church.

Yet despite such pogroms, rebellions, and internal turbulence, Palestine underwent a massive increase in population during the Byzantine period. Archaeological surveys of pottery picked up in the fields of Israel and the West Bank have found around four times the density of Byzantine pottery as that of the Israelite period, implying that the population during Byzantine rule must have been quite significantly higher than during the centuries preceding it. Whole areas of the region never settled before (or since) were cultivated in this period: in the depths of the Negev desert, for example, six Byzantine towns have been excavated standing in what was then cultivated land. It is probably only in the twentieth century that the population of the region began to equal or surpass the exceptional high point reached during the sixth century.

The seeds of the destruction of Byzantine Palestine may well have lain in the scale of this sudden expansion. Excavations at Scythopolis (modern Beit Shean) have shown that while the town's brothels were flourishing, bathing was falling out of fashion: the town's five bath houses, all flourishing during the Roman period, fell into disuse under the Byzantines. This may have been partly due to the influence of the monks, who regarded the baths with horror and heaped praise on those who refrained from washing for the longest possible period: one story of the desert fathers admiringly tells how a wandering monk chanced upon a saintly hermit in a cave in the furthest reaches of the desert, 'and believe me, my brothers, I, Pambo, this least one, smelt the good odour of that brother from a mile away'. Basic norms of hygiene were not just ignored by the monks and their admirers: they were deliberately, piously flouted.

But it was not just a question of fashion; there were structural problems too. The old Roman aqueducts were clogging up, while in Scythopolis the neatly paved drains built during the pagan Empire fell into disrepair and were replaced by open sewers. In all the Byzantine sites excavated in Palestine and Jordan only two lavatories have ever been discovered, and one of those was located directly over a monastic kitchen.

The result of all this was a wave of epidemics throughout the sixth century. The pages of John Moschos contain many references to outbreaks of plague, and the evidence of modern archaeologists has shown that leprosy, smallpox and tuberculosis were rife, while lice proliferated to an extent unknown in almost any other period of Middle Eastern history.

Many historians now believe that it is in the devastating infections and plagues of the late sixth century that the root cause of the rapid collapse of the Byzantine Levant should be sought.

Every morning during my stay in Jerusalem I toured the lanes and alleys of the Old City, searching out fragments of the Byzantine period, often in the company of Bishop Hagop. The Bishop had cheered up somewhat since our first meeting, and was always at his liveliest in the ancient vaulted passageways of the different quarters, pointing out both the architectural remains littered around us and some of the Old City's more unusual modern inhabitants.

'See that blind beggar? Yes, the man in the wheelchair in front of that Crusader arch. He's only blind from nine until twelve. Then he takes off his dark glasses and has another job, as a waiter in a kebab restaurant in the Muslim Quarter. Very good kebabs, too. Over there, that's the Church of St John the Baptist. It's got some lovely Byzantine stonework but the Greeks have gone and put horrible new frescoes in the apse: bright yellows and blues.'

The Bishop shuddered. 'The taste of some of these modern Greeks . . . Have you seen the mosaic they've put up in the Holy Sepulchre? It looks like something out of Walt Disney. Now, look down here. See the tall man selling olive-wood figurines? He's called Isa. For years he used to be a cook. Specialised in making sandwiches: nice dainty ones for wedding parties. He was famous for his special liver sandwiches and soon became the most popular caterer in the Old City. Then someone noticed that the cat population near his house kept declining every time there was a wedding: eight to ten cats went missing whenever a reception was held. News spread about this, but people kept begging him for sandwiches. In the end he couldn't supply the demand: the cat population ran too low and he couldn't produce the goods. So he got into olive wood instead. But at least he was quite humane with the cats. There's a Cypriot monk who makes his unfortunate cats fast in Lent. He locks them up and you can hear them yowling into the night. And it's not just Lent. About once every year he has dreams in which he thinks he is given an exclusive premonition of the coming of the Messiah. So for a fortnight afterwards he makes these poor cats scream all night in expectation of the Second Coming. Terrible noise. Now, see that pillar . . .'

Perhaps the biggest surprise of our walks was discovering quite how little of Byzantine Jerusalem has survived. While in northern Syria hundreds of unnamed and unknown late antique towns and villages still exist virtually intact, in Jerusalem, once probably the most magnificent provincial town in the entire Christian Empire, only desultory fragments of floor mosaic and piles of collapsed pillars remain to hint at what has been lost. Following the trail of John Moschos's writings around the city takes one to a variety of dank cellars and obscure crypts, but even here there is little surviving that is of more than antiquarian interest. Ironically, the only great Byzantine building left in the city is a mosque – the Dome of the Rock – decorated by Byzantine craftsmen for the new

Muslim conquerors in the late seventh century, shortly after the fall of the eastern half of the Empire. Runciman has called the Dome 'the supreme example of the rotunda-style of building in Byzantine architecture'.

Of Constantine's original Holy Sepulchre very little survives. Fragments of its walls are visible through a dark hole in the side of the Syriac chapel, but most of the existing structure is Crusader, with a few later additions from the Ottoman period. The Nea, Justinian's magnificent New Church of Mary, Mother of God, where one of Moschos's friends, Abba Leontios the Cilician, worked for forty years, has also effectively vanished. Fragments of it – mere lumps of wall, along with some strange vaulted substructures – lie scattered around various undercrofts in the Jewish Quarter. Archaeologists have excavated what remains, and seem excited by their discoveries, but it is almost impossible for the layman to imagine that these sad piles of brick and stone once surpassed many of Justinian's surviving churches – Haghia Eirene in Istanbul or San Vitale in Ravenna – still less that the Nea could be mentioned in the same breath as Haghia Sophia, the greatest of all Byzantine buildings.

The Cardo – the great central bazaar of Byzantine Jerusalem – is a similar story. It dominates the portrait of the city on the sixth-century mosaic map discovered at Madaba in Transjordan in 1884, and fragments of it have been discovered all over Jerusalem. Near the Holy Sepulchre, deep within the bowels of an echoing Russian Orthodox complex known as the Alexander Hospice, one can see a hundred yards of its arcades and paving, as well as a modest Byzantine stab at a classical Triumphal Arch. The Cardo resurfaces again for two hundred yards in a hole in the ground in the Jewish Quarter, beside a line of new boutiques selling bronze *menorah*, Israeli flags and Hebrew T-shirts for the American tourists. It then disappears into the side of a restaurant, never to be seen again.

One place where you cannot see the slightest hint of Byzantine work is at a busy road interchange just outside the Damascus Gate. I went there with Bishop Hagop one damp winter's afternoon, after lunching at an Armenian restaurant near the Austrian

Hospice. The Bishop stood on the pavement beside a new plastic bus shelter and asked me what I could see.

'Well . . .' I ventured. 'A bus shelter?'

'Anything else?'

'A couple of manholes?'

'Exactly. A bus shelter and a set of manholes. But nothing else.'

'No,' I agreed. 'So what?'

'This manhole is all that marks the site of one of the greatest Armenian monasteries of the Byzantine period. To the north-east, over by that filling station, were the monastic buildings of St Stephen's, the largest Greek monastery in Jerusalem. The foundations of its abbey church still survive under the chapel of the French École Biblique. But its monastic buildings were considered long lost.'

I mentioned how Sophronius had said the last mass before the fall of Jerusalem in St Stephen's, and asked when the monastery had been discovered.

'Both monasteries – the Greek and Armenian complexes – were discovered when the Israelis were building a dual carriageway to link some of the new West Bank settlements to the Old City: the settlers said they needed a new road which did not pass through Arab neighbourhoods because of *intifada* stone-throwing. The Israeli archaeologists excavated the ruins, took our mosaic to West Jerusalem, then backfilled both sites.'

'Didn't you protest?'

'Protest? We *begged* them to preserve it. But they would not listen. They said their road was more important. All they preserved was one of our burial chambers. It's under this manhole here. Originally they promised access for pilgrims, and lighting as well, but it never materialised. In Jerusalem we Christians are now too small a community to have any influence. We don't have a lobby. We don't even have a vote. As a result, in the space of a few months, two of the biggest monasteries ever discovered in the Middle East have been erased from the face of the earth. A visitor passing this spot today would never know any Christian building – let alone a pair of the most important monasteries in Palestine – had ever been here.'

'They probably didn't have the funds to preserve them,' I said. 'Ruins get bulldozed all over the world.'

'At exactly the same time as the two monasteries were discovered,' answered Hagop, 'builders located the tomb of a fifteenth-century rabbi in the Palestinian village of Silwan, a mile from here. Archaeologically, the site is of no great importance, but tourists are now taken around the tomb, and the impression is given that Jerusalem has always been a Jewish-dominated city. The truth is quite different: for eighteen hundred years the Jerusalem Jewish community was a small minority here. But with the ultimate political status of the town still undecided, it is vital for the Israelis that that truth is suppressed, or at least disguised. Jerusalem is meant to be their eternal capital. These monasteries are evidence of a Christian-dominated Jerusalem. So they were hidden.'

'I'm sure there must have been a good reason for their being bulldozed,' I said. 'I don't believe in conspiracy theories.'

'They promised us a plaque, some sort of memorial,' replied Hagop, scowling. 'Two years later, can you see anything except this manhole? They've still got our mosaic and the bones from the Armenian burial chamber. They're in the storerooms at the back of the Israel Museum. If we don't shout too loud, and behave ourselves, we might get them back. Otherwise we can probably forget it. As for the monastery, we will probably have to wait another century until this road is taken out of commission and we get the site of our shrine back.'

We wandered over the site of the two vanished monasteries, Hagop pointing out the approximate places where various features had stood: a mosaic here, a hospice there, the abbey church here, monastic buildings over there.

'It was a huge complex,' said Hagop. 'From here right over to where that filling station has been built. It was our first Armenian Quarter, another reminder of the continuous Christian presence in this city.'

We headed towards the garage. A little way beyond it stood the École Biblique, where Hagop had promised to help get me a reader's ticket for the library. As we passed the pumps, Hagop suddenly pointed to a sign in the newly planted garden beside the filling station.

'Look!' he said. 'This is new. It must have just gone up.'

We walked closer and read the notice, which was written in Hebrew and English, but not Arabic:

JERUSALEM MUNICIPALITY/MINISTRY OF TRANSPORT
ROAD NUMBER ONE ARCHAEOLOGICAL GARDEN:
FRAGMENTS OF THE THIRD WALL.

'I don't believe it,' said Bishop Hagop.

'What's the Third Wall?' I asked.

'It is the wall built by Herod Agrippa before the Jewish Revolt of 66 A.D. It's an important discovery. Scholars have been arguing for years about where this wall ran, so it's quite legitimate to preserve it. But to keep this when a whole monastic complex has been obliterated before our eyes, right next door to it – that's just nationalistic bigotry. Nothing is erected to commemorate our ruins. There's no mention of them. Nothing. They might as well never have existed. Then they find ten feet of walling from the period of their King Herod and they build a special archaeological garden to preserve it. Do you still call me paranoid?'

Later, in the cuttings library of the *Jerusalem Post* and the archaeological section of the École Biblique, I checked what Bishop Hagop had said.

Like so many apparently trivial disputes in Jerusalem, it turned out that the question of the monastic complex had mushroomed into something of an international scandal. The Christian Churches in the city had been deeply incensed by the authorities' decision to bury a pair of major Christian shrines. They had also been furious at the lack of protection afforded to the ruins, which allowed vandals – allegedly ultra-Orthodox Jewish *haredim* from nearby Mea She'arim, according to the *Jerusalem Post* – to pour tar over a beautiful sixth-century Byzantine mosaic and pile rocks

331

on top of a Christian funerary crypt. Church leaders had given interviews to the international press making clear their view that while finds of importance to Judaism were treated with care and respect, Christian antiquities were being disregarded as part of Israel's campaign to assert its rights to the city. When these interviews had no effect, the heads of all the leading Christian Churches in the Holy Land issued a formal joint statement of complaint about Israeli cultural policies, singling out what they described as Israel's 'depredation' of the Christian archaeological heritage, and threatening to appeal for international protection for their ruins unless 'appropriate and satisfactory measures are taken to preserve our universal Christian heritage'.

According to the official Israeli archaeological report (entitled, significantly enough, *Excavations at the Third Wall*), there were in fact not two but *four* separate monasteries discovered in the excavations north of the Damascus Gate, as well as two hostelries for pilgrims and a large Christian cemetery. Moreover, shortly afterwards, a fifth Byzantine shrine – a small burial chapel decorated with mosaics and rare frescoes – was discovered near the Jaffa Gate during building for the Mamilla Project, a politically motivated scheme intended to 'integrate' the Old City with the new and make it impossible for the two ever again to be divided as they had been from 1948 to 1967, with the Old City going to the Arabs and the New City to the Israelis – a division the Palestinians wish to reinstate. But despite the unprecedented Christian protests, not one of these sites was preserved for posterity. All were reburied, with the exception of the frescoed chapel outside Jaffa Gate, which was bulldozed to make way for nothing more important than an underground parking lot. 'The whole Mamilla Project depends on it [the carpark],' Gideon Avni of the Israel Antiquities Authority told the *Jerusalem Post* by way of explanation.

There is probably nowhere else on earth where the far distant past is so politicised as in the Holy Land. In its 1948 Proclamation of Independence, Israel referred to 'the re-establishment of the Jewish State', thus firmly basing its historic right to exist on the Biblical precedent of the Israelite Kingdom that had thrived in the same area. Since 1967 the same justification has been advanced for the Israeli colonisation of the West Bank and Golan: many of the new Jewish settlements that were set up, such as Shilo, Givon and Katzrin, were deliberately built on sites identified as having originally been colonised by the ancient Israelites three thousand years earlier.

In a situation like this, where contemporary political claims are based on rival interpretations of ancient history, it is almost impossible for archaeologists to remain neutral or objective. There have long been accusations that Israeli archaeologists have a tendency to excavate not so much to illuminate the general history of the region as to uncover their own history, in some cases allegedly digging through and discarding as irrelevant the intervening Turkish, Arab and Byzantine layers. Indeed, to Israel's great credit, many of the fiercest criticisms of this political bias have come from Israeli liberals incensed at what they regarded as the right-wing nationalistic bias of the country's archaeological establishment. In 1992 the Jerusalem-based archaeologist Shulamit Giva accused Israeli Biblical archaeology of being 'a tool in the hands of the Zionist movement [attempting] to find a connection between the ancient history of the Land of Israel and the historic occurrence of the [modern] State of Israel'. Israeli archaeology, she continued, had 'lost its independence as a scientific discipline and become an executive arm of an ideological movement, a nationalist and political instrument which provided "roots" for the new state'.

The distinguished Israeli writer Amos Elon echoed some of Giva's concerns in a long article on politics and archaeology in the *New York Review of Books*. Elon argued that the worst abuses took place in the early years of the Jewish state: 'In the ethnocentric atmosphere of these early years there was a rush to identify Jewish sites, an overemphasis on digging them up, and a tendency to expose to public view the Jewish strata of a site even where other layers may have been historically or artistically more significant or revealing. The task of archaeology was to prove a point about Jews in the Holy Land and not always as it probably should have been, to explore material remains in order to determine the circumstances of ancient cultures and civilisations in a country where they have been so varied and so many.'

Other liberal Israelis have attacked the way the history of the region is presented to tourists. The former Deputy Mayor of Jerusalem, Meron Benvinisti, himself a respected historian of the Crusader period, has attacked the bias in the Tower of David Museum of the History of Jerusalem, the principal museum of the Old City. 'After the Israelite period,' commented Benvinisti, 'the written text informs us that the city was occupied by foreigners. Describing them as foreigners emphasises the exclusivist character of the museum's perspective – only the Israeli-Jewish claim to the city is granted legitimacy. In fact the Israelite period only lasted six hundred years, but all the periods which followed it are represented as a chain of occupations – Persian, Byzantine, Mameluke, Ottoman and British.' Moreover, Benvinisti pointed out that the word 'Arab' does not appear even once in a vast display covering maybe thirty rooms, while the only Arabic name mentioned in the entire complex is that of the conqueror, the Caliph Omar. 'Distorted history is being presented,' he concludes. 'The victor's version of history.'

The archaeologist I most wanted to meet to discuss all this with was Fr. Michele Piccirillo of the Studium Biblicum Franciscanum. Piccirillo is an Italian Franciscan who has lived in Jerusalem since 1960 and who since then has single-handedly rediscovered much of the monastic world described in *The Spiritual Meadow*. In a series of remarkable excavations, he uncovered many previously unknown Byzantine monasteries, chapels, churches and villas dating mainly from the sixth to the eighth century, and in the process brought to light a breathtaking treasury of late antique floor mosaics, including some of the finest mosaic work ever discovered in the Levant. I had seen some of them as I passed through Jordan on my way to Israel, for the finest set of all lies around Madaba and Mount Nebo, immediately above the Allenby Bridge, the frontier post leading into the West Bank. There is little of the ascetic spirit that is visible in Walid Jumblatt's mosaics from

Porphyreon. Instead Piccirillo's mosaics are animated by a remarkable classical *joie de vivre* that hints at a revival of Hellenistic taste
– if not a wholesale classical renaissance – in the period immediately after Justinian: leopards chase stags through swirls of
acanthus; personifications of the seasons sit enthroned with crown
and sceptre, looking on as shepherds process through scrolls of
vine branches; satyrs with flutes lead a Bacchic procession while
cupids swoop above the orange trees.

But the importance of these new discoveries goes beyond mere
aesthetics and art history. Perhaps their most unexpected aspect
is the astonishing degree of continuity they reveal. According to
Piccirillo, the Arab conquest of the seventh century is archaeologically invisible: the rulers changed, but life went on exactly as
before. Indeed much of the finest 'Byzantine' work he has dug up
dates from the period immediately *after* the Arab Conquest, when
order was better kept, trade was flourishing and the area was
released from the crippling taxes imposed by the Byzantine exchequer. 'The archaeologist who searches for a break between the
pre- and post-Muslim conquest searches in vain,' wrote Piccirillo
in *The Mosaics of Jordan*, the book which sums up his life's work.
'Archaeology demonstrates an uninterrupted continuity between
the two periods.'

There are reasons for this. Just as Angle and Saxon mercenaries
were drafted into Western Europe to defend Rome's northern
borders before the barbarian invasions that brought down the
western half of the Roman Empire, so Christian Arab tribes were
drafted in by Byzantine rulers to defend the eastern frontiers
several centuries before Mohammed. Justinian, for example, had
an alliance with two of the Christian Arab tribes: the Banu Ghassan
and the Banu Taghlib, both of whom he settled within the boundaries of the Christian Empire. By the time of the Arab conquests,
therefore, Arabs already made up a significant minority within
the eastern provinces of the Byzantine Empire.

Piccirillo's work has, however, implied that the Arab infiltration of Palestine must have been even more gradual than
had previously been recognised; so slow, in fact, that the
conquest seems to have brought little immediate change in the

racial composition of the inhabitants of the country. After the conquest, the local population soon adopted the Arabic tongue and over the centuries many converted to Islam, but the conquerors' armies were not large and initially provided little more than a military caste superimposed on the existing population. There was no wholesale exchange of population. The Palestinians we see today – and especially the Palestinian Christians – are therefore likely to be the descendants of roughly the same mix of peoples Moschos saw on his travels through this region in the seventh century: an ethnically diverse blend of the many races that have passed through this area since the earliest periods of prehistory.

Piccirillo's evidence is very important, for official Israeli histories still paint a picture of pillaging nomad conquerors sweeping in from the desert, massacring or wiping out the indigenous peoples and leaving the area a depopulated desert – until the birth of the Zionist movement in the nineteenth century. Despite the fact that no serious historian, in Israel or elsewhere, would even begin to try to defend such a crude distortion of Palestine's medieval history, this version still possesses a curious half-life in government propaganda. *Facts About Israel*, for example, is an information book produced by the Israeli Ministry of Foreign Affairs which is prefaced by a fifteen-page account of 'the history of the Land of Israel'. Here, following an extremely detailed account of the Biblical Israelite kingdoms, fourteen hundred years of the region's Islamic history is written off in a small section entitled 'Arabs in the Land of Israel':

> Arab migration in and out of the country started at the time of the Arab conquest of the Land in the seventh century, fluctuating thereafter with economic growth and decline . . . Towards the end of the nineteenth century, when increased Jewish development stimulated economic and social revival in the Land, many Arabs from surrounding countries were attracted to the area by its employment opportunities, higher wages and better living conditions.

336

I rang Piccirillo and arranged to come around for tea that afternoon. We sat in his small cell in the Studium Biblicum Franciscanum and talked for a long time about his work.

'All the sites I have excavated,' he said, 'call into serious question the old view that the Arab invasions resulted in the destruction of Christian buildings, that the Arabs persecuted the Christians and prohibited the building of new churches. The sheer number of Christian mosaics dating from the Ummayad period constitutes *very* strong evidence not only for the continuity of the Christian presence but also for the tolerance of the new Islamic rulers.'

I asked him about the accusations I had heard of bias in the Israeli archaeological establishment. He was quite clear in his response. Whatever the situation in the early years of the state, he said, current Israeli archaeological methods were thoroughly professional. In his opinion the historical sites of Israel were excavated impartially, without regard to religion. But he was equally adamant about the serious disparity in the presentation of those finds.

'The conservation of Christian remains is systematically less good than the treatment accorded to Jewish remains,' he said. 'Of course conservation is a problem everywhere. But here, where it so easily becomes a political issue, the Israelis should be doubly careful. The fact is that the Holy Land has many communities. Each has its rights, and if a state wants respect it should respect others.'

'How does this neglect show itself?' I asked.

'Synagogues they look after beautifully,' said Piccirillo. 'They cover them with shelters and stop people standing on the mosaics. But newly excavated churches or monasteries they can quite easily rebury, as they did with those outside the Damascus Gate. They would never dream of doing that to a synagogue, and the religious establishment would never let them. With Christian buildings, if they don't bulldoze them, they leave them just as they find them. In Jordan every single mosaic I have excavated is now under specially built shelters, even in specially built museums. But there are churches with good mosaics open to the air all over Israel.'

'Does that matter?' I asked.

'It matters very much. If these Christian sites are not guarded they can get attacked.'

Only a few days before there had been a report in the *Jerusalem Post* of an assault on an unguarded Byzantine church at Mamshit, near the Israeli nuclear facilities at Dimona. 'The vandals, suspected *haredim*, pulled apart colourful mosaics and shattered columns that held up the church's ceiling,' read the report, which said the incident was one of a series over the previous fortnight which had included the vandalising of another Byzantine church at Sussita on the Golan Heights. The *haredim* who were apparently responsible were said to be against archaeological excavations in general, and so were not setting out specifically to target Christian sites; nevertheless, Christian sites did figure on their hit lists.

'But you see,' continued Piccirillo, 'it's not just a matter of protecting from vandals. A mosaic . . .' He broke off and searched for words: 'A mosaic which is not looked after is like a rosary whose string is cut. Once one or two tesserae have gone, the whole mosaic falls apart. In a short time everything – *everything* – is lost.'

JERUSALEM, 14 NOVEMBER

One of the most depressing aspects of Israel and the West Bank is the degree of separation between the two peoples who share the Holy Land. Israelis employ Palestinian labour to do the jobs too badly paid, too dirty or too boring to attract their own compatriots. Palestinians work on production lines, clean the streets, wash the dishes. But beyond that there is no contact and few friendships. There are no mixed dinner parties; intermarriage is virtually unknown. The few places where Palestinians and Israelis meet side by side on equal terms – such as in prayer at the Tomb of the Patriarchs in Hebron – are famous for their tensions rather than for playing any part in bringing together the two mutually antagonistic peoples. The divide appears to be too deep to be bridged.

All this is in stark contrast to the situation during the early Ottoman period, when Palestine, like everywhere else in the Middle East, saw a degree of religious interaction unimaginable today. In Syria I saw that cooperation still surviving in Cyrrhus and Seidnaya, and I was interested to find out if anything of the sort had survived in the Holy Land, if there was anywhere where shrines were places of interaction between the two communities, rather than battlegrounds.

In the École Biblique I had found a book by J.E. Hanauer published in 1907 entitled *Folklore of the Holy Land: Muslim, Christian and Jewish*. It mentioned a shrine in the village of Beit Jala, beside Bethlehem, which at the time was frequented by all three of Palestine's religious communities. Christians regarded it as the birthplace of St George, Jews as the burial place of the Prophet Elias, Muslims as the home of the legendary saint of fertility known simply as Khidr, Arabic for green. According to Hanauer, in his day the monastery was 'a sort of madhouse. Deranged persons of all the three faiths are taken thither and chained in the court of the chapel, where they are kept for forty days on bread and water, the Greek priest at the head of the establishment now and then reading the Gospel over them, or administering a whipping as the case demands.' In the 1920s, according to Taufiq Canaan's *Mohammedan Saints and Sanctuaries in Palestine*, nothing seemed to have changed, and all three communities were still visiting the shrine and praying together. What, I wondered, happened now?

I asked around in the Christian Quarter in Jerusalem, and discovered that the place was very much alive. With all the greatest shrines in the Christian world to choose from, it seemed that when the local Arab Christians had a problem – an illness, or something more complicated: a husband detained in an Israeli prison camp, for example – they preferred to seek the intercession of St George in his grubby little shrine at Beit Jala rather than praying at the Holy Sepulchre in Jerusalem or the Church of the Nativity in Bethlehem. But what of Muslims and Jews? Did they still attend? Beit Jala lay a short distance from Jerusalem, so I drove over to try to find out. By pure good fortune I happened to arrive at the same time as the shrine's Greek Orthodox custodian.

Fr. Methodius – grey-bearded, blue-robed, with a small black chimneypot hat – slammed the door of his Subaru station wagon and locked it with a click of the remote-control bleeper. Then he looked over to the door of his church, and frowned.

There, waiting patiently by the door of the Church of St George, were two Muslim women in white headscarves. One was holding a fine damask veil, the other a small rectangular prayer mat. To one side stood three unshaven Palestinian labourers, each grasping a lead. On the end of each lead was a small, bow-legged, rather scraggy-looking sheep. Fr. Methodius took the gifts from the women with a peremptory nod, and handed the sheep over to the doorkeeper – an ancient hunchbacked Arab in a dirty *keffiyeh* – who led them away to a shed by the monastery gate.

'I'm afraid I won't have time to sacrifice these sheep until Monday,' said Fr. Methodius to the labourers, a little curtly. 'Come back at four if you want to collect the blood.'

The labourers shuffled off backwards towards the road, bowing gratefully, like schoolboys thankful to be dismissed from the head-master's study. Methodius signalled to me to follow him into the church, and pointedly closed the door behind us.

'Look at this!' he said, holding the prayer mat at arm's length, as if it might somehow infect him. 'It's got a picture of Mecca embroidered on it! You tell me: what can we do with it? And this veil? What's the price of this? Ten shekels? Never mind. Those sheep: that's something.'

'Do you get many Muslims coming here?' I asked.

'Many? We get hundreds! Almost as many as the Christian pilgrims. Often when I come in here I find Muslims all over the floor, in the aisles, up and down' – he made a rocking gesture with his hand – 'bottoms in the air, prayer mats on the floor: yes – in an Orthodox church!'

He snorted into his beard. 'You see, like us they believe this church marks the site of St George's birthplace. And St George is a great saint for them also.'

'And Jews?' I asked. 'Do they come and pray here too?'

'In the old days the Palestinian Jews would come,' replied Fr. Methodius. 'But modern Israelis would never come to such a shrine.'

He led me up to an icon hanging from a pillar in the nave. Beneath the sepia smudge of smoke stains and the clustering silver-work I could just make out the familiar classical face: the young Byzantine cavalryman with his golden breastplate and spear, mounted high upon a white charger.

'All the Arabs – Christian and Muslim alike – call him "Khidr" – the Green One. The Palestinians think St George can help give women babies or bring good crops to their fields or healthy lambs to their sheep. And if they get what they want, then they all come back again and give me these . . .' he stuttered as he searched for the word: '. . . these . . . these . . . rugs.'

'Or a sheep.'

'Yes; that's better. But of course I get to keep only a very small portion. The rest goes to the poor, while the donor takes the blood and smears it on his doorpost. That's the tradition.'

'It sounds very pagan.'

'It may well be,' said Fr. Methodius, his face puckering into a frown.

It was all very curious: Orthodox priests merrily slaughtering sheep, and doing so in homage to St George. Not the way, perhaps, that the Knights of the Garter might expect their patron saint to be venerated. After all, the English have always liked to believe that they have something of a monopoly on St George. If the Victorians had no qualms about proclaiming that God was an Englishman, then few had any doubts at all about claiming for England the country's own patron saint. What English schoolboy did not know the battlecry 'God for Harry, England, and St George'? Did the saint's body not lie in Windsor Castle? Was not his flag the national banner, the linchpin of the Union Jack?

However, no one can travel for very long around the Middle East, particularly among the Christian Arabs, without quickly realising that the English are not the only people to claim St George as their own. The English may fondly believe that they have got their patron saint safely stashed away in St George's Chapel in Windsor, but this will come as news to the nine monasteries on Mount Athos, the thirty-five other churches in Greece, the twenty-four churches and monasteries on Crete and the Greek islands, the six churches on Cyprus, the fifteen churches in Egypt, the five churches in Israel and the West Bank, the citadel in Aleppo and the two monasteries in northern Iraq which also claim the honour of possessing part or all of the ubiquitous and clearly many-boned St George.

In fact the veneration of St George originated in the Byzantine Levant and did not become popular in England until returning Crusaders brought the saint's cult back with them. In 1348 Edward III made St George the patron of the Knights of the Garter, and it was around this time that George seems to have replaced Edward the Confessor as England's national saint.

Although most scholars now tend to accept that St George probably *was* a historical figure, solid facts about England's patron saint are hard to come by. He appears to have been a Christian legionary from Palestine who was martyred for refusing to worship the old pagan gods, probably during the reign of Diocletian (284–305 A.D.). He may or may not have been the unnamed martyr mentioned as suffering a particularly horrible death in the eighth book of Eusebius's *Ecclesiastical History*, but what *is* clear is that his cult was a very early one, and that it originated in Lydda, now the Tel Aviv suburb of Lod, the Heathrow of the Holy Land, directly under the flightpath of jets heading into Ben Gurion Airport. Nothing else can be said with certainty; already in the sixth century St George was referred to as 'that Good Man whose deeds are known to God alone'.

But lack of facts never stopped medieval hagiographers from assembling impressively detailed saints' *Lives*, and the cult of St George spread with astonishing speed, gathering odd stories and enveloping pagan legends as it went. By the time of Jacobus da Voragine's *The Golden Legend*, written in Genoa around 1260, St George's life-story had become one of the longest epics in medieval hagiography, revolving around the dragon whose breath could 'poison everyone who came within reach'.

What is intriguing about the cult of St George as it is practised today in Beit Jala is the extraordinary degree to which it still resembles the form the cult took *before* it came to acquire all the late medieval accretions that fill out the pages of *The Golden Legend*. On the one hand, then as now, St George is seen as a fertility symbol, a sort of baptised Green Man; on the other he is the Soldier Saint, the combater of demons and the divine champion against the power of evil.

The myths of St George-Khidr have spread across the width of Asia, and from Persia eastwards their links to Christianity have been long forgotten: outside Delhi I was once taken to a cave where Muslim Sufis would go to fast for forty days in order to summon up Khidr, the Green Sufi. Yet it seems that there is nowhere in the East where it is quite as easy to summon up Khidr as in his birthplace at Beit Jala.

'Ask anyone,' said Fr. Methodius when I questioned him on the matter. 'Stop anyone in the street outside and ask if they have seen St George. They will all have stories. Don't take my word for it: go out and see for yourself.'

We left the church and I did as he suggested. The first person we came across was an elderly Muslim gentleman named Mansour Ali. I asked him whether he had ever seen St George.

'Of course,' he said. 'I live just around the corner, so I see him frequently – he is always coming and going on his horse.'

'You see this in dreams?'

'No, when I am awake, in daylight. Khidr is not dead. Whenever we have problems he comes and helps us.'

'In what way?'

'Well, last year I asked him to find work for my children. Within two weeks both my sons had good jobs.'

'For other people he has worked bigger miracles,' said the old doorkeeper, who had shuffled up and begun eavesdropping on the conversation. 'Last month there was a big man from Ramallah. He was very sick: he'd had a stroke and couldn't speak. Half his body had stopped. Well, he came here and took some of the oil from the lamp which burns in front of the icon of St George. Two weeks later he came back with a pair of sheep, completely cured. In fact he wouldn't stop chattering until we locked him out of the church.'

Later, back in the monastery courtyard, I asked Methodius: 'Do you really believe all this talk of miracles?'

He stroked his beard. 'It is according to your faith,' he said after a while. 'If you don't have faith in St George, nothing will happen. If you really believe, then maybe you will be healed.'

'And do you believe?' I asked.

'Well, I'll tell you the greatest miracle,' said Methodius. 'I live here alone: there are no other monks here, and there are no other Christians in the village round about. That doorkeeper – he's a Muslim. So is my sacristan. There are mosques all around: listen – can you hear? That's the call to evening prayer. '

Methodius pulled out his bleeper and unlocked the car. 'There are plenty of Hamas people in Beit Jala,' he said, opening the door of the Subaru. 'And however well Christians and Muslims used to get on, since the rise of Hamas in the last couple of years things have become a little strained. But I'm quite safe, and so is the whole monastery. I sleep easy at night. Now, there aren't many places you could say that of in Israel or the West Bank these days, are there?'

That night, in my rooms in Jerusalem, I thought back to my first stay on the West Bank in the summer of 1990, when I had heard a story that illustrated as well as any the tensions in the occupied region. The story had been told to me in the village of Biddya, and concerned Abu-Zeid, the corrupt village *mukhtar* (mayor) installed by the Israeli military authorities to rule the village for them.

Seven times the villagers had attempted to rid themselves of the hated collaborator, and the story of his eventual demise had rapidly turned into something of a folk tale across the West Bank. I had been wanting to get to Biddya to try to seek out a relatively trustworthy account of the story ever since I had first started hearing heavily elaborated versions of it in the coffee houses of Ramallah, but it was not easy. The village was nearly always under curfew, most recently as punishment for a Molotov cocktail lobbed at a passing Israeli patrol. But at six one morning I had been rung up by my contact in the village, a Palestinian landowner named Usamah, and told that the curfew had been lifted until noon. He said I should get ready; he would pick me up at seven.

We drove out of Ramallah, past an avenue of Israeli army checkpoints – little birds' nests of Uzis and razor wire – and out into the West Bank countryside: low, dry, rolling slopes; silvery olive groves; villages of old stone houses sheltering under the lee of the steeper hills. Only a mile before Biddya did the scene change. Turning the bend of a dry *wadi*, we saw Settlement Ariel ahead of us: a modern Western town with shopping arcades, sports centres and supermarkets. No Palestinian, either Christian or Muslim, ever needed to bother applying to live in Ariel: its houses were available only to Jewish settlers. When local Palestinian labourers at the settlement were forced to wear large badges reading 'Foreign Worker', some liberal Israeli commentators went as far as drawing comparisons with the race laws of Nazi Germany. The badges were later removed.

'That was my grandfather's land,' said Usamah as we passed beneath the settlement. 'It has belonged to this village since the time of the Canaanites. But the Israelis took it 1977. We've never received any compensation.'

Ariel, Usamah explained, was now home to eight thousand Israelis, but was projected ultimately to house a hundred thousand – a gloomy prospect for Biddya, which, sited precariously beneath the town, looked certain to have all its remaining land requisitioned for new housing estates from which Palestinians would be banned. This year, said Usamah, a further series of olive groves separating the village from the settlement had been seized and bulldozed to provide room for a thousand new houses being built for Soviet Jews fleeing a resurgent Russian racism. Yet again it was the Palestinians who were being made to pay the price for European anti-Semitism.

'A Russian can come to my land tomorrow and have more

right to it than me, my wife or my children,' said Usamah. 'Now the cultivated land has all been taken, and nearly all the olives cut down. Every year they take a little bit more. They think that if they can take it piece by piece there will be no trouble.'

In the end, however, Biddya had not stood by and waited for the slow extinction that was being imposed on it. On the outbreak of the *intifada* Palestinian flags had been raised on the power lines, demonstrations had been mounted, stones thrown. Faced with this defiance, the Israelis could have placed the village under rigorous curfew. This would have limited the trouble but would have been time-consuming, expensive and have tied up large numbers of troops. Far less effort was the option of controlling the village through a client *mukhtar* who, in return for power over the village, would keep order for his Israeli masters.

For seven years Abu Zeid had ruled Biddya as a tyrant, but since his demise the Israelis had been forced to rule the village directly. Neither method had managed to subdue Biddya, but together they had succeeded in ruining it. Of a total population of 3,300, more than five hundred villagers – most of the younger generation – were currently in prison, and forty families had had their houses destroyed. Moreover, after every incident the army made a point of cutting down an olive grove: so far two thousand trees had gone, and only a few remained. Ninety per cent of the village's income used to come from its olives, and it is now bankrupt.

Usamah's uncle, Tariq, was part of the large Nasbeh clan that had ruled Biddya until the Israeli military authorities deposed them. We found him in the walled garden of the family's ancestral house, tending his old musk roses under a trellis of tumbling vines. Usamah had sent word that we were coming, and his aunt, Um-Mohammed, had prepared breakfast for us. She was a big woman and wore a big blue dress, trussed at the waist. At her command we sat on stools, nibbling from the avalanche of olives, mountains of humus and several low ranges of feta cheese she had spread out for our pleasure.

While we ate, Tariq began. 'Abu-Zeid – God burn his bones! – was a very clever man.' He rearranged his shift and twirled his worry beads around his index finger. 'Ya Allah! No one knew how to extort money like him.'

'How did he do it?' I asked.

'The wild dog!' said Um-Mohammed. 'He tried everything.'

'It's true,' said Tariq. 'My great-great-great-grandfather brought Abu-Zeid's Negro forebears here from the Hijaz to be our house-slaves. This was his way of getting revenge.' Tariq shook his head sadly. 'He did everything he could to ruin this village. He would threaten to build a road through someone's house, then collect bribes to stop it. Once he cut off everyone's water and electricity and demanded 500 dinars [£700] from every family before he would reconnect it.'

'Tchk!' said Um-Mohammed, spitting on the ground. 'That was nothing. It was what he did with our land that made us hate him.'

'My younger brother was in prison for throwing stones,' explained Tariq. 'Abu-Zeid came to our house and offered to get his sentence reduced. He asked my father to put his thumbprint on some papers. It was only later that we discovered that he had tricked my father into signing away 110 dunums of our land west of the village. Ariel has an industrial park there now.'

'Abu-Zeid tricked all of us,' said Um-Mohammed. 'Like a mad dog he bit everyone around him.'

'We got a petition signed by every family in the village and took it to the Military Governor. He was a good man, and I think he would have replaced Abu-Zeid. But the settlers at Ariel blocked it. Abu-Zeid was their man. After our petition failed, Abu-Zeid arranged the killing of the old man who had organised the petition. We knew then that we had to destroy Abu-Zeid before he destroyed the village.'

'We are under military occupation,' said Usamah. 'We have no courts or civil authorities to look after our interests. This is what the occupation has reduced us to.'

'At that time we knew nothing about killing,' said Tariq, 'so we hired a Bedouin to do it for us. The Bedouin collaborate with the Israelis and are allowed to join the army and possess weapons. But they will kill anyone if they are paid. My brother knew this killer from Kafr Qasim. After we hired him, this man waited for

Abu-Zeid and shot him with an Uzi. He took fourteen bullets in the stomach. But he didn't die. The Israelis took him to a new hospital in Jerusalem and gave him a new plastic stomach. After a month he was back. The Bedouin is still in prison.'

Tariq popped an olive into his mouth. 'After the Bedouin failed, we vowed to finish Abu-Zeid ourselves. Our first attempt was very amateur. We tried to run him over. The first time we used a car, but he clung onto the bonnet. When the car crashed against the wall, the driver was killed but Abu-Zeid was unhurt. The next time we used a big lorry. That put Abu-Zeid in hospital – he lost his left leg – but although both his younger sons were killed, Abu-Zeid lived.'

'We didn't give up, though,' said Usamah. 'We sent a boy to buy two grenades on the black market in Tel Aviv. When he got back he experimented with one in a cave. It seemed easy to operate, so the next day he threw the other at Abu-Zeid. It sailed through the window of his car, but it was faulty and didn't blow. After that the Israelis gave Abu-Zeid many more weapons and rebuilt his house so that it was like a fortress.'

'Abu-Zeid went crazy,' said Usamah. 'He destroyed the houses belonging to everyone he thought of as an enemy. Then he bought two huge Rottweilers. He used to hobble around the village on his wooden leg, patrolling with the dogs, his brother and his two remaining sons. They beat anyone they found in the streets after dark.'

'Abu-Zeid promised, "Before the next olive season I will have destroyed this village completely,"' said Tariq. 'People said he had gone insane. He blew up the olive press we had been given by the Jordanians before 1967, then began systematically cutting down the olive trees of those he didn't like. But he didn't run away. He knew we would try again, and wherever he went we would find him and kill him.'

'The fifth attempt was a mass attack,' said Usamah. 'The *intifada* was at its height and the *shabab* [young men] had formed hit squads. On 6 March at eight o'clock the *shabab* attacked his house with molotov cocktails. Their object was to blow him up by igniting the gas canisters he kept in his garage. But they didn't know that the Israelis had given the garage new metal doors. As they tried to break in, Abu-Zeid hobbled up onto his roof and began picking them off with his gun. After he had killed four, the village imam broadcast an appeal for help on the mosque loudspeakers. The whole village rushed into the street and joined in. There must have been seven hundred people out there.'

'But we didn't get anywhere,' said Tariq gloomily. 'While we all went off to evening prayers, one of Abu-Zeid's sons slipped out the back and ran to Ariel. When prayers were over, we managed to get into the garage and blow up his bulletproof car. But before we could do anything more the settlers arrived. They were all armed, and began firing into the crowd. Later, when the army came, they put the village under curfew, arrested a hundred people and demolished . . . I don't know how many houses.'

'Ya Allah!' said Um-Mohammed, who had reappeared with a little bowl of humus. 'There wasn't a woman in the village who wouldn't have gladly strangled Abu-Zeid after that.'

'It's true,' said Tariq, raising his eyebrows and giving his beads a twirl. 'But we thought he would not suspect this. So on the sixth attempt we dressed up one of my nephews as a Palestinian woman and sent him off to Abu-Zeid's house with a basket of fruit on his head. Abu-Zeid was sitting outside with Zeid, his eldest son. My nephew put the basket down, pulled out a pistol from under the figs and fired six shots from twenty metres. He hit both men and killed Zeid, but he only succeeded in taking off Abu-Zeid's left arm and wounding him in one lung. Abu-Zeid was fifteen days in intensive care and they had to give him a new arm and a mechanical lung. By this stage he was more like a robot than a man. But within a month he was back.'

'Some in the village believed that Abu-Zeid was some kind of *djinn*,' said Um-Mohammed. 'We thought he would never die.'

'He escaped us six times. *Six times!* But we got him in the end.'

'I saw it with my own eyes,' said Um-Mohammed, rearranging her white calico *chador*. 'It was a few days before the olive season. I was coming back from my brother's house early in the morning when I noticed Abu-Zeid's car coming along the Ariel road. He turned a corner and saw that there was a roadblock. At the same time two *shabab* leapt out from behind a wall and – *pfoo!* – peppered his car with Uzi guns.'

'The Israelis had given him bulletproof windows,' said Tariq, 'but he had left them open.'

'Abu-Zeid tried to reverse and escape, but he hit a wall and they got him all the same.' Um-Mohammed's face exploded into a broad grin. 'He died in great pain. I was so happy.'

'The village gathered around and one of the old men said that they should pour gasoline over the car and burn it, otherwise the settlers might take him away to Tel Aviv and bring him back to life with one of their machines. After his earlier escapes they were worried he might survive even thirty bullets in the chest.'

'But do you know the strange thing?' said Um-Mohammed, scooping up some humus on a piece of pitta bread and popping it into her mouth. 'Because he was half Negro, the smoke was as black as pitch. The place where he died, nothing grows there now.'

'So you understand now why we were so pleased when we finally got him on the seventh attempt?' asked Tariq.

'After we killed him and made a fire of his body, the *Yahoodi* [Jewish] settlers saw the black smoke and came running again. But they were too late. There was only a burned skull, a leg bone, a fire-blackened lung machine and a great pile of plastic sludge that had been his stomach. All they could do was put it all in a sack and give it to his wife. '

'She threw it onto a rubbish tip,' said Um-Mohammed. 'Abu-Zeid had another woman in Kifl Harith. His wife hated him as much as the rest of us.'

'The army put the village under curfew for two weeks,' said Tariq. 'We couldn't even harvest our trees. But no one minded. Inside every house it was like a holiday. People were singing and dancing.'

'Even in the prisons there was rejoicing,' said Usamah. 'All Abu-Zeid's old enemies – there were about two hundred of them in jail at that time – they had a big party also.'

The curfew was due to resume in less than ten minutes. I got up and said my goodbyes, while Usamah hurried me out to the car. We drove out of the village and past the gates and guntowers of Ariel. Under the razor wire, the settlers' bulldozers were at work clearing Biddya's olive groves.

'It was a great day for the village when we killed Abu-Zeid,' said Usamah. 'But in the long run, what difference does it make?'

He stopped the car by a pile of uprooted olive trees and got out, indicating that I should do the same: 'Such trees are 150 years old – three times the age of the State of Israel,' he said, pulling out a clod of earth from the roots and crumbling it in his hands. 'Generation after generation our people have come three times a year to dress, fertilise and harvest these trees. All our life, all our traditions, are connected to such trees. But now they bring their powerful machines from the USA and destroy our inheritance in fifteen minutes. Like us, these trees have deep roots. Look how strongly these roots bond the trees to the soil! But now they are uprooted, and with or without Abu-Zeid, if the settlers get their way we will be next. Sooner or later they will expel us all. It is only a matter of time.'

'The Americans would never let them,' I said.

'Wouldn't they?' replied Usamah.

'You want Utopia?' said Mayor Ron. 'I got Utopia! Look!'

Ron Nachman, the Mayor of Settlement Ariel, called to his secretary. Seconds later she appeared with the official photograph album.

'Ariel was my idea,' explained Mayor Ron. 'In 1977 nobody lived here. There was nothing. Look: here – nothing except a few old trees. Here's me in the first tent . . . and that's the luxury caravan we moved into a little later. Here are the watertanks and the bulldozers. You see these boulders? That's the supermarket now. And over there? Those stones? That's now a lawn.'

The secretary took the album and Mayor Ron settled down behind his desk. Above his head was a plaque:

For representing the people of Judaea, Samaria and
Gaza.
For reclaiming our Biblical roots in Eretz Israel.
For courage and conviction and deep vision.
Presented by Americans for a Safe Israel, April 1990.

'I give people the chance to participate in the greatest adventure,' said the Mayor, 'the building of a new town from scratch
– from nothing! Developing a new society for all our tomorrows.'

Mayor Ron clearly knows the reputation he has for public
relations. He is still a young man, and exudes energy and dyna-
mism. He talks fast, in flawless American.

'Friend, I'll tell you something. Do you know what the Arabs
used to ask me? "Ron," they would say, "why do you come to
this bare mountain?" I said, "Wait five years – you'll see what we
can do with this land."'

'Do you have problems with your Palestinian neighbours?' I
asked.

'The Arabs don't have a problem with Jews,' replied Mayor
Ron. 'They have problems with Arabs – with the PLO terrorists.
The PLO are enforcing a rule of terror around here – anyone who
cooperates with us is as good as dead – even the *mayor* of an
Arab village near here was gunned down by PLO terrorists, d'you
know that? Friend, let me tell you: these Arabs don't want peace
with Israel – they want a piece *of* Israel.'

Mayor Ron smiled a winning breakfast-cereal smile. 'But I guess
you're asking about me personally. No – I don't have anything
against Arabs at all. I'm no racist: I have an Arab cleaning lady.'
He leaned forwards on his desk: 'That's right – *an Arab cleaning
lady*. She is alone with my babies. I can't say everyone would trust
an Arab like that.'

Mayor Ron paused to let the full implications of his liberalism
sink in. 'You know, William, I am deeply proud of what we've
built here. A nice town, a clean town, full of nice people. We
accept everybody. Already we are the fastest-growing town in
Israel. The land is there. All we suffer from is lack of housing. If

we can overcome that, soon we'll be a town of a hundred thousand, and stretch for eight miles over these hills.'

He pointed to an aerial photograph of the area tacked to the wall beside his desk. 'Go on! Walk around! See it for yourself. This is a free country, a democracy – the *only* democracy in the Middle East!'

Outside, tanned, healthy children were racing around the crazy paving on BMX bikes. Long lines of supermarkets, cafés, shops and jeans stores were spread out across a plaza; Kenny Rogers was piped through the Tannoy. Beyond the swimming pool and the ranks of gleaming station wagons in the parking lot, the bare hills of the West Bank stretched into the distance.

The children seemed less keen on Ariel than their Mayor. 'Boring' was the opinion of most of the teenagers I spoke to, 'no nightlife'; but there was no shortage of enthusiasm among the adults. I ended up talking to Dina Salit, who had emigrated five years earlier from Canada. We sipped cappuccinos and picked at chocolate croissants, and while we sipped and nibbled, Dina enthused.

'My husband and I are very happy here, very happy indeed. I mean, if we had just gone to Tel Aviv, we might as well have stayed in Montreal. But here we are making a truly Zionist statement, doing something, you know, totally different. I mean, how many people get the chance to be in on the building of a new town?' Dina beamed at me. 'Here you feel that your presence really makes a difference. Here you feel . . . valued.'

'Yes?'

'*Deeply* valued. Howard is the director of a security company, so he feels valued too.'

'And what about the Arabs?' I asked.

'Before the *intifada* we made friends with several A-rabs,' Dina said, drawing out the first syllable. 'To me, as a Canadian, that was a miracle. I didn't know it could be done. I mean, you know, *A-rabs*. But all the same we did used to have some of the A-rab construction workers in for coffee. I'm not saying we were best friends, that it was a love affair, but it was OK.'

'Has the *intifada* changed everything?'

353

'Yes and no. We don't have A-rabs in for coffee any more, but you know, the political scene is seldom a topic of conversation here. We're all much more concerned about gossip, or street cleaning,' Dina giggled. 'That's a *much* greater problem!'

I paid the bill, and Dina walked me over to the Ariel bus stop. As we strolled, I asked: 'So what would you say to those Israelis who would give away your settlement and the rest of the West Bank in return for peace?'

'I've never heard any A-rab say they want Judaea and Samaria only,' she replied. 'For them it's only the first step. They want to drive the Israelis into the sea. Everyone knows that. I won't be taken in by that terrorist Arafat – forget it!'

She paused, and in the silence I could hear the strains of Kenny Rogers still drifting over the shopping arcade.

'Arafat and his terrorists are playing political games – and we're talking people's homes. You know what that means? *People's homes.*'

THE ANGLICAN HOSTEL, NAZARETH, 20 NOVEMBER

Around 570 A.D., after he was first professed as a monk at the Abbey of St Theodosius, John Moschos withdrew into the wilderness and spent ten years in the remote cave monastery at Pharan, to the north of Jerusalem.

Pharan, the modern Ein Fara, is reputedly the oldest abbey in Palestine. It was founded in the early fourth century by the great Byzantine hermit St Chariton, who, it is said, settled here in a cave above a pool of pure spring water. There he gathered a community of like-minded ascetics around him, living a life of silence, self-abnegation and severe fasting, interspersed with long hours of prayer. Two hundred years later, Moschos appears to have been drawn to the site less by its antiquity than by the wisdom of its then *hegumen*, Abba Cosmas the Eunuch. In a crucial passage in *The Spiritual Meadow*, Moschos credits Cosmas with first giving him the idea to collect the sayings of the fathers: 'Whilst he [Abba Cosmas] was speaking to me about the salvation of the soul, we came across an aphorism of St Athanasius, Archbishop of Alexandria. And the elder said to me, "When you come across such a saying, if you have no paper with you, write it on your clothing" – so great was the appetite of Abba Cosmas for the words of our holy fathers and teachers.' It was advice that was eventually to lead Moschos to compiling *The Spiritual Meadow*, and so to preserve the otherwise largely unrecorded history of the monks of Byzantine Palestine.

By a remarkable coincidence, at the beginning of this trip, on Mount Athos, I had met a monk who claimed to have been the last hermit to have lived in the very same cave as Moschos at Ein Fara. Fr. Alexandros was a tall, rubicund figure with a faded serge cassock, a short Orthodox pigtail and a grey beard, matted and tangled like John the Baptist's on some early Byzantine icon. I had stumbled across him on a walk one afternoon, soon after digging out the manuscript of *The Spiritual Meadow* from the library at the Monastery of Iviron. He lived alone in a small wooden hut in a clearing in the forest, high above Karyes. It was an idyllic place, a bright and silent retreat, fringed with lilies and ilex and commanding an astonishing view down over the silver domes of the Russian Skete to the deep, fragmented blue of the Aegean far below. But this, Fr. Alexandros told me, was not his home, nor where he longed to be: he had moved to this Greek hilltop only a decade before, after being driven out of his hermitage in the Holy Land.

For most of his adult life, he explained, he had followed the ways of the desert fathers in the cave at Ein Fara, a millennia and a half after St Chariton first founded the monastery. But Fr. Alexandros had been the last of the line. About ten years after the Israeli conquest and occupation of the West Bank, he had begun to receive death threats which he believed came from a group of Israeli zealots who had established a settlement nearby. Then one day in the winter of 1979 his spiritual father and distant neighbour, a Greek monk named Philloumenos, was hacked to death in his cell at Jacob's Well near Nablus; someone had poisoned his dogs, attacked him with an axe, then incinerated his remains with a grenade. Shortly afterwards, Fr. Alexandros returned from a trip to Jerusalem to find his cave-chapel desecrated and his books and possessions scattered and burned. The pulpit in the chapel had been axed into a hundred pieces. The hermit fled, caught ship to Athens, and had eventually found his way to Athos. The cave and spring had apparently since been wired off and absorbed into a new settlement.

Like many hermits, Fr. Alexandros was a deeply eccentric man, a holy fool who talked to his pet owl, fed the lizards, and claimed to receive occasional visits from angels. He was a man whose statements could not, perhaps, be taken entirely at face value. I was therefore a little surprised to discover, on my visit to the Greek Orthodox Patriarchate in the Old City of Jerusalem, that much of what he had said had indeed been true. A bearded Greek Metropolitan who had known both Philloumenos and Alexandros showed me a file full of reports and correspondence about the desecration of the cave of St Chariton and the violent murder in Jacob's Well. A mentally ill Israeli from Tel Aviv had been charged with the Jacob's Well murder, I learned, as well as with two other killings. I was even directed to the Martyrion at the Orthodox Seminary on Mount Zion where Fr. Philloumenos's shattered skull and axe-cloven bones lay on permanent – if rather grisly – display, dressed in his old habit, awaiting potential canonisation.

'He *is* a saint,' I was assured by Fr. Aristopoulos, the earnest young monk who showed me into the Martyrion. 'Fr. Philloumenos received many telephone calls from the Jewish zealots saying he must leave Jacob's Well, that it was their holy place, not ours. After his dogs were poisoned the Patriarch said that he should come away and live in Jerusalem where it was more safe, but every time Philloumenos refused. He was saying vespers when the killer found him and started to chop at him with the axe.'

'He didn't kill him outright?'

'No,' replied the monk, 'but with many cuts: hands off, then feet, then legs. In pieces. Very nasty. Only at the end he threw the grenade.' Fr. Aristopoulos crossed himself in horror. 'But you know, when they held a small service for him four years after his death, they exhumed his relics and found that his body was uncorrupted.'

'But how could it be uncorrupted,' I asked, 'when he had already been chopped up and incinerated?'

'Well not *totally* uncorrupted,' admitted the monk. 'But it was still a very miraculous preservation. After this there were miracles – including healing of the sick – and many visions of Fr. Philloumenos. Some I have seen myself.'

'You've seen Fr. Philloumenos?'

'In my dreams I have seen him,' said Aristopoulos. 'Also I have smelt him.'

'I don't understand,' I said. 'I thought you said his body hadn't corrupted.'

'No, no,' said Fr. Aristopoulos. 'It was a good smell. During the Gulf War the Greek Consulate ordered all Greeks to go home. The seminary was closed and all the students left. I was here alone. I locked up the chapel and for three months I stayed upstairs in my room with my gasmask because of Saddam's Scud attacks. Then in March, when the war was over, I came and unlocked the door and walked in here for the first time since the New Year. It was as if the church was full of incense: a heavy smell, so nice, so sweet. It was coming from Fr. Philloumenos.'

So this, I thought, was how miracle stories began.

I told Fr. Aristopoulos about my meeting with Fr. Alexandros and his story of the assault on his cave. Aristopoulos replied that attacks on Church property were far from unusual. During the Six Day War, he said, the room in which we were standing had been attacked by a lone Israeli soldier who had fired off several shots at the iconostasis before being wounded – so at any rate claimed Fr. Aristopoulos – by a miraculous ricochet from an icon of the *Theotokos*, the Holy Virgin.

Checking these stories in the more sober *Jerusalem Post* archives and with the different Church authorities in Jerusalem, I found that from the early 1970s to the mid-1980s there had indeed been a wave of attacks on Church property. A Jerusalem church, a

Baptist chapel and a Christian bookshop had all been burned to the ground, allegedly by ultra-Orthodox *haredim*, while students from a nearby *yeshiva* had committed serious vandalism at the Dormition Abbey. There had also been a series of unsuccessful arson attacks on the Anglican church in West Jerusalem (the old wooden doors had had to be changed to steel to thwart repeated attempts at igniting them), as well as on two churches in Acre (a Greek Orthodox church in the Old City and a Protestant chapel in the new Israeli suburbs) and an Anglican church in Ramleh.

In addition to this, the Protestant cemetery on Mount Zion – already damaged between 1948 and 1967 when it stood in the no-man's land between Israel and Jordan – had been further desecrated no fewer than eight times. I visited it afterwards: the tombstones had almost all been shattered, metal crosses lay twisted in their sockets, and some of the sepulchres had been broken open; the one standing mausoleum was riddled with bulletholes. As Canon Naim Ateek of St George's Anglican Cathedral in Jerusalem put it after he had spent half an hour listing all the incidents of desecration he knew about: 'Israel would like to give the impression that it champions religious tolerance, but the whole country was built on the usurpation and confiscation of Christian and Muslim land. To this day the confiscation and desecration of Church land and buildings continues.'

Canon Ateek's views are widely held by the Palestinian Christians I talked to in Jerusalem, but there is another side to the story. The Israeli authorities have always roundly condemned the vandalism of Church property and assisted the churches to recover from any serious damage. While ultra-Orthodox Jewish *haredim* remain the chief suspects for most desecrations – and their presence is further indicated by the nature of the Hebrew graffiti sprayed on several of the desecrated sites – their involvement is rarely proven, while in some cases, such as the desecration of the cave of St Chariton, it is not impossible that the attack could equally well have been carried out by disgruntled Arabs. Moreover, while Christian institutions still tend to suffer from abusive graffiti – when Archbishop Desmond Tutu recently visited Jerusalem, for example, the gates of St George's were daubed with 'Go home dirty black Nazi pig' – the wave of arson and vandalism that took place during the seventies and early eighties now largely seems to have ceased, and there has been only one major arson attack in recent years: the gutting of a church in Tiberias.

Certainly, none of these unconnected incidents in any way proves the Palestinian Christians' contention that there is a concerted campaign to drive them out of their ancestral homes. But what they do undoubtedly reveal is a degree of prejudice and intolerance in Israel reminiscent of several other Middle Eastern countries – notably Turkey – where a religiously homogeneous majority is able to lord it over a relatively powerless minority community. Few Western Christians are aware of the degree of hardship faced by their co-religionists in the Holy Land, and the West's often uncritical support of Israel frankly baffles the Palestinian Christians who feel their position being eroded year by year. As Fr. Aristopoulos at the Martyrion put it: 'Had we been Jews and our churches been synagogues, the desecration we have suffered would have caused an international outcry. But because we are Christians no one seems to care.'

The day after I saw Fr. Philloumenos's axe-cleaved remains, I found a Christian Palestinian driver, Sami Fanous, who agreed to take me to see the cave at Ein Fara. I very much wanted to see the ruins of the *lavra* where Philloumenos used to visit his friend Fr. Alexandros, and where, fourteen hundred years earlier, John Moschos had retired to spend a decade of his life in silent meditation.

Since Alexandros's departure, the new Israeli settlement of Pharan had absorbed the cave, the spring and much of the surrounding countryside, and to get to the ruins we had first to get into the settlement. At its entrance, a massive yellow-painted electric steel gate blocked the road; on either side tangles of razor wire led off across the hills as far as the eye could see. Sami stopped the car and we were questioned by the guard. I showed him the monastery marked on a map, and he went off to a sentrybox with my passport. There he conferred with someone on a telephone. He replaced the receiver and came back to tell us to wait. After twenty minutes, the telephone rang, permission was granted, and we were waved through.

The path to the monastery led off from the bottom of one of the settlement's housing estates. I left Sami with his car and headed off down into the valley on foot. All around, the hillsides were hard and dry: compressed beds of geological strata rolled off in great undulating contortions into the distance; there was no tree, and barely a blade of grass visible in the whole great panorama. As I descended into the *wadi*, however, the path turned a corner, and far below, at the lowest point in the valley, there appeared a small oasis: a patch of the densest woodland made up of ferns, pines and palms. From where I was standing I could not see the spring itself, but I could clearly hear it. The distant sound of the running water filled the silence of the *wadi*, echoed and amplified as it bounced off the walls of the ravine. It was an unseasonably hot day, and I shouldered my pack and stumbled down the path towards the sound.

Arriving at the bottom, I took off my shoes and bathed my feet in the clear, cold water. Despite the heat, the area around the spring was cool, shady and peaceful. As I sat there I thought how easy it was to understand why Moschos had chosen this spot to spend his years as a hermit: in such a place, it seemed to me, it must have been easy to foster the great monastic virtues of gentleness, balance, lack of haste and clarity of spirit. All around the spring, peppering the cliffs of the ravine, were the mouths of the caves that had once been filled with Moschos's fellow hermits, men like Abba Paul, 'a holy man of great humility . . . I don't know whether I ever met his like in all my life'; or Abba Auxanon, 'a man of compassion, continence and solitude who treated himself so harshly that over a period of four days he would eat only a twenty-four *lepta* [ha'penny] loaf of bread; indeed sometimes this was sufficient for him during a whole week.' These caves had also been home to Abba Cosmas the Eunuch, Moschos's spiritual father. Moschos only sketches his Abbot fairly briefly in the *Meadow*, but we learn that he apparently had the power to heal the sick, and that even by Byzantine standards he was famous for his ascetic self-control: 'on the eve of the holy Lord's day, he would stand from vespers to dawn singing and reading, in his cell or in church, never sitting down at all. Once the sun had risen and the appointed service had been sung, he would sit reading the holy Gospel until it was time for the Eucharist.'

Other than the bare hermits' caves, only a little survived of the monastery that Moschos had known. There were some crumbling cell walls, a cistern, a few stretches of Byzantine stonework, the odd staircase and a little sagging terracing where the monks had once, presumably, grown vegetables. A Byzantine mosaic was said to survive in the cave church at the top of the honeycomb of interconnected caverns, but it was impossible now to reach it without a rope or a ladder. After an hour poking around, clambering into some of the more accessible cave-cells, I set off up the hill again.

I was halfway up the path when I was met by Sami, my taxi driver. He was clearly very frightened. In my absence, he explained, he had been interrogated by the settlement's security guards. They had confiscated his ID card, and he was now terrified of being detained or arrested. 'Don't say I'm a taxi driver,' he begged. 'Say I'm your friend.'

We got back to the car and drove to the main gate, where a different guard was now on duty. He called for the head of security on his walkie-talkie, and told us to move the car off the road and to wait.

'There are many Arab terrorists in this area,' he said by way of explanation.

We waited for nearly an hour before the head of security turned up. He was a small, tough-looking man in khaki fatigues. A pistol was tucked into his belt and in his hands he held an assault rifle. He cross-questioned me for thirty minutes, examining my maps, my paperback of *The Spiritual Meadow* and my passport over and over again. What was I doing? Was the driver my friend? Where was this monastery I kept referring to? Was it an Arab monastery?

And who was John Moschos? Was he an Arab too? Did I have other Arab friends? Had my Arab friends asked me to do anything for them in the settlement? He then returned to the sentrybox and read my passport details down the telephone to someone. He made several more phone calls and conferred for a further fifteen minutes on the walkie-talkie. Finally he came over and returned my passport and Sami's ID.

'There has been a misunderstanding,' he said gruffly as the steel gate rolled back. 'You can go now.'

But he didn't apologise.

NAZARETH, 22 NOVEMBER

Before I left Jerusalem I had bought a bus ticket to the Egyptian border. From there I planned to make my way to Alexandria. The bus was due to leave in two days' time, but before I left Israel I had a promise to keep.

On my last day in Beirut I had promised to visit Kafr Bir'im, the village from which the Christian Palestinian family I had met in the Mar Elias refugee camp had fled in 1948. The Daous had felt they would be safer if they temporarily left their homes, and as a result of that decision had spent forty-six years in exile in a succession of squalid refugee camps. I wanted to know what would have happened to them if they had decided to stay. Would their life have been any easier in the new State of Israel?

In a general sense I already knew the answer. Compared to their compatriots who fled or were expelled – or indeed those on the West Bank who had been conquered by the Israelis in 1967 and were still under military rule twenty-seven years later – the Palestinian Christians who had stayed on and become citizens of Israel in 1948 had been very lucky. They had Israeli passports, and could vote in Israeli elections. They had access to Israeli edu-cational facilities, enjoyed Israeli civil justice and could even, if they so wished, join the Israeli army. True, there were complaints about land expropriation and discrimination: the councils of Arab towns were said to receive less than a third of the funds available to those with Jewish populations. Yet compared to the dismal fate of those who still languished in refugee camps, the Israeli Arab Christians had been very fortunate indeed. Unlike their counterparts on the West Bank, relatively few have emigrated, and since the foundation of Israel their numbers have quadrupled, from the thirty-four thousand left in their homeland in 1949 to around 150,000 today.

But what I wanted to compare with what I had heard in Beirut was more specific: the fate of the Daous' neighbours in Kafr Bir'im who had stayed on. Samira Daou had told me that when Israeli planes had bombed Kafr Bir'im, her friends and neighbours had taken shelter in the nearby town of Jish. What had happened to them?

After leaving Ein Fara, I got Sami to drive me through the occupied West Bank, past Biddya and Ariel, to Nazareth in northern Israel. Then this morning, after breakfast, we set off north again towards Jish. The drive led past the Sea of Galilee, with its ancient Byzantine churches clustering around the shore, and up, over stark hillsides of black volcanic stone, on towards the north and the Lebanese border.

The countryside was dotted with Israeli *kibbutzim* energetically scratching a living from the harsh soil. But as we drove, Sami pointed out the sites of some of the 385 Palestinian villages – many of them Christian – which had preceded such Israeli settlements in Galilee, until they were systematically depopulated and destroyed by the Jewish Haganah during the war of 1948. It was the cactus plants that always gave the old villages away: however efficiently the Israelis had bulldozed the buildings and erased the Palestinian communities from the map, the old villages' cactus hedges had deep roots, and kept sprouting again and again to mark the sites of the former garden boundaries and the shadows of former fields.

'That was the village of Faradi,' said Sami at one stage, pointing to a few blocks of stone and some cactus plants by the side of the road at the bottom of a hill. 'Now the Kibbutz of Farud farms that land.'

As we climbed the hill, Sami's battered old Mercedes labouring behind a convoy of slow military trucks, the kibbutz's cowsheds and farm buildings came into view, their solar panels glinting in the morning light. Beyond, the low hills and plains of Galilee spread out before us. Despite the mass immigration of the 1920s and thirties, in 1948 the Jews had still formed less than a quarter of the population of this area, and the displacement of the Arab majority had been achieved only by a process which Yigal Allon, the commander of the Jewish military forces in Galilee (and later Deputy Prime Minister of Israel), himself described as 'cleansing'. 'We saw a need to clean the Inner Galilee,' he wrote in his memoirs, 'and to create a Jewish territorial succession in the entire area of Upper Galilee. We therefore looked for means to cause the tens of thousands of sulky Arabs who remained in Galilee to flee ... Wide areas were cleansed.'

In the process of this 'cleansing' of the Galilee, the Christian Palestinians had offered less resistance than the Muslims, and consequently were better treated. Moreover, Israel was careful not to offend public opinion in the Christian West by over-zealous 'cleansing' in the more famous Christian towns and villages; indeed, special instructions were issued by Ben Gurion himself not to loot Christian holy places such as Nazareth. As the Brigade Commander who captured the city later wrote: 'The conquest of Nazareth has political importance – the behaviour of the [Israeli] occupation forces in the city could serve as a factor in determining the prestige of the young state abroad.'

In nearby Beit Shean (then known by its Arabic name Beisan) the inhabitants were divided in two: Muslims were bussed across the Jordan into exile, while the Christians were given the option of fleeing to Nazareth. Canon Naim Ateek was eleven when he was expelled from his family home in Beisan. 'When the Israeli army came into the town there was no resistance,' he had told me when I had visited him at St George's. 'Then quite suddenly a fortnight later we were given two hours to pack up and leave: the soldiers came around from house to house and said, "If you don't leave we will kill you." We were allowed to take only what we could carry.' Ten years later, in 1958, when travel restrictions on the Israeli Arabs were lifted, Ateek's father took the family back to see their old house. They knocked on the door, but were sent roughly away by a Polish man armed with a rifle. They never went back again.

An hour's drive beyond Nazareth, the road turned a corner and we found ourselves looking down over thick conifer forests to the tower blocks of Safad. 'Before 1948 it was a mixed town,' said Sami. 'There were Muslims, Jews and Christians. Now it's exclusively Jewish. The Christians and the Muslims were driven out by force and were never allowed back again. My mother had cousins there, but most of her family were killed when the Haganah bombarded the Arab part of the town with mortars. A few made it to Lebanon, but we haven't heard from them since the invasion of '82. We don't know whether they are alive or dead.'

Jish lay a short distance beyond Safad, a little higher into the hills. It was a scrappy-looking place, the few old stone houses surrounded by many more new bungalows, the minaret of a mosque and the spires of two churches. Unsure where to begin my enquiries, I asked an Arab woman in a pinafore the way to the priest's house. I was directed a short distance down the street.

The door was opened by Fr. Bishara Suleiman, the Maronite parish priest. He was a tall man with a short clipped goatee beard, and he spoke excellent English (and French, as I later discovered: he had studied theology at the Sorbonne). Unusually for a Middle Eastern clergyman he was dressed not in formal black robes, but in a T-shirt and slacks. I explained the reason for my visit to the town, and he immediately invited me in. At the same time he called to his nephew, John Suleiman, to go and fetch some of the old men from Kafr Bir'im.

We took seats on a balcony, looking out onto the village's olive groves. Fr. Suleiman's wife produced a thermos of strong Turkish coffee from the kitchen, and while we sipped the scalding liquid I asked the priest if he would tell me the full story of what had happened to Kafr Bir'im after the Daous had left it in 1948. Would they have been better advised to stay?

'Very few of our villagers did flee in '48,' said Fr. Suleiman. 'We had always had good relations with the Jews and the British: so much so that in 1936 [during the Palestinian revolt] we were accused of collaboration and had to beg the British to protect us. They sent some Tommies who set up camp on the edge of the village, and after that we had no trouble. We had always helped the Jews entering Palestine from Lebanon, and we thought that if there was any trouble they would help us. That was why most of the villagers stayed on, despite all the stories we heard about Deir Yassin and other massacres nearer here.'

'Such as?'

'The Haganah massacred seventy Arab prisoners at Ein al-Zaytun near Safad. They tied their hands behind their backs. Then they shot them. But we thought nothing like that would happen here, partly because we were Christians and partly because we had always been friendly towards the Jews.'

At this moment Fr. Suleiman's nephew returned with the old village schoolmaster of Bir'im, Elias Jacob.

Elias was a thin, wizened old man. At seventy-five he was a little uncertain on his legs, but still absolutely clear in his mind. He was, said Fr. Suleiman, the best authority on the history of Kafr Bir'im; and as if to prove it, Elias produced from his pocket a slip of paper on which were written the main dates and facts of the story. He didn't want anyone getting anything wrong, he said. He took a seat, threw back a small cup of Turkish coffee, and at Fr. Suleiman's invitation began to talk.

'The Haganah soldiers arrived in our village on 29 October 1948,' he said, checking the date against his notes. 'Most of us remained in our houses, but the old men and the priest received the troops at the entrance of the village with a white flag. We offered them bread and salt, the symbol of friendship and peace.'

'Were they equally friendly?' I asked.

'They were,' said the old man. 'They were very good, very polite. We gave them food and they occupied some houses. They stayed for fifteen days. Then on 13 November 1948 an order arrived that we all had to leave.'

'Were you surprised?'

'We were amazed. At first we refused to go. But then a new officer arrived and he was very different. He said we had twenty-four hours to get out. Then we were afraid. He gave no reasons. He just said that we had to be five kilometres from the village or we would be shot.'

As Elias was speaking we were joined on the balcony by another old man, Wadeer Ferhat. He was a big, high-spirited man with a huge walrus moustache. When he discovered what we were talking about he began shouting in a series of angry outbursts of guttural Arabic. Sami translated.

'Mr Wadeer says that they threw the people out from their homes into the countryside. They had no tents. Some found shelter in caves. Everyone else just squatted under trees or in the fields. It was November, but much colder than this year. By December there was thick snow. He said several babies died from exposure.'

Wadeer continued shouting, hands flying in the air in a series of graphic gestures.

'He says he was thirty-five at the time, but that both his parents were very old, over seventy. He says that they cried for many days because they had lost their homes and their land.'

'What Wadeer has not said,' pointed out Elias Jacob, calmly consulting his fact sheet, 'was that before we left, each of the 1,050 villagers was given a number, granting them Israeli citizenship. We tidied and cleaned our houses because we thought we would soon be allowed back. After a time the Minister for Minorities, Mr Bichor Shitrit, came here. He saw that we were living under trees and ordered that we be given the houses here in Jish which had been vacated by fleeing Muslims. He said that we should wait for just fifteen days, and after that, when the area was calm, we could go back to Kafr Bir'im. In the meantime he allowed a few old men to stay in the village to guard the houses and the crops.'

'What happened then?' I asked.

'Six months later the old men were ordered out of the village, and it became clear that we were not going to get our houses back. So we decided to take the matter to the Israeli High Court.'

'The people of Bir'im have never resorted to violence,' said

Fr. Suleiman. 'We have always fought by law and by Christian principles.'

'In 1953 we finally won the case,' continued Elias. 'The court ordered that the evictions were unjust and said we should all be allowed back to our homes and to farm our fields.'

'So why aren't you back there now?' I asked.

'Because the next day the Israeli army declared the area a military zone and banned us from entering it. That afternoon they destroyed Kafr Bir'im by aerial bombardment. We had won the case, but they tricked us all the same. There was nothing we could do.'

Wadeer frowned and banged his fist on the table. Again Sami translated: 'He says all the villagers went up onto that hill and watched the bombing of their homes. They call it the Crying Hill now, because everyone from Kafr Bir'im wept that day. Everything they owned was still in those houses.'

'My father told me they didn't know what was going to happen until they heard the planes begin their bombing,' said Fr. Suleiman. 'It was 16 September 1953. They thought it was going to be the day they returned to their homes. But it was the day we lost them – and our fields – for ever.'

'I had built a house with my own hands,' said Elias. 'It had five rooms. But I lived in it only five months. Everything went. My furniture, cupboards, beds, icons. Worst of all, I lost my books.'

'I remember my father telling me what a wonderful village it was,' said Fr. Suleiman. 'The climate was very good. The soil was fertile. The air was fresh . . .'

'There were figs, olives, grapes, apples, springs of fresh water . . .' said Elias.

'And many wells,' added Wadeer in Arabic. 'I can see the whole village very clearly when I close my eyes. I remember every house, every building.'

'But when the Israeli air force began bombing there was nothing we could do,' said the old teacher. 'We could do nothing – nothing but go up to the hill and spend the whole day weeping like children.'

'We were betrayed,' said Wadeer.

'We still feel betrayed,' added Fr. Suleiman.

A silence fell over the balcony.

'So what happened to your land?' I asked eventually.

'In 1949 they gave some of our fields to a new kibbutz, Kibbutz Bar'am,' said the teacher, consulting his precious list of facts and figures. 'The kibbutz was built on 350 dunums of our land. Then in 1963 they established Moshav Dovev, with another two thousand dunums.'

'The site of the village is now a National Park,' said Fr. Suleiman. 'At the entrance to it they have put up a sign saying that "Bar'am Antiquities" date from the Second Temple Period. It's true that there are the ruins of a Roman-period synagogue in the middle of our village, but the sign gives the impression that the remains of our houses are all Roman ruins. The schoolchildren who are taken around it think that our old buildings – our stables and schools and houses – are like the ones you see at Pompeii.'

'We've been edited out of history,' said the old teacher. 'They don't admit to our existence. Or to the existence of our fathers and grandfathers and great-grandfathers.'

'I and my father dug a well,' said Wadeer. 'Now there is a sign there saying that it was built by someone called Yohanan of Bar'am at the time of the Romans.'

'Who is Yohanan of Bar'am?'

'Apparently a leader of the Jewish Revolt in 66 A.D.,' said the teacher. 'Though we in the village had never heard of him until the park was built.'

'They've made it as if my well is part of ancient Jewish history,' said Wadeer. 'But I dug that well with my own labour!'

'Another man, a friend of mine called Farah Laqzaly, made a sculpture of the Madonna,' said Elias. 'I remember seeing him making it. But now they say it is centuries old. They took it to Kibbutz Sasa and put it on display.'

'If the village is now a park, does that mean I could go and visit it?' I asked.

'Of course,' said Fr. Suleiman. 'And we will come too. No one from Bir'im misses a chance to return.'

Everyone rose. Wadeer and Fr. Suleiman's nephew John went in the priest's old station wagon, while Sami and I followed with Elias the schoolteacher. It was a short drive from Jish to Kafr Bir'im, less than ten minutes.

At the entrance to the park new Israeli flags were flying above a neat parking lot. In it sat two enormous tour buses. A large sign next to the ticket office, did indeed read BAR'AM ANTIQUITIES, just as Fr. Suleiman had said. In English and Hebrew – though not in Arabic – it told the ancient Jewish history of the site. No mention was made of the medieval and modern Arab history of the ruins, and there was no reference to the bombing of the village in 1953. The brochure available at the ticket office was a little more forthcoming, remarking at the end of a long description of the synagogue that 'until 1948 Bar'am was a Maronite Christian village. During the War of Independence, the villagers were evacuated and the site is now under the auspices of the National Parks Authority.'

Fr. Suleiman shrugged when I showed him the leaflet. 'Of course they do not tell the truth of what really happened to us,' he said, adding proudly and without irony, 'But at least they don't make me pay to get in. It's because I'm a priest, you see.'

Meanwhile the two old men were already halfway across the ruins. Far from being depressed at seeing the flattened remains of their childhood village, they were almost skipping with excitement: 'It always makes us happy to breathe the air of Bir'im,' said Wadeer.

'The Daous' house stood over there,' said Elias, pointing to some foundations sticking out of the carefully manicured grass. 'The family of Ghattas lived beside them in that house, beside the pine trees. After 1948 two of their boys ended up in Brazil, where they became famous footballers. You haven't heard of Rai and Socrates? They played in the World Cup. Now, see over there, where those American tourists are standing? Yes, those two with the baseball caps. Those are the ruins of the old synagogue. And over here: that's our church. It was the one building the Israelis left standing when they flattened our homes.'

'And those gothic arches?' I asked. 'To the side of the church. Are they Crusader?'

'No, no,' said Elias, frowning. 'Those arches are all that remains of my school. This was my classroom.'

Elias stood in the middle of what was now a carefully tended patch of grass. 'For four years I taught in here, from 1944 to 1948. This was the door. The blackboard was here. But that was forty-five years ago now.'

Wadeer began rattling away in Arabic; this time it was Fr. Suleiman who translated.

'He says he was taught in here. In his day it was a Jesuit school. The teacher afterwards became the Maronite Patriarch, Cardinal Kreish. He was very strict. He would beat the children with a canvas shoe and sometimes also with a stick.'

Wadeer walked over to the corner of the plot, making whacking gestures with his wrist.

'He says the stick was kept here. Everyone in the class tasted the stick. No one dared to play tricks.'

Fr. Suleiman had got out his keys and was now opening the door into the churchtower. We all followed him up the winding stairs. Halfway up, Wadeer began to gesture excitedly at the wall of the staircase.

'Look! Look!' he said. 'Yes, here: here is my name. I was fifteen when I wrote that.'

At the top, a grille in the roof looked down into the nave below. Through it you could see two graves.

'That was the grave of the parish priest,' said Fr. Suleiman. 'They let us bury him here in 1956. It was the first time we had been allowed back into the village since the bombing. The military gave us authorisation, as long as we didn't take more than three hours.'

'Between 1948 and 1967 there were soldiers everywhere,' said Elias. 'We were not allowed to come here at all.'

'Once my goats escaped and came here,' said Wadeer. 'I came to get them back and was caught. They took me to the military tribunal in Nazareth. I spent a month in prison and had to pay a large fine.'

'Now it is much better,' said Fr. Suleiman. 'If we pay, we can come as often as we like. And they let us use the church for free on Easter, Christmas, Palm Sunday and Pentecost. Also for burials. They do not charge us for that.'

All six of us were now standing against the parapet looking out over the countryside around us.

'When we come here we are happy,' said Elias. 'All the old memories come back. We remember many things: the streets, the homes, the neighbours. Everything. My house was over there, at the end of the village to the right. But it was completely destroyed.'

'Over there,' said Wadeer, pointing to the horizon, 'that is the hill where we stood when they destroyed the village.'

'See through those trees?' said Fr. Suleiman, pointing into the distance. 'That is Kibbutz Bar'am. And over there, to the north? That's Moshav Dovev. They took two parts of our land, but this, to the south: that is free. Where the forest is now growing, that used to be our fig trees and our vineyards. There are ten thousand *dunums* which are not used. That is all we want.'

'It would be so easy,' said Elias. 'We don't even need ten thousand *dunums*. Five thousand *dunums* would do. We would accept anything.'

We began to file down the stairs. The priest closed and locked the door behind us.

'But, you see, they are worried it would be a precedent,' said Fr. Suleiman as we walked back to the carpark, past the American tourists who were now eating a picnic at a wooden table by the ticket office. 'They say that once you let one Arab back, you admit that the others have rights too. That is why, despite everything, they dare not give us back what is ours. Israel says it is a democracy, and it is true. But it seems that for us Palestinians there is no justice.'

'We've told the government that Kafr Bir'am is like a house of three rooms,' said Elias, looking back at his old village. 'One is now the kibbutz. One is the moshav. One is empty. We don't ask much. But that we must have.'

VI

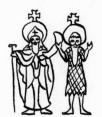

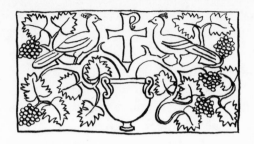

HOTEL METROPOLE, ALEXANDRIA, EGYPT,
1 DECEMBER 1994

I am sitting writing in the first-floor breakfast room of the Hotel Metropole. At the far side of the room waiters in white jackets and black bow ties hover at the edge of the parquet floor; a classical frieze of naiads and centaurs runs along the dado overhead. Pale warm winter sun streams in through the open shutters; outside you can hear the rattle and clang of the trams and the clip-clop of horse-drawn cabs passing up the Grand Corniche. The sky is clear, the wind is high, and beyond a shivering screen of palms the Mediterranean stretches out into the distance.

After the incessant tensions and hatreds of Israel, the glib self-righteousness of the settlers and the bleak despair of the Palestinians, Alexandria feels refreshingly detached from the troubles of the Middle East; indeed it feels detached from the Middle East altogether. The cafés with their baroque mirrors and gleaming tables have a vaguely French or Viennese air to them, while the façades of the townhouses with their stained tempera and shuttered windows are strikingly Italianate. But, if anything, the city feels Greek. Alexandria was, after all, founded by a Greek and remained a Greek-dominated town until the 1950s, when Nasser expropriated the Greeks' banks and businesses and expelled the families who owned them. The Jews, the French and the English were thrown out at the same time, leaving the city – always

375

something of a European expatriate exiled on the coast of Africa – a cold cadaver, its magnificent art deco buildings still intact but emptied of the men and women who built and owned them, a city 'clinging to the minds of old men like traces of perfume on a sleeve: Alexandria the capital of Memory'.

I first came to Alexandria through the pages of Lawrence Durrell's *Alexandria Quartet*. A bound volume of the four novels has accompanied me all the way through this journey, and has formed a welcome counterpoint to the sometimes grim otherworldiness of the monasteries I have visited on the way. During long monastic mid-afternoons, when the sun beat down on the dust-dry guest rooms and nothing stirred, with no noise to break the slow intake and recoil of the cell's faded curtains, how reassuring it could be to set aside the *Sayings of the Desert Fathers* and sit reading instead of brothels and dancing girls, of corrupt merchants and voluptuous landowners, 'libertines who were prepared to founder in the senses as deeply as any Desert Father in the mind', as Balthazar puts it in *Justine.*

From my table I can see across Saad Zagloul Square to the Hotel Cecil, where Justine first makes her appearance 'amid the dusty palms, dressed in a sheath of silver drops, softly fanning her cheeks with a little reed fan'. The gilded birdcage lift is still there; potted palms still frame the great marble staircase in the lobby. But the cast is impossibly different from the bright thirties figures with whom Durrell peoples his novels. There are no beautiful Jewish women with dark gloves and skimpy cocktail dresses; no pashas or beys arriving for secret assignations in their great silver Rolls-Royces; no Armenian bankers discussing intrigues amid the potted palms. Instead Alexandria is now, for possibly the first time in its history, a truly Egyptian city, looking more towards the deserts of the south than to the wider Mediterranean world.

Deserted by its entrepreneurs – its Greeks and Jews and Armenians – impoverished by nationalisation and decades of corrupt state socialism, Alexandria is now full of Egyptian holidaymakers dressed in their village *gelabiyas* and turbans. *Mukhtars* from the delta – rough-skinned, unshaven – sit cross-legged on the esplanade nibbling nuts or watching through clouds of smoke as the barrow-vendors fry whitebait or grill their corncobs. The old art deco mansions of the seafront have been divided up into decrepit hotels and poky flats. There is laundry hung out to dry on each collapsing balcony, and brickwork showing through the leprous stucco. Below, under the flapping awnings of the cafés, *fellahin* women with tattoos on their faces sit nibbling at sticky pastries.

The shops and hotels may still recall the multinational Levant of the late Ottoman Empire – Épicerie Ghaffour, Cinéma Metro, Hotel Windsor, Maison Paul, Bijoux Youssouffian – and some of the most famous names are still extant: the Trianon, even Pastroudis (where the fictional Nessim would drink coffee with Justine, and where, in reality, Cavafy would sip coffee with E.M. Forster). But, like everywhere else in the old Ottoman world, the multinational has given way to the mono-ethnic, the cosmopolitan to the narrowly national, and all these establishments are now Egyptian-owned and now have a specifically Egyptian – not an international – flavour.

You have to look quite hard to find any last remnants of the old order lurking in the backstreets of the town. At the synagogue, now heavily guarded by paramilitary Egyptian police, Joe Harari, the elderly custodian, opened the great double doors to reveal the echoing emptiness of the vast neo-classical prayer hall.

'Over a thousand people could fit in here,' said Joe. 'And this was just one of fifteen synagogues in Alexandria.'

Each of the one thousand seats had a nameplate on the back, but now only sixty Jews are left in Alexandria, a city that once, in the early centuries A.D., had the largest Jewish population in the world. Moreover, there is no rabbi, and as these last survivors are almost exclusively old women, there are not enough men left to form a *minyan* (quorum). So the synagogue remains unused, except by a family of pigeons roosting above the *bema*.

'Israel took all our young men,' said Joe as we sat drinking coffee in his office afterwards. Above his head, flanking the framed photographs of President Mubarak and the Lubavitch Rebbe, were wooden plaques recording the names of the synagogue's donors:

Mme Esther Hopasha, L.E.5,000; Jacques Riche, L.E.200; Emilio Levi, L.E.50 . . .

'Now there is peace,' said Joe, 'maybe some of them will return.'

'Did you ever consider emigrating?' I asked.

'I was born in Alex,' replied the old man. 'My mother is from Alex. All my life I have lived in Alex. I was married here. I've seen Israel for one week only, when I was taken there by Sadat. Why should I go?' The old man gestured at the streets behind him: 'This is my home,' he said.

'What do you miss most of the old days?' I asked.

'Family,' he replied. 'Sisters, cousins, friends. When they had to leave, everyone cried. My sister had to sell her house in one week. She was alone – her husband was away – so she had to manage by herself, with two small children. Of course she got a very bad price. She left with just two suitcases. Almost everything was left behind. Now one of her sons in the States is Vice President of . . . of . . . something beginning with tri. Trident? Tristar?' Joe beamed proudly.

'Israel was necessary, maybe,' he added. 'But because of it Alexandria can never be as before.'

'You should have seen it,' agreed Olga Rabinovitch, who had just walked into the office and had overheard Joe's last remark. Olga was a thin, elegant old lady with brightly rouged lips. She must once have been very beautiful. This, I thought, was what Justine would look like now if she had stayed on in Alexandria.

'Ahh,' she sighed, sitting down. 'When I was young – sixteen, seventeen, eighteen – the operas came from France. The theatre, the ballet . . .'

'Edith Piaf visited once,' said Joe.

'And the streets!' said Olga. Her right hand caressed the thin string of seed pearls hung around her neck. 'You should have seen the shops. You should have seen Sharif Street in the thirties!'

'The beautiful women . . .'

'The most lovely women in the world.'

'. . . with beautiful dresses and jewellery . . .'

'What luxury there was!'

'There used to be so much work. So much prosperity . . .'

'Of course, it's changed completely.'

'For a start, in the old days the Egyptians were not much in evidence here.'

'The kind of people you see on the Corniche. They would not have been there.'

'They were living in the suburbs. This area was like a European colony.'

'Now anyone who is not an Egyptian is like a fly in the milk.'

'It's a complete change.'

'All the beautiful old villas with trees and flowers – they've destroyed everything to build these . . . awful, *awful*, ugly buildings.'

'When I go around now, I get lost.'

'To live here now you have to stay at home,' said Joe, toying with his coffee cup. 'Just to look at the streets makes me sad.'

'Some of the Egyptians are very nice,' said Olga. 'But they are the old ones. Brought up with Europeans.'

'And they don't go out much.'

'You know I live in a home for old ladies now?' said Olga. She sounded bewildered by the information, as if she had just woken up there for the first time that morning. 'It is called the Casa di Riposo – run by the Italian sisters. I left my apartment: it was too big and my servant got sick. The home is very nice, very clean. But I have nothing to do.' She crossed her legs: 'I sold everything. Except a portrait of myself when I was young.'

'She was so beautiful,' said Joe. 'You cannot imagine.'

'Everyone looks at it and says, "Oh, how beautiful!" But look at me. You wouldn't know now, would you?'

Olga looked at me. Again she asked, this time almost surprised: 'Would you?'

Five minutes' walk from the synagogue, opposite the Metro Cinema, lies the Élite Café. Its octogenarian owner, Miss Christina – all kaftan and coloured beads – is one of Alexandria's few remaining Greeks.

'Alexandria was a Greek town,' she said, sitting down at a table near the window. 'But few of us are left. Every year, little by little, we get smaller. In twenty years no one will be left.'

Miss Christina gestured to the dance floor at the back of the café: 'See over there?' she said. 'When I was young we used to have a Greek dance-band at the back here. We were dancing until two, three o'clock in the morning. Going out, eating breakfast at the Cecil, then off somewhere else.'

'But no longer.'

'No!' Miss Christina laughed. 'Things are very calm now. The Egyptians don't dance. They are very polite. They like their families. They go to bed early. And the Greeks who are left are not much better.'

'No?'

'No. The Greeks here are not so rich or so interesting. They are neither industrialists nor poets. They're just shopkeepers. None have ... you know, pictures by Picasso or Cézanne or anything nice like that. All the old families – the Dositsas, the Antoniadis, the Sakalaritas – they've all gone.'

Miss Christina shrugged her shoulders. 'Now books are my greatest friends here. Even if they have given me cataracts from reading by bad light in bed.'

I asked whether the change in Alexandria had happened slowly.

'Phh!' spluttered Miss Christina, raising her eyebrows. 'It happened overnight. After Nasser threw the Europeans out everything ground to a halt: the Italian opera, the French concerts, the theatre. Before that Alexandria was like Paris. It was the most creative town – all these different cultures collaborating and mingling with each other: conferences, lectures, galleries ... This was the café of the artists. They would all come here. Particularly the writers and the poets.'

'Lawrence Durrell?'

'No, I never met him. But I liked *Justine*. I think it's a good portrait. In fact I have a cat named Justine. But she is very old now.'

'What about Cavafy? Did you know him?'

'Yes, Cavafy I knew very well! Of course, as he died in '33, he was an old man when I was a young girl. But he used to come here every day. We have five of his original manuscripts, including "The God Abandons Antony".'

'So your family knew him very well?'

'His house was just around the corner, in rue Lepsius, and I suppose we did see quite a lot of him. He loved this area. There was a brothel immediately below his rooms – the English used to call it rue Clapsius – the Patriarchal Church was nearby and the Greek Hospital was opposite. He used to say that the area had everything he ever needed in life: "Where could I live better? Below, the brothel caters for the flesh. And there is the church which forgives sin. And there is the hospital where we die."'

Miss Christina smiled. 'That's his portrait,' she said, pointing to a framed photograph at the back of the café. It showed a willowy young man in a three-piece suit with round Aldous Huxley spectacles, a centre parting and a rather anxious expression.

'He was a perfect gentleman: very well dressed,' said Miss Christina. 'But he was very serious. Never smiled. People used to try and talk to him but he always wanted to be alone. Perhaps he was thinking too much.'

Miss Christina sipped her coffee. 'Sometimes he could be very gloomy. He was unhappy whenever he looked in a mirror and saw himself getting older. Every night he would rub cream into his face to try and stop the wrinkles. I think he was afraid of death. But for all that, no one would dispute that he's the best poet in Greek this century.'

'Was he kind to you?'

'To me, yes. When he came here I would always give him a sweet-smelling flower, the *fouli*, a cousin of jasmine. I think he liked that. But in general he did not like women. It was because of his mother.'

'What do you mean?'

'He was the last of eight boys. His mother wanted very much a girl, so she dressed him as one, in little girlie dresses, caressing him very much: "Oh, my sweet boy! My sweet sweet Costakis! Oh, my darling." So he became a homosexual.'

Miss Christina lowered her voice and bent closer to me: 'He

wrote many poems about the bodies of young boys. But he was very careful. He did not expose himself.'

'Expose himself?'

'I mean he never published these homosexual poems,' hissed Miss Christina.

'Why?'

'Because,' said Miss Christina, 'he was absolutely terrified of what his mother might say.'

ALEXANDRIA, 5 DECEMBER

One morning in the first year of the twentieth century a donkey-herder was driving a mule train through the outskirts of Alexandria when the frontmost ass suddenly disappeared into the ground in front of him.

Such events are not uncommon in Alexandria: no other city in the world is given such frequent reminders of the cavernous chambers and unexplored treasures that lie buried just beneath its streets. Only recently a wedding was celebrated in the city centre near the supposed site of the Soma, the lost tomb of Alexander; the pavement opened beneath the bride and she was never seen again.

For centuries Alexandria was not just the capital of Egypt, she was the Queen of the Mediterranean, the greatest port of the classical world. 'She is undoubtedly the first city of the civilised world,' wrote Diodorus of Sicily in the first century B.C., 'certainly far ahead of the rest in elegance and extent and riches and luxury.' Her villas and temples, palaces and monuments, churches and colonnaded avenues extended for many miles beyond the limits of the modern city – and yet not one building of this legendary Alexandria survives today above the ground; everything is hidden beneath the mundane surface of the modern streetscape. Under the city's cheap hotels and bare-shelved shops, its brothels and seedy restaurants, lie many of the greatest buildings of antiquity: the Caesarium, where Cleopatra committed suicide; the Pharos lighthouse (one of the Seven Wonders of the World); the Great Alexandrian library with its seven hundred thousand scrolls; the Mouseion; the Serapium; the tomb of Alexander. All have disappeared, utterly and completely, so that at street level only a handful of fallen pillars and broken capitals remain to mark the site of some of the most magnificent buildings the world has ever seen.

Yet, subtly, the ancient city continues to make its presence felt. Every so often the earth will give way and some unsuspecting Alexandrian will plummet into the cellars of a lost temple or a forgotten palace crypt. Certainly when, in 1900, the donkey disappeared into the ground, the muleteer knew exactly what to do. The authorities were summoned, and they in turn summoned the archaeologists. In a short time work had begun on uncovering one of the most extraordinary complexes of catacombs to survive from the ancient world.

I walked over there this morning from my hotel. Off the back-streets of the town, in a narrow lane blocked by donkey carts and lined with teashops full of old men with hubble bubbles, a low-roofed roundhouse gives onto a circular flight of stairs. The shaft corkscrews downwards for turn after turn, until it leads quite suddenly into a honeycomb of underground chambers. These rock-cut caverns with their flat limestone divans were feasting rooms where bereaved families would meet to toast the memory of dead relatives; though the catacombs were long forgotten, even to legend, the broken fragments of the pots and plates left over from these feasts have given the area its modern Arabic name, Kom el Shogafa, the Mound of Shards.

From the feasting halls, the galleries lead down again, deeper into the ground, darker, further from the light. Down here in the partially flooded depths of the complex lie the burial chambers themselves. What is so odd about this part of the catacomb is less the size or magnificence of the mortuary chambers than the bizarre nature of their decoration. At first sight this decoration appears merely standard Pharaonic: a pair of Egyptian papyrus capitals lead into an inner chamber where the jackal-headed figure of Anubis stands over a recumbent mummy, holding in his hand the bloody heart of the dead man; to one side falcon-headed Horus looks on, impassive.

But the more closely you look, the odder the reliefs become. Flanking the pillars on either side are a pair of medallions sculpted with Greek Gorgon heads, below which rises, in high relief, a pair of very Roman bearded serpents from whose powerfully piled coils emerge the suggestively phallic pinecone sceptre of Dionysus and the serpent wand of Hermes. More confusingly still, on either side of the entrance door stands a single figure. To one side is Anubis again, still with his dog's head, but now dressed up as a Roman legionary with breastplate, short sword, lance and shield; flanking him is an image of the Nile god Sobek, who, despite being a crocodile, has also been squeezed into a legionary's uniform. Whole cultures are colliding here: it seems that the Graeco-Egyptian burial syndicate who commissioned this strange complex would think nothing of being buried in Greek sarcophagi and guarded by Egyptian gods in Roman military uniform.

This subterranean tomb, at first sight merely eerie, is in fact vastly important. A random quirk of fate has left this small upper-middle-class burial chamber as the sole object in the entire city that looks now almost exactly as it would have done to an ancient Alexandrian; it is, therefore, one of the only indicators of the mood of Alexandria at a time when that city was about to become the intellectual capital of Christianity. That mood, as is indicated by the strange syncretic catacomb sculptures, was one of exceptional intellectual tolerance and experimentation: it was a city where, even in death, the inhabitants would attempt to fuse opposites, to reconcile two entirely different artistic traditions and religious pantheons, to mix deities as lightly as Durrell's Alexandrians would mix their cocktails.

This, then, was the heady world into which, in the late first century A.D., Christianity was about to be thrown – and from which the religion would emerge with its theological underpinnings and its artistic iconography altered for ever.

Alexandria was the scholarly capital of the late classical world. Situated at the meeting place of trade routes linking both Asia and Africa with Europe it was quite natural that the city should be a centre of intellectual ferment. Indian *sadhus* wandered its streets, debating with Greek philosophers, Jewish exegetes and Roman architects. It was here that Euclid wrote his treatise on geometry, that Eratosthenes measured the diameter of the world (he was only fifty-four miles out), that Ptolemy produced his astonishing maps and that a great team of seventy-two Hellenistic Jews produced the *Septuagint*, the first Greek translation of the Old Testament.

The same spirit of breezy internationalism that guided the scholars of Alexandria also informed its mystics and its priests. Religions in Alexandria were notoriously porous, ideas and images from one faith trickling imperceptibly into another: the Alexandrian god Serapis, for example, combined elements of the Egyptian cults of both Osiris and Apis, grafted onto that of Greek Zeus.

The arrival of Christianity from Palestine at first merely added to the mix. In the second century, Clement of Alexandria regarded pagan Greek philosophy as divinely inspired, and wrote of Christ driving his chariot across the heavens like the Sun God; indeed many pagans (including the young Tertullian) believed, perhaps correctly, that the Alexandrian Christians actually worshipped the sun, meeting as they did on Sunday, and praying to the east, where the sun rises. Other Alexandrian Christians undoubtedly worshipped Serapis. As late as the early fifth century a pagan philosopher from Alexandria, Synesius, was chosen to be a bishop although he was not even a baptised Christian. He accepted on the condition that though he might 'speak in myths' in church, he should be free to 'think as a philosopher' in private. It was this cross-fertilisation of Christianity with Alexandrian Greek philosophy that drew the developing Christian doctrines away from the strictly Jewish traditions which had given them birth, and which raised the religion – initially a simple series of precepts addressed to the poor and illiterate – to the level of high philosophy.

The evidence of the confusion that resulted from this promiscuous conjunction can be seen most clearly in the Alexandrian Graeco-Roman Museum. Here, in gallery after gallery, there is an easy drift of pagan and Christian motifs, styles, subjects and iconographies. The *ankh*, the Pharaonic symbol of life, appears on early Christian Alexandrian gravestones transformed into an ambiguous looped cross. The image of Isis nursing Horus is reused in the Christian era unchanged, but now depicts the Virgin suckling the Christ child. A sword-wielding Anubis, holding the heart of a corpse, sprouts wings and turns into St Michael weighing the souls of the dead. Apollo raises a lamb over his shoulders and becomes the Good Shepherd. The Romano-Egyptian image of a mounted Horus in Roman military uniform lancing the Seth-crocodile transforms itself into St George on his charger spearing the dragon. Dionysian vine scrolls tangle around scenes of the vintage; the same scrolls, hastily baptised with a cross, tangle on unchanged into the Christian era as a Eucharistic symbol. Nereids and victories swoop down from capitals and turn into angels midflight; pagan deities – Osiris and Aphrodite, Orpheus and Dionysus, Leda and the Zeus-Swan – survive into an afterlife as demons and godlings, removed from the centre of shrines but lurking still unvanquished at the back of Alexandrian churches, as in the dark recesses of Egyptian folk memory, peeping down from architraves or glaring maliciously from the metopes or dadoes.

Amid this fizz of dissolving philosophies, this iconographic metamorphosis, there is a thrilling feeling of being present at the birth of medieval art. On all sides one can hear the soft ripping of gossamer as old pagan images emerge from the Alexandrian chrysalis transformed into the conventional Christian symbols, the same symbols and images that will carry on reappearing in gospel books and altarpieces, stained glass and frescoes, diptychs and triptychs, fixed and immutable for centuries to come.

This afternoon, after a siesta, I returned to the garden of the Graeco-Roman Museum. There I sat in the shade of an orange tree, surrounded by fragments of Byzantine sculpture, reading John Moschos's account of the now buried city from which these sculptures had come.

Moschos and Sophronius spent so much time in Alexandria that in one of his books, Sophronius, a native of Damascus, actually refers to 'us Alexandrians'. The two monks probably paid their first visit to the city in the winter of 578–9, at the very beginning of their travels. They may have had the same weather I am having now: crisp, sunny days growing slowly colder and shorter. Nearly thirty years later the two monks returned, this time by sea, as refugees fleeing the sack of Antioch by the marauding Persian army. On both occasions, Alexandria was their base for an extensive exploration of the monasteries of desert Egypt, reaching, on their second trip, as far south as the Great Oasis.

During this second Alexandrian period, the two monks appear to have based themselves in the city on and off for the seven years between 607 and 614 A.D. During this period Sophronius seems to have been suddenly struck down with blindness, then equally suddenly cured during a visit to the Shrine of Saints Cyrus and John at Menuthis (the shrine's own name eventually came to replace Menuthis, so that for the last thousand years the place has been known as Abukir). In gratitude for his miraculous healing, Sophronius wrote a book containing stories of some of the shrine's more remarkable cures, in the process of which he allows us an intriguing peek into what was contained in a Byzantine doctor's bag: if Sophronius is to be believed, a standard prescription was a compote of Bithynian cheese, wax, and roast crocodile.

Following Sophronius's cure, the two monks began to campaign energetically against the Monophysite leanings of the local Egyptians, tendencies that had already begun to lead to a schism between mainstream Orthodoxy (identified with Egypt's Greek-speaking, Alexandrian-based upper class) and the indigenous Coptic-speaking Egyptians (the word Copt simply deriving from the Greek term for a native Egyptian, *Aiguptios*).

Finally, however, in the spring of 614, the Persian army caught up with the two monks. As the Persians breached the walls of the city and put it to the sword, Moschos and Sophronius were again forced to take ship. This time they were accompanied by John the Almsgiver, Alexandria's Orthodox Patriarch, whose biography Sophronius was later to write. In a state of some distress, the party stopped off in Cyprus, where the heartbroken Patriarch died. The boatload of refugees finally reached the safety of the walls of Constantinople some time later, probably towards the end of the year 615.

The burning city they left behind had clearly changed dramatically since the prosperous, free-thinking days of the second and third centuries A.D. This was not just because Alexandria was already full of penniless refugees fleeing the earlier Persian assault on Palestine; the change was more profound. For in Alexandria the triumph of Christianity had been effected by hordes of often fanatical Coptic monks who would periodically sweep down from their desert monasteries, attacking the pagans and their shrines, and burning any temples left undefended; in 392 A.D. they finally succeeded in burning the Serapium, and with it the adjacent Alexandrian library, storehouse of the collected learning of antiquity.

The houses of the city's pagan notables were ransacked in the monks' search for idols; no one was safe. The most notorious outrage was the lynching of Hypatia, a neoplatonic philosopher of the School of Alexandria and a brilliant thinker and mathematician. She was pulled from her palaquin by a lynch-mob of monks, who stripped her, then dragged her naked through the streets of the town before finally killing her in front of the Caesarion and burning her body.

This murder was applauded by the monastic chroniclers. 'Hypatia was devoted to her magic, astrolabes, and instruments of music,' wrote Bishop John of Nikiu. 'She beguiled many people through her satanic wiles. [After her murder] all the people surrounded the Patriarch Cyril [who had instigated the mob] and

388

called him "the new Theophilus" for he had [completed the work of Patriarch Theophilus who had burned the Serapium and] destroyed the last remains of idolatry in the city.' The pagans, understandably, were less enthusiastic: 'Things have happened the like of which haven't been seen through all the ages,' wrote one distraught student to his mother in Upper Egypt. 'Now it's cannibalism, not war.' 'If we are alive,' commented another, 'then life itself is dead.'

Nevertheless, there are hints that the intellectual spirit in the city had not died completely. According to Moschos's near-contemporary, the historian Ammianus Marcellinus, 'even now in that city the various branches of learning make their voices heard; for the teachers of the arts are somehow still alive, the geometer's rod reveals hidden knowledge, the study of music has not yet dried up and some few still keep the fires burning in the study of the movement of the earth and stars. The study of medicine grows greater every day, so that a doctor who wishes to establish his standing in the profession can dispense with the need for any proof, by merely saying that he trained at Alexandria.' This seems to have been true: it was in Alexandria that Caesarius, brother of the theologian Gregory of Nazianzen, obtained the qualifications that won him the post of Byzantine Court Physician.

Certainly Alexandria seems to have brought the scholar in Moschos to the fore, and his account of his time in the city depicts him and Sophronius (who was, after all, a Sophist, a teacher of philosophy and rhetoric) engaged in high-minded intellectual pursuits. In one story the pair are attending lectures at the university by Theodore the Philosopher; in another talking to the calligrapher and book illuminator Zoilus the Reader; on yet another occasion, in a charming picture of bookish Byzantine life, they are visiting a bibliophile named Cosmas the Lawyer.

'This wondrous man greatly benefited us,' wrote Moschos, 'not only by letting us see him and by teaching us, but also because he had more books than anybody else in Alexandria and would willingly supply them to those who wished. Yet he was a man of no possessions. Throughout his house there was nothing to be seen but books, a bed and a table. Any man could go in and ask for what would benefit him – and read it. Each day I would go in to him.'

The most intriguing story of all, however, concerns a visit to another scholar friend. The tale is set one hot summer afternoon sometime in the late 580s, with Moschos and Sophronius sheltering from the midday heat in the shade of the monumental *tetrapylon* at the centre of Alexandria. The monks had set out to visit another bibliophile friend, Stephen the Sophist, but Stephen's maid had shouted out of the top window that her master was fast asleep. So while they waited for the Sophist to finish his siesta, the pair amused themselves by eavesdropping on a conversation between three blind men who were also taking advantage of the *tetrapylon*'s shade. They were passing the time by telling each other how they had lost their sight, and the last of the men told a strange and macabre story which Moschos records.

Before he lost his sight, said the blind man, he had been a grave-robber. One day he saw a richly-decked-out corpse being taken through the streets of Alexandria for burial in the Church of St John, and he had made up his mind to plunder the grave. When the funeral had finished, the man broke into the sepulchre and began to strip the tomb. Suddenly he gave a start: the dead man appeared to sit up before him and stretch out his hands towards the grave-robber's eyes. It was the last thing, said the blind man, that he ever saw.

Later on, Moschos heard a similar story about another grave-robber who had broken into a rich girl's tomb in the depths of the night. Again the corpse seemed to come to life, only this time the girl grabbed the robber: 'You came in here when you wanted to,' she said, 'but you will not go out of here as you will. This tomb will be shared by the two of us.' The corpse refused to let the robber go until he promised to repent and become a monk. In shock, the man agreed.

When I first read these stories I had assumed them to be pious superstition, like many of Moschos's other tales. But this afternoon, reading *The Spiritual Meadow* in the museum garden, I suddenly understood where such tales originated. For from the first century A.D. through to the early Byzantine period, it was the custom in Egypt to bury those who could afford it in mummy cases onto which were bound superb encaustic (hot wax) portraits of the deceased; in some cases – there are two fine examples in the Graeco-Roman Museum – full-length pictures were painted onto the mummy's winding sheet itself.

These mummy portraits throw a reflected beam of light on the lost world of classical portraiture, vanished now but for a few frescoes at Pompeii, and more importantly form a bridge between the painting of antiquity and the panel-painted icons of Byzantium. It can be no coincidence that the oldest icons in existence are to be found in St Catherine's Monastery in the Sinai, and that they are painted in the same encaustic technique as their Alexandrian mummy-portrait predecessors. If, as Otto Demus observed, 'the icon is the root-form of the European picture', then in these Graeco-Egyptian mummy-portraits we see the immediate genesis of the icon.

But it is as works of art that the mummy portraits are most striking. They are so real that you can almost hear the sitters speak – as Moschos's grave-robbers seem to have discovered. Even today, behind glass in a museum, the portraits are so astonishingly lifelike that they can still make you gasp as you find yourself staring eyeball to eyeball with a soldier who could have fought at Actium, or a society lady who may have known Cleopatra. There is something deeply hypnotic about the silent stare of these sad, uncertain Graeco-Roman faces, most of whom appear to have died in their early thirties. Their fleeting expressions are frozen, startled, as if suddenly surprised by death itself; their huge eyes stare out, as if revealing the nakedness of the departed soul. The viewer peers at them, trying to catch some hint of the upheavals they witnessed and the strange sights they must have seen in late antique Egypt. But the smooth neo-classical faces stare us down.

Perhaps the most disconcerting thing about these portraits is that they appear so astonishingly familiar: the colours and technique of some of them resemble Frans Hals, others Cézanne, and two thousand years after they were painted the faces still convey with penetrating immediacy the character of the different sitters: the fop and the courtesan, the anxious mother and the tough man of business, the bored army officer and the fat *nouveau-riche* matron, hung with gold, dripping with make-up. Indeed, so contemporary are the features, so immediately recognisable the emotions that play on the lips, that you have to keep reminding yourself that these sitters are not from our world, that they are masks attached to Graeco-Egyptian mummies, covering the desiccated corpses of people who possibly saw the world through the glass of an initiate in the cult of Isis, who maybe married their brother or sister (as late as the third century Diocletian was still trying to outlaw incest in Egypt) and who perhaps studied in the great Alexandrian library before it was burned to the ground by the howling monks of the Egyptian deserts.

As André Malraux put it, these mummy portraits 'glow with the flame of eternal life'. Certainly it is easy to imagine their effect on John Moschos's nervous grave-robbers breaking into a necropolis at night: no wonder they thought the dead had risen.

This evening, my final one in the city, following Miss Christina's directions I found my way along the tramlines to the gathering place of the last Greeks in Alexandria.

The Greek Club consisted of an empty hall, opening onto a trellised courtyard where twenty or thirty elderly Greek couples sat playing backgammon and poker. From the bar, tinned Greek music wafted out into the night. There I found Nicholas Zoulias, the President of the club and an old friend of Miss Christina. Soon a circle had gathered around our table as the old people began to pour out their memories of pre-war Alexandria. They were the same stories I had already heard in the synagogue and the Élite Café: how Alexandria had once been the Paris of the East, the diamond of the Mediterranean, how lively the place had been, how prosperous and creative; and also how little remained of what once was. But what I had not heard before, nor expected, was how little these old men thought of Greece. They regarded Alexandria, their own personal city state, as the apogee of civilisation, and looked on modern Greece as some sort of ill-mannered *parvenu*.

'Alexandria was always more sophisticated than Athens or Saloniki,' explained Nicholas Zoulias, lighting a cigarette. 'One hundred years ago, when Athens was still a village, Alexandria was a cosmopolitan city.'

'Everything you wanted was here,' agreed Taki Katsimbris.

'We don't like the Greeks,' said Michael Stephanopoulos. 'To be honest, I can't live there more than fourteen days.'

'Athens is just the nightclub of Europe,' said Zoulias, sucking his teeth in contempt. 'Nothing more.'

'The Greeks in Greece are more rough than we are,' said Michael.

'They don't know languages as we do,' said Zoulias. 'French, Arabic, English . . .'

'They are as rough as Turks,' said Michael. 'In Greece, if you ask what time it is, they don't answer.'

'If you ask an address in Greece, they will say they don't know. Here they will show you. They'll take you there.'

'They don't have a tradition of hospitality.'

'We are different from them,' said Zoulias. 'We have different food, different speech, different morals . . .'

'We are more like the Egyptians,' said Taki. 'We have the same mentality as them.'

'Many of our grandmothers would wear the veil.'

'They even used to pray like the Egyptians: with a carpet on the floor.'

'What's the difference between Christianity and Islam? It's the same God.'

'But there is nothing like that in Greece. They are very . . . narrow-minded over there. They think only they know what is right.'

'Greece is part of Europe,' said Zoulias, 'and they now have a very . . . automatic way of living. They have speed. They are always running. Here we have an easy way: *wahde wahde* – step by step.'

All the other old men nodded in agreement.

393

'Here the automobiles are slow,' said Michael. 'The railway is slow . . .'

'And slowly we are dying out,' added Taki.

No one disagreed with what he had said. I asked: 'How long will your community last?'

'Five, ten years at most,' said Zoulias.

'There are only five hundred of us left.'

'All the young are going to Athens. As soon as they finish school.'

'They say they get bored here. They say there are no jobs for them.'

'When Nasser nationalised our factories he signed our death warrant.'

'Many who were rich became beggars. He took everything we had.'

'But they found it easy to get jobs in Greece. Because of their skills and languages. So everyone went.'

'As Nasser had taken everything, they had no reason to stay.'

'When I was a boy there used to be two hundred thousand Greeks in Egypt. Two hundred thousand! Even ten years ago there were five thousand. Now there's just us.'

'We've got ten years. Maximum.'

'Unless those who left come back.'

'I don't think they will,' said Michael.

The old men shook their heads. Taki took a gulp of *arak*. 'They'll stay in Greece.'

'Leaving Alexandria without any Greeks.'

'After 2,300 years.'

'They won't come back.'

'No.'

'But who can say?' said Zoulias, lighting a cigarette. 'Who can say?'

I knew we were in for trouble the minute I saw the taxi.

It was a sort of prehistoric ancestor of the Peugeot, with a patchwork of repainted bumps and scars that gave it a vaguely scaly appearance, like a large lizard or a small dinosaur. The man who was to drive this beast was even less prepossessing. Ramazan was a Bedu from the Sinai. He wore a faded denim waistcoat over an off-white shift, and around his head he wrapped a red and white *keffiyeh*; his chin was darkened by a wispy stab at a beard.

We loaded my rucksack into the boot, and Ramazan turned the ignition. The Peugeot bucked, coughed and staggered like a disgruntled camel. Ramazan tried the ignition a second time, with equally disappointing results. He then got out and did to the car what Bedu tend to do to disgruntled camels who behave in a similar manner. He beat it on its side, kicked its chassis, then whispered some encouraging words into its bonnet. On the third attempt the car hiccupped grudgingly into life and we juddered drunkenly out of the hotel carpark.

I had arrived in Cairo off the Alexandrian train the day before, and had immediately set about trying to obtain permission to visit Asyut, the province in Upper Egypt where the majority of Egypt's Copts have always lived; it also contains the Great Oasis, modern Kharga, the southernmost point reached by Moschos on his travels.

The area has been closed to foreigners since its resurgent Islamic movement began widening its scope from taking occasional pot-shots at the local Copts – whom they have been shooting on and off since the founding of the Muslim Brotherhood in 1928 – to targeting foreign tourists as well. In the process they came close to destroying Egypt's tourist industry, and as a result foreigners have now been banned from the vicinity of Asyut. But journalists have occasionally been allowed into the area to report on the government's (often heavy-handed) attempts to quell the Islamist uprising. I therefore went straight to the Egyptian Press Centre, presented my credentials and duly made an application, in triplicate. I was told to return in a week. Rather than hang around Cairo, waiting for bureaucrats to shuffle my papers and rearrange their red tape, I decided to take the opportunity to visit two important Byzantine sites that I had always wanted to see.

The first was St Antony's, the birthplace of Christian monasticism and the greatest monastery in Byzantine Egypt. The second was the lost city of Oxyrhynchus, once one of Byzantine Egypt's most important provincial towns and subsequently the site of the discovery of the greatest treasure trove of Byzantine documents ever uncovered. Its ruins lay on the way to St Antony's, and when I looked at the map it seemed as if it would be easy to take it in on the way. What I did not take into account was Ramazan's driving. For five minutes the taxi juddered along at ever lower speed through the empty early-morning streets of Cairo. Then it finally stalled at a set of traffic lights. 'No problem,' said Ramazan, ducking to avoid the outsized pink velvet love-heart dangling from his mirror. 'No problem at all.'

As the cars behind hooted angrily, Ramazan disappeared behind the bonnet with a length of metal tubing. There followed the sound of hammering and a strong reek of diesel. Early attempts at reigniting the engine came to nothing, and Ramazan began to look a little worried. But quite suddenly, without anyone apparently turning the ignition key, the car bucked into life and off we set again.

The incident had taught Ramazan a lesson. Henceforth traffic lights were obstacles we carefully ignored, and we shot through all the others we came to with impressive gusto. At any other time of day Ramazan's tactics would have been suicidal. At 5.30 in the morning they were merely very frightening. Bar a couple of scratches on the boot – souvenirs of a brief clinch with a truck carrying watermelons – we emerged from Cairo remarkably unscathed, and headed off southwards, driving parallel to the Nile through the pretty villages of the fertile valley.

Here and there, groups of early risers were sitting outside under the vine trellising of the tea houses smoking the first hubble-bubble of the day; a few women were washing clothes by the canals. Through this pastoral scene Ramazan passed like a rugby player in a ballet. He clearly believed that the key to avoiding further stalling lay in keeping the car travelling at some speed. With this in mind he raced along, cutting into the opposite lane, swerving around bends, one minute narrowly avoiding killing two farmers chatting in the middle of the road, the next coming within inches of knocking down a fat sheikh in a blue shift ambling along on a donkey. In this manner we headed down the Nile, the world's most peaceful river transformed before my eyes into the setting for a one-man dragster rally.

Ramazan's driving may have been terrifying, but it got us to our destination in record time. After two hours' racing down the narrow strip of cultivation that flanks the banks of the Nile we reached Behnasa, the medieval Arab village which grew up on the edge of Oxyrhynchus's ruins. Passing through the village – in the process of which Ramazan came close to overturning an old horse-drawn brougham full of heavily veiled village women – we juddered out of the cultivation into the desert, searching for the ruins marked on my map. We drove into the dunes, then drove back again. The Western Desert stretched all around us, flat, inhospitable and echoingly empty. There were no temples, no pillars, no colonnaded streets, nothing at all except for a single small, mud-brick tomb belonging to a medieval Sufi sheikh.

It was while walking back from the tomb, baffled by the total absence of any visible remains, that I noticed for the first time what I was standing on. Every time my foot touched the ground, the sand appeared to crunch beneath my weight. Bending down, I looked more closely at the surface. The dunes all around were littered with pot shards: handles of amphorae, small roundels of red Samian-ware dishes, the decorated bases of cups, jugs, mugs and bowls. But it was not just pieces of pottery: fragments of brilliant aquamarine Byzantine glass glinted in the winter sun; beside them lay small lumps of slag and smelting clinker, fragments of jet, amber and garnet, pieces of bone and the shells of mussels and oysters.

I walked and walked for the rest of the morning, but the soft crunch underfoot did not stop: the midden extended for many miles. The town of Oxyrhynchus had clearly disappeared, destroyed – presumably – by generations of Nile floods and the robbing of the villagers of Behnasa; but its middens remained: epic drifts of Pharaonic, Graeco-Roman and Byzantine rubbish, left where it had been dropped by the street cleaners nearly two thousand years ago. I was standing on one of the great rubbish dumps of the ancient world.

Pulling at an amphora handle jutting out of the ground, I broke a Byzantine pot, and its contents, a pile of chaff winnowed, perhaps, while Justinian still ruled the Empire, floated away in the winter breeze.

The rubbish dumps of Oxyrhynchus first came to the attention of the outside world in 1895 when reports reached the British archaeologists Bernard Grenfell and Arthur Hunt that the area had begun to yield an extraordinary number of papyrus fragments. What the two men found when they visited the site, however, surpassed their wildest expectations.

'The papyri were, as a rule, not very far from the surface,' wrote Grenfell in the *Journal of the Egypt Exploration Fund* the following year. 'In one patch of ground, indeed, merely turning up the soil with one's boot would frequently disclose a layer of papyri ... I proceeded to increase the number of workmen gradually up to 110, and, as we moved northwards over other parts of the site, the flow of papyri soon became a torrent which it was difficult to cope with ...'

What was written on the papyri was every bit as remarkable as the sheer quantity of texts uncovered. On the second day of the excavations Dr Hunt was examining a crumpled fragment which had just been produced by the workmen. It contained only a few legible lines of text, but one of these contained the very rare Greek word '*karphos*', which means 'a mote'. Immediately Hunt made the connection with the verse in St Matthew's Gospel about the mote in your brother's eye and the beam in your own, but with a thrill he realised that the wording on the fragment differed significantly from that of the Gospel. The fragment turned out to be part of a lost collection of *The Sayings of Jesus*, which predated by hundreds of years any New Testament fragment then extant.

By the end of the first season Grenfell and Hunt had discovered an entire library of lost classics: a forgotten song by Sappho; fragments of lost plays by Aeschylus and Sophocles; the earliest papyrus of St Matthew's Gospel then known; a leaf of a previously unknown book of New Testament Apocrypha, *The Acts of Paul and Thecla*. They also unearthed great quantities of historical documents such as the report of an interview between the Emperor Marcus Aurelius and an Alexandrian magistrate, as well as an entire archive of Byzantine correspondence and administrative documents.

This last discovery was not a great cause of excitement to the Victorian excavators, brought up as they were with Gibbon's magisterial contempt for the late Roman Empire. Nevertheless, a century later, these documents are now usually regarded as the most important of all the finds from the site. For in the administrative flotsam from a provincial Byzantine town on the very edge of the Empire, we come closer to the lives of ordinary Byzantines than from any other surviving contemporary source; it casts a bright beam of light on the private life of the world John Moschos knew as he travelled through the last days of the Eastern Empire.

Before setting off on this journey, I had spent a week in the London Library poring through some of the 142 volumes of the Oxyrhynchus papyri that have so far been edited, translated and published. Taken together they provide a uniquely detailed picture of a late antique city: reading them is like opening a shutter onto a sunlit Byzantine street and eavesdropping on the gossip, the scandals and the secret affairs of the people milling about below.

It is the extraordinary randomness of the fragments that forms much of their fascination: we may have lost every one of the seven hundred thousand scrolls of high philosophy and world history stored in the great library of Alexandria, but in obscure Oxyrhynchus we meet the forgotten vendors in the street, the sleepy nightwatchmen on their shift, the disgruntled school-teachers in their classrooms, even the city's teenage girls creeping back from assignations with their lovers. A shoemaker promises to water the tree that stands outside his house. A husband writes to his wife asking her to come to him and 'bring the old cushion that is in the dining room'. A father writes to his son to complain that he has not kept in touch ('I have been much surprised, my son, at not receiving hitherto a letter from you to tell me how you are. Please answer me with all speed, for I am quite distressed . . .'). An indignant son complains to his father that he has been misrepresenting him ('You wrote to me: "You are staying in Alexandria with your paramour." Tell me then, who *is* my paramour?'). A pained lover in desperation scribbles down a spell or a prayer: 'Make her to be sleepless, to fly through the air, to love me with a most vehement love, hungry, thirsty and without sleep until she comes and melts her body with mine . . .'

Some of the most interesting Oxyrhynchus fragments read like pages of tabloid journalism. In one fragment a respectable matron writes to her husband in horror at the promiscuity of their children: 'If you want to know about the harlotries of your daughters, ask the priests of the church, not me, how they leaped out saying, "We want men" and how Lucra was found with her lover, making a whore of herself.'

In another fragment a wife writes to the Oxyrhynchus magistrate to complain about her husband's mistreatment of her and her family: 'Concerning all the insults uttered by him against me. He shut up his own slaves and mine with my foster daughters for seven days in his cellars, having insulted his slaves and my slave Zoe and half killed them with blows. Then he applied fire to my foster daughters, having stripped them quite naked which is contrary to the laws. He also said to the same foster daughters, "Give up all that is hers" . . . He persisted in vexing my soul about my slave Anilla, saying "Send away this slave." But I refused to send her away, and he kept saying, "A month hence I will take a mistress." God knows this is true . . .'

Walking around the midden mounds, I looked over to the green of the cultivation around Behnasa, under whose houses the city centre of Oxyrhynchus had once stood. Somewhere over there must have been the stall of Aurelius Nilus, the egg seller. In one of the Oxyrhynchus papyri he makes a solemn declaration that he will only sell his eggs in the forum and cease to operate on the black market. Somewhere by those palm trees may have been the mansion of Aurelia Attiaena. She walks into history in a fragmentary piece of papyrus bitterly complaining about the treatment she received from her husband: '. . . A certain Paul, coming from the same city, carried me off by force and compulsion and cohabited with me in marriage . . . a female child by him . . . but when soldiers were billeted in my house he robbed them and fled, and I was left to endure insults and punishments to within an inch of my life . . . Then, once more giving way to recklessness, and having a mistress again installed in his house, he brought with him a crowd of lawless men and carried me off. He then shut me in his house for days. When I became pregnant he again abandoned me, cohabiting with his mistress, and now tells me he will stir up malice against me. Wherefore I appeal to my Lord's staunchness to order him to appear in court that he might be punished for his outrages towards me.'

It was disgust with such violent sensuality and grasping materialism that led St Antony, a semi-literate Egyptian farmer from the nearby town of Beni Suef, to reject the world and set off into the desert. As I followed his route through the Eastern Desert in Ramazan's stuttering car later that afternoon, I thought of the untold consequences for the history of the Christian world that St Antony's actions would have.

St Antony first fled to the site of the present monastery in the late third century A.D. in an effort to escape the attentions of a stream of adoring Graeco-Roman intellectuals from Alexandria. Through no apparent fault of his own, the saint had became the darling of Alexandria's fashionable intelligentsia, who revered him for his earthy asceticism and his reputed power over demons. Like modern London literati falling over themselves to become the biographers of Premiership footballers, these Alexandrian sophisticates had turned up in streams at St Antony's cave, causing the baffled hermit – a painfully shy man who had retreated into the sand dunes with the express purpose of avoiding other human beings – to flee from his admirers further and further into the desert.

When his fan club pursued him to the site of the present monastery, located as it was in the middle of some of the most inhospitable sand-wastes in the entire Middle East, the saint realised that he was never going to shake off his followers. He decided instead to organise them into a loose-knit community of hermits, over which he kept watch from a cave a safe distance further up the mountain.

So was born Christian monasticism; and with incredible speed the idea spread. By the early fifth century some seven hundred monasteries filled the desert between Jerusalem and the southern border of the Byzantine Empire; they flourished to such an extent that travellers reported that the population of the desert now equalled that of the towns: 'The number of monks is past counting,' wrote Rufinus of Aquileia after his visit to Egypt only twenty-one years after the death of Antony. 'There are so many of them that an earthly Emperor could not assemble so large an army. For there is no town or village in Egypt which is not surrounded by hermitages as if by walls; while other monks live in desert caves or in even more remote places.'

The story of St Antony's life, which was written within a year of his death by Athanasius, the Bishop of Alexandria, was soon translated into Latin by Evagrius of Antioch for 'the brethren from overseas'; within twenty years it was being read and copied in distant Gaul. Not long afterwards, St Augustine, sitting in Hippo in North Africa, records that he was profoundly moved by a story he heard that two secret policemen from Trier (now part of Germany), having read *The Life of St Antony*, decided to leave their comfortable posts to become monks in Egypt. A century later monasticism was flourishing all over the West, and had become especially popular in Italy and southern France. By 700 it had reached even the Highlands of Scotland: around that time an image of St Antony under a palm tree was sculpted by Pictish monks on the windswept promontory of Nigg near Inverness, hundreds of miles beyond the Roman Empire's northernmost border.

The Monastery of St Antony – which, unlike most of its medieval Western imitators, is still flourishing – lies in the desert some three hundred miles south-east of Cairo, fifty miles inland from the barren shores of the Red Sea. Even today when the monastery is linked to the outside world by a tarmac road, the drive is a long and dispiriting one, through a desolate wasteland: flat, shimmering with heat during the day, icily cold at night, impossibly inhospitable. Yet until forty years ago St Antony's could only be reached by a three-week journey, and it depended for all its supplies on a monthly camel caravan.

The monastery is so well camouflaged against its khaki backdrop that it is almost invisible until you drive up directly underneath it. Then, less than half a mile from your destination, the whole complex comes slowly into focus: out of the sand rises a loop of camel-coloured walls pierced by a series of pepperpot mud-brick bastions. Above these stand two enormous towers – the gatehouse and the Byzantine keep – beyond which you can see the tops of dusty palm trees shivering in the desert wind.

Inside the walls, the monastery looks more like some African oasis village than it does Tintern, Rievaulx, Fountains or any of the great medieval monasteries of Europe. Streets of unglazed mud-brick cottages with creaking wooden balconies lead up to a scattering of churches and chapels; occasionally a small piazza filled with a sway of date palms breaks the spread of cells. Over everything tower the wall turrets and the great castellated mud-brick keep. It is a deeply suggestive spread of buildings – to the European eye like some nineteenth-century Orientalist's fantasy – but to the Byzantines it must have sent out a very different message.

For the monastery's simple mud-brick buildings were constructed in the fourth century in a manner as crude and earthy as the buildings of Byzantine Alexandria must once have been refined and beautiful. This contrast was not accidental. St Antony and the monks who followed him into the Egyptian desert were consciously rejecting everything that Alexandria stood for: luxury, indulgence, elegance, sophistication. Instead they cultivated a deliberate simplicity – sometimes even a wilful primitiveness – and their way of life is reflected in their art and their architecture.

In contrast to medieval Western monks, the Egyptian desert fathers also tended to reject the concept of learning, the worship of knowledge for its own sake. St Antony was particularly scathing about books, proclaiming that 'in the person whose mind is sound there is no need for letters', and that the only book he needed was 'the nature of God's creation: it is present whenever I wish to read His words'. Many of St Antony's Coptic followers emulated his example, preferring a life of hard manual labour and long hours of prayer to one of study. A millennium of classical literary culture came to be forgotten as the works of Homer and Thucydides went unread for the first time; in the words of a monastic chant to the Virgin, 'the many tongued rhetors have fallen as silent as fishes.' As late as the mid-nineteenth century, this attitude to the classics seems to have lingered in Coptic monasteries: when the British bibliophile the Hon. Robert Curzon visited the Monastery of Deir el-Suriani in the Wadi Natrun, he discovered manuscripts of lost works of Euclid and Plato serving as stoppers in jars of monastic olive oil.

Modern Egyptian monks tend to be literate – in fact the majority are university graduates – but their energy is still consciously channelled away from scholarly study and into prayer and agriculture. The monks rise at three in the morning – just as the Cairo nightclubs and casinos are beginning to empty – and spend the next five hours praying together under frescoes of the desert fathers in the ancient early Byzantine abbey church. There then follows a day of gruelling physical activity as the monks attempt, with a certain degree of success, to get the desert around the monastery to flower.

Indeed they are such enthusiastic students of arid farming techniques that yesterday evening after vespers – the one period of the day when the monks are free to mill around – I saw several groups of fixated novices poring over seed catalogues and the latest issue of some obscure farming magazine – *Irrigation Today* or *Bore Hole Weekly* or some such – as excitedly as a gaggle of teenage schoolboys with their first girlie glossy. Because of this agricultural bent, conversation at mealtimes can turn surprisingly technical. Yesterday, when St Antony's Guest Master, Fr. Dioscuros, brought me my supper, he produced a single boiled egg with as much flourish as a Parisian restaurateur might present some incredibly *recherché* piece of *nouvelle cuisine*. Then he waited while I tasted it.

'Very good,' I said, trying to rise to the occasion. 'It must be the most delicious boiled egg I've ever tasted.'

'That's hardly surprising,' replied Fr. Dioscuros. 'It's an Isa Brown.'

Isa, the Arabic form of the name Jesus, is a common name among Copts, so I asked if the egg were named after some pioneering Coptic hen-breeder.

'No, no,' replied the Guest Master, looking at me as if I were some sort of halfwit. 'Not Isa – I.S.A.: *Institut de Sélection des Animaux* near Paris – the most famous poultry centre in the world. Fr. Abbot visited it two years ago. Now all our animals are from the most modern and superior breeds.'

This obsession with state-of-the-art chicken-farming techniques is one of a number of ways in which the modern world has begun to knock at the gates of St Antony's. The abbey has recently abandoned candles in favour of its own electrical generator, and Fr. Dioscuros turned out to have a portable phone tucked away amid the folds of his habit. More radically, the increase in the number of Coptic pilgrims visiting St Antony's has forced the monks finally to abandon their age-old practice of winching visitors into the abbey by a rope (a practice which began in the sixth century A.D. when Byzantine Egypt first began to be assaulted by Bedouin war bands) in favour of the relatively up-to-date option of a front gate.

Nevertheless, these concessions apart, the monks remain wonderfully Dark Age in their outlook and conversation. Exorcisms, miraculous healings and ghostly apparitions of long-dead saints are to them what doorstep milk deliveries are to suburban Londoners – unremarkable everyday occurrences that would never warrant a passing mention if foreigners did not always seem to be so inexplicably amazed by them.

'See up there?' said Abuna Dioscuros as I was finishing my egg. He pointed to the space between the two towers of the abbey church. 'In June 1987 in the middle of the night our father St Antony appeared there hovering on a cloud of shining light.'

'You saw this?' I asked.

'No,' said Fr. Dioscuros. 'I'm short-sighted.'

He took off his spectacles to show me the thickness of the glass. 'I can barely see the Abbot when I sit beside him at supper,' he said. 'But many other fathers saw the apparition. On one side of St Antony stood St Mark the Hermit and on the other was Abuna Yustus.'

'Abuna Yustus?'

'He is one of our fathers. He used to be the Sacristan.'

'So what was he doing up there?'

'He had just departed this life.'

'Oh,' I said. 'I see.'

'Officially he's not a saint yet, but I'm sure he will be soon. His canonisation is up for discussion at the next Coptic synod. His relics have been the cause of many miracles: blind children have been made to see, the lame have got up from their wheelchairs . . .'

'All the usual sort of stuff.'

'Exactly. But you won't believe this' – here Fr. Dioscuros lowered his voice to a whisper. 'You won't believe this, but we had some visitors from Europe two years ago – Christians, some sort of Protestants – who said they didn't believe in the power of relics!'

The monk stroked his beard, wide-eyed with disbelief. 'No,' he continued. 'I'm not joking. I had to take the Protestants aside and explain that we believe that St Antony and all the fathers have not died, that they live with us, continually protecting us and looking after us. When they are needed – when we go to their graves and pray to their relics – they appear and sort out our problems.'

'Can the monks see them?'

'Who? Protestants?'

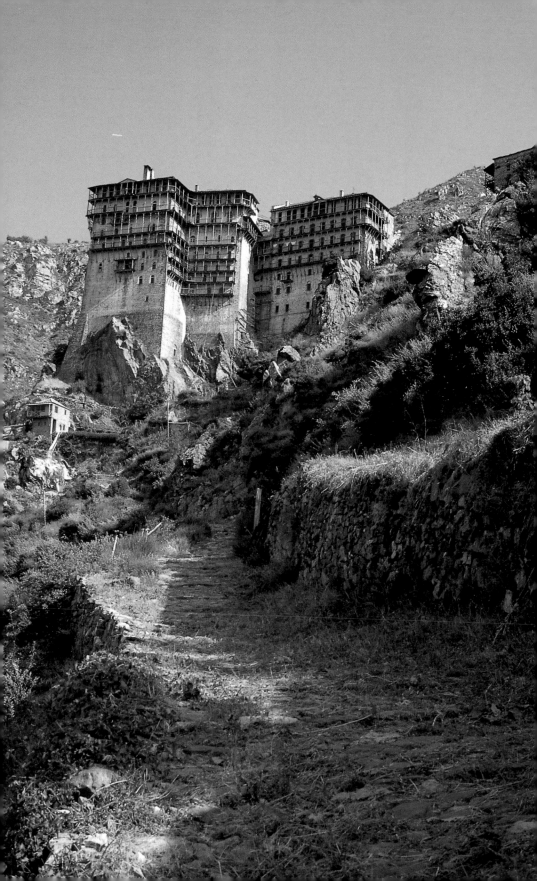

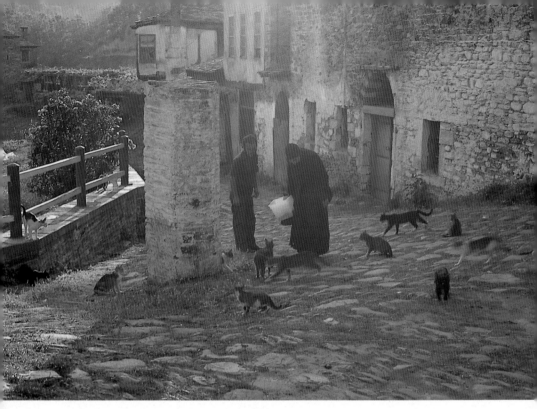

Above Fr. Christophoros and his cats, Monastery of Iviron, Mount Athos.

Previous page The Monastery of Simopetra, Mount Athos.

Below Haghia Sophia and Haghia Eirene, Istanbul.

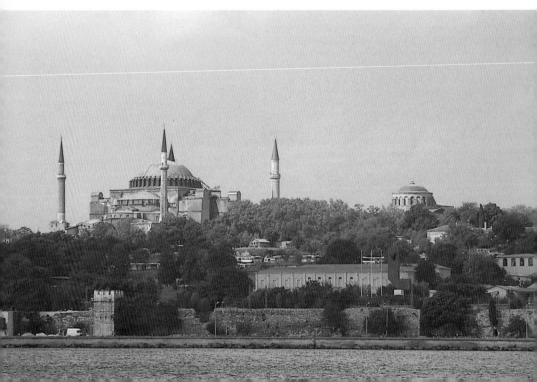

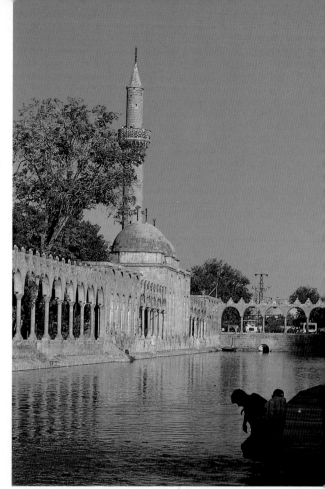

Right The Fishponds
of Abraham, Urfa
(Edessa).

Below Qala'at Semaan,
the Basilica of St
Symeon Stylites, Syria.

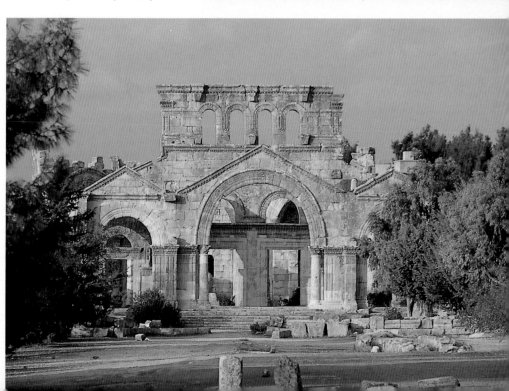

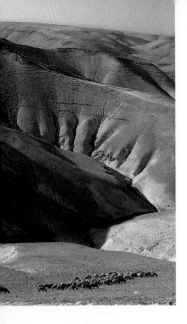

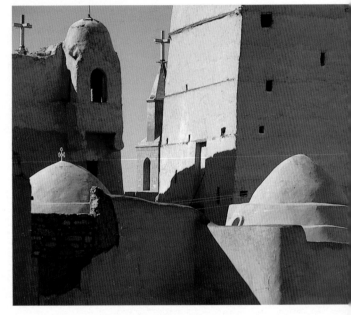

Above A flock of sheep in the wilderness of Judaea.

Right The ancient fortress, Monastery of St Antony, Egypt.

Below The necropolis of Bagawat, the Great Kharga Oasis.

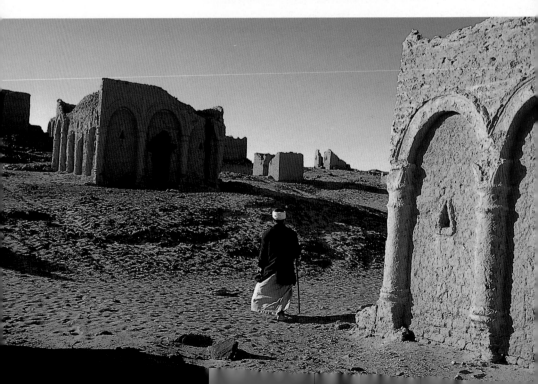

'No. These deceased fathers.'

'Abuna Yustus is always appearing,' said Fr. Dioscuros matter-of-factly. 'In fact one of the fathers had a half-hour conversation with him the day before yesterday. And of course St Antony makes fairly regular appearances – although he is very busy these days answering prayers all over the world. But even when we cannot see the departed fathers we can always feel them. And besides, there are many other indications that they are with us.'

'What do you mean?' I asked. 'What sort of indications?'

'Well, take last week for instance. The Bedouin from the desert are always bringing their sick to us for healing. Normally it is something quite simple: we let them kiss a relic, give them an aspirin and send them on their way. But last week they brought in a small girl who was possessed by a devil. We took the girl into the church, and as it was the time for vespers one of the fathers went off to ring the bell for prayers. When he saw this the devil inside the girl began to cry: "Don't ring the bell! Please don't ring the bell!" We asked him why not. "Because," replied the devil, "when you ring the bell it's not just the living monks who come into the church: all the holy souls of the fathers join with you too, as well as great multitudes of angels and archangels. How can I remain in the church when that happens? I'm not staying in a place like that." At that moment the bell began to ring, the girl shrieked and the devil left her!' Fr. Dioscuros clicked his fingers: 'Just like that. So you see,' he said. 'That proves it.'

ST ANTONY'S, 11 DECEMBER

The Guest Master has installed me in an ageless egg-domed mud-brick cell. Although it is only 9 p.m., the monastery generator has just been turned off for the night, and I am writing this on a rickety table by the flickering light of a paraffin lamp.

I spent the day reading a book lent to me by Fr. Dioscuros: *The*

Life of St Antony by Athanasius, the early-fourth-century Bishop of Alexandria. Athanasius's *Life* is probably the most influential work of Christian hagiography ever written, and it was the ultimate model for a thousand subsequent saints' *Lives* written across the Christian world in the centuries which followed: the Venerable Bede, for example, drew heavily on Athanasius's exemplar when writing his *Life of St Cuthbert.* Nevertheless, to the modern reader it is a grim, humourless and rather offputting text, too much concerned with ascetic self-torture and the saint's alarming victories over the demon hordes. At one point Athanasius has Antony's cell overwhelmed by an invasion of devils in animal form, so that it sounds rather like feeding time at London Zoo: 'The demons breaking through the building's four walls were changed into the form of beasts so that the place was filled with the appearance of lions, bears, leopards, bulls and serpents, asps, scorpions and wolves ... and the brothers [who came once a month with provisions for him] heard tumults, and many voices and crashing noises like the sound of weapons; and at night they saw the mountain filled with beasts.'

Although this sort of thing clearly appealed to Athanasius's contemporaries, I found that St Antony's charm and power is communicated far more effectively in the simple aphorisms attributed to him in *The Sayings of the Desert Fathers.* Here he emanates wisdom and good rustic common sense, encouraging his followers to live simply, not to fuss unnecessarily and to ignore the opinions of the world. There are two I particularly like:

'Abba Pambo asked Abba Antony: "What ought I to do?" and the old man said to him: "Do not trust in your own righteousness, do not worry about the past, but control your tongue and your stomach."'

And again:

'When Abba Antony thought about the depth of the judgements of God, he asked, "Lord, how is it that some die when they are young, while others drag on to extreme old age? Why are there those who are poor and those who are rich? Why do wicked men prosper and why are the just in need?" He heard a voice answering him, "Antony, keep your attention on yourself; these things are according to the judgements of God, and it is not to your advantage to know anything about them.'"

The Coptic monks who live in St Antony's today manage successfully to combine the severity of their founder's way of life with the calm wisdom that emanates from his *Sayings*. Those I have talked to are kind, gentle men, much more modest and reasonable than the bristling Greek brigands of Mar Saba or their sometimes fanatical brethren on Mount Athos. This evening I had a long conversation with Fr. Dioscuros in the refectory of the guest quarters. As the last light was fading gradually from the sky outside, I asked him about his motives for becoming a monk and why he had left the comforts of Alexandria for the harsh climate of the desert.

'Many people think we come to the desert to punish ourselves, because it is hot and dry and difficult to live in,' said Fr. Dioscuros. 'But it's not true. We come because we love it here.'

'What is there to love about the desert?'

'We love the peace, the silence. When you really want to talk to someone you want to sit together in a quiet place and talk, not to be in the midst of a crowd of other people. How can you talk properly in a crowd? So it is with us. We come here because we want to be alone with our God. As St Antony once said: "Let your heart be silent, then God will speak."'

'But you do seem to want to punish yourselves deliberately: the hot, coarse robes you wear, the long Lenten fasts you all undertake . . .'

'Ah,' said Fr. Dioscuros, 'but you see fasting is not punishment. It is a tool, not an end in itself. It is not easy to communicate with God on a full stomach. When you have had a big meal you cannot concentrate your mind. You want to go to sleep, not to sit in church praying. To pray successfully it is better to be a little hungry.'

'But doing without possessions: isn't that a punishment?'

'No, it's a choice. For myself I have begun to get rid of many of the things which clutter up my cell. Last week I threw out my chair. I don't need it. Now I sit on the floor. Why should I bother with extra food, with spare clothes, with unnecessary furniture?

All you need is a piece of bread and enough covering for the body. The less you have, the less you have to distract you from God. Do you understand?'

I smiled, uncertainly.

'Well, just look around this room. When I am in here I think that the chair is in the wrong place, I must move it. Or maybe that the lamp is out of oil, I must fill it. Or . . . or that that shutter is broken and I must get it mended. But in the desert there is just sand. You don't think of anything else; there is nothing to disturb you. It should be the same in a monk's cell. The less there is, the easier it is to talk to God.'

'Do you find it easy?'

'It is never easy, but with practice I find it less difficult,' said Dioscuros. 'The spiritual life is like a ladder. Every day if you are disciplined and make the effort you find you will rise up, understand a little better, find it a little easier to concentrate, find that your mind is wandering less and less. When you pray alone in your cell without distraction you feel as if you are in front of God, as if nothing is coming to you except from God. When you succeed – if you do manage to banish distractions and communicate directly with God – then the compensation outweighs any sufferings or hardships. You feel as if something which was dim is suddenly lighted for you. You feel full of light and pleasure: it is like a blinding charge of electricity.'

'But you don't have to come to the middle of the desert to find an empty room free of distractions. You can find that anywhere: in Cairo, or Alex, or London . . .'

'What you say is true,' said Fr. Dioscuros with a smile. 'You can pray anywhere. After all, God is everywhere, so you can find him everywhere.' He gestured to the darkening sand dunes outside: 'But in the desert, in the pure clean atmosphere, in the silence – there you can find *yourself*. And unless you begin to know yourself, how can you even begin to search for God?'

Unlike the other monasteries I have visited on this journey, St Antony's is bursting with young monks, and there are no worries about its imminent extinction; indeed, it is many centuries since it has been so full and so active. The same is true of many of the Egyptian desert monasteries: since the current Coptic Pope, Shenoudah III, assumed office in 1982, there has been a massive revival of monasticism in Egypt, and many ancient monastery ruins, abandoned for hundreds of years, are being brought back into use. Nevertheless, for all this activity, there are some very dark clouds on the horizon, and after I had spent a few days at St Antony's the monks began, very hesitantly, to talk about their worries for the future.

The Copts have suffered petty discrimination for centuries, but the recent revival of Islamist insurgency in Upper Egypt has made their position more dangerous, and their prospects more uncertain, than they have been for years. In April 1992 fourteen Copts in Asyut province were gunned down by the Islamist guerrillas of the *Gema'a al-Islamiyya* for refusing to pay protection money. There followed a series of crude bombs outside Coptic churches in Alexandria and Cairo. Finally in March 1994 armed militants attacked the ancient Coptic monastery of Deir ul-Muharraq near Asyut; two monks and two lay people were shot dead at the monastery's front gate. After centuries of deliberate isolation the world is suddenly pressing in on the Coptic monks in the most alarming fashion.

Like the Suriani in Turkey, the Copts are very reluctant to talk about their worries; hundreds of years of living as a minority under Muslim rule has taught them to keep their heads down. 'We have some small problems,' was all Abouna Dioscuros would say when I referred to the attack on Deir ul-Muharraq soon after my arrival. Slowly, however, the monks have begun to be a little more forthcoming. This morning I tackled one of the older fathers on the subject. To begin with he just looked down at his shoes.

Then, plucking up his courage, his fears came pouring out.

'Deir ul-Muharraq is only the latest massacre,' he said. 'In the last few years many churches were burned, many of our priests and laymen were killed. Every day there are death threats. Around Asyut the *Irhebin* [terrorists] walk into the houses of the Copts. They take money and belongings and if the Copts resist they shoot them dead. The Government does nothing. The police arrest no one, though they know very well who does this. When the *Gema'a* murdered fourteen Copts in one hour in 1992, the government just said: "This is Upper Egypt. Probably it is only a feud. Probably it is two families squabbling: nothing more." Only now, in the last few months, when the *Gema'a* has begun attacking tourists and government ministers, are they taking this threat seriously. Maybe they have left it too late. If they had tackled the problem when it began, all would have been well. But because it was just the Copts who were suffering they did nothing. Now it is out of hand. The *Irhebin* are everywhere.'

Other monks I talked to muttered about the oppressive Hamayonic Laws, the old Ottoman legislation, still extant in Egyptian law, which requires a special decree from the President himself if a Christian wishes to build or even repair a church: technically, the monks should seek a special decree from President Mubarak himself if they wish to repair even a broken lavatory.

'The government does nothing for us,' said one monk, who begged me not to mention his name. 'In Egypt the authorities are very bad to the Copts. No senior policemen are Copts. No judges are Copts. There is no justice for our people. The *Irhebin* know they can attack the Copts and nothing will happen to them. That is why our people are very frightened. That is why we are all afraid.'

Historically, of course, the monks of Egypt have often had to face violence. In Robert Curzon's classic nineteenth-century travel book *Visits to Monasteries in the Levant*, he remarks that 'all [Egyptian monasteries] are surrounded by a high strong wall, built as a fortification to protect the brethren within, and not without reason, even in the present day ... [Many times] I have been quietly dining in a monastery when shouts have been heard, and shots have been fired against the stout bulwarks of the outer walls, which, thanks to their protection, had but little effect in altering the monotonous cadence in which one of the brotherhood read a homily of St Chrysostom from the pulpit provided for that purpose in the refectory.'

Only on one occasion did the strong walls of St Antony fail to protect the brethren within. Sometime in the first decade of the sixteenth century a tribe of Bedouin besieged, attacked and eventually took the monastery, killing most of the monks, camping in its buildings and turning the fourth-century Church of St Antony into their kitchen. There they lit their fires with ancient scrolls and documents from the monastic library; the smokestains still remain amid the ancient frescoes of the church's roof, a daily reminder of the dangers that lurk outside the monastery walls.

In John Moschos's day St Antony's was also threatened by nomadic raiders. Remote as it was from the protection of Egypt's Byzantine garrison, it presented an inviting target to tribesmen in search of plunder. In *The Spiritual Meadow* Moschos retells a story told to him by a 'pagan Saracen' who was hunting in the vicinity of the monastery when he

> saw a monk on the mountain above St Antony's holding a book and reading. I went up to him intending to rob him; perhaps to slay him also. As I approached him, he stretched out his right hand towards me saying: 'Stay!' And for two days and two nights I was unable to move from that spot. Then I said to him: 'For the love of the God whom you worship, let me go!' He said, 'Go in peace,' and it was only thus, with his blessing, that I was able to leave the spot to which his powers had rooted me.

Other monks were less lucky. Between Moschos's first visit to Egypt in the 580s and his return nearly thirty years later, the entire fabric of the eastern Byzantine Empire had begun to crumble. The four monasteries of the Wadi Natrun had been burned and ravaged by the pagan Mazices and the 3,500 monks who lived there had been scattered around the Levant; Moschos was to meet refugees from the monasteries in both Gaza and Alexandria, and according to another source, the *Ethiopian Synaxarium*, many other homeless Wadi Natrun exiles took refuge behind the ramparts of St Antony's.

The Egyptian section of *The Spiritual Meadow* grimly reflects the anarchy of the period and is full of tales of 'barbarians' burning monasteries and leading great caravans of monks stumbling off to the slave markets of the Hejaz. In one story Moschos tells of a Patriarch of Alexandria whose secretary stole some gold from him; in his flight he was captured by 'barbarians' who carried him off into slavery – until the saintly Patriarch forgave him and agreed to ransom him from captivity. Another tale tells of a friend of Moschos who was taken captive but somehow managed to escape and make his way to the *lavra* of Monidia, where Moschos found him full of wise spiritual advice. A third tale tells of a monk who meets three Saracens travelling with a Byzantine prisoner:

> [The prisoner] was an exceptionally handsome young man, about twenty years old. When he saw me, he began crying to me to take him away from them. So I started begging the Saracens to let him go. One of the Saracens answered me in Greek: 'We are not letting him go.' So I said: 'Take me and let him go, for he cannot endure servitude.' The same Saracen replied, 'We are not letting him go.' Then I said to them for the third time, 'Will you let him go for a ransom? Hand him over to me and I will bring whatever you demand.' The Saracen replied: 'We cannot give him to you because we promised our priest that if we took a good-looking prisoner, we would bring him to the priest to be offered as a sacrifice. Now be off with you, or we will cause your head to roll on the ground.'
>
> Then I prostrated myself before God and said: 'O Lord God, our Saviour, save your servant.' The three Saracens immediately became possessed of demons. They drew their swords and cut each other to pieces. I took the young man to my cave and he no longer wished

to leave me. He renounced the world – and after completing seven years in the monastic life, went to his rest.

Yet then as now, the monks seemed to believe that their sufferings were permitted by God for a reason, and that good would come out of disaster.

'God is most easily discernible in times of trouble,' explained Fr. Dioscuros. 'When your troubles cease, then you leave God. But in difficult times men go to God for help.'

'So are you saying that God allows suffering to remind us that He is still there?'

'No,' replied Fr Dioscuros, 'that is not what I meant. But thanks to God good can come out of evil. Christianity in Egypt – our Coptic Church – grew out of the terrible persecutions of Diocletian. The blood of martyrs nourishes the seed of belief.'

Fr. Dioscuros held up the wickerwork Coptic pectoral crucifix that was suspended by a leather thong around his neck. 'What is Christianity,' he said, 'without the Cross?'

That evening, at Fr. Dioscuros's invitation, I attended vespers with the monks.

Walking into the great abbey church was like entering a tunnel. Outside the monastery compound was all bright glare; inside, past the long lines of monastic sandals left mosque-like at the porch, it was so dark that the sanctuary candles and oil lamps blazed like fireflies in the soupy stygian gloom. The darkness drained the church of colour, the shadows of its rigorously simple lines appearing stern and impressive in the glimmering half-light.

As my eyes adjusted, I took in the number of monks drawn up in ranks at the front of the nave. So far in my stay I could not have seen more than a dozen of the brethren. Although I knew the monastery to be bursting with new recruits, the echoing monastic quiet conspired to make St Antony's feel strangely deserted: after the bustle and noise of Alexandria and Cairo, here one could

415

hear every shutter creak as it was blown in the wind, every snatch of whispered monastic dialogue echoing around the ancient mud walls.

Now, as if from nowhere, at least sixty monks had materialised in the nave and all were chanting loudly in a deep, rumbling bass plainchant quite different from the elusive, bittersweet melodies of Gregorian Chant or the angular, quickfire vespers of the Greeks. Individually the gentlest of men, the Copts at prayer made a massive, dense, booming sound, each stanza sung by the monastic cantor echoed by a thundering barrage of massed male voices. The wall of sound reverberated around the church, bouncing off the squinches of the dome, crashing onto the mud-brick roof then down again like a lead weight into the nave. Yet despite its heaviness, there was nothing harsh or brutal about the Coptic chant, the swelling notes of the refrain resolving to give the whole threnody a tragic, desolate air, as if all the distilled deprivations of generations of monks were being enunciated and offered up, at once an agonised atonement for the sins of mankind and an exorcism forestalling the terrors of the night to come.

The service – like all the liturgies of desert Egypt – was conducted in Coptic, a direct descendant of the ancient tongue of the Pharaohs. The same tongue that had sung the praise of the Christian God in this church for more than one and a half thousand years had been used in the great Pharaonic temples of Thebes to praise Isis and Horus for the three thousand years preceding that: of the sacred tongues of the world, only Sanskrit has a comparable antiquity. It is a strange and exotic language whose elliptical conflation of syllables sounded as though they had been specially designed for the uttering of incantations: 'In the name of the Father and the Son and the Holy Ghost, for ever and ever, Amen,' became '*Khenevran emeviot nem ipshiri nembi ebnevma esoweb enowti enowti ami . . .*'

There was a moment of silence as the monks marched from the middle of the nave, through the swirling incense, to a long lectern near the sanctuary where a line of ancient bound vellum lectionaries lay open. There the brethren split into groups. Quietly at first, those on the north began singing a verse of the psalm of the day, those to the south answering them, the volume gradually rising, the stiff, illuminated pages of the service books all turning together as the chant thundered on into the late evening, accompanied now by an occasional clash of cymbals or an ecstatic ringing of triangles. As the service progressed and the tempo of the singing rose, novices swung their thuribles and the great cumulus clouds of frankincense coagulated into a thick white fog in the body of the nave.

Gradually, as the liturgy stretched on into its third hour, the fog of incense grew so thick that the monastic presence at the front of the nave became dim. From my place at the rear all I could see was the distant image of a line of dark figures standing at the lectern, and a little behind them a gaggle of novices in white *gelabiyas* prostrating themselves on the ground. Around me a group of large, black-clad peasant women from Upper Egypt arranged themselves in a circle, earnestly scribbling prayers and petitions onto scraps of paper. Their children and grandchildren were then dispatched to post them in the letterbox attached to the velvet-covered shrine of St Antony. At the very back of the nave another small group of Coptic pilgrims were now circling the icons, touching the face of a saint then kissing his fingers, or attempting to use saliva to stick piastre coins onto the glass of the icon-frame.

As I watched the pilgrims at work, I found myself increasingly distracted by the various images and icons of St Antony which dotted the church. Although they clearly dated from many different periods, their iconography was fixed and consistent. St Antony was shown as an old man whose white beard stretched down to his knees. He was barefoot and wore only a simple monastic habit, belted at the waist; in some icons the habit appeared to be made of animal pelts. Often the saint was shown in the company of his friend St Paul the Hermit: while St Antony was held by the Copts to be the first monk, St Paul was said to be the first hermit. When the two were shown together they were always accompanied by a raven who, according to St Jerome's version of the legend, diligently brought a loaf of bread every day to their cave. In some icons the two men were also accompanied by a pair of lions, again

417

a reference to St Jerome's *Life of St Paul the First Hermit*, which tells how the lions helped St Antony bury his friend:

> Even as St Antony pondered how he was to bury his friend, two lions came coursing, their manes flying from the inner desert, and made towards him. At the sight of them, he was at first in dread: then turning his mind to God, he waited undismayed, as though he looked on doves. They came straight to the body of the Holy Paul, and halted by it wagging their tails, then couched themselves at his feet, roaring mightily; and Antony knew well they were lamenting him, as best they could. Then, going a little way off, they began to scratch up the ground with their paws, vying with each other to throw up the sand, till they had dug a grave roomy enough for a man . . .

The reason for my particular interest in the icons of St Antony was that during the Dark Ages the saint was also a favourite subject for the Pictish artists of my native Scotland, as well as for those across the sea in Ireland. The Celtic monks of both countries consciously looked on St Antony as their ideal and their prototype, and the proudest boast of Celtic monasticism was that, in the words of the seventh-century Antiphonary of the Irish monastery of Bangor:

> This house full of delight
> Is built on the rock
> And indeed the true vine
> Transplanted out of Egypt.

Moreover, the Egyptian ancestry of the Celtic Church was acknowledged by contemporaries: in a letter to Charlemagne, the English scholar-monk Alcuin described the Celtic Culdees as '*pueri egyptiaci*', the children of the Egyptians. Whether this implied direct contact between Coptic Egypt and Celtic Ireland and Scotland is a matter of scholarly debate. Common sense suggests that it is unlikely, yet a growing body of scholars think that that is exactly what Alcuin may have meant. For there are an extraordinary number of otherwise inexplicable similarities between the Celtic and Coptic Churches which were shared by no other Western Churches. In both, the bishops wore crowns rather than mitres and held T-shaped Tau crosses rather than crooks or croziers. In both the handbell played a very prominent place in ritual, so much so that in early Irish sculpture clerics are distinguished from lay persons by placing a clochette in their hand. The same device performs a similar function on Coptic stelae – yet bells of any sort are quite unknown in the dominant Greek or Latin Churches until the tenth century at the earliest. Stranger still, the Celtic wheel cross, the most common symbol of Celtic Christianity, has recently been shown to have been a Coptic invention, depicted on a Coptic burial pall of the fifth century, three centuries before the design first appears in Scotland and Ireland.

Certainly there is a growing body of evidence to suggest that contact between the Mediterranean and the Celtic fringe was possible. Egyptian pottery – perhaps originally containing wine or olive oil – has been found during excavations at Tintagel Castle in Cornwall, the mythical birthplace of King Arthur. The Irish Litany of Saints remembers 'the seven monks of Egypt [who lived] in Disert Uilaig' on the west coast of Ireland. But the fullest account of direct contact is given by none other than Sophronius himself. In his *Life of John the Almsgiver* (the saintly Patriarch with whom he and Moschos fled Alexandria in 614 A.D.), Sophronius tells the story of an accidental voyage to Britain – more specifically, in all likelihood, to Cornwall – undertaken by a bankrupt young Alexandrian aristocrat to whom the Patriarch has lent money:

> We sailed for twenty days and nights [reported the man
> on his return] and owing to a violent wind we were
> unable to tell in what direction we were going either
> by the stars or by the coast. But the only thing we
> knew was that the steersman saw [an apparition of] the
> Patriarch [John the Almsgiver] by his side, holding his
> tiller and saying to him: 'Fear not! You are sailing quite
> right.' Then, after the twentieth day, we caught sight of
> the islands of Britain, and when we had landed we found

a famine raging there. Accordingly, when we told the chief man of the town that we were laden with corn, he said, 'God has brought you at the right moment. Choose as you wish either one "nomisma" for each bushel or a return freight of tin.' And we chose half of each. Then we set sail again and joyfully made once more for Alexandria, putting in on our way at Pentapolis [in modern Libya].

I was still thinking over all these curious links joining the Celts with the Copts when vespers finally drew to a close. There was a last procession of the monks around the nave, then slowly the brethren began to file out of the doors into the fresh air and pale evening light.

As I stood outside the church, Fr. Dioscuros came over and introduced me the Abbot. As we chatted, I happened to mention how St Antony had once been a highly revered and much sculpted figure in my home country. Surprised, the Abbot questioned me closely about the Pictish images of his patron saint, and I described to him the scene shown on a particularly beautiful seventh-century Pictish stone from St Vigeans (near Dundee) which illustrates the scene in St Jerome's *Life of St Paul the First Hermit* where the two saints meet for the first time. They eat together but cannot agree which of them should break the bread. Each defers to the other, until finally they 'agreed that each should take hold of the loaf and pull towards himself, and let each take what remained in his hands'. In the Pictish version of the scene, the two saints are shown in profile as they sit in high-backed chairs facing each other, with one hand each stretched out to hold a round loaf. It was a very different image, I said, from any I had seen in the monastery, all of which showed St Antony standing full-frontal, staring into the eyes of the onlooker, in the classic Byzantine manner.

'You are wrong,' said the Abbot, smiling enigmatically. 'We have your image as well. Come, I will show you.'

We walked through the darkening monastery, the Abbot leading, staff in hand. As we made our way through the maze of mud-brick buildings, monks would emerge rustling from the shadows to touch the Abbot's feet. Eventually we arrived at a stucco-covered building. The Abbot drew a bunch of keys from his habit, selected one and turned it in the lock. The door was stiff, but he pushed it open and led me inside.

The library was narrow, long and ill-lit. On either side stretched glass cabinets, seven shelves high, stacked with a riot of heavy old liturgical books, leather-bound folios and great rolls of charters and manuscripts. Without hesitation, the Abbot walked straight over to a pillar in the middle of the room. On it was hung a framed picture.

'Here,' said the Abbot.

My heart sank. I had dreamed of stumbling across some ancient but unnoticed Coptic icon, a copy of which might have made its way to Dark Age Scotland, there to inspire the Pictish images of St Antony and St Paul I knew so well. But the picture at which the Abbot was pointing was not only a conventional Byzantine-inspired image of a full-frontal standing figure, it was also clearly very late: perhaps seventeenth or eighteenth century.

'But that's just St Antony,' I said. 'It's not Paul and Antony breaking bread. It's not in profile. It's not even . . .'

'Not the main picture,' replied the Abbot gently. 'Look at the side panel.'

I looked where he was pointing. There, under the outstretched arm of the saint, a much smaller scene had been painted. Two figures, immediately recognisable as Paul and Antony, sat facing each other in a cave under a hill, on top of which grew a palm tree. Both figures had one arm outstretched to grasp a round loaf of bread with a line down its centre. It was exactly the image sculpted by the unknown Pictish artists in seventh-century Scotland.

What was more exciting still, the image showed every sign of being closer to the original iconography of the scene than that sculpted on the Pictish stone. There, the two saints sit facing each other in high-backed chairs, unnaturally close. But in the image in the library, the two saints are correctly shown to be in St Paul's cave, each sitting on a rock ledge. Their close proximity, almost head to head, is due to the narrowness of the cave. The oddness of the Pictish scene results from the sculptor moving the saints from the constriction of their cave but otherwise maintaining the original composition.

The only conceivable explanation of the similarity of the two scenes – one in Scotland, one in Egypt, whole continents apart – is that the icon in the library must be a late copy of a much older Coptic original, an earlier version of which had somehow made its way from Egypt to Dark Age Perthshire, either by trade, pilgrimage or in the hands of wandering Coptic monks. Another piece in the unlikely jigsaw linking the deserts of Coptic Egypt with the bleak snowfields of early medieval Scotland had fallen into place. I beamed at the Abbot, immensely pleased.

It was my last evening in the abbey. On the way back to the guest rooms, prompted by the Abbot, I dropped into the abbey church to pray for St Antony's blessing on the last and probably the most dangerous section of this pilgrimage: the journey through Upper Egypt, past the fundamentalist strongholds of el-Minya and Asyut, then on through the Western Desert to the Great Kharga Oasis. I sat in front of the tomb for twenty minutes before heading back to my cell. There I opened this diary, lit the paraffin lamp and wrote into the night.

HOTEL WINDSOR, CAIRO, 15 DECEMBER

A party of Coptic pilgrims took me as far as a filling station outside Suez. After standing there for half an hour with outstretched hand, I was picked up by a *servis* taxi on its way to Cairo.

My companions were a group of drunken Egyptian construction workers. They begged me to change my itinerary: 'Meester! You go Hurghada! Nice! Too much *arak*! Too many girlses! Too many boyses! Nice! Not expensive!' They passed a bottle of *arak* around the taxi, smoked incessantly and told smutty stories about their time at a beach resort on the Red Sea coast. There was much miming of outsized breasts and suggestive waggling of first fingers, followed by gales of laughter. They sung along to wailing Egyptian disco music ('*Isk Isk Iskanderiyaaa . . .*'), stopping only to urinate into the open desert. For five hours I sat in the back, frowning like an outraged Mother Superior.

The *servis* dropped me at a traffic island in the middle of the smoggy, hooting, ill-tempered Cairo traffic. After five days in the calm and quiet of monastic seclusion, I was horrified by everything I saw. Cairo suddenly seemed to be a nightmare vision of hell on earth, fly-blown and filthy, populated entirely by crooks and vulgarians, pimps and pickpockets, a city of seedy degenerates hustling and haggling their way to the fires of Gehenna.

When I had unpacked my rucksack in the comforting quiet of the Hotel Windsor, I opened at random my copy of *The Sayings of the Desert Fathers*. My eye fell on an aphorism of St Antony: 'Just as fish die if they stay too long out of water, so the monks who loiter outside their cells or pass their time with men of the world lose the intensity of inner peace. So like a fish going towards the sea, we must hurry to reach our cell, for fear that if we delay outside we will lose everything we have gained.'

I made up my mind not to linger in Cairo, and to get away as quickly as possible to the troubled desert monasteries of Upper Egypt. Besides, I reminded myself, I had already spent over a month in Cairo earlier in the year.

I had visited Cairo for the first time in early March when The *Sunday Times* had flown me there to interview President Mubarak. The paper's Washington correspondent had passed on to London a leak he had received from contacts in the CIA. Apparently the Agency was gravely concerned that Mubarak's moderate and secular regime was about to fall. I was dispatched to Cairo with a view to recording the run-up to the expected Islamic revolution.

At the time, the CIA assessment did not seem to be over-alarmist. In the spring of 1992, severe cracks in Mubarak's regime had begun to appear. It was at this time that the *Gema'a al-Islamiyya* first began making the headlines with a series of murderous attacks: in April, the fourteen Coptic Christians massacred for refusing to pay protection money; in June, the same group shot down Dr Farag Foda, a secular writer who had dared to condemn the movement in print. At the same time hit-and-run attacks on foreign tour-groups began in earnest, killing eight and wounding nearly a hundred tourists. The following year, in the summer of 1993, the Islamic militants began a series of assassination attempts against the Prime Minister and two other prominent government ministers, all three of whom were wounded. In November the militants hatched a plot – uncovered in advance by the security forces – to blow up Mubarak himself.

By the beginning of 1994 tens of thousands of Islamic activists had been arrested under emergency regulations, while around 330 people had been killed in the accelerating cycle of violence which had developed between the police and the militants. Cassandras among the foreign press began making comparisons with Iran in the period leading up to the Islamic Revolution, or the crisis in Algeria, where around four thousand people had been killed in the previous two years. Others speculated on an unstoppable Islamic fundamentalist wave gathering force along the shores of the Mediterranean, poised – so they said – to sweep away every secular Arab government from Casablanca to Baghdad.

I spent all of March in Cairo investigating the situation. What I found was very different from what the CIA assessment had led me to expect. In Europe and America analysts may have been fretting over Reuters reports of bombs and death threats, but in Cairo the buses continued to run, the shops were open and spring was in the air. The situation in Egypt appeared far more threatening when viewed from the newsrooms of Fleet Street or the conference halls of the Pentagon than it did from the calm and shady banks of the Nile. The tourist fatality rate was still lower than that in, say, Florida. The militants seemed by all accounts to be poorly trained and lightly armed; moreover, they had only limited popular support.

Mubarak was not personally unpopular – he was certainly not

in the situation of the Shah of Iran in 1979 – and it seemed most unlikely that he was in imminent danger of being overthrown by any sort of revolution, Islamic or otherwise. Commentators in Cairo were genuinely baffled when they read some of the grimmer prophecies then being made in the Western press – as indeed was President Mubarak himself: 'It is a PROPAGANDA!' he boomed during our interview when I mentioned the reports suggesting that his regime was tottering. 'A BIG propaganda! I wonder why, whenever some small, small incident takes place here in Egypt, in the foreign media [I read articles claiming] "there is no stability" or "regime is shaking". Even in your *Sunday Times* they were writing this. I was wondering, where are they getting these informations? I was wondering,' and here he leaned forward conspiratorially, 'maybe they are taking their informations from the fundamentals.' When I told him the source of our information his face darkened, adding that the Americans had never understood the Middle East, and probably never would. (At the request of the horrified Interior Minister, I later removed this quote from the published interview.)

In fact, far from tottering, Mubarak's regime seemed that March to be successfully digging in. Everyone I talked to in Cairo repeated the same thing: that since the government crackdown the previous year, things had become much better. The violence – though still extremely bad – was now mainly limited to a few towns and villages in Upper Egypt. As for the conventional wisdom that Mubarak was alienating large swathes of the population by the heavy-handedness of his measures, that was not the story you heard on the streets. While no one denied that the police were capable of behaving extremely roughly with suspects, people complained less about the abuse of human rights than about the fact that the crackdown had been so long delayed.

'The government always knew who the *Gema'a al-Islamiyya* people were,' I was told by Boutros Gabra, a Coptic goldsmith. 'As long as they just shot up a few Copts, the government was happy to tolerate them. Only when they started attacking foreigners and threatening tourism did the government take the necessary steps.'

Nevertheless, while an Islamic revolution appeared improbable, there did seem to be a considerable likelihood that Mubarak's regime would allow – indeed was already allowing – a slow Islamicisation of the country in an effort to appease the more moderate elements of the religious right wing. The censorship powers of the Sheikhs of Al-Ahzar University, the senior Islamic authority in Egypt, had recently been widened. More and more hardline Islamic preachers were appearing on government television, some openly attacking Christianity on the air. Even the vaguest outlines of Christian religious teaching had been taken off the curriculum in government schools, while in many places Coptic schools had had to raise walls around themselves for protection. According to the government's own statistics, mosque building had accelerated dramatically – some 125,000 unauthorised *masjids* had been erected in the last decade alone – but in the same period the Hamayonic Laws had been used to deny permission for the building of more than a handful of churches.

Off the record, many Copts argued that Mubarak's government deliberately turned a blind eye to a culture of anti-Christian discrimination and intolerance, thus indirectly fostering the climate that encouraged anti-Coptic violence. Certainly, whether by accident or design, in the last two decades Copts appeared to have been weeded out of all positions of influence, as army generals, university professors, police officers and senior Cabinet Ministers: although the Copts made up at least 17 per cent of the Egyptian population, not one of the country's provincial governors was a Copt, and Copts made up less than 1 per cent of MPs in the Egyptian National Assembly. As a result of all this there had been two major Coptic migrations: terrorised Coptic farmers from Upper Egypt were selling up their farms and making for the relative anonymity of the cities, while at the same time the urbanised Coptic middle class was emigrating in search of better opportunities and less discrimination abroad. It was estimated that in the past ten years as many as half a million Coptic professionals had left the country, mainly for Australia, Canada and the US.

More worrying still, an increasing number of ordinary Muslim Egyptians seemed to be convinced that a degree of peaceful

Islamicisation – fewer nightclubs, more veils, less alcohol, more *Sharia* law – would act as a panacea for their many problems. It was probably here – in the gradual fundamentalist annexation of Egyptian public life – and not in terrorism or revolution, that the real danger for Egypt's future lay. As a Sheikh I talked to put it: '*Inshallah* the tide of feeling is so strong that no one can oppose it now. We don't need or want violence. The majority are already calling for a society based on the Holy Koran. Until this latest violence the government was moving in the right direction by itself.'

One interview I had in March left a particularly vivid impression on me. It was with a man who was in the process of getting divorced. The bizarre feature of the case was that the couple concerned – Dr Nasr Abu Zaid and his wife Dr Ibthal Yunis, both elderly academics at Cairo University – were very happily married, but were having divorce proceedings forced on them against their will by hardline Islamists who had never even met them.

When the case was first brought to court, most of middle-class Cairo assumed the charge was a joke. Only later did it become apparent that there was in fact an obscure law allowing a complete stranger to initiate divorce proceedings against a married couple on the grounds of incompatibility. The fundamentalists' case was based on their claim that Dr Nasr Abu Zaid's academic writings, which strongly attack the political manipulation of the Koran, show him to be an atheist, and thus an apostate. His wife was a Muslim; *ergo* the two were incompatible.

Although the fundamentalists lost the first round of the case, the affair showed quite how far their writ now ran, and how successfully they have managed to infiltrate Egyptian institutions. The Sheikh who first attacked Dr Abu Zaid, a heavily-bearded TV preacher named Dr Abdul Shaheen, was not openly a member of the Muslim Brotherhood, but was Chairman of the ruling party's Religious Affairs Committee. The university, far from helping Dr Abu Zaid in his fight against this medieval obscurantism, bowed to fundamentalist pressure and turned down his application for promotion. Neither the Student Union nor the University Staff Club uttered a word in Dr Abu Zaid's support; both institutions, it turned out, had effectively been taken over by the Muslim Brotherhood.

I went to see Dr Abu Zaid at the university. A shy, retiring and rather rotund figure, I found him in a corner room of the old colonial Arts Faculty building, protected by a bodyguard.

'I could have simply stated that I was a good Muslim, made a profession of faith and the case would have been dropped,' said Dr Abu Zaid. 'I *am* a practising Muslim, but I was determined not to back down and allow these people to manipulate Islam for their own ends. This was a battle which had to be fought.'

'Do you ever wish you had backed down?' I asked, looking at his guard.

'No,' replied Dr Abu Zaid. 'After Dr Farag Foda was declared an apostate and shot dead by these terrorists, my wife and I have had to live in fear of our lives. But if I was able to choose again, I would still fight on. What is going on in Egypt is a battle between those Muslims who defend the future and those who want to drag us back into the past. More and more people want to take the easiest solution: to smoke the opium of fundamentalism. Someone has to stand up and have the courage to show that in that direction only disaster lies.'

Dr Abu Zaid talked at length about his fight with the fundamentalists, about their attempts to censor his writing and suppress his work. Before I left I asked: was he hopeful for the future?

'For the immediate future,' he said, 'no: I am not hopeful. I don't fear revolution – that is very unlikely. It is the so-called moderates I worry about. They want to suppress rational thought; they won't let anyone oppose them. In the long term history shows that freedom and truth will prevail. But in the short term I think things will get much worse before they get better.'

We walked together through the corridors of the university, shadowed by the bodyguard. As we walked Dr Abu Zaid pointed out how many of the female students now wore the veil.

'My generation has witnessed many ups and downs,' he said. 'After the dreams and hopes of Nasser's revolution in 1952 there have been so many disappointments: the defeat by Israel in 1967, the assassination of Sadat, the Israeli invasion of Lebanon, the

Iran–Iraq war, Desert Storm, the anarchy in Algeria. All of this is stored in the memories of our people.'

He turned to face me. 'After all that,' he said, 'you tell me: would *you* be optimistic?'

In the Byzantine period, Cairo was a small and relatively unimportant riverside fortress guarding the route from Alexandria to the provincial cities upstream. It was known as Babylon-in-Egypt.

The town receives only a couple of passing mentions in the pages of *The Spiritual Meadow*, both times in reference to a prophecy that Moschos's friend Abba Zosimos the Cilician would one day become its Bishop (he did). Few other sources are much more forthcoming, though *The Chronicle of John, Bishop of Nikiu* does describe its surrender to the Muslim General Amr in 641 A.D., when the defenders, deserted by their generals, handed over the fortress – and all the weapons and munitions contained within it – in return for their lives.

It was the Muslims who turned this previously obscure fortress into the first city of Egypt, and the Christians were never as dominant an element in the population of Cairo as they had been in Alexandria; indeed it was only in the eleventh century that the Coptic Patriarch deigned to move his cathedral from Alexandria (by then reduced to little more than a fishing village). Today Cairo has a large Coptic population, possibly numbering as many as three million out of the total of fifteen million, but the Copts lie scattered about the poorer suburbs – where, as fate would have it, the more aggressive fundamentalist factions can also be found.

This afternoon I set out to visit two Coptic churches which had been damaged in the course of the accelerating conflict between the local Copts and their Islamist neighbours. In one case a bomb had been let off outside the church porch; the other had been attacked when a Muslim mob, whipped up by a fundamentalist demagogue, spilled out of a mosque calling for infidel blood. Neither was a major incident, but I only realised quite how frightened the Copts were when, at both churches, those in charge initially denied that there had been any trouble at all, and only admitted the truth when I produced press cuttings outlining what had happened.

Menas, the Coptic taxi driver at the Hotel Windsor, drove me up to the district of Shubra. The streets were wide and the houses were high and brown. Overnight the weather had turned wet, and the air came cold through the open window. The sky was grey and there was mud on the road. Men zigzagged between puddles, their woollen winter *gelabiyas* hitched up to their shins, revealing woolly longjohns beneath. They all had scarves wrapped around their heads.

An armed guard stood outside the Church of el-Adra (the Virgin). He directed me to the office of the priest. Fr. Mark Bishara had a grey beard and wore a domed Coptic hat. As soon as I asked him about the bomb which had gone off outside his church, he rose and began nervously ushering me out of the room.

'This bomb is forgotten,' he said.

'But was it a big bomb? Was anyone killed?'

'It was nothing,' said the priest, by now propelling me towards the door. 'Only two or three were injured. I can't remember the details. No, please, I do not want to talk about it. The matter is finished.'

'Was anyone arrested?'

'The man responsible was captured. I think so.'

'So the government is helping you?'

'Let me not answer, please,' said the priest, half closing the door and looking out through the crack. 'It would not be suitable to write about this matter. It is not good for us. We have no problem. We are very friendly with the Muslims. The government is very well equipped to deal with everything. I have much work, I am sorry . . .'

And with that the door slammed shut. I walked around the church compound, amazed by the priest's behaviour. What was he so afraid of? As I wandered about I heard children chanting, and following the sound I came to a modern building behind the church. It held a line of classrooms, and inside several lay people were teaching small children Bible stories and Coptic hymns. One of the classes was just finishing, and when the children had dispersed I approached the teacher to ask if he could tell me anything more about the blast. Like the priest, he looked very uncomfortable, but did say that the bomb had been hung on the church gate during a service, and that it went off as the congregation trooped out. Luckily it had been a very crude device, and no one was killed, though there had been many injuries. I asked the man if he was worried that the church might be bombed again.

'Only God knows,' he replied.

'Have these attacks made many Copts want to leave Egypt?'

'Yes,' he said. 'Five or six of my own friends have emigrated, not just because of the terrorists, but to find work. In Egypt it is more difficult for Christians to get good jobs than it is for Muslims. For this reason many, many Christians – the clever ones – are going to Canada and Australia. They think it is better for their children.'

'Will you go too?'

'No,' replied the man firmly. 'It is important to remain. We should stay and do our best to defend our religion.'

As I was leaving the church compound, Fr. Bishara hurried out of the door of his office and called after me.

'I'm sorry,' he said gently, reaching for my hand. 'I am a priest. If you want to learn to pray, I can help. If you want to go to Heaven, I can help. But if you want to talk about politics . . .'

He shrugged his shoulders. 'I think you have not spent long in Egypt,' he said. 'When you have been here longer, you will understand.'

From Shubra, Menas drove me to the distant suburb of Ein Shams, now one of Cairo's main Islamist strongholds. As we drove, the houses got poorer and the people more bedraggled-looking. Brick tenements hung with laundry gave way to a shanty-town sprawl. Rubbish was piled on the hard shoulder of the road. It began to drizzle, and the vendors lining the roadside began to strap umbrellas to their fruit barrows. Others – beggars, sweet-sellers and newsboys – cowered in the doorways of cafés, looking out onto the muddy streets. In one doorway I saw an old man emptying out the water from a leaky shoe. Nearby, ragged street children were playing football, using puddles as goalposts.

The drizzle turned to rain and the rain to a downpour. The badly drained streets filled with water as puddles grew into ponds. At one flooded junction, two donkey-carts were ferrying pedestrians across a small newly formed lake.

After much hunting down narrow lanes, we eventually found the Church of St Michael and the Virgin. The priest was not in, and instead I was shown in to meet his wife, who politely offered me tea. But like everyone else that day, she looked suddenly panic-stricken when I tried to turn the conversation towards the attack on the church.

'There is no problem,' she said. 'It is very nice here. Very nice Muslims.' She giggled nervously.

'But didn't a mob of Muslims attack the church only recently?'

'Yes,' replied the woman. 'But do not write this.'

'What happened?' I asked.

'Nothing. The Muslims came to the church. But the police were stronger.'

'Was there firing?'

'No.'

'But I read in the newspapers that several people were killed.'

'A little firing. Maybe. But in the street. Not in the church.'

I felt brutal forcing the woman to say what she wanted to keep hidden, but I really needed to know what had happened. 'How many people attacked the church?' I asked.

'Not many.'

'Roughly?'

'Four hundred. Five hundred. My husband telephoned the government and the police came.'

'They wanted to burn the church,' said a voice from the door. It was the old man who had shown me into the priest's house. He was about seventy, with a greying toothbrush moustache. He had been listening to the woman floundering, and decided to speak up. 'It was a Friday, after Muslim prayers. They came from the Adam Mosque in Ibrahim Abdel Ghazi Street. After prayers had finished, an *Irhebi* in the congregation took the microphone from the imam. He told the people to go to the church and burn it, and to kill policemen. Some good Muslims in the mosque came and told us what was happening, so we had time to lock the gates.'

'Were they armed?'

'They had guns. Many kinds of gun. And some of the *Irhebin* had bombs.'

'Home-made?'

'Yes. Not professional bombs. They threw them over the fence. They didn't make a big fire, just broke one or two windows. Many children were here having lessons. They were afraid and were crying. The teachers took them into the church and made them sing hymns, but still they could hear the chanting outside.'

'What were they chanting?'

'"*Islamaya Islamaya la Mesihaya wa la Yahoudaya . . .*" It means "Islam Islam, no Christians, no Jews." Over and over again they were shouting it. Also "*Islam el Haq!*" – "Islam is the truth" and "Kill the Christians, Kill the Christians."'

'When we heard this we were all praying,' said the priest's wife. 'But we had confidence that God would help us. My husband was calling the police and Pope Shenoudah. We were not frightened.'

'And the police came quickly?'

'Yes,' said the old man. 'In two big trucks. When the Muslims saw them they ran away. For a month afterwards there were policemen standing every metre along the road.'

'Do you think it could happen again?'

'We hope it will not,' said the woman. 'Afterwards many Muslims telephoned us to say how sorry they were.'

'But none visited us,' said the man. 'Like us, the Muslims are afraid of the *Irhebin*.'

As we drove back to the hotel in the rain, I asked Menas

why the Copts had been so unwilling to talk openly about their troubles.

'They are afraid,' he said. 'They know the government says there is no problem, so they say that too.'

'But isn't that counterproductive?'

'We don't like to create problems with the Muslims. At the moment our life is not too bad. To shout out our complaints will do us no good. The Christians in Europe will not help. Nor will the Americans. There is no one to help us. So we keep quiet. We have no option but to get on as best we can.'

He frowned: 'To be honest,' he said, 'the people are afraid. The Father in the church was afraid. If the government does not like what we are saying, it can be very cruel with us, in many ways: with work, with business, with our families, with our children in schools. They can make our life hell. For this reason the people are not telling you the clear situation.'

He slowed the car to drive through a deep puddle covering the entire width of the road. When we had safely reached the far side he said: 'This is not your problem. It is our problem. You make a book then you go home. But we have to stay here. I know you are trying to help. But you must be very careful. If you are not, you could do us great harm.'

That evening, for the third time since my return from St Antony's, I visited the Press Centre to find out whether my application to visit Upper Egypt had yet been approved.

Predictably, I was informed that no decision had so far been reached. As no decision seemed likely in the near future, I decided to play my trump card. Opening my bag, I presented the bureaucrats with a transcript of my March interview with President Mubarak. Highlighted on the last page was the following exchange:

W.D.: What would you tell people who want to visit Egypt? Is it safe for them to return?

MUBARAK: It is VERY safe. We have so many tourists already.

W.D.: So I could go to Asyut?

MUBARAK: Of course. You can go tomorrow! Some of the people in Asyut are criminals and fundamentals. But the majority of the people in Asyut are very good peoples. VERY GOOD PEOPLES. You can go anywhere. No problem. Do not worry about these so-called terrorists.

At first the transcript caused suspicion, then bewilderment, followed shortly afterwards by a fluster of manic activity. When it was verified that I had actually seen the President and that he had given me his personal permission to visit Asyut, my hotel telephone number was taken and I was told that I would have an answer first thing in the morning.

That call has just come through. A government car will come to pick me up at the hotel early tomorrow morning. There was no problem, said the official; I could go anywhere I liked.

My initial jubilation was, however, tempered by the knowledge that this time tomorrow I will be heading towards Asyut – and into the waiting arms of the *Gema'a al Islamiyya*. But beyond Asyut, *inshallah*, lies the Great Kharga Oasis, the Alcatraz of Byzantium, and still one of the most isolated spots in Egypt. It was the ultimate destination of John Moschos's travels, and will be mine too.

HOTEL CASABLANCA, ASYUT, 18 DECEMBER

The journey to Asyut started promisingly. At six in the morning a black government Mercedes drew up outside my hotel; inside were a chauffeur and an interpreter (or rather minder) named Mahmoud. The chauffeur loaded my grubby rucksack into the beautifully hoovered boot. The Mercedes purred into life and we set off through the early-morning traffic in rather different style to my last trip in Ramazan's battered Peugeot.

435

For the first hundred miles there was not the slightest indication of trouble. It was a perfect cold, sharp winter's morning. We followed the same road through the peaceful mud-brick villages of the Nile Valley, with their hookah-smoking farmers and trellised tea houses, the edges of the villages punctuated by mud-brick pepperpot pigeon towers. The road was raised on a brick embankment with bright green paddy fields stretching off on either side. In a few areas the winter crop had already been harvested, and as we passed we could see white egrets standing out against the black alluvial mud.

Village labourers were trooping into the fields, silhouetted as they filed along irrigation dykes, hoes balanced over their shoulders. There were no other cars, though as we neared the larger towns, the roads would clog up with an armada of donkey-carts, or occasionally an old village bus rattling over the railway crossings. Sometimes the Mercedes would have to edge its way through a herd of leathery water buffaloes or a nuzzle of sheep being led into market by long-robed peasants, heavily swathed against the morning chill. Kingfishers hovered above the irrigation runnels. Scenes of Biblical calm surrounded us on all sides. It was impossible to imagine that we were heading into a civil war.

Only after we passed the market town of el-Minya did the atmosphere begin to change. We began to pass police checkpoints – at first every five miles or so, but then more frequently. At the same time the big black Mercedes began to attract more and more attention. People stared at us as we passed; few of them were smiling.

By the time we got to the town of Mallawi the police were everywhere. Sandbag emplacements dotted the rooftops; haphazard brick fortifications guarded the police stations and banks. Not only the police were armed: perhaps one in ten of the local population carried assault rifles as they inspected their fields or drove into town to go shopping, the barrels of the Kalashnikovs poking out of the car windows. Mahmoud, who had started the journey full of soothing words about the Western press exaggerating the problems in the region, began for the first time to look nervous.

To distract myself, I concentrated my attention on the region's history. Every ten miles or so we would pass the ruins of some major Byzantine city or monastery: Hermopolis, the Monastery of the Pulley, Antinoe, Deir al Barsha, Bawit. I pulled out my copy of *The Spiritual Meadow*, finding it some comfort that Moschos had had the same problems when he passed through here in the first decade of the seventh century.

Then as now, Upper Egypt was lawless bandit country, where the traveller proceeded at his own risk. Although subject to frequent armed incursions from Nubia and the deserts to the south, the region seems only to have been defended by a half-hearted regiment of part-time *limitanei* (border troops), who did not apparently take their military duties very seriously. Among the papyri from Oxyrhynchus were discovered the family papers of one Flavius Patermuthis, who describes himself with engaging frankness as a 'soldier of the regiment of the Elephantine, by profession a boatman'. In a similar vein, John Moschos met a pious soldier who used every day to sit weaving baskets and praying from dawn until the ninth hour (3 p.m.), then put on his uniform and went on parade. This carried on for eight years, during which time his commander seems to have been quite unsurprised by his behaviour.

Slack discipline among the *limitanei* exacerbated the region's security problems. When he came to Antinoe, Moschos visited Phoebamon the Sophist, who told him the following story:

> In the district around Hermopolis there was a brigand chief whose name was David. He had rendered many people destitute, murdered many others and committed every kind of evil deed. One day while he was engaged in brigandage on the mountain [behind Hermopolis], together with a band of more than thirty robbers, he came to his senses. Conscience-stricken by his evil deeds, he left those who were with him and went to a monastery.
>
> He knocked at the monastery gate [and in due course] the porter emerged and asked what he wanted. The robber chief replied that he wanted to become a monk,

so the porter went inside and told the Abbot. The Abbot came out and when he saw that the man was advanced in age, he said to him: 'You cannot stay here, for the brethren labour very hard. They practise great austerity. Your temperament is different and you could not tolerate the rule of the monastery.' The brigand said he could put up with these things, but the Abbot was persistent in his conviction that the man would not be able to. Then the brigand said to him: 'Know, then, that I am David the robber chief; and the reason I came here was that I might weep for my sins. If you do not accept me, I swear to you and before Him who dwells in Heaven, that I will return to my former way of life. I will bring those who were with me, kill you all and even destroy your monastery.' When the Abbot heard this, he received him into the monastery, tonsured him and gave him the holy habit. Thus he began spiritual combat [against the demons and devils of temptation] and he exceeded all the other members of the monastery in self-control, obedience and humility.

'There were about seventy persons in that monastery,' adds Moschos, 'and David benefited them all, providing them with an example.'

I was still reading about Moschos's journey through the badlands of Upper Egypt when the car was brought to a halt at a heavily guarded checkpoint some fifty miles north of Asyut. From slits in the brick turret surmounting the police bunker, the barrels of three machine guns covered the three approaches to the road junction. An officer barked into his walkie-talkie; a pair of conscripts paced nervously around the bunker, fidgeting with the safety catches of their ancient Enfield rifles. One of them looked no older than sixteen. His boots were old and scuffed, and one of them had no laces. He was clearly very frightened.

Mahmoud got out and talked to the two boys, offering them imported American cigarettes. By the time he returned to the car he had discovered why we had been held up.

'They say that it is too dangerous to go on without a guard,' he said. 'The police killed seven militants last weekend. Then yesterday the militants ambushed and killed three policemen not far from here. The militants need to get another four before they get even. Until then the whole district is on alert. They say we'll have to wait here until someone is free to escort us on.'

'How bad do they say the situation is around here?' I asked.

'They say it is very bad,' replied Mahmoud, shaking his head gravely. 'Very bad indeed.'

Our escort drove up less than fifteen minutes later. I had expected a single conscript with an old gun; what we got, rather alarmingly, were six heavily armed paramilitary policemen in a souped-up Japanese pick-up. We had to struggle to keep up. Every time we neared a village, the pick-up driver increased his speed, while one of the guards would flick off his safety catch, balance on the back-flap and search the rooftops for snipers. Before long we turned off the main Upper Egypt road and headed into the town of Sanabu. This was the place that the *Gema'a al-Islamiyya* had attacked two years before, initiating the current campaign. Two convoys of armed activists had swooped down early in the morning. By the time they withdrew, seven Coptic farmers had been hunted down and murdered in their fields; seven others were shot dead in the streets. I had read brief agency reports on the massacre, but wanted to know more. What had precipitated the attack? Had it been completely unexpected?

We drove fast through the narrow streets of the old town, our escort frantically scouring the rooftops and windows for guerrillas, their rifles raised and their fingers on the triggers. It occurred to me, not for the first time, that there could not be a better way of attracting the attention of the *Gema'a al Islamiyya* than to travel in a black government limousine with an escort of trigger-happy paramilitaries. If it hadn't been for the difficulty of getting through the police roadblocks, it would surely have been safer to have come anonymously in Ramazan's beaten-up old Peugeot, and perhaps to have pulled on one of his dirty old *gelabiyas* while I was about it. As it was, any self-respecting *Gema'a* active service unit must now have been alerted to the fact that a foreigner was in the area, charging around Sanabu in a ludicrously opulent government Mercedes.

Eventually we came to a halt at a makeshift roadblock in a small square at the centre of the town. The roadblock was made up of a pair of logs balanced on two battered old oildrums. Behind it stood a line of tall men in *gelabiyas* and white turbans, each holding a gun. Behind the men rose the façade of a Coptic church.

'These are village guards,' explained Mahmoud. 'Come on. If you want to do an interview, make it quick.'

I jumped out of the car and was ushered hurriedly into the priest's house beside the church. The paramilitaries stayed outside with their guns levelled, but the leader of the village guards came into the presbytery with Mahmoud and me. With his scarf and dark glasses removed I saw that he was a surprisingly old man, at least sixty. He kissed the priest's hand and sat down beside him. When the two men had introduced themselves, using Mahmoud as an interpreter, I asked them about the events which had led up to the massacre. Slowly the story emerged. It was a tale of almost Sicilian viciousness.

It had all begun several years before, when a Copt decided to sell his house. One of the leading Muslim families in the village, who also happened to be local commanders of the *Gema'a*, had wished to buy it. But they had offered an insultingly low price, and were outbid by a relatively wealthy Copt named Munir who owned the local garage. Gemal Haridi, the head of the Muslim family, made it clear that if he was magnanimous enough to let the sale go ahead between the two Copts, his family would at least expect a considerable cut of the purchase price. Munir refused to pay. Two weeks later, Munir's son, an engineer aged twenty-five, was shot dead as he bent under the bonnet of a car in his father's garage. In the same attack Munir was shot in the foot. He had to have the foot amputated. But he still refused to pay.

Haridi then got some *Gema'a al Islamiyya* hitmen to murder another relative of Munir who worked in Asyut. The assassins ambushed him as he was walking to work at the Asyut Medical Centre. They were armed with long sickles and killed him by holding him down and cutting off his head. Then they cut his body to pieces. Still Munir remained intransigent: he would not pay a piastre to men who had killed his son and his cousin. The Copts of Sanabu were proud of his resistance, and many others also stopped paying Haridi protection money. Haridi beat up several Copts as a warning. There was no change. Slowly the tension rose. Haridi encouraged the local Muslims to spit at the Copts when they passed them in the street; the Copts sneered back. Haridi decided that the Copts were getting above themselves. They needed to be taught a proper lesson.

Early in the morning of 24 April 1992, Gemal Haridi gathered together a small task force of his extended family and a group of *Gema'a* henchmen from Asyut. He equipped them all with automatic weapons and they hijacked several cars on the main Asyut–Cairo highway. Then they split up. One convoy attacked the fields near the Coptic hamlet of Manshit Nasser, where all the Coptic villagers were engaged in the harvest. The Muslims hunted the harvesters through the stooks and haystacks. Seven Copts were killed, all members of a single family whose fields happened to lie nearest the road. The second convoy, led by Haridi, drove into the town centre of Sanabu. At point-blank range, they shot the Coptic doctor as he opened up his surgery. They killed the Coptic headmaster, hunting him through the school before gunning him down in front of his pupils, riddling his body with more than eighty bullets. Then they killed five Coptic shopkeepers in their shops, before jumping back in their cars and heading on to Asyut. It all took less than an hour.

'I heard the shots as I was getting dressed,' said Amba Dawood, the priest. 'We had been expecting violence, so I was not surprised. From all over the town you could hear the sound of screaming.'

'Every family who had lost one of their members was crying,' said Abdil Mesiyah Tosi, the head of the village guards.

'What about the police?'

'They came, but it was too late,' said Tosi. 'They knew Haridi had already killed three people and was demanding money, but before this they had not intervened at all or offered us protection. By the time they came everything was over.'

'Had you done anything to protect yourselves? Bought guns or anything?'

'No,' said the priest. 'We have always believed that God will retaliate for us.'

'And does He?'

'Of course. Gemal Haridi is in jail now. The other big *amir* of the terrorists in this area, Arafa Mahmoud, was killed by the police one year ago. They ambushed him as he was coming out of a mosque. When they tried to arrest him he resisted, so they shot him dead.'

'So are your relations with the local Muslims improved at all?'

'The majority of Muslim families here are fanatics,' said Tosi. 'After the massacre they did not even come to see what had happened to us.'

'But it is a little better now,' said the priest. 'Since Arafa was killed and Haridi put in jail they have become a little more friendly. These two men were scaring the Muslims and telling them not to deal with the Copts.'

'And the government?' I said. 'Is it helping?'

'Now the government is doing everything possible to crush the *Gema'a*,' said the priest. 'The only trouble we have is when we request to repair our church. I applied to make improvements to it three years ago and still the government has not given us permission. No acknowledgement. Nothing. When the sheikhs ask for something for their mosques the government gives them whatever they want. They are trying to appease the Muslims. But with the Copts they don't even respond.'

'But do you think the worst is over?'

The two men hesitated.

'No,' said Tosi. 'In this village it is a little better, but beyond here it is still very bad. We are still very scared to go to Deir ul-Muharraq, for instance. Many fanatics are living there.'

'It has become a feud between the local Muslims and the police,' explained Amba Dawood. 'If they have the chance, any of the people in that area will try to kill a policeman. In that area there are still shootings every day.'

'So are the Copts leaving?' I asked.

'A few have gone to Cairo,' said the priest. 'But the rest of us are staying.'

'This incident has increased our resolve to stay and fight,' said Tosi. 'This is our country. We will stay here for ever.'

Back on the main road, our escort drove into a lay-by and stopped. The leader, a young major, spoke earnestly into his walkie-talkie. Mahmoud got out and asked what was happening. They explained that as we wanted to go to Deir ul-Muharraq, they needed more guards. Mahmoud returned looking anxious.

'I don't understand what has happened,' he said. 'I last came here three years ago with a party of twenty foreign journalists. Then we went anywhere we liked without an escort. Now they are worried that six guards are insufficient.'

I felt more exposed than ever sitting up on the embankment in our black government limousine. Mahmoud clearly felt the same, and after a couple of minutes he remarked: 'The terrorists hide in canebrakes like these and shoot at passing police convoys. I don't like it.'

To pass the time until our second escort arrived, I went up to the Major and talked to him. He was from Alexandria, he said, and didn't like it in Upper Egypt. The people were very primitive, without any manners or education. I asked him about the *Gema'a*. Thankfully, he said, they had no heavy weapons: no grenades or mortars. Nor were they good fighters. When confronted they always ran away. The problem was that they were invisible. Some were educated, some were small landowners, others were just simple farmers. A few had beards but many had shaved them off. They were always young; otherwise they were indistinguishable from any other locals.

'You never know when something will happen,' he said. 'It can be just like now, very quiet, and suddenly two of your men will be dead. Yesterday afternoon, three of the local policemen were killed on this road just half a mile up there. Earlier in the month one of my boys was gunned down a mile to the south. There is no warning, just a shot and then the peace returns. The worst of it is that you never know when it will happen.'

I went back and waited inside the car. After what felt like an age, but in reality was probably no more than twenty minutes, our new escort arrived and we headed on, now sandwiched between two pick-ups bristling with armed men. A little way along the highway we turned off down a narrow mud track, towards a great plantation of palm trees. Before long the fortified walls of the Coptic Abbey of Deir ul-Muharraq, the Burned Monastery, reared up out of the palms.

The monastery is supposed to mark one of the resting places of the Holy Family on their flight into Egypt, but six months before our visit it had become famous for a less uplifting event.

'This was where Amba Benjamin was standing when the *Gema'a* opened fire,' said Amba Beiman, the monk who met us at the monastery gate. He pointed to a patch of dust at his feet. 'And over here, this was where Amba Agabios fell.'

The old monk bristled through his thick black beard as he pointed out the lines of bulletholes in the plaster of the monastery wall. 'We had a tip-off from one of our tenants that something of the sort was being planned,' he said. 'He had heard his nephew discussing plans to attack the monastery and he came here one night to warn us. Three times we begged the police to give us a guard, but they didn't take any action. Now the terrorists have won martyrs' crowns for Amba Benjamin and Amba Agabios.'

Mahmoud, who had been scanning the surrounding palm trees, hurried us into the monastery and porters closed the great iron-clad gates behind us.

'We monks don't search for martyrdom,' said Amba Beiman. 'But we welcome it if it comes.'

He led us into the monastery. Like a Crusader castle, it was defended by not one but three rings of walls.

'It was Lent, and none of the fathers would normally have left the monastery gates,' said Amba Beiman. 'But Amba Benjamin had come out to talk to a layman who wanted to get married here. Amba Agabios had followed him to tell him that the Abbot

444

had asked him to lead prayers the next day. The gunmen were waiting in a car in the shadows when they opened fire. The layman was shot too, as was a thirteen-year-old boy. He just happened to be passing at the wrong moment.'

The monk shook his head. 'We gave them all nice funerals,' he said.

At this point Mahmoud spoke up: 'Forgive me for asking, Father,' he said. 'I have never been in a monastery before. Do monks weep when one of you dies?'

'Of course,' said Amba Beiman. 'We are human beings. But we live in contemplation. Our senses are especially delicate. Anything can hurt us. Something like this is terrible for us.'

'Aren't you afraid that the *Gema'a* might come back?' I asked.

'We lost two good fathers in the attack,' said Amba Beiman. 'But we trust in God.'

'And do none of the monks want to move to a safer area, if only for the time being?'

'No,' replied Amba Beiman. 'This is a holy place for us. There have been Christians here ever since the Holy Family took shelter here from King Herod. In dreams some of the fathers still see the Holy Family wandering around here. As monks we should overcome evil, not let evil overcome us. This is a place of visions: we cannot ever leave it.'

By now the sun was sinking low in the sky. Mahmoud urged me to hurry up: he didn't want to be on the roads after dark. But before we left, Amba Beiman insisted on taking us into the innermost courtyard to show us the high castellated keep that the Byzantine Emperor Zeno had built to defend the monks from Bedouin attacks in the fifth century A.D.

'We Copts have always been attacked for our faith,' said Amba Beiman. 'Compared to some of those attacks, this trouble is nothing.'

'What sort of attacks are you thinking of?' I asked, alarmed.

'Oh, the massacres of the Emperor Diocletian, for instance,' replied Amba Beiman. 'Now there was a *real* persecution.'

The twilight was giving way to darkness by the time we drove into Asyut, sandwiched between our two escorts. Armed soldiers, heavily swathed against the cold, stood at every junction. Paramilitary police sat in open pick-ups scanning the passers-by. Plainclothes security men stood around with walkie-talkies, clutching machine guns and signalling to police snipers on the rooftops. The town felt like an armed camp.

The police had already arranged a hotel for us. Our escort fanned out and Mahmoud and I bolted from the car into the hotel. That night we slept with three armed men guarding the lobby. The journey and the tension had exhausted me, but I slept calm in the knowledge that the difficult part of the journey was nearly over. Only one last stretch of road remained.

HOTEL OASIS, KHARGA, 20 DECEMBER

Asyut was known in Byzantine times as Lycopolis. The Byzantines regarded it as the back of beyond, the Siberia of the Empire. As such it was a suitable place of exile for those who fell foul of the Emperor or his consort. John of Cappadocia, Justinian's rapacious Praetorian Prefect (known as 'The Scissors' in reference to his tax-collecting methods), was exiled here after incurring Theodora's displeasure; more humble offenders would be dispatched to spend the rest of their lives in forced labour in the Eastern Desert, mining porphyry and granite at the quarry of Mons Porphyrites.

But it was not quite the end of the known world. Beyond Lycopolis lay one last outpost of Byzantine rule, the most distant and inaccessible spot in the entire Empire. To this place the most dangerous criminals and subversives were dispatched. In Byzantium, no crime was taken more seriously than advocating heresy, and it was thus to the Great Oasis, modern Kharga, that Nestorius, one of the most reviled heretics in Byzantine history, was banished after his disgrace at the Council of Ephesus in 431 A.D. John Moschos knew this and includes a story about Nestorius's exile in *The Spiritual Meadow*. Possibly it was his notoriety that attracted Moschos to Lycopolis. Possibly the monk in Moschos was drawn to this place of ultimate spiritual exile, the very last outpost of Christendom. Whatever the motivation, despite the extreme danger inherent in such a journey, Moschos and Sophronius chose to travel to this most isolated oasis settlement, deep in the desert that formed the southern boundary of the Empire.

It was to be the last trip that the friends would make of their own volition. For me too this was to be the end of my journey. At 5.30 a.m. I packed my bags, paid the bill and set out for the last time in Moschos's footsteps.

Our convoy left Asyut at dawn. Mist from the Nile swirled through the riverside streets, deserted except for a scattering of heavily muffled sentries warming their hands at makeshift bonfires. It was still dark and still exceptionally cold. Toad-like armoured personnel carriers and light tanks had been deployed at most of the town's principal road junctions. I had not seen such armour since leaving eastern Turkey, and the sight of it brought back memories of Diyarbakir and the Tur Abdin three months previously.

Despite a similar feeling of political disintegration and, for the local Christians, a sense of siege, the two situations were in fact very different. Indeed the problems faced by the Christians right across the Middle East had proved surprisingly diverse. When I began this journey I had expected that Islamic fundamentalism would prove to be the Christians' main enemy in every country I visited. But it had turned out to be more complicated than that.

In south-east Turkey the Syrian Christians were caught in the crossfire of a civil war, a distinct ethnic group trodden underfoot in the scrummage between two rival nationalisms, one Kurdish, the other Turkish. Here it was their ethnicity as much as their religion which counted against the Christians: they were not Kurds

447

and not Turks, therefore they did not fit in. In Lebanon, the Maronites had reaped a bitter harvest of their own sowing: their failure to compromise with the country's Muslim majority had led to a·destructive civil war that ended in a mass emigration of Christians and a proportional diminution in Maronite power. The dilemma of the Palestinian Christians was quite different again. Their problem was that, like their Muslim compatriots, they were Arabs in a Jewish state, and as such suffered as second-class citizens in their own country, regarded with a mixture of suspicion and contempt by their Israeli masters. However, unlike most of the Muslims, they were educated professionals and found it relatively easy to emigrate, which they did, *en masse*. Very few were now left. Only in Egypt was the Christian population unambiguously threatened by a straightforward resurgence of Islamic fundamentalism, and even there such violent fundamentalism was strictly limited to specific Cairo suburbs and a number of towns and villages in Upper Egypt, even if some degree of discrimination was evident across the country.

But if the pattern of Christian suffering was more complex than I could possibly have guessed at the beginning of this journey, it was also more desperate. In Turkey and Palestine, the extinction of the descendants of John Moschos's Byzantine Christians seemed imminent; at current emigration rates, it was unlikely that either community would still be in existence in twenty years. In Lebanon and Egypt the sheer number of Christians ensured a longer presence, albeit with ever-decreasing influence. Only in Syria had I seen the Christian population looking happy and confident, and even their future looked decidedly uncertain, with most expecting a major backlash as soon as Asad's repressive minority regime began to crumble.

Outside Asyut, we passed through a thin strip of arable land: the farmers were rising now, old men on donkeys disappearing down lanes, women carrying panniers of dung on their heads as they walked in pairs down avenues of palm trees. Soon after that we crossed an invisible boundary and left the cultivation for the desert. There our escort turned back, and we pulled in to say goodbye.

'From here it should be safe,' said the Major. 'As long as you reach Kharga by nightfall.'

Ahead of us stretched an apparent infinity of empty desert. The dunes were made not of sand but of a white powder so fine, so light, so easily blown into the atmosphere by the slightest breeze, that the desert seemed to steam like a white swamp. From that swirling surface the powder rose, fugging the atmosphere, obscuring the sun, blowing onto the road and dusting the car bonnet and windscreen.

The desert played tricks with our senses. In such a place it was impossible to verify the size of any object that might break this white madness. Outcrops of rock might be pebbles, boulders or small mountains. At one point, shortly after leaving our escort, we came across a group of workers who were labouring to mend a stretch of road badly damaged by a freak storm that had hit Asyut a month earlier. From a distance the men appeared like giants; as we got nearer they shrunk to dwarves. Only as we passed alongside them were we able to judge their true height with any certainty.

In the entire journey only one geological feature broke the formless hallucination through which we passed. This was the massive faultline which ran straight through the middle of the wasteland. For hundreds of miles the desert extended onwards, completely flat. Then it hit the faultline – a near-vertical cliff-face a thousand feet high – before continuing at the new lower level, as resolutely horizontal as before. It was an extraordinary sight and must have been even more dramatic for travellers like Moschos and Sophronius who passed this way on foot, striding wearily over the sand dunes, the hoods of their habits wrapped over their mouths to keep out the choking white dust.

The face of the cliff was pitted with caves, and I wondered whether any contained a spring that might have allowed monks to live there. It was certainly the sort of remote, suggestively apocalyptic location which would have appealed to the imaginations of the Coptic monks. It made me think of a gruesome story told by the hermit Paphnutius:

> I thought one day that I would go into the inner desert
> to see whether there were any monks beyond me. So I

walked on for four days and four nights, and did not eat bread or drink water. On the last day I came to a cave, and when I reached it, I knocked on the door for about half the day. No one answered me, so I imagined that there was no one there. I looked inside and I saw a brother sitting down, silent. So, I grasped his arm and his arm came away in my hands and was like this earthly dust. I touched his whole body and found that he was dead, and indeed had been dead for many years. And I looked and saw a sleeveless tunic hanging up, and when I touched this, it too fell apart and turned to dust. And I stood and prayed and I took off my cloak, and I wrapped him up. I dug with my hands in the sand and buried him, and I came away from that place . . . [That evening I was still walking when] the sun was beginning to set. I looked up and saw a herd of antelope coming from a distance, and in their midst was a monk. And when he approached me he was unclothed, and his hair concealed his nether parts, serving for clothing around him. And when he reached me he was very afraid, thinking I was a spirit, for many spirits had tried him . . .

After winding our way down the face of the cliff, nothing else broke the relentless white emptiness of the desert until, in the middle of the afternoon, we saw the first hint of green on the horizon. We were held up for a quarter of an hour at an army checkpoint, and shortly afterwards entered the date palm plantations that today, as in Byzantine times, mark the edge of the Great Oasis.

Kharga still feels like the end of the earth. In the 1950s Nasser attempted to move some of the population of the Nile valley to this place, and for ten years much energy was expended in trying to make Kharga into a prosperous and innovative new town. It came to nothing. The city was too isolated and too remote. Since the Second World War it has rained only once in Kharga, for ten minutes, in the winter of 1959. The population, lured there by the promise of grants and tax breaks, slowly drifted back to their homes by the Nile. After Nasser's death the political urge vanished too, the tax breaks dried up and Kharga was left a bleak, empty monument to the clumsiness of central planning, a maze of silent roundabouts, derelict factories and empty apartment blocks.

The vast 1950s Kharga Oasis Hotel is a witness both to Nasser's hopes and, in its terrible emptiness, to their spectacular disappointment. After we had checked in, Mahmoud and I went to eat lunch in the dining hall. There we sat next to the only other guests staying in the hotel. They were engineers refurbishing the huge Kharga prison which, they whispered, was Egypt's principal depository for political prisoners. As in Byzantine times, the Oasis had proved to have only one real use: hermetically sealed by the wastes surrounding it on every side, its isolation and bleakness still made it an ideal place to hide the embarrassing and banish the unwanted. Only the cast has changed, with communists and militant Islamists now filling the cells once occupied by Nestorian heretics.

After lunch, I gave Mahmoud the slip and walked out alone to the place where I wanted to end my pilgrimage, alone. Two miles outside the town, amid the date palms on the edge of desert, there stood the ruins of an ancient Pharaonic temple to the god Amun. In Byzantine times the old Pharaonic priests had been expelled and the site taken over by monks. They erased some of the more erotic of the Pharaonic sculptures and erected in their place a series of pious Greek inscriptions, punctuated here and there with crosses. These were intended to keep away the families of demons the monks believed to have inhabited the temple under its previous management. The ruined temple is almost certainly the site of the Lavra of the Great Oasis which Moschos mentions as having been sacked in a nomad raid immediately before his visit:

> When the Mazices came and overran all that region, they came to the Great Oasis and slew many monks, while many others were taken prisoner. Among those taken captive at the Lavra of the Great Oasis were Abba John, formerly lector at the Great Church of Constanti-

nople, Abba Eustathios the Roman and Abba Theodore, all of whom were sick. When they had been captured, Abba John said to the barbarians: 'Take me to the city and I will have the Bishop give you twenty-four pieces of gold.' So one of the barbarians led him off and brought him near to the city. Abba John went to the Bishop and began to implore him to give the barbarian the twenty-four pieces of gold, but the Bishop could only find eight. He gave these to Abba John, but the barbarian would not accept them. The men of the fortress had no choice but to hand over Abba John, who wept and groaned as he was carried off to the barbarians' tents.

Abba Leo [an old friend of Moschos] happened to be in the [oasis's] fortress at that time. Three days later, he took the eight pieces of gold and went out to the barbarians. He pleaded with them in these words: 'Take me and these eight pieces of gold, and let those three monks go. They are sick and cannot work for you so you will have to kill them. But I am in good health and I can work for you.' So the barbarians took both him and the eight pieces of gold, letting the other monks go free. Abba Leo was carried off by the barbarians and when he was exhausted and could go no further, they beheaded him. Thus did Abba Leo fulfil the scripture: *Greater love hath no man than to lay down his life for his friends.*

Overlooking the monastery ruins, on top of a low hill a short distance out into the desert, lay the Coptic necropolis of Bagawat. I walked over there in the bright red evening sun. The necropolis was like a Byzantine village sitting amid the dunes: long streets of simple *café-au-lait* mud-brick tomb-houses and chapels: some flat-topped, others with domes, a few decorated with blind arcading or naïve frescoes, many severely plain. Some of the tombs had clearly held the bodies of saints or holy men, for their walls were marked with pious Byzantine graffiti: 'Pray for the soul of Zoe',

'Blessings on Theophilus', 'Remember Menas'. But the tombs had decayed in the winds of 1,500 winters, so that the brick was cracked and brittle, and many of the buildings were left like skeletons, without a roof or a back wall. Many had been attacked by tomb-robbers, and deep pits had been dug to reveal the hidden burial chambers. Others had collapsed altogether. The whole complex was windswept and eerie, and a gathering breeze wailed through the broken doorways.

These tombs, I realised, must have been the last thing that John Moschos saw before he left the Great Oasis on the Alexandria road, *en route* to his final exile in Constantinople. Sitting there, looking out over the temple-monastery where his friend Abba Leo had lived before being carried off into slavery, Moschos must have known that his whole world was crumbling. But I wondered whether even he realised the extent to which he was witnessing the last days of the golden age of the Christian Middle East.

Soon after his return to Alexandria, the city was to fall to the Persians. Briefly recovered by the Byzantines, it fell again in 641 A.D., this time to the Muslims. Islam has held it – and most of the rest of the Middle East – ever since. The Christian population that Moschos knew and wrote about – the monks and the stylites, the merchants and the soldiers, the prostitutes and the robber chiefs – all the strange and eccentric characters who wander in and out of the pages of *The Spiritual Meadow*, were conquered and subjugated, their numbers gradually whittled down by emigration, intermarriage and mass apostasy. With occasional intervals of stasis, such as the early Ottoman period, that process has persisted ever since, greatly accelerating in this century. It is a historical continuum that began during the journeys of Moschos and the final chapter of which I have been witnessing on my own travels some fourteen hundred years later. Christianity is an Eastern religion which grew firmly rooted in the intellectual ferment of the Middle East. John Moschos saw that plant begin to wither in the hot winds of change that scoured the Levant of his day. On my journey in his footsteps I have seen the very last stalks in the process of being uprooted. It has been a continuous process, lasting nearly one and a half millennia. Moschos saw its beginnings. I have seen the beginning of its end.

So, as the sun sank down behind the date palms of the oasis, I thought of Moschos standing on this hillside amid these tombs at the end of the world, fretting about the heretics and brigands on the road ahead, checking in his bag to make sure his roll of notes and jottings was safe, then turning his back on this last crumbling outpost of the Christian Empire, and tramping on over the dunes to catch up with the tall, ascetic figure of Sophronius.

I left them there, and wandered back down the hill alone. As I walked, I realised I had now been on the road for more than five months. I had left Scotland in midsummer. Next week would be Christmas. On the front of my diary was a damp-ring left by a glass of ouzo I drank on the Holy Mountain. Inside were stains from a glass of tea knocked over in Istanbul. Some sugar grains from the restaurant in the Baron Hotel have stuck to the pages on which are scribbled my notes from Aleppo. Around these marks, this book is filled with a series of names, places and conversations, some of which even now seem strangely odd and distant.

As I was standing there a flight of brilliant white ibises passed overhead, circling down to roost at the pool beside the old temple. I pulled up the collar of my jacket and headed back out of the desert into the oasis, ready now for the journey home. Darkness was drawing in, and behind me at the top of the hill a chill wind was howling through the tombs.

GLOSSARY

LIST OF BIBLIOGRAPHICAL
SOURCES

INDEX

GLOSSARY

Agah: Kurdish chieftain or commander. A term of respect. (Pronounced Aah)

Amir: (lit. 'rich') Muslim nobleman or commander.

Apophthegmata: (or Apophthegmata Patrum), a collection of sayings of the desert fathers.

Archimandrite: Abbot of an Orthodox monastery or the superior of a group of monasteries.

Arianism: An early Christian heresy, named after Arius of Alexandria (*c.* 250–336 A.D.), which denied the true divinity of Christ. Arianism became popular in parts of the early medieval West, notably in Visigothic Spain. When Islam first erupted from Arabia, many early Byzantine theologians, including St John of Damascus, believed that the new faith was merely an exotic strain of Arianism.

Assyrian Christians: Name given to members of the East Syrian or Nestorian Church (q.v.). The name derives from the mistaken belief of early Anglican missionaries that the Nestorians were descendants of the ancient Assyrians.

azan: The Muslim call to prayer.

Ba'ath Party: Arab nationalist party, founded by the Michel Aflaq, a Syrian Christian. Different (and mutually hostile) incarnations of the Ba'ath Party are currently in power in both Syria and Iraq.

bema: The elevated platform at the front of a synagogue; also the sanctuary of an Eastern Christian church.

burka: Muslim women's body covering. Generally refers to something more substantial and voluminous than a simple headscarf.

chador: (lit. 'sheet') Muslim women's veil. Can involve anything from a headscarf to a fully-fledged tent. Similar to *hijab* (q.v.) and *burka* (q.v.).

chi-rho: The monogram of Christ, made up of the two Greek letters *chi* and *rho*. Probably introduced by Constantine the Great after his vision before the battle of the Milvian Bridge (312 A.D.).

chrysobul: An Imperial Byzantine letter or diploma granting privileges.

Named after the golden seal of the Emperor with which such an ordinance was impressed.

coenobitic: The centralised form of Byzantine monasticism, involving a communal life for the monks under the rule of an Abbot, as opposed to the decentralised, idiorrhythmic system, where a group of hermits would live largely independent lives, subject only to the vague strictures of a committee (the *epitropeia*), and meeting only once a week for the Divine Liturgy on Sundays. While a form of idiorrhythmic monasticism was the norm among Celtic monks, it was the coenobitic model that really took off in the West, and almost all modern Western monasteries are coenobitic.

Copt: A native Egyptian Christian. The Coptic Church broke off from the Orthodox mainstream after rejecting the theological decisions of the Council of Chalcedon (451 A.D.). Its Orthodox enemies accused it of indulging in the Monophysite heresy (q.v.), something modern Copts deny.

diamonitirion: The monastic passport necessary to enter and stay upon Mount Athos.

djinn: According to Islamic tradition, a djinn is an invisible spirit, composed of flame, often (though not necessarily always) mischievous.

dormition: In Eastern Christian Churches, the Falling Asleep (*dormitio*) of the Blessed Virgin. Corresponds to the Assumption in the West.

dunum: Traditional Palestinian unit of land measurement. One dunum = 919 square metres, 1/11 of a hectare or 0.23 acres.

exo-narthex: The outer narthex or porch of an Orthodox church.

fellahin: Egyptian peasant farmers. Plural of *fellah*.

flabella: Ceremonial liturgical fan. Now usually a stave topped with a metal disk decorated with images of angels. In some cases small bells can be attached to the disk, in which case the flabella is shaken during the most solemn parts of the liturgy to symbolise the participation of the angels. Flabellae were common in Anglo-Saxon England and Celtic Ireland, but died out in the West before the Norman Conquest. Their use has continued only in the Eastern Churches.

gavour: Infidel.

gelabiya: Long Arab gown. Alternative rendering of *jellaba* (q.v.).

Gema'a al-Islamiyya: (lit. 'The Islamic Party' in Arabic) Fundamentalist Muslim guerrilla organisation fighting to turn Egypt into an Islamic Republic. Operates mainly in Upper Egypt and the poorer Cairo suburbs.

Gnostics: Late antique heretics claiming knowledge of hidden spiritual mysteries. Christian gnosticism had its roots in trends of thought already present in esoteric pagan religious circles. Gnosticism took many different forms, but the most popular Gnostic sects were those that followed the teachings of Valentius, Bardaisan and Marcion.

grimoire: A book of spells.

Haganah: (lit. 'defence' in Hebrew) Left-wing Jewish paramilitary organisation operating illegally in British Mandate Palestine from 1920 onwards. Came out into the open in 1948 as the principal Zionist army fighting for the creation of Israel. As well as winning a remarkable victory against the different Arab armies which invaded Palestine on the British departure, the Haganah was responsible for formulating and carrying out 'Plan Dalet', which led to the expulsion of most of the Palestinian population from their ancestral homes and villages.

Haredim: Ultra-Orthodox Jews.

Hegumenos: Archimandrite (q.v.) or Abbot of a coenobitic (q.v.) Orthodox monastery.

Hezbollah: (lit. 'The Party of God') Militant Islamist organisation. Most notorious as the Iranian-backed terrorist outfit responsible for kidnapping the Western hostages and masterminding the hit-and-run guerrilla operations against the Israeli occupation forces in the south of Lebanon. But it is also now a registered democratic party representing the Shia community in the Lebanese parliament, and runs widespread humanitarian and educational projects alongside its paramilitary activities.

hijab: Muslim women's veil or body covering. Same as *chador* (q.v.).

hypocaust: Roman (and Byzantine) under-floor heating system.

iconoclasm: The period of Byzantine history, from 725 to 842 A.D., when the veneration of icons was outlawed and all sacred images were ordered to be destroyed.

iconoclast: One who destroys images and icons. An opponent of iconodules (q.v.).

iconodule: Worshipper of images. An opponent of iconoclasts (q.v.).

iconostasis: The screen separating the chancel from the main area of a Byzantine church. Corresponds to the English rood-screen, except that the Byzantine version is almost always decorated with a number of icons.

inshallah: God willing (in Arabic.)

intifada: The popular Palestinian uprising against the Israeli occupation of the West Bank and Gaza Strip.

irhebi: Terrorist (in Arabic.)

jellaba: Long Arab gown. Alternative rendering of *gelabiya* (q.v.).

katholikon: The principal church of an Orthodox monastery.

keffiyeh: Checkered Arab headscarf. Particularly associated with the Palestinians.

khatchkar: An intricately carved Armenian cross-slab.

kibbutz: An Israeli collective, usually (though now not always) agriculturally based.

Kyrie: (lit. 'Lord' in Greek) The petition ('Lord have mercy') at the beginning of the Divine Liturgy in the Eastern and Roman Churches.

lavra: (sometimes also spelled *laura*) Today *lavra* is a title that can be given to any large Orthodox monastery, but originally it referred specifically to those organised on the idiorrhythmic method: a collection of detached monks' cells clustered around a monastic church. The monks would generally meet only once a week when they would celebrate the Sunday liturgy together; otherwise they lived as semi-independent hermits.

limitanei: Byzantine border troops.

loukoumi: A sticky rosewater confection beloved of Orthodox monks. The Greek version of Turkish Delight.

Magister Militum: Byzantine provincial military governor.

Malfono: Teacher (in Turoyo).

Maronite: An Eastern Christian Church, originally based in Syria, though for many centuries located mainly in Lebanon. The Maronites look to an obscure fourth-century Syrian hermit, St Maron, as their founder. Although it seems certain that the Maronites once subscribed the Monothelite heresy (q.v.), they have been in full communion with Rome since the Crusader period, and today their Patriarch has the rank of Cardinal; but they still use the ancient Antiochene rites.

masjid: Mosque.

medresse: An Islamic college.

mihrab: Prayer niche in mosques, indicating the direction of Mecca.

minyan: The minimum quorum of adult males without which Jews may not celebrate the more solemn prayers and rituals in a synagogue.

misericord: Projecting ledge on the hinged seat of a Western choirstall serving as a support to a standing singer. They are often beautifully carved and decorated.

Monophysite: (lit. 'one nature') The belief that there is only one divine nature in the person of Christ, as opposed to the Orthodox position that Christ has a double nature, at once human and divine. Monophysitism was declared heretical at the Council of Chalcedon (451 A.D.), after which the Coptic, Syrian and Armenian Churches all separated from the rest of the Christian community. Today all these Churches regard the term Monophysite as pejorative, and claim it represents a misunderstanding of their theology.

Monothelite: A compromise definition of the nature of Christ suggested by the Emperor Heraclius in 638 A.D., in an attempt to end the split between Orthodox and Monophysites which was then threatening to break apart the Empire. The definition maintains that Christ has one divine energy and one will. Rejected out of hand by all the parties it was trying to reconcile, the only sect to subscribe to the doctrine were the unfortunate Maronites, who thus came to be regarded as heretics by both the Monophysites and the Orthodox. Persecuted accordingly, the Maronites fled to the heights of Mount Lebanon, where they still remain.

moshav: A small collective farm in Israel.

muezzin: Muslim prayer leader. In the old days used to chant the *azan* (q.v.) from the minaret five times a day, but a bit of an endangered species since the advent of the cassette recorder.

Mukhabarat: Secret police (in Arab countries).

Mukhtar: (lit. 'the man chosen' in Arabic) Village headman.

narthex: Railed-off western portico or antechamber to the main body of an Orthodox church, for the use of women, penitents and catechumens.

Nestorian: An adherent to the doctrines of Nestorius, Patriarch of Constantinople in 428 A.D., who asserted that Christ had two quite distinct divine and human persons, as opposed to the Orthodox position that the incarnate Christ was a single person, at once God and man. Nestorianism was characterised by the rejection of the term *Theotokos* (q.v.). Nestorius was expelled from the Orthodox Church at the Council of Ephesus (431 A.D.) and his followers declared heretics. Modern Nestorians revere the memory of Nestorius but deny that their Church was founded by him, claiming instead that their traditions go back to the apostle Addai who led a mission to Edessa and the Persian Empire soon after Christ's death. They therefore prefer to be known as the Church of the East, the Assyrian Church or the East Syrian Church. Once a major religious force in Asia, with churches dotting the Silk Route from Eastern Turkey to China, the Nestorian Church is now small and internally divided. It is based mainly in Iraq, where its adherents suffer from persecution, although refugees have spread the faith to Syria, India, England, Australia and the US.

nomisma: A Byzantine unit of currency, roughly equivalent to ten pence.

Panaghia: (lit. 'the All-Holy' in Greek) Orthodox honorific for the Virgin Mary.

Pantocrator: (lit. 'All Mighty' in Greek) The image or icon of Jesus ruling as Christ the King, generally placed in the apse or dome of an Orthodox church.

Sassanian: (or Sassanid) The dynasty which ruled the Persian Empire from 211–651 A.D. In the early seventh century the Sassanians invaded and occupied most of the Byzantine Levant, sacking Antioch, Jerusalem and Alexandria, until being driven back and defeated by the Byzantine Emperor Heraclius in 651 A.D.

servis: A shared taxi in Arab countries.

shabab: (lit. 'young men' in Arabic) Now generally used in the English-language press to refer to the young stone-throwers of the Palestinian *intifada* (q.v.).

shalwar: Baggy 'Turkish' trousers (or 'Allah catchers').

simandron: The wooden stick 'rung' in Eastern Christian monasteries to summon the faithful to prayer. Introduced after the advent of Islam, when Christians were forbidden from ringing bells.

skete: A minor monastery or large hermitage.

stylite: Byzantine monk or hermit who, following the example of St Symeon Stylites, chose to live on top of a pillar. St Symeon originally mounted his pillar to stop pilgrims attempting to pluck hairs from his cloak or person, but subsequent stylites chose to live up pillars as a specific form of rigorous asceticism which symbolised their attempt to come as close to God as was humanly possible. Stylitism spread as far north as Georgia and as far west as Trier, but it remained most popular in the vicinity of Antioch where, in the fifth and sixth centuries A.D., pillars dotted most of the highest hilltops.

Suriani: The name given to the Syrian Orthodox (q.v.) community in Turkey and Syria.

Syrian Orthodox: At the Council of Chalcedon in 451 A.D., the Church of Antioch was condemned for Monophysitism (q.v.). It broke from the orthodox mainstream and set up a new hierarchy of its own. Surviving persecution first by the Byzantine Emperors, then by a succession of Muslim rulers, the remnants of the Church still survive in eastern Turkey, Syria and parts of southern India. It is also known as the Jacobite Church, while in Turkey and Syria its members are referred to as the Suriani (q.v.).

Tau cross: T-shaped bishop's staff used in Eastern (and Celtic) Churches.

tell: (Arabic) A mound or tumulus covering an archaeological site.

tetrapylon: A ceremonial arch with openings on all four sides.

Theotokos: (lit. 'The Mother of God' in Greek) A title of the Virgin Mary adopted at the Councils of Ephesus and Chalcedon (431 and 451 A.D. respectively) as an assertion of the doctrine of the divinity of Our Lord's person.

wadi: Arabic for valley. A riverbed or gorge, usually dry except in the wet season.

wahde: Arabic for 'gently'.

Yezidis: A rare and esoteric religion, perhaps originally an offshoot of some Gnostic Christian or heretical Muslim sect. Yezidis believe that Lucifer, having extinguished the flames of hell with the tears of his penitence, has been forgiven by God and reinstated as the Chief Angel. Now known as Malik Tawus, the Peacock Angel, he superintends the daily running of the world. Abused as devil-worshippers by their enemies, the Yezidis get on surprisingly well with the Syrian Orthodox, in whose villages many of the Turkish Yezidis live, and whose saints the Yezidis also venerate. The Yezidis can also be found in Georgia, Armenia and Iraq.

BIBLIOGRAPHY OF PRINCIPAL
SOURCES

GENERAL

A.J. Arberry, *Religion in the Middle East* (Cambridge, Cambridge University Press, 1969)

Aziz S. Atiya, *A History of Eastern Christianity* (London, Methuen, 1968)

Norman H. Baynes, 'The "Pratum Spirituale" ', in *Orientalia Christiana Periodica* xiii (1947), pp. 404–14, reprinted in Baynes, *Byzantine Studies* (1955), pp. 261–70

Robert B. Betts, *Christians in the Arab East* (London, SPCK, 1979)

Peter Brown, *The World of Late Antiquity* (London, Thames & Hudson, 1971)

Peter Brown, 'A Dark Age Crisis: Aspects of the Iconoclast Controversy', in *English Historical Review* cccxlvi (January 1973), pp. 1–34

Peter Brown, *The Making of Late Antiquity* (Cambridge, Mass., Harvard University Press, 1978)

Peter Brown, 'Late Antiquity', in Paul Veyne (trans. Arthur Goldhammer), *A History of Private Life: From Pagan Rome to Byzantium* (Cambridge, The Belknap Press of Harvard University Press, 1987)

Peter Brown, *Power and Persuasion in Late Antiquity: Towards a Christian Empire* (Wisconsin, Wisconsin University Press, 1992)

Averil Cameron, *The Mediterranean World in Late Antiquity, A.D 395–600* (London, Routledge, 1993)

Henry Chadwick, 'John Moschos and his Friend Sophronius the Sophist', in *Journal of Theological Studies* xxv, pt 1 (April 1974)

Kenneth Cragg, *The Arab Christian: A History in the Middle East* (London, Mowbray, 1992)

E. Follieri, 'Dove e quando morì Giovanni Mosco?', in *Rivista di Studi Bizantini e Neoellenici* 25 (1988), pp. 3–39

David Fromkin, *A Peace to End All Peace: The Fall of the Ottoman Empire and the Creation of the Modern Middle East* (New York, Avon Books, 1989)

J.F. Haldon, *Byzantium in the Seventh Century: The Transformation of a Culture* (Cambridge, Cambridge University Press, 1990)

Judith Herrin, *The Formation of Christendom* (Oxford, Blackwell, 1987)

Albert Hourani, *Minorities in the Arab World* (Oxford, Oxford University Press, 1946)

Albert Hourani, *A History of the Arab Peoples* (London, Faber & Faber, 1991)

Irmgard Hutter, *Early Christian and Byzantine* (London, Herbert Press, 1988)

A.M.H Jones, *The Later Roman Empire* (Oxford, Blackwell, 1964, 2 vols)

Walter E. Kaegi, *Byzantium and the Early Islamic Conquests* (Cambridge, Cambridge University Press, 1992)

Ernst Kitzinger, 'The Cult of Images in the Age Before Iconoclasm', in *Dumbarton Oaks Papers* 8 (1954)

Ernst Kitzinger, 'Byzantine Art in the Period Between Justinian and Iconoclasm', in *Berichte Zum XI Internationalen Byzantinisten Kongress* (1960)

Ernst Kitzinger, *Byzantine Art in the Making* (London, Faber & Faber, 1977)

Jules Leroy, *Monks and Monasteries of the Middle East* (London, Harrap, 1963)

Cyril Mango, *Byzantium: The Empire of the New Rome* (London, Weidenfeld & Nicolson, 1980)

Cyril Mango, *The Art of the Byzantine Empire 312–1453* (Toronto, Toronto University Press, 1986)

Cyril Mango, *Byzantine Architecture* (London, Faber & Faber, 1986)

Peter Mansfield, *A History of the Middle East* (London, Viking, 1991)

John Moschos (trans. John Wortley), *The Spiritual Meadow* (Kalamazoo, Cistercian Publications, 1992)

John Julius Norwich, *Byzantium: The Early Centuries* (London, Viking, 1988)

Philip Pattendon, 'The Text of the *Pratum Spirituale*', in *Journal of Theological Studies* 26 (1975)

David Talbot Rice, *Art of the Byzantine Era* (London, Thames & Hudson, 1963)

Lyn Rodley, *Byzantine Art and Architecture: An Introduction* (Cambridge, Cambridge University Press, 1994)

Steven Runciman, *Byzantine Civilisation* (London, Edward Arnold, 1933)

Christoph von Schörnborn, *Sophrone de Jerusalem: Vie monastique et confession dogmatique* (Paris, 1972)

Jean-Pierre Valonges, *Vie et mort des Chrétiens D'Orient* (Paris, Fayard,1994)

Kallistos Ware, *The Orthodox Way* (Oxford, Mowbray, 1979)

Timothy Ware, *The Orthodox Church* (London, Pelican, 1963)

Bat Ye'or, *The Dhimmi: Jews and Christians Under Islam* (Cranbury, Farleigh Dickinson/Associated University Presses, 1985)

Bat Ye'or, *The Decline of Eastern Christianity: From Jihad to Dhimmitude* (Cranbury, Farleigh Dickinson/Associated University Presses, 1996)

CHAPTER 1

Robert Byron, *The Station, Athos: Treasures and Men* (London, Duckworth, 1928)

Robert Curzon, *Visits to Monasteries in the Levant* (London, John Murray, 1849)

John Julius Norwich and Reresby Sitwell, *Mount Athos* (London, Hutchinson, 1966)

Virginia Surtees, *Coutts Lindsay* (Norwich, Michael Russell, 1993)

CHAPTER II

Alexis Alexandris, *The Greek Minority of Istanbul and Greek–Turkish Relations 1918–1974* (Athens, Centre for Asia Minor Studies, 1992)

Percy George Badger, *The Nestorians and their Rituals* (Reprint: London, Darf Publishers, 1987)

Gertrude Bell, *The Churches and Monasteries of the Tur Abdin* (Reprint: London, Pindar Press, 1982)

Sebastian Brock (trans.), *The Syriac Fathers on Prayer and the Spiritual Life* (Kalamazoo, Cistercian Press, 1987)

Peter Brown, 'The Rise and Function of the Holy Man in Late Antiquity', in *Journal of Roman Studies* lxi (1971)

Robert Browning, *Justinian and Theodora* (London, Thames & Hudson, 1971)

Vahakhn N. Dardarian, *The History of the Armenian Genocide* (Oxford, Berghahn Books, 1995)

Leslie A. Davis, *The Slaughterhouse Province* (New York, Aristide D. Caratzas, 1989)

Glanville Downey, *Constantinople in the Age of Justinian* (New York, Dorset Press, 1960)

Glanville Downey, *A History of Antioch in Syria* (Princeton, Princeton University Press, 1961)

Egeria, (trans. George E. Gingras), *Diary of a Pilgrimage* (New York, Newman Press, 1970)

Eusebius, *The History of the Church* (London, Penguin, 1965)

Clive Foss, 'The Persians in Asia Minor and the End of Antiquity', in *English Historical Review* 90 (1975), pp. 721–47

John Joseph, *Muslim–Christian Relations and Inter-Christian Rivalries in the Middle East: The Case of the Jacobites in an Age of Transition* (New York, State University of New York Press, 1983)

J.N.D. Kelly, *Golden Mouth: The Story of John Chrysostom – Ascetic, Preacher, Bishop* (London, Duckworth, 1995)

Michael Lapidge (ed.), *Archbishop Theodore* (Cambridge, Cambridge University Press, 1995)

Samuel N.C. Lieu, *Manichaeism* (Manchester, Manchester University Press, 1985)

H.F.B. Lynch, *Armenia: Travels and Studies* (Reprint: Beirut, Khayats, 1990)

H.J. Magoulias, 'The Lives of Byzantine Saints as a Source for the History of Magic: Sorcery, Relics and Icons', in *Byzantion* 37 (1967), pp. 228–69

Marlia Mundell Mango, 'The Continuity of the Classical Tradition in the Art and Architecture of Northern Mesopotamia', in Nina G. Garsoian, Thomas F. Matthews and Robert W. Thomson (eds), *East of Byzantium: Syria and Armenia in the Formative Period*, Dumbarton Oaks Symposium 1980 (Washington, Dumbarton Oaks, 1982)

Philip Mansel, *Constantinople: City of the World's Desire, 1453–1924* (London, John Murray, 1995)

John Moorhead, 'The Monophysite Response to the Arab Invasions', in *Byzantion* 51 (1981)

J. Naayem, *Les Assyro-Chaldéens et les Armeniens massacrés par les Turcs* (Paris, Bloud & Gay, 1920)

Carl Nordenfalk, 'An Illustrated Diatessaron', in *Art Bulletin* 50 (1968)

Carl Nordenfalk, 'The Diatessaron Once More', in *Art Bulletin* 55 (1973)

Andrew Palmer, *Monk and Mason on the Tigris Frontier: The Early History of the Tur 'Abdin* (Cambridge, Cambridge University Press, 1990)

Oswald H. Parry, *Six Months in a Syrian Monastery* (London, Horace Cox, 1895)

John A. Petropulos, 'The Compulsory Exchange of Populations: Greek–Turkish Peacemaking, 1922–1930', in *Byzantine and Modern Greek Studies* 2 (1976)

Procopius (trans. G.A. Williamson), *The Secret History* (London, Penguin, 1966)

Kurt Rudolph (trans. Robert McLachlan Wilson), *Gnosis* (Edinburgh, T&T Clark, 1983)

Steven Runciman, *The Medieval Manichee* (Cambridge, Cambridge University Press, 1947)

J.B. Segal, 'Mesopotamian Communities from Julian to the Rise of Islam', in *Proceedings of the British Academy* 41 (1955), pp. 109–39

J.B. Segal, *Edessa: The Blessed City* (Oxford, Oxford University Press, 1970)

T.A. Sinclair, *Eastern Turkey: An Architectural and Archaeological Survey* (London, Pindar Press, 1990, 4 vols)

R.S. Stafford, *The Tragedy of the Assyrians* (London, George Allen & Unwin, 1935)

J.M. Thierry and Patrick Donabedian, *Les Arts Armeniens* (Paris, Mazenod, 1988)

Pierre Vidal-Naquet, *A Crime of Silence: The Armenian Genocide* (London, Zed Books, 1985)

Gary Vikan, 'Art, Medicine and Magic in Early Byzantium', in *Dumbarton Oaks Papers* 38 (1984)

Christopher J. Walker, *Armenia: The Survival of a Nation* (London, Croom Helm, 1980)

W.A. Wigram, *A History of the Assyrian Church 100–640 A.D.* (London, SPCK, 1910)

W.A. Wigram, *The Cradle of Mankind: Life in Eastern Kurdistan* (London, A&C Black, 1914)

W.A. Wigram, *The Assyrians and their Neighbours* (London, G. Bell & Sons, 1929)

CHAPTER III

Willi Apel, *Gregorian Chant* (London, Burns & Oates, 1958)

Sebastian Brock, 'Early Syrian Asceticism', in Brock, *Syriac Perspectives on Late Antiquity* (London, Variorum Reprints, 1984)

Peter Brown, 'Sorcery, Demons and the Rise of Christianity', in *Witch-*

craft, *Confessions and Accusations* pp. 17–45 (Cambridge, Cambridge University Press, 1970)

Peter Brown, 'The Saint as an Exemplar in Late Antiquity', in *Representations* 1 (1983), pp. 1–25

E.A. Wallis Budge, *The Monks of Kublai Khan* (London, Religious Tracts Society, 1928)

Ross Burns, *Monuments of Syria* (London, I.B. Tauris, 1992)

Robert Doran (trans.), *The Lives of Simeon Stylites* (Kalamazoo, Cistercian Press, 1992)

Han J.W. Drijvers, 'The Persistence of Pagan Cults and Practices in Christian Syria', in Drijvers, *East of Antioch: Studies in Early Syriac Christianity* (London, Variorum Reprints, 1984)

W.H.C. Frend, 'The Monks and the Survival of the East Roman Empire in the Fifth Century', in *Past and Present* 54 (1972), pp. 3–24

Nicholas Gendle, 'The Role of the Byzantine Saint in the Development of the Icon Cult', in *The Byzantine Saint*, ed. S. Hackel, pp. 181–6, supplementary to *Sobornost* 5 (1981)

Hermann Gollancz (ed. and trans.), *The Book of Protection, Being a Collection of Charms* (London, Henry Frowde, 1912)

Henry Hill, 'The Assyrians: The Church of the East', in Hill (ed.), *Light From the East: A Symposium* (Toronto, Anglican Diocese of Toronto, 1988)

Dom. Anselm Hughes, (ed.), *Early Mediaeval Music up to 1300* (Oxford, Oxford University Press, 1949)

Huneberc of Heidenheim (trans. Talbot), 'The *Hodoeporicon* of St. Willibald', in Talbot, *Anglo-Saxon Missionaries* (1954), pp. 151–77

Hugh Kennedy, 'The Last Century of Byzantine Syria: A Reinterpretation', in *Byzantinische Forschungen* 10 (1985), pp. 141–83

Hugh Kennedy, 'Antioch and the Villages of Northern Syria', in *Nottingham Mediaeval Studies* 32 (1988), pp. 65–90

Patrick Seale, *Asad: The Struggle for the Middle East* (London, I.B. Tauris, 1988)

Georges Tate, 'La Syrie a l'Époque Byzantine', in *Syrie: Memoire et civilisation* (Paris, Flammarion, 1994)

Theodoret of Cyrrhus (trans. R.M. Price), *A History of the Monks of Syria* (Kalamazoo, Cistercian Press, 1985)

Colin Thubron, *Mirror to Damascus* (London, Heinemann, 1967)

J. Spencer Trimingham, *Christianity Among the Arabs in Pre-Islamic Times* (Beirut, Librairie de Liban, 1979)

A. Voobus, *A History of Asceticism in the Syrian Orient* (Louvain, 1960)

Egon Wellesz, *Eastern Elements in Western Chant* (Oxford, Oxford University Press, 1947)

Egon Wellesz, *A History of Byzantine Music and Hymnography* (Oxford, Oxford University Press, 1949)

CHAPTER IV

Robert Fisk, *Pity the Nation: Lebanon at War* (London, André Deutsch, 1990)

David Gilmour, *Lebanon: The Fractured Country* (London, Martin Robertson, 1983)

Charles Glass, *Tribes with Flags: A Journey Curtailed* (London, Secker & Warburg, 1990)

Charles Glass, *Money For Old Rope* (London, Picador, 1992)

Elinor A. Moore, 'Severus of Antioch and the Law School of Beirut', in Moore, *The Early Church in the Middle East* (Beirut, Aleph, 1946)

Matti Moosa, *The Maronites in History* (New York, Syracuse University Press, 1986)

Jonathan Randal, *The Tragedy of Lebanon* (London, Chatto & Windus, 1983)

Kamal Salibi, *The Modern History of Lebanon* (London, Weidenfeld & Nicolson, 1965)

Kamal Salibi, *A House of Many Mansions: The History of Lebanon Reconsidered* (London, I.B. Tauris, 1988)

Anthony Sampson, *The Arms Bazaar* (London, Hodder & Stoughton, 1977)

Ze'ev Schiff and Ehud Ya'ari (trans. Ina Friedman), *Israel's Lebanon War* (London, George Allen & Unwin, 1985)

Colin Thubron, *The Hills of Adonis: A Journey in Lebanon* (London, Heinemann, 1968)

CHAPTER V

Said K. Aburish, *The Forgotten Faithful: The Christians of the Holy Land* (London, Quartet, 1993)

Karen Armstrong, *A History of Jerusalem: One City, Three Faiths* (London, HarperCollins, 1996)

Naim Stifan Ateek, *Justice and Only Justice: A Palestinian Theology of Liberation* (New York, Orbis, 1989)

Dan Bahat, *The Illustrated Atlas of Jerusalem* (Jerusalem, Carta, 1989)

E.A. Wallis Budge, *St George of Lydda* (Oxford, Oxford University Press, 1930)

David Burrell and Yehezekel Landau, *Voices from Jerusalem: Jews and Christians Reflect on the Holy Land* (New Jersey, Paulist Press, 1992)

Taufik Canaan, *Mohammedan Saints and Sanctuaries in Palestine* (London, Luzac & Co., 1927)

Derwas J. Chitty, *The Desert a City* (Oxford, Blackwell, 1966)

Saul P. Colbi, *Christianity in the Holy Land* (Tel Aviv, Am Hassefer, 1969)

Frederick C. Conybeare (trans.), 'Antiochus Strategos' Account of the Sack of Jerusalem in 614 A.D', in *English Historical Review* 25 (1910), pp. 502–17

Cyril of Scythopolis (trans. R.M. Price), *The Lives of the Monks of Palestine* (Kalamazoo, Cistercian Publications, 1991)

Norman G. Finklestein, *Image and Reality of the Israel–Palestine Conflict* (London, Verso, 1995)

David Gilmour, *Dispossessed: The Ordeal of the Palestinians* (London, Sidgwick & Jackson, 1980)

David Grossman, *The Yellow Wind* (London, Jonathan Cape, 1988)

David Grossman, *Sleeping on a Wire* (London, Jonathan Cape, 1993)

J.E. Hanauer, *Folklore of the Holy Land* (London, Duckworth, 1907)

Yizhar Hirschfeld, *The Judaean Desert Monasteries in the Byzantine Period* (New Haven, Yale University Press, 1992)

David Howell, 'Saint George as Intercessor', in *Byzantion* xxxix (1969), pp. 121–36

Walid Khalidi (ed.), *All That Remains: The Palestinian Villages Occupied and Depopulated by Israel in 1948* (Washington, Institute of Palestine Studies, 1992)

Benny Morris, *The Birth of the Palestinian Refugee Problem, 1947–1949* (Cambridge, Cambridge University Press, 1987)

Jerome Murphy-O'Connor, *The Holy Land* (Oxford, Oxford University Press, 1980)

F.E. Peters, *Jerusalem* (Princeton, Princeton University Press, 1985)

Michele Piccirillo, *The Mosaics of Jordan* (Amman, American Centre of Oriental Research, 1993)

Michele Piccirillo, 'The Christians in Palestine during a Time of Transition: 7th–9th Centuries', in Anthony O'Mahony (ed.), *The Christian Heritage in the Holy Land* (London, Scorpion Cavendish, 1995)

Michael Prior and William Taylor, *Christians in the Holy Land* (London, World of Islam Festival Trust, 1994)

John H. Melkon Rose, *The Armenians of Jerusalem* (London, Radcliffe Press, 1993)

Edward Said, *The Question of Palestine* (London, Vintage, 1992)

Edward Said, *The Politics of Dispossession: The Struggle for Palestinian Self-Determination 1969–1994* (London, Chatto & Windus, 1994)

Colin Thubron, *Jerusalem* (London, Heinemann, 1969)

Yoram Tsafrir (ed.), *Ancient Churches Revealed* (Jerusalem, Israel Exploration Society, 1993)

Peter Walker, 'Jerusalem and the Holy Land in the Fourth Century', in Anthony O'Mahony (ed.), *The Christian Heritage in the Holy Land* (London, Scorpion Cavendish, 1995)

Keith Whitelam, *The Invention of Ancient Israel: The Silencing of Palestinian History* (London, Routledge, 1996)

John Wilkinson, *Jerusalem Pilgrims Before the Crusades* (Jerusalem, Ariel, 1977)

CHAPTER VI

Nils Aberg, *Occident and Orient in the Art of the Seventh Century* (Stockholm, Wahlstron & Widstrand, 1943–7, 3 vols)

Athanasius, *The Life of Antony* (New York, Paulist Press, 1980)

Alexander Badawy, *Coptic Art and Archaeology: The Art of the Christian Egyptians from the Late Antique to the Middle Ages* (Cambridge, Mass., MIT Press, 1978)

Roger S. Bagnall, *Egypt in Late Antiquity* (Princeton, Princeton University Press, 1993)

Alan K. Bowman, *Egypt After the Pharaohs, 332 B.C.–A.D. 642* (London, British Museum Publications, 1986)

A.J. Butler, *Ancient Coptic Churches of Egypt* (London, Henry Fowden, 1884, 2 vols)

A.J. Butler, *The Arab Conquest of Egypt* (Oxford, Oxford University Press, 1902)

Luciano Canfora, *The Vanished Library* (London, Hutchinson, 1989)

B.L. Carter, *The Copts in Egyptian Politics* (London, Croom Helm, 1986)

Euphrosyne Doxiadis, *The Mysterious Fayum Portraits: Faces from Ancient Egypt* (London, Thames & Hudson, 1995)

P.M. du Bourguet (trans. Caryll Hay-Shaw), *Coptic Art*, (London, Methuen, 1971)

E.M. Forster, *Alexandria: A History and Guide* (London, Michael Haag, 1982)

G. Fowden, 'Bishops and Temples in the Eastern Roman Empire, A.D. 320–435', in *Journal of Theological Studies* xxix, pt 1 (April 1978)

Michael Gough, *The Origins of Christian Art* (London, Thames & Hudson, 1973)

Bernard P. Grenfell, 'Oxyrhynchus and its Papyri', in *Egypt Exploration Fund Journal* (1896–7)

Wilfred Griggs, *Early Egyptian Christianity* (Leiden, E.J. Brill, 1990)

Michael Haag, *Discovery Guide to Egypt* (London, Michael Haag, 1990)

H. Hondelink, *Coptic Art and Culture* (Cairo, Shoudy Publishing House, 1990)

Walter Horn, 'On the Origin of the Celtic Cross', in Horn, Jenny White Marshall and Grellan D. Rourke (eds), *The Forgotten Hermitage of Skellig Michael* (Berkeley, University of California Press, 1991)

John of Nikiu (trans. R.H. Charles), *The Chronicle of John of Nikiu*, (London, Text and Translation Society, 1916)

Jill Kamil, *Coptic Egypt* (Cairo, The American University of Cairo Press, 1987)

J.W. McPherson, *The Moulids of Egypt* (Cairo, NM Press, 1941)

Otto Meinardus, *Monks and Monasteries of the Egyptian Deserts* (Cairo, The American University of Cairo Press, 1961)

Otto Meinardus, *Christian Egypt: Ancient and Modern* (Cairo, French Institute of Oriental Archaeology, 1965)

Otto Meinardus, *Christian Egypt: Faith and Life* (Cairo, French Institute of Oriental Archaeology, 1970)

G.R. Monks, 'The Church of Alexandria and the City's Economic Life in the Sixth Century', in *Speculum* 28, pp. 349–62

Cecil Mowbray, 'Eastern Influence on Carvings at St Andrews and Nigg, Scotland', in *Antiquity* x (1936), pp. 428–40

Elaine Pagels, *The Gnostic Gospels* (New York, Random House, 1979)

Robert K. Ritner, 'Egyptians in Ireland: A Question of Coptic Peregrinations', in *Rice University Studies* 62 (1976), pp. 65–87

Erwin Rosenthal, 'Some Observations on Coptic Influence in Western Early Medieval Manuscripts', in *Homage to a Bookman: Essays on Manuscripts, Books and Printing Written for P. Kraus on his Sixtieth Birthday* (Berlin, 1967)

Norman Russell (trans.), *The Lives of the Desert Fathers: The Historia Monarchorum in Aegypto* (Oxford, Mowbray, 1981)

George Scott-Moncrieff, *Paganism and Christianity in Egypt* (Cambridge, Cambridge University Press, 1913)

Sophronius the Sophist, 'The Life of St John the Almsgiver', in Elizabeth Dawes and Norman H. Baynes (trans. and ed.), *Three Byzantine Saints* (Oxford, Blackwell, 1948)

Helen Waddell, *The Desert Fathers* (London, Constable, 1936)

Edward Wakin, *A Lonely Minority: The Modern Story of Egypt's Copts* (New York, William Morrow, 1963)

Benedicta Ward (trans.), *The Sayings of the Desert Fathers* (Oxford, Mowbray, 1975)

Barbara Watterson, *Coptic Egypt* (Edinburgh, Scottish Academic Press, 1988)

Klaus Wessel, *Coptic Art* (London, Thames & Hudson, 1965)

INDEX

480